Autism and Child Psychopathology Series

Series Editor

Johnny L. Matson, Baton Rouge, LA, USA

More information about this series at http://www.springer.com/series/8665

Johnny L. Matson
Editor

Handbook of Childhood Psychopathology and Developmental Disabilities Assessment

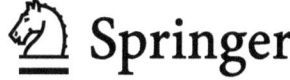

Editor
Johnny L. Matson
Department of Psychology
Louisiana State University
Baton Rouge, LA, USA

ISSN 2192-922X ISSN 2192-9238 (electronic)
Autism and Child Psychopathology Series
ISBN 978-3-319-93541-6 ISBN 978-3-319-93542-3 (eBook)
https://doi.org/10.1007/978-3-319-93542-3

Library of Congress Control Number: 2018953172

© Springer International Publishing AG, part of Springer Nature 2018
This work is subject to copyright. All rights are reserved by the Publisher, whether the whole or part of the material is concerned, specifically the rights of translation, reprinting, reuse of illustrations, recitation, broadcasting, reproduction on microfilms or in any other physical way, and transmission or information storage and retrieval, electronic adaptation, computer software, or by similar or dissimilar methodology now known or hereafter developed.
The use of general descriptive names, registered names, trademarks, service marks, etc. in this publication does not imply, even in the absence of a specific statement, that such names are exempt from the relevant protective laws and regulations and therefore free for general use.
The publisher, the authors, and the editors are safe to assume that the advice and information in this book are believed to be true and accurate at the date of publication. Neither the publisher nor the authors or the editors give a warranty, express or implied, with respect to the material contained herein or for any errors or omissions that may have been made. The publisher remains neutral with regard to jurisdictional claims in published maps and institutional affiliations.

This Springer imprint is published by the registered company Springer Nature Switzerland AG.
The registered company address is: Gewerbestrasse 11, 6330 Cham, Switzerland.

Contents

History and Overview of Childhood Assessment 1
Johnny L. Matson and Esther Hong

Diagnostic Classification Systems 13
Fabiana Vieira Gauy, Thiago Blanco-Vieira,
and Marina Monzani da Rocha

Interview and Report Writing 35
Amie E. Grills, Eleanor Castine, and Melissa K. Holt

Intelligence Testing 59
Abigail Issarraras and Johnny L. Matson

Adaptive and Developmental Behavior Scales 71
Jasper A. Estabillo and Johnny L. Matson

Academic Assessment 83
George H. Noell, Scott P. Ardoin, and Kristin A. Gansle

Neuropsychological Testing 103
Peter J. Castagna and Matthew Calamia

**The Assessment of ADHD in Persons
with Developmental Disabilities** 127
Pamela McPherson, Michelle Yetman, Claire O. Burns,
and Bob Wynn

Assessment of Autism Spectrum Disorders 151
Leland T. Farmer, Michelle S. Lemay, and Robert D. Rieske

Assessing Bipolar Disorder and Major Depression 169
Johnny L. Matson and Claire O. Burns

Assessment of Anxiety Disorders.......................... 189
Paige M. Ryan, Maysa M. Kaskas,
and Thompson E. Davis III

Posttraumatic Stress Disorder.............................. 207
Jennifer Piscitello, Adrienne Anderson, Sabrina Gretkierewicz,
and Mary Lou Kelley

Tics and Tourette's Syndrome.............................. 227
W. Jason Peters and Johnny L. Matson

Aggression and Conduct Disorders.......................... 245
Laura C. Thornton and Paul J. Frick

Behavioral Assessment of Self-Injury........................ 263
Timothy R. Vollmer, Meghan Deshais, Kimberly N. Sloman,
and Carrie S. W. Borrero

Assessment of Pica....................................... 289
Abigail Issarraras and Johnny L. Matson

Social Skills.. 301
Elizabeth K. Wilson, Kaitlin A. Cassidy, Delaney J. Darragh,
and Jacob L. DeBoer

Communication Disorders................................. 313
W. Jason Peters and Johnny L. Matson

Sleep Disorders: Prevalence and Assessment in Childhood....... 331
Catherine Winsper

Pain... 359
Soeun Lee, Lara M. Genik, and C. Meghan McMurtry

Eating Disorders.. 391
Pamela McPherson, Hannah K. Scott, Astik Joshi,
and Raghu Gandhi

Assessment of Pediatric Feeding Disorders................... 415
Kathryn M. Peterson, Vivian F. Ibañez, Caitlin A. Kirkwood,
Jaime G. Crowley, and Cathleen C. Piazza

Assessment of Obesity.................................... 433
Sarah Mallard Wakefield, Joshua Sanderson,
and Pamela McPherson

Assessment of Toileting Problems........................... 453
Esther Hong and Johnny L. Matson

Assessment of Fine and Gross Motor Skills in Children.......... 467
Maya Matheis and Jasper A. Estabillo

Index... 485

Contributors

Adrienne Anderson Louisiana State University, Baton Rouge, LA, USA

Scott P. Ardoin Department of Educational Psychology, University of Georgia, Athens, GA, USA

Thiago Blanco-Vieira Department of Psychiatry, UNIFESP, São Paulo, Brazil

Child and Adolescent Mental Health Specialization Course (CESMIA), Federal University of São Paulo (UNIFESP), São Paulo, Brazil

Carrie S.W. Borrero Kennedy Krieger Institute, Baltimore, MD, USA

Claire O. Burns Louisiana State University, Department of Psychology, Baton Rouge, LA, USA

Matthew Calamia Louisiana State University, Department of Psychology, Baton Rouge, LA, USA

Kaitlin A. Cassidy Louisiana State University, Department of Psychology, Baton Rouge, LA, USA

Peter J. Castagna Louisiana State University, Department of Psychology, Baton Rouge, LA, USA

Eleanor Castine Department of Counseling Psychology and Applied Human Development, Boston University, School of Education, Boston, MA, USA

Jaime G. Crowley University of Nebraska Medical Center's Munroe-Meyer Institute and Department of Pediatrics, Omaha, NE, USA

Marina Monzani da Rocha Mackenzie Presbyterian University, São Paulo, Brazil

Delaney J. Darragh Louisiana State University, Department of Psychology, Baton Rouge, LA, USA

Thompson E. Davis III Louisiana State University, Department of Psychology, Baton Rouge, LA, USA

Jacob L. Deboer Louisiana State University, Department of Psychology, Baton Rouge, LA, USA

Meghan Deshais Caldwell University, Caldwell, NJ, USA

Jasper A. Estabillo Louisiana State University, Department of Psychology, Baton Rouge, LA, USA

Leland T. Farmer Idaho State University, Department of Psychology, Pocatello, ID, USA

Paul J. Frick Louisiana State University, Baton Rouge, LA, USA

Australian Catholic University, Brisbane, Australia

Raghu Gandhi University of Minnesota, Minneapolis, MN, USA

Kristin A. Gansle School of Education, Louisiana State University, Baton Rouge, LA, USA

Fabiana Vieira Gauy Department of Psychology, University of São Paulo (USP), São Paulo, Brazil

Instituto Brasiliense de Terapia Cognitivo-Comportamental (IBTCC-DF), São Paulo, Brazil

Lara Genik University of Guelph, Department of Psychology, Guelph, ON, Canada

Sabrina Gretkierewicz Louisiana State University, Baton Rouge, LA, USA

Amie E. Grills Department of Counseling Psychology and Applied Human Development, Boston University, School of Education, Boston, MA, USA

Melissa K. Holt Department of Counseling Psychology and Applied Human Development, Boston University, School of Education, Boston, MA, USA

Esther Hong Louisiana State University, Department of Psychology, Baton Rouge, LA, USA

Vivian F. Ibañez University of Nebraska Medical Center's Munroe-Meyer Institute and Department of Pediatrics, Omaha, NE, USA

Abigail Issarraras Louisiana State University, Department of Psychology, Baton Rouge, LA, USA

W. Jason Peters Louisiana State University, Department of Psychology, Baton Rouge, LA, USA

Astik Joshi Louisiana State University, Health Sciences Center, Shreveport, LA, USA

Maysa M. Kaskas Louisiana State University, Department of Psychology, Baton Rouge, LA, USA

Mary Lou Kelley Louisiana State University, Baton Rouge, LA, USA

Caitlin A. Kirkwood University of Nebraska Medical Center's Munroe-Meyer Institute and Department of Pediatrics, Omaha, NE, USA

Soeun Lee University of Guelph, Department of Psychology, Guelph, ON, Canada

Michelle S. Lemay Idaho State University, Department of Psychology, Pocatello, ID, USA

Maya Matheis Louisiana State University, Department of Psychology, Baton Rouge, LA, USA

Johnny L. Matson Louisiana State University, Department of Psychology, Baton Rouge, LA, USA

Pamela McPherson Northwest Louisiana Human Services District, Shreveport, LA, USA

C. Meghan McMurtry Department of Psychology, University of Guelph, Guelph, ON, Canada

Pediatric Chronic Pain Program, McMaster Children's Hospital, Hamilton, ON, Canada

Department of Paediatrics, Western University, London, ON, Canada

Children's Health Research Institute, London, ON, Canada

George H. Noell Louisiana State University, Department of Psychology, Baton Rouge, LA, USA

Kathryn M. Peterson University of Nebraska Medical Center's Munroe-Meyer Institute and Department of Pediatrics, Omaha, NE, USA

Cathleen C. Piazza University of Nebraska Medical Center's Munroe-Meyer Institute and Department of Pediatrics, Omaha, NE, USA

Jennifer Piscitello Louisiana State University, Baton Rouge, LA, USA

Robert D. Rieske Idaho State University, Department of Psychology, Pocatello, ID, USA

Paige M. Ryan Louisiana State University, Department of Psychology, Baton Rouge, LA, USA

Joshua Sanderson Louisiana State University Health New Orleans, LA, USA

Hannah K. Scott Louisiana State University, Health Sciences Center, Shreveport, LA, USA

Kimberly N. Sloman Florida Institute of Technology, Melbourne, FL, USA

Laura C. Thornton Boys Town National Research Hospital, Omaha, NE, USA

Timothy R. Vollmer University of Florida, Department of Psychology, Gainesville, FL, USA

Sarah Mallard Wakefield Texas Tech University Health Sciences Center, Lubbock, TX, USA

Elizabeth K. Wilson Louisiana State University, Department of Psychology, Baton Rouge, LA, USA

Catherine Winsper University of Warwick, Coventry, UK

Bob Wynn Louisiana State University Health Sciences Center, Shreveport, LA, USA

Michelle Yetman Louisiana State University Health Sciences Center, Shreveport, LA, USA

About the Editor

Johnny L. Matson is Professor and Distinguished Research Master in the Department of Psychology at Louisiana State University, Baton Rouge, LA, USA. He has also previously held a professorship in psychiatry and clinical psychology at the University of Pittsburgh. He is the author of more than 800 publications including 41 books. He was the Founding Editor-in-Chief of two journals: *Research in Developmental Disabilities* (Elsevier) and *Research in Autism Spectrum Disorders* (Elsevier). Dr. Matson is currently the Editor-in-Chief for the *Review Journal of Autism and Developmental Disorders* (Springer).

History and Overview of Childhood Assessment

Johnny L. Matson and Esther Hong

The history of childhood assessment is of fairly recent origin. The beginnings can be traced to the development of intelligence testing. Most notable was the work of Binet in Paris. The goal of the Binet-Simon Intelligence Test was to ascertain which children had major deficits in cognitive development. This information was used to place children with marked cognitive deficits in separate classes. Building on this work, Terman developed the Stanford-Binet intelligence test in California. With these developments, the new field of formal childhood assessment quickly emerged.

The development of mental health-based assessments for children came along later. One of the earliest studies on child mental health was described by Long (1941). This paper consisted of a community survey of mental health issues of children and adolescents. Early reports also included the evaluation of mental health issues in school settings (Wickman, 1928). As with the mental health literature in general, the number of studies in this area has increased dramatically over time. Beginning with papers published in the 1950s, Roberts, Attkisson, and Rosenblatt (1998) reviewed 52 studies on the prevalence of mental health disorders in children and adolescents. Especially in more recent studies, the *Diagnostic and Statistical Manual of Mental Disorders* (DSM) criteria were frequently used for case identification. These authors also addressed the question of whether rates of child and adolescent psychopathology are increasing. They did not see a trend of that nature. However, the rates of psychopathology did differ based on the scale used. Obviously then, the specific measure used became important, not only with respect to specificity and sensitivity but in incidence and prevalence of various childhood mental health disorders as well. Perhaps one approach in mitigating these issues in both research and clinical practice is to focus on using multiple measures across multiple informants. This issue, in fact, became a focus for a number of clinicians.

Meyer and colleagues (2001) pointed out that for clinical psychologists, assessment is among the most important professional tasks that are performed. This statement is undoubtedly true for other professional groups. Psychological tests based on these authors' review of more than 125 meta-analyses and 800 data sets described those various tests as valid and comparable to medical tests. They also concluded that psychological tests add additional data and enhance information

J. L. Matson · E. Hong (✉)
Department of Psychology, Louisiana State University, Baton Rouge, LA, USA
e-mail: ehong1@lsu.edu

obtained via interview. Therefore, given the high rates of psychopathology in children (often reported to be 14–25%) and the value of specific mental health measurement techniques, their use is certainly warranted. We now turn to a brief overview of different types of assessment.

Methods of Assessment

Structured Interviews The development and use of interviews based on standardized questions, typically using a branching tree system of yes or no responses, was quite popular in the 1980s and 1990s (Hodges, 1993). These detailed assessment systems, typically based on DSM criteria, were particularly popular among researchers. Among the most commonly described systems in the research literature have been the Child and Adolescent Psychiatric Assessment (CAPA; Angold, Prendergast, Cox, & Harrington, 1995) and the Schedule for Affective Disorders and Schizophrenia for School-Age Children (Kiddie-SADS; Puig-Antich & Chambers, 1978).

The Kiddie-SADS, or K-SADS, is perhaps the best known of these diagnostic instruments falling under the category of structured interviews. Chambers et al. (1985) described the test-retest reliability of the scale with 52 children and adolescents between 6 and 17 years of age. The scale has also been successfully used with preschoolers (i.e., 1.5–5 years old) in the assessment of oppositional defiant disorder, attention deficit hyperactivity disorder (ADHD), anxiety disorder, mood disorder, and elimination problems. In most cases, these structured interviews were completed by mental health workers with a bachelor's or master's degree, under the supervision of a child psychiatrist or a clinical child psychologist. Based on the items endorsed by the parent or caretaker, the licensed professional provides a final DSM diagnosis (Birmaher et al., 2009).

Another one of these structured scales, the Interview Schedule for Children and Adolescents (ISCA) is described by Sherrill and Kovacs (2000). The scale was initially the Interview Scale for Children (Kovacs, 1985), but was broadened to include young people from 8 to 17 years of age. This measure has five sections, which includes a section on the symptoms and signs of various disorders such as mood (i.e., depressed, manic, hypomanic), anxiety, and cognitive problems (e.g., negative self-esteem and impaired concentration). Other problems assessed include neurovegetative functioning, such as a marked change in appetite, sleep and fatigue, and toileting issues. From a methodological standpoint, mental states, behavioral observations, clinical impressions, and developmental milestones are also evaluated. As with many of these semi-structured assessment systems, an open-ended interview on the nature of the problem and history is also included. The parent is interviewed first, followed by a separate interview with the child.

The Child Assessment Schedule (CAS) is another of these methods (Hodges, McKnew, Cytryn, Stern, & Kline, 1982). These authors established good psychometrics with 63 children. The standardized questions are geared to making a DSM diagnosis across 11 content areas. Most of these scales employed small sample sizes when their psychometrics were established. One can assume this was due to the very labor-intensive nature of the development and evaluation of these measures.

The Diagnostic Interview for Children and Adolescents (DICA) was initially developed in the early 1980s and was based on a very popular set of diagnostic criteria at the time, the Feighner Research Criteria (Reich, 2000). Also included was the World Health Organization's International Classification of Diseases (ICD) criteria (Herjanic & Reich, 1982; Reich, Herjanic, Welner, & Grandhy, 1982). The test was designed to assess ADHD, oppositional disorder, conduct disorder, depression, generalized anxiety disorder, separation anxiety disorder, and simple phobias in children and adolescents between 6 and 18 years of age. Reich (2000), in a very nice overview of the scale and its evolution, concluded that the DICA is a reliable tool for assessing childhood psychopathology in research and clinical settings. Having said that, the DICA has many of the same shortcomings as other structured interviews.

Most notably, Reich (2000) stated that it can take 2–4 weeks to train a rater and is time-consuming to administer. This author also pointed out that the length of administration may become boring to some clients, and clients may answer "no" simply to speed up the time of administration.

The Diagnostic Interview Schedule for Children (DISC) is one of the more extensively studied of the structured interviews for children and adolescents (Costello, Edelbrock, Kalas, Kessler, & Klaric, 1982). This measure has been sponsored by the National Institute for Mental Health. Over time, the test has been modified (Shaffer, Fisher, Lucas, Dulcan, & Schwab-Stone, 2000). Topics covered are generalized anxiety disorder, panic disorder, eating disorder, elimination disorder, depression, ADHD, and conduct disorder. A format for phone interviewing has been developed along with computer scoring. Some discrepancies have been reported and possible explanations have been mentioned also. Bidaut-Russell et al. (1995) note that a possible reason for adolescent discrepancies included parental denial, problems being trivialized by parents, and the fact that parents may forget about symptoms or may misread problems.

Structured interviews have received a good deal of attention from mental health researchers, particularly in the 1980s and 1990s. The big strength of this assessment approach is the standardization of questions. However, it may be a less flexible method than some other approaches. The biggest drawbacks however are the large amount of time needed to train interviewers and, of course, the considerable length of time required for administration. Thus, while these methods still command a good deal of attention in university settings, they are infrequently used in most clinical settings.

Observations Directly evaluating a child or adolescent's behavior in real time is another approach that has been in common use since the late 1960s. Some observations are free form, but most of the existing research describes much more structured techniques. Usually, a group of 1–5 "target behaviors" are defined and assessed with the goal of recording data throughout the treatment. Thus, the focus of this methodology has traditionally been on evaluating treatment outcome while structured interviews are primarily used for diagnosis. One system involves counting behaviors for the entire day. This approach would be appropriate for low-rate, high-intensity behaviors (e.g., lengthy, aggressive outbursts which occur 2–4 times per week). Far more common is the use of time sampling, since most childhood problem behaviors tend to be much less intrusive and also much more frequent. Thomas, Becker, and Armstrong (1968) described a time-sampling method for classroom disruptions of 28 elementary school students who were 6–7 years old. Observations were conducted by one to three observers from 9:15 A.M. to 10:00 A.M. each school day. Ten children were randomly selected and assessed for disruptive behaviors. Rates of target behaviors under the categories of gross motor, noise, verbalization, orienting, aggression, and other tasks were counted. Childhood behaviors were divided into 2-min segments, with a time-sampling method of 10-s intervals. A behavior could be rated as occur or does not occur during each of these intervals.

Buell, Stoddard, Harris, and Baer (1968) described a somewhat different approach. They used observations to assess motor and social deficits of a 3-year-old girl. Target behaviors were rated using time sampling and included touching objects, verbalizations, using her name, parallel play, cooperative play, baby talk and hand flapping, and playing on outdoor equipment. Any behaviors that occurred during consecutive 10-s intervals were rated by two independent raters. Then, the rate of agreement between raters was calculated.

In another study, two fourth-grade students with autism spectrum disorder (ASD) were assessed for academic engagement and peer interactions in a social skills classroom setting (Dugan et al., 1995). Time sampling was again the assessment method of choice. Conversely, Marcus and Vollmer (1995) assessed disruption (i.e., getting out of a chair at school without permission) in a 5-year-old girl with a history of disruptive behavior. In addition, compliance was rated and defined as complying with teacher's instructions within 5 s, stating "finished" to the instructor, and completing tasks independent of instruction. Time samples of 10-s intervals were used, with two observers present and independently recording behaviors. Handheld computers were used to record data.

Magee and Ellis (2000) assessed a 7-year-old boy diagnosed with ADHD and an 8-year-old boy diagnosed with moderate intellectual disabilities. Target behaviors in this study included out-of-seat behavior, yelling, inappropriate language, object destruction, object mouthing, and aggression. Data were collected via a time-sampling procedure using 10-s intervals.

These examples provide a good idea regarding how much of the observational data are collected. Short intervals of 10 s are common, and data are generally collected in naturalistic settings versus therapy rooms. Having said that, most of these procedures would easily translate to a therapy setting at a mental health clinic and to home settings.

When multiple behaviors are recorded, keeping up with the process and accurately entering data can be daunting. Note that Marcus and Vollmer (1995) used a handheld computer to assist with data recording. In the past, more rudimentary methods were used to assist in counting behaviors. Mattos (1968), for example, described using a handheld digital counter to count behaviors. These counters typically fit nicely into the palm of one's hand and have small plungers that when pressed record the response on a small display. Similarly, Worthy (1968) described a portable timer that could fit in an observer's pocket. This was a device that would make an audible sound at the start and end of an observation period, thus eliminating the need to look at a watch.

A considerable amount of time and effort has been put into the development of observation systems for children and adolescents. The bulk of these observations involve tailoring a few specific behaviors which are counted in small intervals, typically using occur/does not occur in small time intervals. These behaviors tend to be externalizing versus internalizing behaviors since the former are easier to observe and count. These observational methods are used extensively by a broad range of professionals including clinical and school psychologists, social workers, child psychiatrists, and applied behavior analysts.

Checklists Along with observational methods, checklists have become a staple in the assessment of mental health problems of children and adolescents in research and clinical practice. These scales were initially very broad-based, but over time, the number of scales has expanded dramatically. In addition, scales have become much more specialized. Now, there are multiple scales that are specific to ADHD, anxiety, phobias, depression, ASD, and a host of other disorders. A more extensive discussion of the specific scales and problem behaviors that are available will follow later in a second section labeled, "Areas of Assessment." These scales can be used as screeners to help establish if a disorder is present, to assess severity of symptoms, and to aid in diagnosis.

Jensen and Watanabe (1999) noted that many studies have attempted to establish the efficacy of standardized tests by comparing them to DSM criteria. Standardized tests that closely matched DSM criteria were deemed to be the better test. To some extent, this approach may be a chicken and egg phenomenon. Does the DSM criteria best reflect the disorder, or is it the test? A more parsimonious approach may be to see various methods as complimentary rather than trying to establish arbitrary "gold standards."

Bird et al. (1990) addressed another important methodological issue in childhood mental health assessment. They reported that about 50% of the child population met the criteria for DSM-III diagnoses. These numbers do appear to be excessive. An important approach then in establishing more conservative criteria may be to use multiple assessment methods and ensure that the young person meets criteria on general diagnostic measures. This method would result in more stringent criteria and fewer false positives.

Following this formulation, a number of studies have been published looking at the implications of using multiple informants. Jensen, Traylor, Xenakis, and Davis (1998) compared parent report to child report. The authors also wished to look at potential gender differences with children (45 girls and 55 boys). Using the Child Behavior Checklist (CBCL) and the Hopkins Symptom Checklist, mothers rated children as more impaired on mental health symptoms than fathers did. Phares and Compas (1992) also addressed ratings of mothers versus fathers. They made the important point that fathers are markedly underrepresented compared to mothers in ratings of child mental health services. Further, in a broad ranging review on the topic, the authors concluded that parent psychopathology is a risk factor for their children. These authors also noted that externalizing behaviors of the father are a particular risk factor for externalizing behaviors of their children.

Verhulst and van der Ende (1991) also evaluated differences among raters: adolescents (132 14-year-olds), parents, and teachers. These researchers found that the reliability was higher for externalizing versus internalizing behaviors. Kerr, Lunkenheimer, and Olson (2007) also noted stability of ratings for externalizing behaviors over time. In their study, mother, father, lab worker, and teacher ratings of 240 children between the ages of 3 and 5 years old were made. The authors stressed the importance of employing multiple raters, especially fathers, since their input is uncommon. In addition, the researchers pointed out that different raters provide unique contributions with respect to the behaviors children display.

De Los Reyes and Kazdin (2005) provided a lengthy and detailed discussion of rater discrepancies when assessing child mental health issues. They underscored that there is no simple gold standard or anchor measure of child psychopathology. We would add that symptom agreement across raters and scales is the best option in establishing a reliable and valid diagnosis. This approach might be referred to as a consensus model. As with most of the papers reviewed, the authors note that more is better with respect to the number of scales and informants that are employed. This consensus is tempered somewhat by Loeber, Green, and Lahey (1990). They point out that all raters are not equal. In the congregate, children are the least accurate reporters, followed by parents. They suggested that, at least in their study, teachers provided the most accurate ratings. The importance of these methodological issues is underscored by how heavily clinicians and researchers have come to rely on formal childhood assessment methods. This statement is particularly true for assessment scales used to aid in diagnosis. A range of disorders now use these measures to assist in diagnosis. Some examples of these follow next.

Areas of Assessment

From a historical perspective, mental health assessment has progressed from general measures of psychopathology to the use of measurement scales of specific forms of psychopathology. A brief review of some of these measures and how they are used follows.

General Psychopathology Early efforts to better evaluate child mental health issues focused on broadband measures. Steinhausen (1987), for example, described the development of the Children's Global Assessment Scale. The emphasis for this measure was on establishing one broad severity rating of psychopathology with scores ranging from 0 to 100. This model really never caught on, however. A much more successful approach has been developed by Achenbach and Edelbrock (1981, 1983, 1986) using the CBCL.

The CBCL has forms for parent, teacher, and clinician and is arguably the most popular of the psychopathology measures for children and adolescents (Dutra, Campbell, & Westen, 2004). The scale has 118 items on behavior problems and 20 more items on social competence. Diagnostic categories are broken into externalizing and internalizing disorders. Among the diagnostic categories are aggression, delinquency, ADHD, schizophrenia, anxiety, depression, social withdrawal, and somatic complaints. Within a few years, the CBCL was so well-respected that it was used as an anchor measure in the development of other childhood psychopathology measures, such as the Childhood Psychopathology Measurement Schedule (Malhotra, Varma, Verma, & Malhotra, 1998). Initially developed in the United States, it also found an audience in many other countries such as Holland, Thailand, Chile, and Puerto Rico (Bird, Gould, Rubio-Stipec, Staghezza, & Canino, 1991).

Jensen et al. (1996) compared the CBCL to the DISC. They found that the CBCL checklist was equal to the DISC structured interview for aiding in diagnosis. Further, the CBCL requires a lot less specific training and takes much less time to administer than structured interviews, adding to its popularity.

Most general measures of child and adolescent psychopathology have been normed on youth with typical intellectual functioning. However, there has been a recognition that persons with intellectual disabilities also may have mental health concerns. Symptoms, particularly for the most severely cognitively impaired, may differ to some extent from the general population. As such, having norms specific to children with intellectual disabilities is important. Aman, Tasse, Rojahn, and Hammer (1996) described one measure developed to address this concern. The scale is the Nisonger Child Behavior Rating Form (Nisonger CBRF). These authors noted that the rate of emotional disorders is higher in persons with intellectual disabilities compared to the general population. In their study, 369 children and adolescents between 3 and 16 years of age were evaluated. These individuals had IQs between 55 and 70. The Nisonger CBRF has 71 items, which are rated on a 4-point scale by parents and teachers. The following behavior problems are assessed: antisocial behavior/defiance, hyperactivity/inattention, withdrawal/depression, negative self-image/self-injury, and anxiety. Two social factors are also included: compliance/self-control and positive/adaptive behavior. Good psychometrics were reported.

Specialized Mental Health Scales Given the success of the general, broadband measures of psychopathology, the next aspect in the evolution of assessment scales for children and adolescents measures specific to individual disorders. Typical of this trend are measures of ADHD. Swanson et al. (2012) described the history of two of the best-known measures on the topic, the strengths and weaknesses of ADHD-Symptoms and Normal-behavior (SWAN) and the Swanson, Nolan, and Pelham (SNAP) test. The SWAP items were originally based on DSM-III criteria (APA, 1980) and then revised when the DSM-III-R (APA, 1987) and DSM-IV (APA, 1994) emerged. Another very popular measure of ADHD is the Conners' Rating Scale (Conners, 1995). These measures, as well as other measures for ADHD, were arguably the most extensively studied in regard to specific types of childhood psychopathology early in the development of normed scales. These scales are widely used in research and in clinical practice.

Another topic that has received a good deal of attention in the assessment of childhood mental health is the assessment of anxiety. Wood, Piacentini, Bergman, McCracken, and Barrios (2002) described one example of this trend, the Anxiety Disorders Interview Schedule for Children (ADIS-C; Silverman & Nelles, 1988). This measure, which was normed on 8- to 17-year-olds, determines social phobias, separation anxiety, generalized anxiety, and panic disorder.

Another of these anxiety scales is the Child Anxiety Impact Scale-Parent Version (CAIS-P; Langley, Bergman, McCracken, & Piacentini, 2004). Their study established norms for this scale, which has school, social, and home/family subscales. The scale correlates with a number of other measures of social anxiety. Similarly, Birmaher et al. (1997) described the Screen for Child Anxiety Related Emotional Disorders (SCARED). The SCARED is an 85-item test that was given to 341 outpatient children and adolescents who were 9–18 years of age. Ratings were on a three-point scale based on the behavior that occurred over the last 3 months. Three hundred parents of these children were also assessed on the SCARED. These authors concluded that the SCARED could serve as a screener for anxiety disorders across five categories: panic/somatic, general anxiety, separation anxiety, social phobia, and school phobia. The authors' prediction proved to be accurate, since this measure is widely used by mental health professionals at the time this chapter was written.

Chorpita, Moffitt, and Gray (2005) described a test that is used to assess anxiety and depression, the Revised Children's Anxiety and Depression Scale (RCADS). This approach is a natural progression from tests specific to anxiety since there is considerable overlap between these two disorders in adults and in younger people. In this study, 513 children and adolescents consecutively referred to a university mental health clinic were assessed. Conditions evaluated with this 47-item scale include panic disorder, obsessive-compulsive disorder, social phobia, separation anxiety, generalized anxiety disorder, and major depression. The authors concluded that this scale and other measures developed in this area have considerable clinical utility.

Measures designed specifically to measure childhood depression began to develop in earnest in the 1980s. Helsel and Matson (1984), for example, described the development of psychometrics for Kovacs and Beck's scale (1997), the Children's Depression Inventory (CDI). Similarly, Reynolds, Anderson, and Bartell (1985) described the development of the CDI, which has largely been used in school settings, and reported good psychometrics for this measure.

Other problems of childhood development are also important to assess and may affect mental health. One example is feeding problems. Borowitz and Borowitz (2018), for example, noted that upwards of half of typically developing children have issues with feeding, while for developmentally disabled children, the rates can approach 80%. The assessment of diet, swallowing skills, and sensory issues are among the topics which must be addressed. Another issue that has been studied is chronic illness (Bruce & Fries, 2003). These authors described the Health Assessment Questionnaire (HAQ). Bruce and Fries (2003) stated that this scale is one of the most frequently employed in practice and is often cited by researchers, particularly with respect to the topic of rheumatic disease. Topics covered in this test include the person's level of disability, a pain/discomfort index, an evaluation of drug side effects, and dollar costs of care. Multiple measures for childhood health are available. The Arthritis Impact Measurement Scales (Meenan, Gertman, Mason, & Dunaif, 1982) is yet another example of this trend.

Another topic that has taken on increasing significance in the development of scaling methods for child mental health has been the focus on comorbid psychopathology. This topic is typically defined as the co-occurrence of two or more mental health disorders in the same person. Matson and Nebel-Schwalm (2007) provided one example of this trend. They noted that in the field of ASD, the co-occurrence of intellectual disabilities, mood disorders, phobias, anxiety, and psychosis are common. Major developments have obviously occurred in this area. These scaling methods have implications for differential diagnosis, which will be briefly discussed next.

Diagnosis

The history of mental health diagnosis predates the development of the assessment methods we have previously discussed. As Cantwell (1996) points out, the DSM evolved out of the United States census of 1840. The focus early on was on adult mental health needs, which grew dramatically when World War II was fought. Veterans hospitals in the United States and elsewhere saw the large-scale need for mental health services, and of course, assessment and diagnosis were major components of this strategy. It was not until the 1970s however that the move to include childhood disorders began to really gain momentum.

The DSM-III (APA, 1980) proved to be a watershed moment in the development of observable symptoms that cut across theories of cause and treatment. According to Cantwell (1996), this was largely due to the development of more rigorous observation-based criteria that had good reliability and validity. He specifically credits the Feighner diagnostic criteria, which were popular at that time. In addition to recognizing more childhood disorders than in the DSM-II (APA, 1968), the DSM-III set the stage for more objective, observable symptoms and for the development of the range of assessment procedures that followed.

It is important to recognize that criteria such as those described in the DSM or ICD should not be used without also including normed scales with established reliability and validity. These psychometric markers are not available for the DSM or ICD independent of these scaling methods. Thus, classification systems such as these provide a guide and should be used in conjunction with established assessment instruments. Also, where possible, multiple methods of assessment should be included.

The development of assessment methods that have acceptable norms, reliability, and validity plays several important roles in differential diagnosis (Mezzich, Mezzich, & Coffman, 1985). Second, they enhance the standardization of the diagnostic process, both across clinicians and across different clients. Third, they are of value in driving conceptual and pragmatic issues regarding differential diagnosis. These data can help in refining symptom profiles for given disorders. Also, they can aid in resetting parameters of given mental health conditions and can assist in establishing where given disorders might overlap, such as generalized anxiety disorders, phobias, and obsessive-compulsive disorder. Thus, diagnostic systems such as the DSM, ICD, and empirically established assessment systems should be viewed as complimentary (Achenbach, 1980). And, while these issues are important, as science goes, these ideas are relatively new since childhood mental health disorders were first recognized in 1968 by the DSM.

Achenbach (1980) provided some cogent arguments about why the identification of childhood mental health diagnosis has lagged so far behind developments in adults. Much of his focus is on differences in how adult and child mental health services are delivered. Children are typically referred by an adult (e.g., parent, teacher, or other caregiver). They need assistance in providing informed consent and may not understand the implications of their treatment. Also, unlike adults, children may not be able to aid in establishing treatment priorities, or if they can, their aid may be limited. Second, the way disorders are expressed in children versus adults may differ. ADHD symptoms would be examples of this point. Additionally, some disorders, such as schizophrenia, have later onset, and thus, a clear childhood equivalent may not be present. As a result, many issues in diagnosis for children and adolescents are unique to this patient group.

As the differential diagnosis of child and adolescent psychopathology has advanced, other aspects of assessment have emerged. One of the biggest issues has been cross-cultural developments of assessment scales (Verhulst & Achenbach, 1995). It is very important to develop assessment methods that have broad applicability across countries and cultures. This approach ensures that a common language of mental health disorders and symptom presentation is available. Common ground allows for better comparisons of new assessment methods, a better understanding of etiology, and a means of assessing the efficacy of various treatments. Also, how problems differ by culture must also be studied and better understood. Issues based on gender, age, and social skills are some of the factors which are salient in this regard. This issue is a big takeaway with respect to the historical development of diagnosis. At the center of the trends in the field, however, is the interface between diagnostic systems and diagnostic methods.

This Volume

This handbook and its companion handbook on treatment is aimed at providing a survey of current mental health practices for children and adolescents. As such, these books should serve as a resource for mental health professionals and mental health professionals in training. This field is expanding rapidly with many new methods for assessment and treatment. There are many assessment methods which have become less useful or obsolete over time. A focus on the empirical literature and sticking with a review of data collection methods that have established reliability and validity is the major emphasis of these volumes. An effort has been made to describe specific methods, by reviewing tests that have documented efficacy. No matter how well-researched a particular test has become, there are always shortcomings. Also, there are always other research questions that need to be answered. Many of these issues are addressed in this volume on the assessment of the mental health needs of children and adolescents. Chapters are organized by type of problem or disorder. Following this model will hopefully aid the clinician and/or researcher in rapidly identifying specific assessment information. Additionally, the hope is that this approach will make it easier to match assessment methods with treatments discussed in the companion volume as well as other texts on the topic and specific empirical studies on assessment and treatment.

References

Achenbach, T. M. (1980). DSM-III in light of empirical research on the classification of child psychopathology. *Journal of the American Academy of Child Psychiatry, 19*, 395–412.

Achenbach, T. M., & Edelbrock, C. S. (1981). Behavioral problems and competencies reported by parents of normal and disturbed children aged four through sixteen. *Monographs of the Society for Research in Child Development, 46*, 1–82.

Achenbach, T. M., & Edelbrock, C. S. (1983). *Manual for the child behavior checklist and revised child behavior profile*. Burlington, VT: University Associates in Psychiatry.

Achenbach, T. M., & Edelbrock, C. S. (1986). *Manual for the Teacher's report from and teacher version of the child behavior profile*. Burlington, VT: University Associates in Psychiatry.

Aman, M. G., Tasse, M. J., Rojahn, J., & Hammer, D. (1996). The Nisonger CBRF: A child behavior rating form for children with developmental disabilities. *Research in Developmental Disabilities, 17*, 41–57.

American Psychiatric Association. (1968). *Diagnostic and statistical manual of mental disorders* (2nd ed.). Washington, DC: American Psychiatric Association.

American Psychiatric Association. (1980). *Diagnostic and statistical manual of mental disorders* (3rd ed.). Washington, DC: American Psychiatric Association.

American Psychiatric Association. (1987). *Diagnostic and statistical manual of mental disorders (3rd ed., rev.)*. Washington, DC: Author.

American Psychiatric Association. (1994). *Diagnostic and statistical manual of mental disorders* (4th ed.). Washington, DC: American Psychiatric Association.

Angold, A., Prendergast, M., Cox, A., & Harrington, R. (1995). The child and adolescent psychiatric assessment (CAPA). *Psychological Medicine, 24*, 739–753.

Bidaut-Russell, M., Reich, W., Cottler, L. B., Robins, L. N., Compton, W. M., & Mattison, R. E. (1995). The diagnostic interview schedule for children (PC-DISC v.3.0): Parents and adolescents suggest reasons for expecting discrepant answers. *Journal of Abnormal Child Psychology, 23*, 641–659.

Bird, H. R., Gould, M. S., Rubio-Stipec, M., Staghezza, B. M., & Canino, G. (1991). Screening for childhood psychopathology in the community using the child behavior checklist. *Journal of the American Academy of Child and Adolescent Psychiatry, 30*, 116–123.

Bird, H. R., Yager, T. J., Staghezza, B., Gould, M. S., Canino, G., & Rubio-Stipec, M. (1990). Impairment in the epidemiological measurement of childhood psychopathology in the community. *Journal of the American Academy of Child and Adolescent Psychiatry, 29*, 796–803.

Birmaher, B., Ehmann, M., Axelson, D. A., Goldstein, B. I., Monk, K., Kalas, C., … Brend, D. A. (2009). Schedule for affective disorders and schizophrenia for school age children (K-SADS-PL) for the assessment of preschool children - a preliminary psychometric study. *Journal of Psychiatric Research, 43*, 680–686.

Birmaher, B., Khetarpal, S., Brent, D., Cully, M., Balach, L., Kaufman, J., & Neer, S. M. (1997). The screen for child anxiety related emotional disorders (SCARED): Scale construction and psychometric characteristics. *Journal of the American Academy of Child and Adolescent Psychiatry, 36*, 545–553.

Borowitz, K. C., & Borowitz, S. M. (2018). Feeding problems in infants and children: Assessment and etiology. *Pediatric Clinics of North America, 65*, 59–72.

Bruce, B., & Fries, J. F. (2003). The Stanford health assessment questionnaire: A review of its history, issues, progress, and documentation. *The Journal of Rheumatology, 30*, 167–178.

Buell, J., Stoddard, P., Harris, F. R., & Baer, D. M. (1968). Collateral social development accompanying reinforcement of outdoor play in a preschool child. *Journal of Applied Behavior Analysis, 1*, 167–173.

Cantwell, D. P. (1996). Classification of child and adolescent psychopathology. *Journal of Child Psychology and Psychiatry, 37*, 3–12.

Chambers, W. J., Puig-Antich, J., Hirsch, M., Paez, P., Ambrosini, P. J., Tabrizi, M. A., & Davies, M. (1985). The assessment of affective disorders in children and adolescents by semistructured interview: Test-retest reliability of the schedule for affective disorders and schizophrenia for school-aged children, present episode version. *Archives of General Psychiatry, 42*, 696–702.

Chorpita, B. F., Moffitt, C. E., & Gray, J. (2005). Psychometric properties of the revised child anxiety and depression scale in a clinical sample. *Behaviour Research and Therapy, 43*, 309–322.

Conners, C. (1995). *Conners' rating scales*. Toronto, CA: Multi-Health Systems.

Costello, A., Edelbrock, C., Kalas, R., Kessler, M., & Klaric, S. A. (1982). *Diagnostic interview schedule for children (DISC)*. Bethesda, MD: National Institute of Mental Health.

De Los Reyes, A., & Kazdin, A. E. (2005). Informant discrepancies in the assessment of childhood psychopathology: A critical review, theoretical framework, and recommendations for further study. *Psychological Bulletin, 131*, 483–509.

Dugan, E., Kamps, D., Leonard, B., Watkins, N., Rheinberger, A., & Stackhaus, J. (1995). Effects of cooperative learning groups during social studies for students with autism and fourth-grade peers. *Journal of Applied Behavior Analysis, 28*, 175–188.

Dutra, L., Campbell, L., & Westen, D. (2004). Quantifying clinical judgment in the assessment of adolescent psychopathology: Reliability, validity, and factor structure of the child behavior checklist for clinical report. *Journal of Clinical Psychology, 60*, 65–85.

Helsel, W. J., & Matson, J. L. (1984). The assessment of depression in children: The internal structure of the child depression inventory (CDI). *Behaviour Research and Therapy, 22*, 289–298.

Herjanic, B., & Reich, W. (1982). Development of a structured psychiatric interview for children: Agreement between child and parent on individual symptoms. *Journal of Abnormal Child Psychology, 10*, 307–324.

Hodges, K. (1993). Structured interviews for assessing children. *Journal of Child Psychology and Psychiatry, 34*, 49–68.

Hodges, K., McKnew, D., Cytryn, L., Stern, L., & Kline, J. (1982). The child assessment schedule (CAS) diagnostic interview: A report on reliability and validity. *Journal of the American Academy of Child Psychiatry, 21*, 468–473.

Jensen, P. S., Traylor, J., Xenakis, S. N., & Davis, H. (1998). Child psychopathology rating scales and interrater agreement: I. Parents' gender and psychiatric symptoms. *Journal of the American Academy of Child and Adolescent Psychiatry, 27*, 442–450.

Jensen, P. S., & Watanabe, H. (1999). Sherlock Holmes and child psychopathology assessment approaches: The case of the false-positive. *Journal of the American Academy of Child and Adolescent Psychiatry, 38*, 138–146.

Jensen, P. S., Watanabe, H. K., Richters, J. E., Roper, M., Hibbs, E. D., Salzberg, A. D., & Liu, S. (1996). Scales, diagnoses, and child psychopathology: II. Comparing the CBCL and the DISC against external validators. *Journal of Abnormal Child Psychology, 24*, 151–168.

Kerr, D. C. R., Lunkenheimer, E. S., & Olson, S. L. (2007). Assessment of child problem behaviors by multiple informants: A longitudinal study from preschool to school entry. *Journal of Child Psychology and Psychiatry, 48*, 967–975.

Kovacs, M. (1985). The interview schedule for children (ISC). *Psychopharmacology Bulletin, 21*, 991–994.

Kovacs, M., & Beck, A. T. (1997). An empirical-clinical approach towards a definition of childhood depression. In J. G. Schulterbrandt & A. Raskin (Eds.), *Depression in childhood: Diagnosis, treatment, and conceptual models* (pp. 1–25). New York, NY: Raven Press.

Langley, A. K., Bergman, L., McCracken, J., & Piacentini, J. C. (2004). Impairment in childhood anxiety disorders: Preliminary examination of the child anxiety impact scale- parent version. *Journal of Child and Adolescent Psychopharmacology, 14*, 105–115.

Loeber, R., Green, S. M., & Lahey, B. B. (1990). Mental health professionals' perception of the utility of children, mothers, and teachers as informants on childhood psychopathology. *Journal of Clinical Child Psychology, 19*, 136–143.

Long, A. (1941). Parents' reports of undesirable behavior in children. *Child Development, 12*, 43–62.

Magee, S. K., & Ellis, J. (2000). Extinction effects during the assessment of multiple problem behaviors. *Journal of Applied Behavior Analysis, 33*, 313–316.

Malhotra, S., Varma, V. K., Verma, S. K., & Malhotra, A. (1998). Childhood psychopathology measurement schedule: Development and standardization. *Indian Journal of Psychiatry, 30*, 325–331.

Marcus, B. A., & Vollmer, T. R. (1995). Effects of differential negative reinforcement on disruption and compliance. *Journal of Applied Behavior Analysis, 28*, 229–230.

Matson, J. L., & Nebel-Schwalm, M. S. (2007). Comorbid psychopathology with autism spectrum disorder in children: An overview. *Research in Developmental Disabilities, 28*, 341–352.

Mattos, R. L. (1968). A manual counter for recording multiple behavior. *Journal of Applied Behavior Analysis, 1*, 130.

Meenan, R. F., Gertman, P. M., Mason, J. H., & Dunaif, R. (1982). The arthritis impact measurement scales: Further investigations of a health status measure. *Arthritis and Rheumatism, 25*, 1048–1053.

Meyer, G. J., Finn, S. E., Eyde, L. D., Kay, G. G., Moreland, K. L., Dies, R. R., & Reed, G. M. (2001). Psychological testing and psychological assessment: A review of evidence and issues. *American Psychologist, 56*, 128–165.

Mezzich, A. C., Mezzich, J. E., & Coffman, G. A. (1985). Reliability of DSM-III vs. DSM-II in child psychopathology. *Journal of the American Academy of Child Psychiatry, 24*, 273–280.

Phares, V., & Compas, B. E. (1992). The role of fathers in child and adolescent psychopathology: Make room for daddy. *Psychological Bulletin, 111*, 387–412.

Puig-Antich, J., & Chambers, W. (1978). *The schedule for affective disorders and schizophrenia for school-age children (kiddie-SADS)*. New York, NY: New York State Psychiatric Institute.

Reich, W. (2000). Diagnostic interview for children and adolescents. *Journal of the American Academy of Child and Adolescent Psychiatry, 39*, 59–66.

Reich, W., Herjanic, B., Welner, Z., & Grandhy, P. R. (1982). Development of a structured psychiatric interview for children: Agreement on diagnosis comparing child and parent interviews. *Journal of Abnormal Child Psychology, 10*, 325–336.

Reynolds, W. M., Anderson, G., & Bartell, N. (1985). Measuring depression in children: A multimethod assessment investigation. *Journal of Abnormal Child Psychology, 13*, 513–526.

Roberts, R. E., Attkisson, C. C., & Rosenblatt, A. (1998). Prevalence of psychopathology among children and adolescents. *American Journal of Psychiatry, 155*, 715–725.

Shaffer, D., Fisher, P., Lucas, C. P., Dulcan, M. K., & Schwab-Stone, M. E. (2000). NIMH diagnostic interview schedule for children version IV (NIMH DISC-IV): Description, differences from previous versions, and reliability of some common diagnoses. *Journal of the American Academy of Child and Adolescent Psychiatry, 39*, 28–38.

Sherrill, J. T., & Kovacs, M. (2000). Interview schedule for children and adolescents (ISCA). *Journal of the American Academy of Child and Adolescent Psychiatry, 39*, 67–75.

Silverman, W. K., & Nelles, W. B. (1988). The anxiety disorders interview schedule for children. *Journal of the American Academy of Child and Adolescent Psychiatry, 27*, 772–778.

Steinhausen, H. C. (1987). Global assessment of child psychopathology. *Journal of the American Academy of Child and Adolescent Psychiatry, 26*, 203–206.

Swanson, J. M., Schuck, S., Porter, M. M., Carlson, C., Hartman, C. A., Sergeant, J. A., … Wigal, T. (2012). Categorical and dimensional definitions and evaluations of symptoms of ADHD: History of the SNAP and the SWAN rating scales. *International Journal of Educational and Psychological Assessment, 10*, 51–70.

Thomas, D. R., Becker, W. C., & Armstrong, M. (1968). Production and elimination of disruptive classroom behavior by systematically varying teacher's behavior. *Journal of Applied Behavior Analysis, 1*, 35–45.

Verhulst, F. C., & Achenbach, T. M. (1995). Empirically based assessment and taxonomy of psychopathology: Cross-cultural applications. A review. *European Child and Adolescent Psychiatry, 4*, 61–76.

Verhulst, F. C., & van der Ende, J. (1991). Assessment of child psychopathology: Relationships between different methods, different informants and clinical judgment of severity. *Acta Psychiatrica Scandinavica, 84*, 155–159.

Wickman, E. K. (1928). *Children's behavior and teachers' attitudes*. New York, NY: Commonwealth Fund.

Wood, J. J., Piacentini, J. C., Bergman, R. L., McCracken, J., & Barrios, V. (2002). Concurrent validity of the anxiety section of the anxiety disorders interview schedule for DSM-IV: Child and parent versions. *Journal of Clinical Child and Adolescent Psychology, 31*(335), 342.

Worthy, R. C. (1968). A miniature, portable timer and audible signal-generating device. *Journal of Applied Behavior Analysis, 1*, 159–160.

Diagnostic Classification Systems

Fabiana Vieira Gauy, Thiago Blanco-Vieira, and Marina Monzani da Rocha

Introduction

What are mental disorders and why do we need diagnostics in mental health sciences are questions that have prompted extensive and complex sociological, biological, and even philosophical dissertations. In this debate there is a tendency toward ideological polarization which intensifies when it comes to the psychic illness of children and adolescents. In this ideological clash, there are two distinct lines of thought: those who argue that diagnostics and classifications are strategies of social control and exercise of the power of science over society, these are the opponents of what is known as the process of medicalization,[1] and those who consider these methods of encoding, defined under the insignia of diagnostics, always existed, despite not being properly named. To neglect them would entail the undue suffering of those that need help.

It is a fact that mental health diagnostics, especially in children and adolescents, involve a delicate process, which needs to be assessed carefully. Considering that we still do not have neuropsychological or biological markers for the respective diseases, clinical assessment is the essential element in the process of diagnosing psychopathologies. Being that this process is dependent on the technical competence of the one performing the assessment, such a privilege implies that diagnostics in mental health is subject to inaccuracies and differences. These weaknesses in terms of consistency and reliability impose onto the diagnostic of the mental health of children and adolescents a significant challenge and result in it often being the object of criticism.

Despite the pertinent criticism that interprets the misguided practices of overdiagnosis and overprescribing, in regard to the issues related to distress in children and adolescents, the diagnostic has important functions that are well recognized: (1) enables the subject in distress to have

F. V. Gauy (✉)
Department of Psychology, University of São Paulo (USP), São Paulo, Brazil

Instituto Brasiliense de Terapia Cognitivo-Comportamental (IBTCC-DF), São Paulo, Brazil

T. Blanco-Vieira
Department of Psychiatry, UNIFESP, São Paulo, Brazil

Child and Adolescent Mental Health Specialization Course (CESMIA), Federal University of São Paulo (UNIFESP), São Paulo, Brazil

M. M. da Rocha
Mackenzie Presbyterian University, São Paulo, Brazil

[1] *Medicalization* is the process whereby human experiences come to be defined or treated as medical in character (Conrad, 2005).

access to the best available therapeutic resources, (2) enables communication between clinicians, (3) alleviates the patient's possible feeling of guilt surrounding his or her own psychopathological condition, (4) enables the bringing together of homogeneous groups, which could be used to conduct scientific research, and (5) assists in health promotion and illness prevention through the elaboration of public policies. In consideration of these views, and from the perspective that a given diagnostic should never be offered unless it ensures the benefit of those who receives it, the adoption of diagnostics as an important clinical resource becomes more acceptable, which for some professionals and researchers is essential.

The different models for classification, which will be addressed throughout this chapter, suffer criticism for being reductionist by nature. In fact, they can be considered reductionists. A diagnostician does not completely translate who the person is, or the environment in which he or she is inserted, nor is that the objective of his work. Probably, there will never be a classification model that on its own is able to take into consideration all the characteristics of a subject or a psychopathological condition in a single nosological reference. However, prompt refusal to use an instrument based on the fact that it has imperfections is frankly wrong. We need to consider the potentials and weaknesses of a given instrument, weigh them, and utilize it with the clarity of its limitations and its function. The limitations that may exist for any instrument can and should be minimized through additional resources such as rating scales, psychological tests, and neuroimaging exams, for example.

It is important to emphasize that a diagnostic label is, in fact, only one facet of a comprehensive diagnostic process (Volkmar & McPartland, 2014). The global diagnostic process is completed within the full understanding of the contexts of the child or adolescent, the child's family and distress, social relations, and the potential psychological weaknesses of the client, as well as the individual's own understanding of the condition and the psychological coping resources that are available.

Jutel (2009) wrote: "The power of diagnosis is remarkable." We agree with and believe in this perspective. Thus, we consider this chapter to be fundamental for anyone whose work involves the mental health of children and adolescents. The objective is for the understanding of the diagnostic resources to enable the clinics to utilize them in a proper, beneficial, and safe manner for all children and adolescents anywhere in the world.

It is a fact that, in general, most children and adolescents are successful in the developmental process, despite the mishaps that may occur along the way. While on this path, a child or adolescent may present difficulties that reflect a variation from normal development (e.g., control of sphincters can occur from 2 to 4 years of age or the defiant behavior in adolescence), or a temporary difficulty (e.g., tantrum at 2 years or drug use in adolescence), not characterizing a clinical psychopathology. However, more recent epidemiological studies have indicated varied rates of prevalence of psychopathology in children and adolescents. Overall, it is estimated that 10–25% of children and adolescents, at a given moment, demonstrate an impairment considered to be clinical or deviant, which requires specialized treatment (Fleitlich & Goodman, 2001; Fleitlich-Bilyk & Goodman, 2004; Merikangas et al., 2010; Paula, Duarte, & Bordin, 2007). In fact, a recent review of the literature indicated that approximately 13.4% of children from around the world exhibit behavioral alterations that would warrant a mental health diagnosis (Polanczyk, Salum, Sugaya, Caye, & Rohde, 2015). In addition, it is estimated that an even higher percentage present subclinical difficulties, which is to say that despite not qualifying as a psychiatric diagnostic, they do significantly affect the life of the child and his or her family.

According to the WHO, by 2020 mental health problems will be listed as one of the top five causes of mortality and morbidity in children (Murray & Lopez, 2002). Precisely due to the high prevalence of behavioral problems, the children population came to represent a recurring demand for mental health services. A study conducted in Brazil by Rios and Williams

(2008) indicates that behavioral problems are more frequent in children of low income, reaching a prevalence of 35%, which indicates how specialized care should be directed to psychopathology in children in low- and middle-income countries (LMICs). In addition to the prevalence rates mentioned, it is cited that retrospective and prospective studies have shown that disorders that begin in childhood and adolescence are predictors of problems in adulthood, which further increases the urgency of interventions for the prevention of illness and promotion of mental health in children and adolescents (Copeland, Shanahan, Costello, & Angold, 2009; Kessler et al., 2005; Mash & Hunsley, 2010; McConaughy & Wadsworth, 2000; Patel, Flisher, Hetrick, & McGorry, 2007; Paula, Duarte, & Bordin, 2007).

We furthermore emphasize that there are still some significant peculiarities in regard to the clinical presentation of mental disorders in childhood and adolescence, which requires a higher level of care from the clinic when elaborating the diagnostic. The following three factors are the most important: (a) the polymorphism of the psychopathological phenotype in childhood and adolescence, (b) the disproportionality of the time in the course of development and between different children and adolescents, and (c) the inaccuracy in the measurement of the degree of impairment and/or suffering in children and adolescents (Rutter, 2011). Literature also indicates a higher prevalence of the clinical pictures between pre-adolescents and adolescents, whose vulnerability is exacerbated by the large biological and psychological variations as well as that of the social context, which occurs in a significant way during this period of development (Fleitlich & Goodman, 2000; Rey et al., 2015). These so-called clinical pictures are maladjusted or deviant responses of exaggerated traits of normal development that results in a behavioral pattern that is atypical, considering age, gender, culture, and socioeconomic factors (Rutter, 2011).

It is known that psychopathological classifications generate direct and indirect costs with significant impacts on personal and family life and in the academic and health institutions as well. In adults, there is extensive documentation on the social costs of mental health problems. The World Health Organization (WHO), in a study on the resources allocated for the mental health of children and adolescents, managed to gather data from only 66 countries, while for the adult population, the same organization has data on 192 countries (Belfer, 2008). Although the data on the costs of mental health problems in childhood and adolescence are limited (Belfer, 2008; Foster & Jones, 2005), a longitudinal study designed to assess the economic impact of these difficulties in 664 children at risk of having behavioral problems in four poor American communities found a direct or indirect cost per child of over US$ 70,000 over a 7-year period (Foster & Jones, 2005).

The first premise in the diagnostics for children and adolescents is that the child is not a miniature adult. Therefore, the simple application of the criteria described for adults cannot be accepted as best practice for the mental healthcare of children and adolescents. This chapter will provide background and history on the various diagnostic systems and how they apply to childhood problems and disorders. The chapter will also discuss how these systems are relevant to the overall assessment process and how they can be integrated.

Background and History on the Various Diagnostic Systems

Initially, the classification models in healthcare have emerged as a statistical survey of the causes of death, which was the case of the International Classification of Diseases (ICD-1), in 1893. Only starting with the sixth revision, in 1948, did this classification of diseases begin to include not only the "mortal" diseases but also the list of diseases in adult psychiatric classifications. There is a record of one census from 1880, in which mental illnesses were divided into seven distinct categories (mania, melancholia, monomania, paresis, dementia, dipsomania, and epilepsy). The transition from a purely statistical model to a clinical model occurred in the twentieth century, when the US Army and the Veterans Association, concerned about their veterans of war, developed one of the most complete categorization of psychiatric illness at that time (Medical 203) to be used in the outpatient clinics. This model influenced the inclusion of this information on mental disorders in ICD-6, in 1948 (Araújo & Neto, 2014; Grob, 1991).

The first edition of the *Diagnostic and Statistical Manual of Mental Disorders* (DSM) came next and was published by the American Psychiatric Association (APA) in 1952. It was the first manual of mental disorders focused on clinical application. The DSM-I basically consisted of a glossary which featured the clinical description of diagnostic categories, grouped into neurotic, psychotic, and character disorders. This version, also influenced by Medical 203, had a psychodynamic perspective, which was a strong line of thought in psychology at the time. Despite being rudimentary, the manual served to motivate a series of reviews on issues related to mental illness. In 1968, the DSM-II was published, developed in parallel with the eighth version of the ICD (ICD-8); it was similar to DSM-I, introducing subtle changes to the terminology and the description of 182 clinical pictures (APA, 1968; WHO, 1965).

Subsequently, the interest and the need to establish criteria to ensure international standardization began to gain force, with the diagnostic criteria being both a tool for the selection of the sample of participants in clinical trials and a way to obtain greater understanding and replication of the studies, with the clinics being left with the task of adapting the research findings to the individual cases (Araújo & Neto, 2014; Taylor & Rutter, 2010).

Under the influence of an atheoretical and scientific perspective, the ICD-9 was published in 1975 and the DSM-III in 1980. The third version of the American manual (DSM III-APA, 1980), introduced major innovations, such as the inclusion of new clinical pictures and a phenomenological perspective, in addition to a multiaxial assessment. Even today this version is considered the most revolutionary American diagnostic classification. It was in this version that terms such as panic disorder and generalized anxiety disorder appeared, which replaced the term anxiety neurosis, while the term manic depressive psychosis was replaced with bipolar mood disorder, for example. Even so, inconsistencies and lack of clarity in the criteria for certain clinical pictures were identified, which, in 1987, led to the publishing a revised version (DSM-IIIR-APA, 1987). A major contribution of the revision was the abolition of a hierarchy of diagnostics, proposed by the DSM-III, and the introduction of the concept of comorbidity in psychiatric disorders that is still maintained.

The tenth version of the ICD (ICD-10), under the influence of the DSM-III, in 1989 proposed a multiaxial assessment of the clinical pictures, and despite defending an atheoretical perspective, it still retains the term neurosis in its classification, when characterizing the clinical pictures of anxiety (WHO, 1992). This is the current version of this model. The fourth version of the DSM came soon after, in 1994, which was revised in 2002 (DSM IV-TR-APA, 2000). The fifth and current version of the DSM was published in 2013, proposing a more dimensional perspective than the previous versions and a reorganization and addition of clinical pictures, which will be discussed later.

Unlike categorical models, which have always had a greater focus on the adult population, in the 1960s a dimensional classification model arose structured for the understanding of clinical pictures in children-juveniles, as proposed by Achenbach (1966). This model was based on empirical dimensional measurements, which differentiates the children's difficulties into "externalizing" and "internalizing" disorders based on empirical population findings. The externalizing syndrome is composed of patterns of overt maladaptive behaviors such as aggressiveness, difficulties with concentration, and delinquent behavior, while the internalizing disorder includes maladaptive private behavior patterns, such as sadness and isolation (Achenbach, 1966).

This dimensional approach is structured by taxonomies derived from multivariate statistical techniques of problems reported by people who have knowledge about the functioning of children and adolescents in different contexts, such as parents, teachers, and the adolescents themselves. It considers that a certain number of traces of independent behaviors exist in children, with varying degrees of severity. With the objective being to find the constructs of patterns of social, emotional, and behavioral problems, the researchers conducted statistical analyses with a large number of assessments of problems presented by children and adolescents. This analysis is known as bottom-up, since the assessment procedures begin with obtaining scores for the problems of the child or adolescent and then group them in rating scales of psychopathology according to the pattern of co-occurrence that was found empirically in the population (Achenbach & Rescorla, 2007). These data are collected from the application of questionnaires such as the Child Behavior Checklist (CBCL), the first instrument proposed for this purpose.

Following another perspective on classification, the National Institute of Mental Health (NIMH) initiated a project in the 1970s, which sought to create a model based on biomarkers. The NIMH's Research Domain Criteria (RDoC) is the result of this project, and its proposal is to structure a classification model of greater reliability and validity, based on empirical data from genetics and neuroscience, while offering a better integration between search results and clinical decision-making. This model, which is still under construction, has conceptualized mental disorders as disorders of the brain circuitry, identifiable by tools of clinical neuroscience, such as electrophysiology, and functional neuroimaging exams and methods to quantify in vivo connections (Insel et al., 2010).

Throughout this process of organizing the classification models, beginning with Medical 203 after the Second World War, the inclusion of the difficulties of childhood and adolescence occurred, despite being rudimentary, only in the 1960s. This is because the understanding of the mental health of children and adolescents is confused with the social and historical recognition of childhood and adolescence itself. According to Ariés (1981), until the seventeenth century, children were still seen as adults, shrunk in size, and there was little concern with the first years of life. At that time, as soon as an individual was able to live without the need for a constant caregiver, he or she joined the adult society – which took place at about 7 years of age. In this way, the only thing that could distinguish the child in medieval iconography was the child's representation as having a small size when compared to the adult. The social changes in the seventeenth and eighteenth centuries would be decisive for the child, or they stopped being placed on the fringes of society and become its centerpiece. This change resulted in the creation of conditions and tools specific to these persons, such as specialized doctors and toys (Ariés, 1981).

The recognition of mental disorders in childhood and adolescence was influenced by four particularly important historic moments in the recognition of these stages of human development. The first was in the 1920s and 1930s, with the advancement of healthcare in England, which profoundly reduced the infant mortality rate and consequently increased the population of children and adolescents. The second involves the process of deinstitutionalization, which occurred around the 1960s, which also included children and adolescents. A third significant historical event concerned with the mental health of children and adolescents was the advent and recognition of psychoanalysis. And, finally, the advent of the diagnostic for autism was instrumental in calling attention to childhood and to promote the need for the establishment of the description of the clinical picture and the diagnostic criteria (Rey et al., 2015).

The little importance given to the mental health in childhood and adolescence until the nineteenth century was also due to, in large part, the belief, even by doctors in general, that until puberty, there were no psychiatric problems. Even after the finding in the nineteenth century that this belief was not true, despite still being considered rare clinical pictures, it was only in 1980 that the theme went on to be included in the scientific and public policy agendas more consistently, especially in low- and middle-income countries (LMICs) (Rey et al., 2015). This delay in the validation of the diagnostics in childhood and adolescence, according to Couto, Duarte, and Delgado (2008), had at least four factors associated with it: (a) the variety of clinical pictures – here are included the amount of disorders, the comorbidity between them, and the variation in the symptomatology due to the developmental phase and the environment in which the child/adolescent is inserted, which presents a challenge to professionals, in regard to the assessment and treatment of the respective clientele; (b) the still recent knowledge in the area, obtained by consistent epidemiological studies only dating back to 1980; (c) the absence, until recently, of data on empirically validated treatments; and (d) the difficulty of including children's mental health in the public healthcare system.

The historical evolution of the psychiatric disorders in the diagnostic manuals is presented in Table 1. It is noteworthy that only starting in the second edition of the DSM (DSM-II), in 1968, and in the ICD-9, in 1975, were certain categories of specific issues or diagnostics usually found in childhood included. However, they were based on theoretical inferences, mainly with a psychoanalytic orientation, while the descriptions were generic, regarding changes in behavior, without using procedures that could be operationalized (Achenbach & Edelbrock, 1978). In ICD-10 and DSM-IV, sessions were definitively introduced that were specifically dedicated to child and adolescent population. It is noteworthy that, in addition to the categorical model of classification of psychopathologies, which is still dominating the mental health field, the dimensional model, which also arose in the 1960s, deserves mention when referring to classification models in childhood and adolescence. Both will be addressed in the following.

Classification Models in Childhood and Adolescence

Following this historical contextualization, we will discuss the current versions in the diagnostic classification with focus on disorders of childhood and adolescence. This section will be divided into (a) categorical criteria models (DSM-5 and ICD-10), (b) dimensional criteria models, and (c) the model for biological markers (RDoC).

Categorical Criteria Models

The models for diagnostic categories are very widespread in mental health services and have the advantage of using criteria and terms that are familiar to specialists, which facilitates the establishment of homogeneous communication. They indicate the diagnostic based on the recognition of the symptoms that occur together, and are prepared by experts in the field. They are described in the *Diagnostic and Statistical Manual of Mental* Disorders (DSM), currently in fifth edition – DSM-5 (APA, 2013) – and in the *Classification of Mental and Behavioral Disorders* of the *International Classification of Diseases and Related Health Problems*, in the 10th edition (ICD-10) (WHO, 1992).

As the DSM-5, the ICD-10 is proposed with a classification model that is essentially descriptive. This is because it is intended to be used by clinics with different theoretical orientations in a comparable manner (Rutter, 2011). However, in the DSM-5, a greater effort to consider the pecu-

Table 1 Historical summary of the inclusion of psychiatric pictures of childhood and adolescence (ICD/DSM)

DSM-I (1952)	CID-7 (1955) CID-8 (1965)	DSM-II (1968)	CID-9 (1975)	DSM-III (1980)	CID-10 (1989)	DSM-4 (1994)
Included mental deficiency.	Included some psychiatric disorders typical of childhood and adolescence (e.g. mental deficiency), but there were no specification of infancy relation of it.	Included a section on the behavioral disorders of childhood and adolescence, listing a variety of "reactions" such as withdrawing, overanxious, runaway, unsocialised aggressive, group delinquent, and hyperkinetic.	Included three specific diagnostic categories of childhood: (313) Disturbance of specific childhood and adolescent affectivity, (314) Hyperkinetic childhood syndrome, and (315) Specific Developmental Delay.	Provided a more comprehensive listing of child psychiatric disorders; Added codings for psychosocial stressors; and Recognised that disorders may persist into adult life.	Inclusion fo two major groups: Psychological developmental disorders and Behavioral and emotional disorders typically beginning in childhood and adolescence.	Inclusion of the section: Disorders typically diagnosed for the first time in childhood and adolescence.

liarities of the diagnostics for the child and adolescent population will be discussed below.

The latest versions of categorical manuals, the DSM-5 and ICD-11, which is expected to be published in the near future, bring together scientific evidence relevant to the nosology and an attempt to provide a more dimensional evaluation of children and adolescents. As in previous versions, the working group was composed of experts from different parts of the world according to the field of practice of each one.

DSM-5

The fifth edition of the DSM (DSM-5) was published in May 2013 and introduced certain changes, starting with the title of the manual which used Arabic numeral system instead of the previous Roman numeral, as well as the break from the multiaxial model introduced in the third edition of the manual. In this edition the personality disorders and mental retardation, which were part of the disorders in axis II, in DSM-III and DSM-IV, were no longer considered to be underlying conditions and joined the other psychiatric disorders in axis I, as well as the other medical diagnostics, from axis III. Despite the removal of the axes, the psychosocial and environmental factors (axis IV) continued to be the focus of attention, although the DSM-5 recommended that the coding of these conditions be performed based on the chapter of the ICD10-CM (Araújo & Neto, 2014).

With regard to childhood and adolescence, rather than separating the disorders that occur in childhood, in this version, the various psychopathologies listed in the manual are presented with emphasis on the different manners in which they may present themselves throughout life. More than in previous versions, the developmental issues and personal variations are included (Kraemer, Kupfer, Narrow, Clarke, & Regier, 2010).

In relation to the child-adolescent population, the main changes were (a) exclusion of section/chapter "disorders initially diagnosed in infancy and childhood/adolescence"; (b) the grouping of "neurodevelopmental disorders," supported by pathophysiological characteristics, characterized by a delay or deviation in the development of the brain influencing phenotypic characteristics; (c) establishment of changes in the diagnostic criteria for attention-deficit hyperactivity disorder (ADHD) and eating disorders; and (d) proposal for a new clinical picture: "disruptive mood dysregulation disorder (DMDD)."

The neurodevelopment disorders constitute difficulties with onset in the developmental period for which the early diagnosis is highly correlated with improved prognoses. Table 2 summarizes the diagnostic categories that correspond to neurodevelopment disorders according to the DSM-5 (APA, 2013).

It is noteworthy that the disorders on the autistic spectrum began to encompass autism, Asperger syndrome, childhood disintegrative disorder, and the pervasive developmental disorders without other specifications, which were pre-

Table 2 Diagnosis categories for neurodevelopmental disorders (DSM-5)

Intellectual disabilities
Intellectual disability (intellectual developmental disorder)
Global developmental delay
Unspecified intellectual disability (intellectual developmental disorder)
Communication disorders
Language disorder
Speech sound disorder
Childhood-onset fluency disorder (stuttering)
Social (pragmatic) communication disorder
Unspecified communication disorder
Autism spectrum disorder (ASD)
Autism spectrum disorder
Attention-deficit hyperactivity disorder (ADHD)
Attention-deficit hyperactivity disorder
Other specified attention-deficit hyperactivity disorder
Unspecified attention-deficit hyperactivity disorder
Specific learning disorder
Specific learning disorder
Motor disorders
Developmental coordination disorder
Stereotypic movement disorder
Tic disorders
Other specified tic disorder
Unspecified tic disorder
Other neurodevelopmental disorders
Other specified neurodevelopmental disorder
Unspecified neurodevelopmental disorder

Source: APA (2013)

sented in different diagnostic categories in the DSM-IV. This junction is based on the principle that these clinical pictures have impairments in common, in terms of communication, social interaction, interest fixation, and repetitive behaviors, beginning in infancy (Gibbs, Aldridge, Chandler, Witzlsperger, & Smith, 2012; Regier et al., 2013; Wing, Gould, & Gillberg, 2011). In this regard, specifically, Wing, Gould, and Gillberg (2011) criticize the fact that the established criteria do not mention a problem that is common for these patients, which is the inability to foresee the consequences of his or actions for himself or for others.

Among the clinical pictures of neurodevelopment disorders, the autism spectrum disorder (ASD) is a diagnostic category that deserves particular attention, being that its incidence has increased over the years. In terms of prevalence, it is estimated that worldwide, there are 52 million cases of ASD, which corresponds to 7.6 cases out of every 1000 or 1 case for every 132 (Baxter et al., 2015). The worldwide increase in the prevalence of ASD is simultaneously associated with several factors, including the adoption of a broader concept of what autism is, the improved detection with the heightened awareness of clinics and the community, as well as the improvement in educational and healthcare policies. Moreover, these numbers indicate that, currently, ASD is much more common than the other diagnoses considered common in childhood, which implies the need for the pediatric clinics to be trained to recognize the clinical picture and perform interventions, with evidence of effectiveness, that are geared toward improving the quality of life of the child and the family.

The diagnostic for ADHD, also included in neurodevelopment disorders, had the following changes: (a) replacement of subtypes, since the term *type* as inattentive, hyperactive, or combined came to be known as *manifestation* predominantly inattentive or hyperactive or combined, (b) change in the criterion for the onset of symptoms from before 7 years of age to before 12 years of age, (c) started to allow the comorbidity with ASD, and (d) better distinction between the conduct disorders and oppositional defiant disorder (Tannock, 2013).

Furthermore, in regard to the main changes introduced by the DSM-5, in the clinical pictures that comprise the *eating disorders*, the biggest change was the replacement of bulimia nervosa with binge eating disorder, characterized by an excessive consumption of calories in a single meal, without compensatory strategies; the revision of the criteria for bulimia and anorexia, in order to better reflect the reality observed in the clinic; and the inclusion of pica, which refers to the ingestion of inadequate liquids or solids (e.g., detergent, foam, feces), with the onset commonly occurring in childhood and often in mental retardation, and rumination, which refers to the process of chewing-regurgitation-chewing (Knoll, Bulik, & Hebebrand, 2010).

And, finally, under disruptive mood dysregulation disorder (DMDD), pathological irritability was included as a distinct diagnostic and no longer as a diagnostic criteria to be included in mood disorders – predominantly bipolar, depression, or dysthymia – in the generalized anxiety disorder and in the oppositional defiant disorder. This new diagnostic comes to counteract the diagnostic of bipolar disorder in childhood (Regier et al., 2013; Stringaris, 2011).

Despite these changes, the current version was met with much criticism. The central issue of discussion was the expansion of the diagnostic criteria, allowing a dramatic increase in the prevalence rates for a variety of clinical disorders (Hebebrand & Buitelaar, 2011; Wing, Gould, & Gillberg, 2011), and a possible greater influence from environmental/cultural factors and the clinical experience of the researcher. In addition, possible commercial-favorable implications are cited in this expansion for the pharmaceutical industry (Hebebrand & Buitelaar, 2011; Kraemer, Kupfer, Narrow, Clarke, & Regier, 2010; Regier et al., 2013). Countering the criticism, Regier et al. (2013), in a study that evaluated the reliability of the diagnostic categories of the DSM-5 for adults and children/adolescents in the United States and Canada, observed that, in the child-adolescent population studied, the changes tested for ADHD showed very good reliability, and the change for ASD showed good reliability. However, other studies will be needed to confirm these data in other populations.

ICD-10

The ICD-10 is a classification resource with an eminently categorical nature, thus providing advantages and disadvantages. In general, the categorical classification schemes tend to take on a greater homogeneity among the individuals belonging to a particular category.

However, even under the categorical perspective, compared to the DSM-IV and DSM-5, the ICD-10 provides a more qualitative nature in the clinical descriptions. Despite including a list of diagnostic criteria, the clinical descriptions comprise the exhibition of the expected symptomatic patterns of manifestation, which permits the clinician to have a more interpretative dimension of the manifestations. Thus, even if it does not strictly adhere to the number of criteria originally identified in the manual, if the clinician considers that the impairment and severity are sufficient, the diagnostic can be given to the patient. Despite often being regarded as an advantage, this implies the loss of a valuable factor in qualifying models, which is the model's reliability (Scott, 2002).

The ICD-10 provides a multiaxial classification in six axes (comparable to what was arbitrated by the DSM-IV). The importance of this classification model entails the possibility of expanding the panorama of the clinician, combining the principal diagnostic with conditions to be managed by different professionals. In addition, the follow-up according to the multiaxial logic allows for the monitoring of the evolution of not only the symptoms but also the quality of life of the patient during the treatment (WHO, 1996). The axes presented by ICD-10 include axis 1, clinical psychiatric syndrome; axis 2, developmental delay; axis 3, intellectual level; axis 4, medical conditions; axis 5, abnormal psychosocial situations; and axis 6, global assessment of functioning. Regardless of the eventual causal link between axis 1 and the other axes, the multiaxial classification is intended to recognize the presence or absence of conditions or situations relevant to the life of the subject under care and not only the presence or absence of disease.

Of particular interest for the mental health of children and adolescents are three groups of disorders: F70–F79 mental retardation; F80–F89 disorders of psychological development, in particular for the F84 group – global developmental disorders; and F90–98 behavioral and emotional disorders with onset usually occurring in childhood and adolescence (Table 3).

As observed, for emotional disorders, the ICD-10 has certain categories specific to childhood, but for most cases, as well as in the DSM, mood disorders – such as the depressive disorder, anxiety disorders, adjustment disorders or panic disorder, and the obsessive-compulsive disorder (OCD) – are diagnosed according to the general criteria, also applied to adults (Scott, 2002).

Of the diagnostics of childhood and adolescence that share criteria with adults, the following are included: F00–F09 organic mental disorders; F10–F19 mental and behavioral disorders due to the use of psychoactive substances; F20–F29 schizophrenia, schizotypal, and delusional disorders; F30–F39 mood disorders; F40–F48 neurotic, stress-related, and somatoform disorders; F50–F59 behavioral syndromes associated with physiological disturbances and physical factors; F60–F69 disorders of personality; and F99 unspecified mental disorders.

The differentiation of specific disorders of childhood in relation to the general is justified, according to the authors of the ICD-10, as it includes conditions with onset usually occurring in childhood, which are usually referred to before adulthood. Therefore, they represent a phenomena closely related with the experiences and psychic processes of the early developmental phases, whereby there is a high degree of specificity for childhood and adolescence (Adornetto, Suppiger, In-Albon, Neuschwander, & Schneider, 2012).

For some of these cases, such as OCD, this is not a significant problem, but, for other disorders, it is, as in the case of the depressive disor-

Table 3 Groups of childhood and adolescence disorders (ICD-10)

F70–F79: Mental retardation	
F70 Mild mental retardation	*F7x.0* No, or minimal, impairment of behavior
F71 Moderate mental retardation	*F7x.* 1 Significant impairment of behavior requiring attention or treatment
F72 Severe mental retardation	F7x.8 Other impairments of behavior
F73 Profound mental retardation	*Fix.9* Without mention of impairment of behavior
F78 Other mental retardation	
F79 Unspecified mental retardation	
F80–F89: Disorders of psychological development	
F80 Specific developmental disorders of speech and language	F80.0 Specific speech articulation disorder
	F80.1 Expressive language disorder
	F80.2 Receptive language disorder
	F80.3 Acquired aphasia with epilepsy [Landau-Kleffner syndrome]
	F80.8 Other developmental disorders of speech and language
	F80.9 Developmental disorder of speech and language, unspecified
F81 Specific developmental disorders of scholastic skills	F81.0 Specific reading disorder
	F81.1 Specific spelling disorder
	F81.2 Specific disorder of arithmetical skills
	F81.3 Mixed disorder of scholastic skills
	F81.8 Other developmental disorders of scholastic skills
	F81.9 Developmental disorder of scholastic skills, unspecified
F82 Specific developmental disorder of motor function	
F83 Mixed specific developmental disorders	
F84 Pervasive developmental disorders	F84.0 Childhood autism
	F84.1 Atypical autism
	F84.2 Rett syndrome
	F84.3 Other childhood disintegrative disorder
	F84.4 Overactive disorder associated with mental retardation and stereotyped movements
	F84.5 Asperger syndrome
	F84.8 Other pervasive developmental disorders
	F84.9 Pervasive developmental disorder, unspecified
F88 Other disorders of psychological development	
F89 Unspecified disorder of psychological development	
F90–F98: Behavioral and emotional disorders with onset usually occurring in childhood and adolescence	
F90 Hyperkinetic disorders	F90.0 Disturbance of activity and attention
	F90.1 Hyperkinetic conduct disorder
	F90.8 Other hyperkinetic disorders
	F90.9 Hyperkinetic disorder, unspecified
F91 Conduct disorders	F91.0 Conduct disorder confined to the family context
	F91.1 Unsocialized conduct disorder
	F91.2 Socialized conduct disorder
	F91.3 Oppositional defiant disorder
	F91.8 Other conduct disorders
	F91.9 Conduct disorder, unspecified

(continued)

Table 3 (continued)

F92 Mixed disorders of conduct and emotions	F92.0 Depressive conduct disorder
	F92.8 Other mixed disorders of conduct and emotions
	F92.9 Mixed disorder of conduct and emotions, unspecified
F93 Emotional disorders with onset specific to childhood	F93.0 Separation anxiety disorder of childhood
	F93.1 Phobic anxiety disorder of childhood
	F93.2 Social anxiety disorder of childhood
	F93.3 Sibling rivalry disorder
	F93.8 Other childhood emotional disorders
	F93.9 Childhood emotional disorder, unspecified
F94 Disorders of social functioning with onset specific to childhood and adolescence	F94.0 Elective mutism
	F94.1 Reactive attachment disorder of childhood
	F94.2 Disinhibited attachment disorder of childhood
	F94.8 Other childhood disorders of social functioning
	F94.9 Childhood disorders of social functioning, unspecified
F95 Tic disorders	F95.0 Transient tic disorder
	F95.1 Chronic motor or vocal tic disorder
	F95.2 Combined vocal and multiple motor tic disorder [de la Tourette's syndrome]
	F95.8 Other tic disorders
	F95.9 Tic disorder, unspecified
F98 Other behavioral and emotional disorders with onset usually occurring in childhood and adolescence	F98.0 Nonorganic enuresis
	F98.1 Nonorganic encopresis
	F98.2 Feeding disorder of infancy and childhood
	F98.3 Pica of infancy and childhood
	F98.4 Stereotyped movement disorders
	F98.5 Stuttering [stammering]
	F98.6 Cluttering
	F98.8 Other specified behavioral and emotional disorders with onset usually occurring in childhood and adolescence
	F98.9 Unspecified behavioral and emotional disorders with onset usually occurring in childhood and adolescence

Source: ICD-10 (WHO, 1989)

der. Considering that the manifestation of depression in a child or adolescent usually will not admit evident melancholic symptoms, and moreover, for changes linked to irritability and temper tantrums, the application of the criteria presented therein is questionable. However, the direct extrapolation of the general diagnostic criteria for children and adolescents should be used sparingly and carefully (Scott, 2002). Another significant element relates to the correlation between the different classification manuals. In the case of anxiety disorders, for example, the correlation coefficient is satisfactory for anxiety disorder and separation anxiety disorder; however, it is poor for phobic disorders (Adornetto, Suppiger, In-Albon, Neuschwander, & Schneider, 2012).

Perspectives on ICD-11

A significant novelty of ICD-11 will be the development of two versions of the chapter on mental and behavioral disorders: one with the clinical description and a diagnostics guide for the disorders and a second version for use in primary care (Bucci, 2014). With respect to diagnostics, changes will be presented relating to sleep disorders, which will receive a specific category, and the disorders related to sexuality, which will be separated from the conditions (non-pathological) related to sexuality (Luciano, 2014). A great effort has been made in order to harmonize the groups of disorders proposed for ICD-11 with those described in the DSM-5. However, it is expected that there will be some differences, especially with regard to diagnostic categories.

Dimensional Criteria Models

The dimensional criteria models are characterized by the use of quantitative procedures to empirically determine which characteristics are present in the various forms of the respective syndrome, the so-called empirical syndromes, in that there is the quantification of behaviors which are considered to be part of a continuum. Statistical techniques, such as factor analysis, are used to make the classification for the grouping of symptoms and/or behaviors into dimensions, including the intensity of the problems identified and the respective variation in each individual. Such a classification uses questionnaires to gather data on the behavior of the child or adolescent who is being evaluated in different environments, from different perspectives, especially that of the parents or guardians, teachers, and the child.

The concept of the syndrome shares the notions of response class or covariance of behavioral responses, which implies that certain behaviors tend to occur together or be related, and may be represented by an infinite number of responses that are topographically different or similar.

A quick review of the literature can indicate how often dimensional assessment systems are used in epidemiological and clinical studies. They are so common that teachers, pediatricians, and other professionals who do not work directly with mental health know them (Hudziak, Achenbach, Althoff, & Pine, 2007). Thus, with the use of dimensional questionnaires, access to standardized information is facilitated, regarding the child's behavior and the comparison between what is observed by the different respondents, which provides greater accuracy and predictive power in the clinical assessment.

One of the most remarkable contributions of the dimensional models for the understanding and classification of psychopathologies, as already mentioned in the historical, was the proposal of the terms "internalizing" and "externalizing" to describe the two large groups of behavioral, emotional, and social problems found in the statistical analyses initially performed by Achenbach (1966). Later, these constraints were confirmed by the same author in different studies and by authors of other dimensional assessment models (Achenbach, Ivanova, Rescorla, Turner, & Althoff, 2016). The problems assessed within these two main areas can be correlated, as they are assessed as patterns of problems in a dimensional profile, which allows the psychopathologies to be viewed from a dimensional perspective, without needing to categorize each child.

Achenbach and Rescorla (2007) present advantages and disadvantages related to this model. On the list of advantages, we can highlight: (a) the ease of the questionnaires in providing information based on the experience with the child for extensive periods and in a variety of situations, which even enables the observation of rare behaviors; (b) the low financial cost and small amount of time spent by the professional to apply the questionnaires; (c) the possibility of evaluating each child in comparison with their peers, using the standardized data; (d) the facility to determine the need for care; (e) the possibility to evaluate before and after the intervention; (f) the possibility to compare the perception of several respondents, who are important, regardless of the accuracy or reliability of the responses; and (g) the possibility to quantify the qualitative aspects of child's behavior, which cannot be immediately accessed by other means. Among the disadvantages, the same authors list: (a) they are subject to systematic errors, such as not measuring the severity of the case, halo effect, logical errors, contrast errors due to comparing the child with some other specific child, and an assessment strictly based on recent events; (b) they are limited to obtaining the perspective of the respondent in the questions that are proposed; and (c) they have difficulty in capturing the subjective experience of the respondent, in that the data are not obtained from direct observation and the misunderstandings may not be clarified.

In consideration of these points, despite all methods being subject to errors, a good clinical assessment requires the combination of assessment tools, including questionnaires, observation, interviews, and tests, should be performed. This is even more important for the child-adolescent population.

Below two dimensional assessment models are presented for demonstration purposes. Other models often used in research and clinical studies around the world include the Behavior Assessment System for Children (BASC; Reynolds & Kamphaus, 1992), the Clinical Assessment of Behavior (CAB; Bracken & Keith, 2004), and the Infant-Toddler Social Emotional Assessment (ITSEA; Carter & Briggs-Gowan, 2006), among others.

Achenbach System of Empirically Based Assessment (ASEBA)

The ASEBA brings together a wide range of inventories that are answered by different respondents in order to perform the assessment of behavioral, emotional, and social problems experienced by the child or adolescent. This assessment system is called "empirically based" due to the way it was prepared, following the bottom-up model. Initially, with the help of professionals and people who live with children and adolescents, a list of behavior complaints that are often observed was prepared. The list has been applied on a large scale in the American population with the aim being to observe the co-occurrence of the problems. In this manner, it was possible to perform statistical analyses that identified the patterns from which the empirically based scales-syndromes were constructed, in order to identify the sets of problems that co-occur (Achenbach & Rescorla, 2000, 2001). Note that in this model, the items were not suggested based on the diagnostic concepts of the specialists (top-down approach) but rather based on the ability to discriminate the children sent to mental health services from those that have similar demographic characteristics, but do not attend these services. Subsequent studies indicated the applicability of this model of syndromes for behavioral, emotional, and social problems in a variety of societies (Rescorla et al., 2012), which confirms the robustness of the model.

For school age children (6–18 years; Achenbach & Rescorla, 2001), three questionnaires are offered by ASEBA: Child Behavior Checklist for ages 6–18 (CBCL/6–18), Teacher Report Form (TRF), and Youth Self-Report (YSR), answered respectively by the parents or guardians, by teachers or faculty member, and by the respective adolescent aged between 11 and 18 years. The responses to the items provided by each informant, on a scale from 0 to 2 (0 = Not true, 1 = Somewhat or sometimes true, and 2 = Very true or often true), allow for the assessment of eight syndrome-scales: anxious/depressed, withdrawn/depressed, somatic complaints, social problems, thought problems, attention problems, rule-breaking behavior, and aggressive behavior. The same scales with the addition of emotionally reactive and sleep problems are encountered in the evaluation made by the guardians and the preschool teachers in the forms prepared for the age group of 1.5–5 years: Child Behavior Checklist for ages 1.5–5 (CBCL/1.5–5) and Caregiver-Teacher Report Form (C-TRF) (Achenbach & Rescorla, 2000).

Seeking to integrate the different paradigms used for assessing psychopathologies and to facilitate the application of the data obtained by using the ASEBA in the formal diagnostic system, the items of the questionnaires were compared with the diagnostics criteria of the DSM-5 by 30 specialists from different places around the world. This analysis resulted in the DSM-5-oriented scales. Considering the school age group, correspondence between items and criteria was found for the following diagnostics: affective problems, anxiety problems, somatic problems, attention-deficit hyperactivity disorder problems, oppositional defiant problems, and conduct problems (Achenbach & Rescorla, 2001). For the preschool age group, the diagnostic indicators for the ASEBA inventories are depressive problems, anxiety problems, autistic spectrum problems, attention-deficit hyperactivity problems, and oppositional defiant problems (Achenbach & Rescorla, 2000). The authors note the caveat that the DSM-oriented scales do not replace the diagnostic, but rather provide evidence to assist the professional in the development of the categorical diagnostic (Achenbach & Rescorla, 2000, 2001).

To facilitate the work of the professional who uses different ASEBA instruments, the Cross-Informant Report was developed. This measure directly compares the responses of up to eight respondents for each of the items and graphically displays the score in each of the scales analyzed. Thus, the analysis of similarities and differences between the scores obtained based on the perception of the different respondents is assessed. This analysis makes it possible to understand how the child's behavior is in the respective environments while interacting with different adults.

It is noteworthy that a perfect correlation between different respondents is not expected. Exactly the opposite would be anticipated: meta-analyses have indicated that the correlation between different respondents in the assessment of emotional and behavioral problems typically ranges from low to moderate (Achenbach, Krukowski, Dumenci, & Ivanova, 2005; Achenbach, McConaughy, & Howell, 1987). Thus, the concern of the professional to come across disparate data should not be to seek what is "right" but rather to work with all the information as subjective truths and parts of the assessment experienced (De Los Reyes, Thomas, Goodman, & Kundey, 2013).

Strengths and Difficulties Questionnaire (SDQ)

The SDQ is a brief behavioral screening questionnaire developed by Robert Goodman in the United Kingdom and adapted for use in several other countries. As with the ASEBA system, three versions of the questionnaire are presented. It can be answered by the parents or guardians, by the teachers, and by the adolescents themselves. In addition, the questionnaires are divided into two age groups: SDQ 2–4 and SDQ 4–17 years.

The elaboration of this instrument was based on the scale of Sir Michael Rutter (1967). Initially, Goodman (1994) added items to the original scale and requested that parents assess their children on a scale of 0 to 2 (0 = Not true, 1 = Somewhat true, and 2 = Certainly true), which is reversed for prosocial items and favorably phrased problem items. The factor analysis of the responses to the questionnaire indicated six dimensions: conduct problems, emotional symptoms, hyperactivity, somatic/developmental, peer relationship, and prosocial behavior. Goodman (1997) used the factors found to devise the SDQ, excluding the somatic/developmental factor. The author prepared five items for each of the factors, getting a 25-item form at the end of the process. The structure of the SDQ is presented in Table 4.

Table 4 Strengths and Difficulties Questionnaire factorial structure

Factor	Examples of items
Emotional symptoms	*Often complains of headaches, many worries, many fears*
Conduct problems scale	*Temper tantrums, often fights, lies, and cheats*
Hyperactivity scale	*Restless, fidgets, easily distracted*
Peer problems scale	*Rather solitary, picked on or bullied, gets on better with adults*
Prosocial scale	*Considerate of other people's feelings, shares, helpful*

Source: SDQ – http://www.sdqinfo.com

Although Goodman (1997) did not prepare the SDQ directly from statistical analyses, following the bottom-up methodology, subsequent analyses have confirmed the factorial structure of the instruments (Goodman, 2001). Currently, there are data obtained with the SDQ for different populations, which allows for the assessment of each child to be made in comparison to others of the same age group and gender of his or her country. In addition, the SDQ also allows for the comparison of the responses given by the respective respondents. The information regarding rules and templates for correction and comparison between respondents are available free on the website http://www.sdqinfo.com.

An interesting feature of the SDQ is the availability of an impact supplement, which can be used to assess the child's overall distress and impairment in the different areas and the weight the child's problem has on the family, facilitating the execution of the qualitative assessment of the problem.

Models for Biological Markers

With the advances in neuroscience and genetics studies, expectations grow for identifying biomarkers associated with the psychopathological disorders (referred to as precision psychiatry). Despite the evidence, they still lack the robustness necessary to establish biomarkers (Franklin, Jamieson, Glenn, & Nock, 2015; Rothenberg, Rhode, & Rothenberger, 2015; Woody & Gibb, 2016).

Rothenberg, Rhode, and Rothenberger (2015), in a review article, commented on the endophenotypes or genetic "markers" that contribute to the development of a mental illness. These factors serve as biological clues of mental disorders and are capable of being measured objectively by endocrine and neurophysiological tests, among others, and could assist in the prevention of psychiatric disorders by identifying risk profiles. It is emphasized that finding biomarkers could be of great assistance to all levels of intervention – from the universal to the very specific.

Below, we will discuss the biomarkers model proposed by the National Institute of Mental Health in the United States, which was briefly mentioned earlier.

Research Domain Criteria (RDoC)

The RDoC is a result of the interest in research seeking biomarkers in psychiatric disorders. This model is based on three assumptions: (a) it conceptualizes mental illnesses as brain disorders or disorders of brain circuit, (b) dysfunction in neural circuits can be mapped by tools of neuroscience such as electrophysiology and functional neuroimages, and (c) the genetic and neuroscience data are biosignatures, which, once identified, can assist in the understanding and intervention for the signs and symptoms of the patient (Carpenter, 2016; Franklin, Jamieson, Glenn, & Nock, 2015; Garvey, Avenevoli, & Anderson, 2016; Insel et al., 2010). Regarding the child-adolescent population, the RDoC aims to dimensionally assess normative and atypical developmental processes and defends the integration of concepts from developmental psychopathology, for considering the dynamic interaction between vulnerabilities (biological and physiological), which are moderated throughout life and have an impact on the expression of clinical pictures (Franklin, Jamieson, Glenn, & Nock, 2015; Garvey, Avenevoli, & Anderson, 2016).

It was structured in order to understand the mechanisms of mental disorders, based on the mapping of a matrix composed of domains, differentiated by a variety of constructs/subconstructs. In each construct, multiple levels of neurobiological markers (gene, molecules, cells, and physiology) are considered as well as the respective behavioral dimensions, in addition to identifying self-reports and paradigms associated with the construct/subconstruct. In the updated version in 2016, the matrix, which is still under construction, there are five domains, namely: (a) negative valence systems, (b) positive valence systems, (c) cognitive systems, (d) social processes, and (e) arousal and regulatory systems. In Table 5 we schematized each domain and its constructs/subconstructs (NIMH, 2016).

To facilitate understanding, take depression as an example. In RDoC, depression can be represented by multiple domains, such as the (a) *negative valence system* (construct: loss), (b) *positive valence systems* (construct: approach motivation/subconstruct: reward valuation/subconstruct: effort valuation/willingness to work/subconstruct: expectancy/reward prediction error/subconstruct: action selection/preference-based decision-making, or (c) *arousal and regulatory systems* (construct: sleep-wakefulness).

Woody and Gibb (2016) performed an analysis of depression, based on the Domain Negative Valence System (construct: loss). When considering, for example, the loss construct, which was defined based on multiple units of analysis, and the developmental and environmental context, the key disruptions for depression are within the limbic-cortical circuits, so that the primary focus will be (a) genetic *level*, those that regulate neurotransmission of monoamines including serotonin and dopamine; (b) *molecular* level, the glucocorticoids, sex hormones, oxytocin, vasopressin, and cytokines; (c) *physiological level*, the autonomic nervous system, hypothalamic-pituitary-adrenal axis, and neuroimmune dysregulation; (d) *behavioral level*,

Table 5 RDoC matrix scheme

Domain	Construct/subconstruct
Domain: negative valence systems	Construct: acute threat ("fear") Construct: potential threat ("anxiety") Construct: sustained threat Construct: loss Construct: frustrative nonreward

Domain: positive valence systems	Construct: approach motivation
	    Subconstruct: reward valuation
	    Subconstruct: effort valuation/willingness to work
	    Subconstruct: expectancy/reward prediction error
	    Subconstruct: action selection/preference-based decision-making
	 Construct: initial responsiveness to reward attainment
	 Construct: sustained/longer-term responsiveness to reward attainment
	 Construct: reward learning
	 Construct: habit

Domain: cognitive systems	Construct: attention
	 Construct: perception
	    Subconstruct: visual perception
	    Subconstruct: auditory perception
	    Subconstruct: olfactory/somatosensory/multimodal/perception
	 Construct: declarative memory
	 Construct: language
	 Construct: cognitive control
	    Subconstruct: goal selection, updating, representation, and maintenance
	    Subconstruct: response selection; inhibition/suppression
	    Subconstruct: performance monitoring
	 Construct: working memory
	    Subconstruct: active maintenance
	    Subconstruct: flexible updating
	    Subconstruct: limited capacity
	    Subconstruct: interference control

Domain: arousal and regulatory systems	Construct: arousal Construct: circadian rhythms Construct: sleep-wakefulness

Domain: social processes	Construct: affiliation and attachment
	 Construct: social communication
	    Subconstruct: reception of facial communication
	    Subconstruct: production of facial communication
	    Subconstruct: reception of non-facial communication
	    Subconstruct: production of non-facial communication
	 Construct: perception and understanding of self
	    Subconstruct: agency
	    Subconstruct: self-knowledge
	 Construct: perception and understanding of others
	    Subconstruct: animacy perception
	    Subconstruct: action perception
	    Subconstruct: understanding mental states

Source: (NIMH, 2016)

heterogeneous list of features (e.g., sadness, anhedonia, morbid thoughts), rumination, and biases in attention and memory; and (e) *self-report level*, the focus will be attributional styles and hopelessness. Among the environmental factors, the severe negative life events – mainly those associated with the loss of relationship or status – are the events of the context considered to be the strongest individual predictor of depression (Woody & Gibb, 2016).

As in the other models, this theory receives criticism for potential biological reductionism and possible ethical issues regarding the implementation of screening programs. Despite the potential of this information, its use is still some time off, even more so when considering the child-adolescent population. What is available today are promising findings; even though there is some information for the multiple levels, the information is still in its infancy (Woody & Gibb, 2016).

Conclusion: How These Systems Are Relevant to the Overall Assessment Process and How They Can Be Integrated

In this chapter, different classification systems have been discussed in diagnostic of childhood and adolescence psychopathology, as well as the respective advantages and disadvantages and their evolution over the years. Despite the existence of different models, it is a fact that a full understanding regarding the etiology of psychopathology is yet to be determined. The current evidence supports the theory that environmental and individual variables interact in complex ways to cause emotional, behavioral, and social difficulties. It is necessary to integrate the various information obtained in the assessment process in order to identify the best diagnosis and course of treatment for a particular patient. Regardless of the model chosen, it must remain clear that we are making clinical decisions for a specific case based on a set of rules prepared in an attempt to understand the human being. Cantwell, in 1966, stated that, at the time, there still was no system of classification of psychopathology that had adequate reliability and validity.

The models proposed in the ICD-10 or in the DSM-5 do include the majority of emotional, behavioral, and social problems that can be experienced in childhood. These systems represent an evolution in the field compared to previous versions. The models continue to be developed based on diagnostic proposals made by specialists in a *top-down* system, with the need for yes/no judgments, with respect to symptom presence, without a possibility of performing a spectral analysis, which would be more consistent with the reality experienced (Achenbach & Ndetei, 2012). The ability to evaluate the diagnostic criteria in a dimensional manner would bring great benefits to the clinician, which in the current model requires the integration of information from different sources (e.g., father, mother, teacher) and decide whether the symptom is present or absent, a task that becomes difficult if we consider that there is no specific diagnostic procedure to be followed.

Certain proposals for the systematization of the assessment procedures following the categorical models of the ICD and DSM have been proposed. Standardized diagnostic interviews (SDIs), such as the Diagnostic Interview Schedule for Children (DISC; Shaffer, Fisher, Lucas, Dulcan, & Schwab-Stone, 2000) and the Development and Well-Being Assessment (DAWBA; Goodman, Ford, Richards, , & Meltzer, 2000) are widely used for diagnosis, especially in research, where standardized procedures are required. In both cases, it is necessary to receive special training in order to conduct the interviews.

It is important to know, however, that the agreement between the SDIs and the clinical assessment is, on average, 39%, according to a meta-analysis performed on data from 38 studies (Rettew, Doyle, Achenbach, Dumenci, & Ivanova, 2009). This datum does not indicate that this type of assessment is not reliable, but rather that it is necessary to consider this information when choosing the assessment process and when interpreting the data obtained from other methods.

On the other hand, the dimensional models depend on the availability of data from a reference sample with the characteristics of the child that we are evaluating. Although the assessment tools developed based on this model have significant data on populations from different parts of the world, extensive research remains to be done in order to make it a global reality. This issue is especially true when we refer to the LMICs. What should be considered a concern, given that the highest rates of psychopathology in childhood are found in these locations.

The dimensional models are often presented as alternatives to the categorical models of psychopathological assessment. The fact that we still haven't found a definite procedure for the assessment and diagnostics of the problems experienced in childhood makes one believe that it might make more sense to work with both approaches. Different types of taxonomies can help us understand more and more about the difficulties experienced in childhood and how to treat them. We believe that this is the current trend when referring to the assessment of psychopathology. The DSM-5 (APA, 2013) itself presented, in its introduction, data that demonstrate the scientific efforts to validate the large groups of internalizing and externalizing disorders, proposed based on a dimensional system (Achenbach, Ivanova, Rescorla, Turner, & Althoff, 2016). In the words of the authors:

> Within both the internalizing group (representing disorders with prominent anxiety, depressive, and somatic symptoms) and the externalizing group (representing disorders with prominent impulsive, disruptive conduct, and substance use symptoms), the sharing of genetic and environmental risk factors, as shown by twin studies, likely explains much of the systematic comorbidities seen in both clinical and community samples. (APA, 2013, p. 13).

Initially, the new version of the DSM-5 was intended to innovate even more, considering its biomarker clusters. However, in spite of the studies being promising, they are still not sufficiently robust to be used broadly in clinical diagnostics and could not be included in the current version of the DSM. Despite the great expectations, sufficient evidence for some biomarkers has still not been met.

It can be concluded that the behavioral, emotional, and social problems experienced in childhood are complex and influenced by multiple factors, such as the onset of the complaint, the course, and the variation in clinical manifestation according to the stage of development. Thus, the use of categorical, dimensional, and eventually biomarker classifications, increasingly complements each other, making the work of researchers and clinicians less arduous while providing better results (Achenbach & Ndetei, 2012; Drotar, 2002).

References

Achenbach, T. M. (1966). The classification of children's psychiatric symptoms: A factor-analytic study. *Psychology Monographs, 80,* 1–37.

Achenbach, T. M., & Edelbrock, C. S. (1978). The classification of child psychopathology: A review and analysis of empirical efforts. *Psychological Bulletin, 85*(6), 1275–1301.

Achenbach, T. M., Ivanova, M. Y., Rescorla, L. A., Turner, L. V., & Althoff, R. R. (2016). Internalizing/externalizing problems: Review and recommendations for clinical and research applications. *Journal of the American Academy of Child and Adolescent Psychiatry, 55*(8), 647–656. https://doi.org/10.1016/j.jaac.2016.05.012

Achenbach, T. M., Krukowski, R. A., Dumenci, L., & Ivanova, M. Y. (2005). Assessment of adult psychopathology: Meta-analyses and implications of cross-informant correlations. *Psychological Bulletin, 131*(3), 361–382. https://doi.org/10.1037/0033-2909.131.3.361

Achenbach, T. M., McConaughy, S. H., & Howell, C. (1987). Child/Adolescent behavioral and emotional problems: Implications of cross-informant correlations for situational specificity. *Psychological Bulletin, 101*(2), 213–232.

Achenbach, T. M., & Ndetei, D. M. (2012). Clinical models for child and adolescent behavioral, emotional, and social problems. In J. M. Rey (Ed.), *IACAPAP e-Textbook for child and adolescent mental health*. Geneva: International Association for Child and Adolescent Psychiatry and Allied Professions.

Achenbach, T. M., & Rescorla, L. A. (2000). *Manual for the ASEBA pre-school forms & profiles*. Burlington: University of Vermont Research Center for Children, Youth, & Families.

Achenbach, T. M., & Rescorla, L. A. (2001). *Manual for the ASEBA school-age forms & profiles*. Burlington: University of Vermont Research Center for Children, Youth, & Families.

Achenbach, T. M., & Rescorla, L. A. (2007). *Multicultural understanding of child and adolescent psychopathology*. New York: Guilford Press.

Adornetto, C., Suppiger, A., In-Albon, T., Neuschwander, M., & Schneider, S. (2012). Concordances and discrepancies between ICD-10 and DSM-IV criteria for anxiety disorders in childhood and adolescence. *Child and adolescent psychiatry and mental health, 6*(1), 40. https://doi.org/10.1186/1753-2000-6-40

American Psychiatry Association [APA]. (1968). *Diagnostic and statistical manual of mental disorders – DSM* (2nd. ed.). Washington: Author.

American Psychiatry Association [APA]. (1980). *Diagnostic and statistical manual of mental disorders – DSM* (3rd. ed.). Washington: Author.

American Psychiatry Association [APA]. (1987). *Diagnostic and statistical manual of mental disorders – DSM* (3rd. ed. Text. Rev). Washington: Author.

American Psychiatric Association (2000), Diagnostic and Statistical Manual of Mental Disorders, Fourth Edition, Text Revision (DSM-IV-TR). Washington, DC.

American Psychiatry Association [APA]. (2013). *Diagnostic and statistical manual of mental disorders – DSM* (5th. ed.). Washington: Author.

Araújo, Á., & Neto, F. (2014). A Nova Classificação Americana Para os Transtornos Mentais – o DSM-5. Revista Brasileira De Terapia Comportamental E Cognitiva, 16(1), 67–82. https://doi.org/10.31505/rbtcc.v16i1.659

Ariés, P. (1981). *História Social da criança e da família*. Trad. Dora Flaksman (2° edição). Rio de Janeiro: LTC.

Baxter, A. J., Brugha, T. S., Erskine, H. E., Scheurer, R. W., Vos, T., & Scott, J. G. (2015). The epidemiology and global burden of autism spectrum disorders. *Psychological Medicine, 45*(3), 601–613. https://doi.org/10.1017/S003329171400172X

Belfer, M. L. (2008). Child and adolescent mental disorders: The magnitude of the problem across the globe. *The Journal of Child Psychology and Psychiatry, 49*(3), 226–236. https://doi.org/10.1111/j.1469-7610.2007.01855.x

Bracken, B. A., & Keith, L. K. (2004). *Clinical Assessment of Behavior (CAB)*. Lutz, FL: Psychological Assessment Resources.

Bucci, P. (2014). Development chapter of ICD-11 for psychiatric disorders-an update to the members of the WPA Letter to the Editor. *Psychiatria Polska, 48*(2), 401–405.

Carpenter, W., Jr. (2016). The RDoC controversy: Alternate paradigm or dominant paradigm? *American Journal of Psychiatry, 173*(6), 562–563. https://doi.org/10.1176/appi.ajp.2016.16030347

Carter, A. S., & Briggs-Gowan, M. J. (2006). *The infant-toddler social and emotional assessment*. San Antonio: Harcourt.

Conrad, P. (2005). The shifting engines of medicalization. *Journal of Health and Social Behavior, 46*(1), 3–14. https://doi.org/10.1177/002214650504600102

Copeland, W. E., Shanahan, L., Costello, E. J., & Angold, A. (2009). Childhood and adolescent psychiatric disorders as predictors of young adult disorders. *Archives of General Psychiatry, 66*(7), 764–772. https://doi.org/10.1001/archgenpsychiatry.2009.85

Couto, M. C. V., Duarte, C. S., & Delgado, P. G. G. (2008). A saúde mental infantil na Saúde Pública brasileira: Situação atual e desafios. *Revista Brasileira de Psiquiatria, 30*(4), 390–398. https://doi.org/10.1590/S1516-44462008000400015

De Los Reyes, A., Thomas, S. A., Goodman, K. L., & Kundey, S. M. A. (2013). Principles underlying the use of multiple informants' reports. *Annual Review of Clinical Psychology, 9*, 123–149. https://doi.org/10.1146/annurev-clinpsy-050212-185617

Drotar, D. (2002). Enhancing reviews of psychological treatments with pediatric populations: Thoughts on next steps. *Journal of Pediatric Psychology, 27*(2), 167–176.

Fleitlich, B. W., & Goodman, R. (2000). Epidemiologia. *Revista Brasileira de Psiquiatria, 22*(Supl II), 2–6.

Fleitlich, B. W., & Goodman, R. (2001). Social factors associated with child mental health problems in Brazil: Cross sectional survey. *Brazilian Medical Journal, 323*, 599–600.

Fleitlich-Bilyk, B., & Goodman, R. (2004). Prevalence of child and adolescent psychiatric disorders in Southeast Brazil. *Journal of the American Academy of Child and Adolescent Psychiatry, 43*, 727–734.

Foster, E. M., & Jones, D. E. (2005). The high cost of aggression: Public expenditures resulting from conduct disorder. *American Journal of Public Health, 95*(10), 1767–1770.

Franklin, J. C., Jamieson, J. P., Glenn, C. R., & Nock, M. K. (2015). How developmental psychopathology theory and research can inform the Research Domain Criteria (RDoC) Project. *Journal of Clinic Child & Adolescent Psychology, 44*(2), 280–290.

Garvey, M., Avenevoli, S., & Anderson, K. (2016). The National Institute of Mental Health Research Domain Criteria and Clinical Research in Child and Adolescent Psychiatry. *Journal of American Academy Child and Adolescent Psychiatry, 55*(2), 93–98.

Gibbs, V., Aldridge, F., Chandler, F., Witzlsperger, E., & Smith, K. (2012). Brief report: An exploratory study comparing diagnostic outcomes for autism spectrum disorders under DSM-IV-TR with the proposed DSM-5 revision. *Journal of Autism and Development Disorders, 42*(8), 1750–1756. https://doi.org/10.1007/s10803-012-1560-6

Goodman, R. (1994). A modified version of the Rutter Parent Questionnaire including extra items on children's strengths: A research note. *Journal of Child Psychology and Psychiatry, 38*, 581–586.

Goodman, R. (1997). The Strengths and Difficulties Questionnaire as a guide to child psychiatric caseness and consequent burden. *Journal of Child Psychology and Psychiatry, 40*, 791–799.

Goodman, R. (2001). Psychometric proprieties of the Strengths and Difficulties Questionnaire. *Journal of the American Academy of Child and Adolescent Psychiatry, 40*, 1337–1345.

Goodman, R., Ford, T., Richards, H., & Meltzer, H. (2000). The development and Well-Being Assessment: Description and initial validation of an integrated assessment of child and adolescent psychopathology. *Journal of Child Psychology and Psychiatry, 41*, 645–655. https://doi.org/10.1111/j.1469-7610.2000.tb02345.x

Grob, G. N. (1991). Origins of DSM-I: A study in appearance and reality [1]. *The American Journal of Psychiatry, 148*(4), 421–431.

Hebebrand, J., & Buitelaar, J. K. (2011). On the way to DSM-V. *European Child & Adolescent Psychiatry, 20*, 57–60.

Hudziak, J. J., Achenbach, T. M., Althoff, R., & Pine, D. (2007). A dimensional approach to developmental psychopathology. *International Journal of Methods in Psychiatric Research, 16*(SI), S16–S23. https://doi.org/10.1002/mpr.217

Insel, T., Cuthbert, B., Garvey, M., Heinssen, R., Pine, D. S., Quinn, K., ... Wang, P. (2010). Research Domain Criteria (RDoC): Toward a new classification framework for research on mental disorders. *The American Journal of Psychiatric, 167*(7), 748–751.

Jutel, A. (2009). Sociology of diagnosis: A preliminary review. *Sociology of Health and Illness, 31*, 278–299.

Kessler, R. C., Berglund, P., Demler, O., Jin, R., Merikangas, K. R., & Walters, E. E. (2005). Lifetime prevalence and age-of-onset distribution of DSM-IV disorders in the National Comorbidity Survey Replications. *Archive of General Psychiatry, 65*, 593–602.

Knoll, S., Bulik, C. M., & Hebebrand, J. (2010). Do the currently proposed DSM-5 criteria for anorexia nervosa adequately consider development aspects in children and adolescents? *European Child & Adolescent Psychiatry, 20*(2), 95–101.

Kraemer, H. C., Kupfer, D. J., Narrow, W. E., Clarke, D., & Regier, D. A. (2010). Moving toward DSM-5: The field trials. *American Journal Psychiatry, 167*(1), 1158–1160.

Luciano, M. (2014). Proposals for ICD-11: A report for WPA membership. *World Psychiatry, 13*(2), 206–208.

McConaughy, S. H., & Wadsworth, M. E. (2000). Life history reports of young adult previously referred for mental health services. *Journal of Emotional and Behavioral Disorders, 8*, 202–215.

Merikangas, K. R., He, J.-P., Brody, D., Fisher, P. W., Bourdon, K., & Koretz, D. S. (2010). Prevalence and treatment of mental disorders among US children in the 2001-2004 NHAES. *Pediatrics, 125*(1), 75–81.

Mash, E. J., & Hunsley, J. (2010). Assessment of childhood disorders. In E. J. Mash & R. A. Barkley (Eds.), *Assessment of childhood disorders* (pp. 3–51). New York: Guilford Press.

Murray, C., & Lopez, A. (2002). *World Health Report 2002: Reducing risks, promoting healthy life*. Geneva: World Health Organization.

National Institute of Mental Health [NIMH]. (2016). RDoC Snapshot: Version 2 (saved10/20/2016). Retrieved from https://www.nimh.nih.gov/research-priorities/rdoc/constructs/rdoc-snapshot-version-2-saved-10-20-2016.shtml

Patel, V., Flisher, A., Hetrick, S., & McGorry, P. (2007). Mental health of young people: A global public-health challenge. *The Lancet, 369*(9569), 1302–1313.

Paula, C. S., Duarte, S. C., & Bordin, I. A. S. (2007). Prevalência de problemas de saúde mental em crianças e adolescentes da região metropolitana de São Paulo: necessidade de tratamento e capacidade de atendimento. *Revista Brasileira de Psiquiatria, 29*(1), 11–17.

Polanczyk, G. V., Salum, G. A., Sugaya, L. S., Caye, A., & Rohde, L. A. (2015). Annual research review: A meta-analysis of the worldwide prevalence of mental disorders in children and adolescents. *Journal of Child Psychology and Psychiatry and Allied Disciplines, 56*(3), 345–365. https://doi.org/10.1111/jcpp.12381

Regier, D. A., Narrow, W. E., Clarke, D. E., Kraemer, H. C., Kuramoto, J., Kuhl, E. A., & Kupfer, D. J. (2013). DSM-5 Field trials in the United States and Canada, part II: Test-retest reliability of selected categorical diagnoses. *American Journal of Psychiatry, 170*(1), 59–70. https://doi.org/10.1176/appi.ajp.2012.12070999

Reynolds, C. R., & Kamphaus, R. W. (1992). *Behavior Assessment System for Children (BASC)*. Circle Pines, MN: American Guidance Service.

Rescorla, L. A., Ivanova, M. Y., Achenbach, T. M., Begovac, I., Chahed, M., Drugli, M. B., ... Zhang, E. Y. (2012). International epidemiology of child and adolescent psychopathology II: Integration and applications of dimensional findings from 44 societies. *Journal of the American Academy of Child & Adolescent Psychiatry, 51*(12), 1273–1283. https://doi.org/10.1016/j.jaac.2012.09.012

Rettew, D. C., Doyle, A., Achenbach, T. M., Dumenci, L., & Ivanova, M. Y. (2009). Meta-analysis of agreement between diagnoses made from clinical evaluations and standardized diagnostic interviews. *International Journal of Methods in Psychiatric Research, 18*, 169–184. https://doi.org/10.1002/mpr.289

Rey, J. M., Assumpção, F. B., Bernad, C. A., Çuhadaroğlu, F. C., Evans, B., Fung, D., ... Schleimer, K. (2015). History of child and adolescent psychiatry. In J. M. Rey (Ed.), *IACAPAP e-Textbook of child and adolescent mental health*. Geneva: International Association for Child and Adolescent Psychiatry and Allied Professions.

Rios, K. S. A., & Williams, L. C. A. (2008). Intervenção com famílias como estratégia de prevenção de problemas de comportamento em crianças: uma revisão. *Psicologia em estudo, 13*(4), 799–806.

Rothenberg, A., Rhode, L. A., & Rothenberger, L. G. (2015). Biomarkers in child mental health: A biopsycho-social perspective is needed. *Behavioral Brain Functions, 11*(1), 31.

Rutter, M. (1967). A children's behavior questionnaire for competency by teachers: preliminary findings. *Journal of Child Psychology and Psychiatry, 8*, 1–11.

Rutter, M. (2011). Research review: Child psychiatric diagnosis and classification: Concepts, findings, challenges and potential. *Journal of Child Psychology and Psychiatry, 52*(6), 647.

Scott, S. (2002). Classification of psychiatric disorders in childhood and adolescence: Building castles in the sand? *Advances in Psychiatric Treatment, 8*(3), 205–213.

Shaffer, D., Fisher, P., Lucas, C. P., Dulcan, M. K., & Schwab-Stone, M. E. (2000). HIMH Diagnostic Interview Schedule for Children version IV (NIMH DISC-IV): Description, differences from previous version, and reliability of some common diagnoses. *Journal of the American Academy of Child and Adolescent Psychiatry, 39*, 28–38. https://doi.org/10.1097/00004583-200001000-00014

Stringaris, A. (2011). Irritability in children and adolescents: A challenge for DSM-5. *European Child & Adolescent Psychiatry, 20*(2), 61–66.

Taylor, E., & Rutter, M. (2010). Classification. In *Rutter's child and adolescent psychiatry* (pp. 177–246). Australia: Blackwell Publishing.

Tannock, R. (2013). Rethinkin ADHD an LD in DSM-5: Proposed changes in diagnostic criteria. *Journal of Learning Disabilities, 46*(1), 5–25.

Volkmar, F. R., & McPartland, J. C. (2014). From Kanner to DSM-5: Autism as an evolving diagnostic concept. *Annual Review of Clinical Psychology, 10*, 193–212.

Wing, L., Gould, J., & Gillberg, J. (2011). Autism spectrum disorders in the DSM-V: Better or worse than the DSM-IV? *Research in Developmental Disabilities, 32*, 768–773.

Woody, M. L., & Gibb, B. E. (2016). Integrating NIMH Research Domain Criteria (RDoC) into depression research. *Current Opinion in Psychology, 4*, 6–12.

World Health Organizadtion [WHO]. (1965). *The ICD-8: Classification of mentl and behavioural disorders.* Genebra: Author.

World Health Organizadtion [WHO]. (1989). *The ICD-9: Classification of mentl and behavioural disorders.* Genebra: Author.

World Health Organization [WHO]. (1992). *The ICD-10 classification of mental and behavioural disorders: Clinical descriptions and diagnostic guidelines.* Geneva: World Health Organization.

World Health Organization [WHO]. (1996). *Multiaxial classification of child and adolescent psychiatric disorders: The ICD-10 classification of mental and behavioural disorders in children and adolescents.* Genebra: Cambridge University Press.

Interview and Report Writing

Amie E. Grills, Eleanor Castine, and Melissa K. Holt

The interview is a critical component of the psychological assessment of a child. In addition to the standard unstructured interview conducted when first meeting new clients, several structured interviews have been developed for use with children and their parents/caregivers.[1] This chapter is designed to introduce and familiarize the reader with techniques appropriate and effective for use during interviews when a child is the identified client, as well as to provide examples of several interviews commonly used in the assessment of children and adolescents. Specifically, we review key components of the first interview, provide information on unstructured and structured interviews, and discuss how to select interview procedures. In addition, we offer considerations in using interview procedures with children who have disabilities as well as other factors related to the use of interviews, such as language dominance. Finally, we close with an overview of report writing. Throughout the chapter, we highlight changes to existing assessments resulting from the recent transition to DSM-5 (APA, 2013) described.

Interviews for Children

Interviews are often the most comprehensive assessment tools for clinicians, allowing for the evaluation and observation of both behavioral and emotional functioning. Historically, reliance was given to caregiver reports, and any information given by the child was considered secondary. In fact, children were rarely included in the interview process due to beliefs that they lacked the cognitive capabilities to give accurate statements about their feelings and behaviors (Edelbrock & Costello, 1990; Herjanic, Herjanic, Brown, & Wheatt, 1975). The seminal work of Lapouse and Monk (1958), as well as Rutter and colleagues (Rutter & Graham, 1968; Rutter, Tizard, & Whitmore, 1970; Rutter, Tizard, Yule, Graham, & Whitmore, 1976, 1977), altered the way in which the reports of youth were perceived, by demonstrating psychometric soundness for child structured interviews. Thus, currently most clinicians consider the child to be an essential informant in the interview process (Chambers et al., 1985; De Los Reyes & Kazdin, 2005; Grills & Ollendick, 2002; Macleod et al., 2017; Moretti, Fine, Haley, & Marriage, 1985; Ollendick & Hersen, 1993).

---

[1] Note: Although interviews are intended to be conducted with any primary caregiver as informant (e.g., parents, grandparents, stepparents, guardian ad litem, etc.), use of the term "parent" will be employed from this point forward for reading ease.

A. E. Grills (✉) · E. Castine · M. K. Holt
Department of Counseling Psychology and Applied Human Development, Boston University, School of Education, Boston, MA, USA
e-mail: agrills@bu.edu

Numerous parent/child interview measures and techniques have now been developed (Frick, Barry, & Kamphaus, 2010; Marin, Rey, & Silverman, 2013). Notably, gathering information from multiple reporters – such as parents and children – helps to provide clarity around the presenting problem, inform treatment, and facilitate communication across clinicians (Leffler, Riebel, & Hughes, 2015). Moreover, teacher and school reports are also often pertinent with child cases, as the child may behave differently in academic settings and/or the parent may be unaware of the child's school behaviors (Karver, 2006; Tripp, Schaughency, & Clarke, 2006).

At a basic level, interviews can be differentiated by the amount of structure utilized to elicit responses, with common differentiations based on the categories of unstructured, semi-structured, and highly structured. Those will be described later in the chapter, but first we provide an overview and considerations for the first interview.

The Initial Interview Regardless of whether unstructured or structured interview formats will dominate the assessment, oftentimes the first interview that occurs is conducted with both the parent(s) and child present. During this interview, basic clinic policies can be covered (e.g., confidentiality procedures), and a general understanding of the concerns that led to the assessment can be discussed. Ideally, this joint session is followed by time spent individually with the child and parent(s) to obtain each perspective unhindered by the others' presence. Even the views and perceptions of younger children are often invaluable and observation of parent-child interactions and/or family dynamics can also be highly informative (e.g., Is the parent paying attention to the child? Does the parent interact with the child or engage the child in discussion?). During the interview the clinician will also have the opportunity to observe and make inferences about the child's thoughts, feelings, and behaviors (e.g., Does the child separate easily from the parent? Does the child have labels and understanding of diverse emotions?). The primary goal of this initial interview is generally to gather as much information as possible about the child's history, presenting problems, and the environment in which these difficulties exist. Many clinicians find use of a comprehensive developmental history form, completed prior to the first meeting, to be helpful (see Appendix A for an example). This form can then be reviewed by the clinician with subsequent questions asked for clarification as needed. In addition, parent and teacher forms (e.g., Child Behavior Checklists, Achenbach, 2001; Behavior Assessment System for Children, Third Edition, Reynolds & Kamphaus, 2015) can be included in a preinterview packet completed before the clinic visit and examined for noted areas of concern for follow-up during the interview.

Rapport with the clinician is of utmost importance as the nature of this relationship will set the tone for the rest of the interview, assessment, and/or therapy contact. Preschool children tend to warm up quickly and respond well to an interviewer who is friendly and supportive (Bierman & Schwartz, 1986). Children in grade school may be more intimidated by the interview experience and may need to be eased into the process. This can be accomplished by inviting the child to explore the toys in the room or discussing "fun topics" (e.g., friends, sports, hobbies) rather than immediately sitting down and commencing with the interview. Adolescents may appear more standoffish and are generally more responsive to open communication and honesty (LaGreca, 1990). In addition, adolescents typically ask more questions about confidentiality issues that should be clarified with all parties prior to continuing the assessment (LaGreca, 1990).

The clinician should prepare by making sure the setup of the room where the interview will take place is "child friendly" (e.g., smaller chairs for young children, appropriate decorations, and toys/activities), as the room is often the first impression the child and his or her parents will have of the assessment experience. The room should feel welcoming to the family without too much clutter or bright/noisy objects which can be tempting distractions, particularly for a child who is restless or hyperactive (Thompson & Rudolph, 2000), and could hinder successful interview completion. The ability of the child to feel comfortable in the environment can improve rapport and ease him or her into the assessment process.

Once adequate rapport has been established, the goal becomes investigation of the child's presenting problems. While any one interview type might be sufficient, intermixing is also common. For example, an unstructured interview format could be used to determine specific diagnostic considerations and modules from a structured interview could then follow as needed. Conversely, a highly structured interview could be conducted to screen for potential psychopathology with an unstructured interview subsequently conducted for clarifications and to gather additional information (e.g., on the course of the disorder). As noted below, with structured interviews, the questions asked are primarily diagnostic. If the interview format is unstructured, the topics of discussion pertain to factors that appear to be relevant and immediate to the child. Generally, topics discussed here include, but are not limited to, symptom presentation, severity of symptoms, duration and onset of problems, somatic concerns, stressors, as well as individual and environmental strengths (Greenspan & Greenspan, 2003). During this discussion, the clinician should be attuned to the child's temperament, attitude, willingness to cooperate, language difficulties, observable emotional change during topic transitions, and nonverbal behaviors suggestive of distress (Sattler & Hoge, 2006). Further, the clinician should be aware of normative developmental domains (e.g., language, cognitive, and social; Bierman & Schwartz, 1986; Greenspan & Greenspan, 2003; Herba, Landau, Russell, Ecker, & Phillips, 2006; Wareham & Salmon, 2006), in order to accurately distinguish between what is severely deviant from normal and what is maladaptive at a stage-specific level and can be self-corrected with age (Sattler & Hoge, 2006). This will also assist the clinician in determining areas in need of further evaluation.

Suggested communication skills that help maintain rapport and facilitate discussion are verbal and nonverbal acknowledgments of the child's thoughts or feelings, descriptive statements that are nonevaluative, reflective statements, statements of positive evaluation, questions, and summary statements which indicate to the child that you have been listening and paying attention (Sattler & Hoge, 2006). The interviewer can also ascertain the child's level of understanding by asking for summarizations of the questions being asked in the child's own words. Avoidance of critical statements and use of praise for the client's discussion can also be used to maintain good rapport and cooperation. Although similar communication approaches are also appropriate during parent interviews, parents frequently require less prompting as they have often sought the assessment.

For children experiencing difficulty sustaining focus or cooperation during the interview process, Sattler and Hoge (2006) also recommend summarizing the discussion up to the point of withdrawal and then rephrasing the question, using hypothetical questions and scenarios, or presenting acceptable alternatives. Techniques such as these have been found to be most effective with younger children who are either not willing to participate or are showing difficulty communicating their experiences (Wesson & Salmon, 2001). Depending on the developmental level of the child, play-oriented interview techniques can also be introduced at these times. For example, therapy games (e.g., thinking, feeling doing), drawing activities (e.g., draw your and tell a story about it), stories (e.g., told to solve hypothetical problems), and use of toys (e.g., dolls whose actions the therapist can ask the child to describe) can be introduced (Bierman & Schwartz, 1986; Priestley & Pipe, 1997; Reid, Grills, Mian, Merson, & Langer, 2017; Salmon, 2006; Wesson & Salmon, 2001). Similarly, the therapist can engage the child in conversation while also participating in parallel play (e.g., shooting baskets on a mini hoop, building with blocks). These techniques can also be used when sensitive and painful topics become the focus of the interview. If the child begins to experience distress, the clinician should not necessarily move away from the topic but rather could try utilizing a different interview tool or discussing the distress (depending on the child's developmental level). Indeed, experienced clinicians become adept at identifying and subtly probing areas of distress and then helping the child reconstitute. An interview should not be confused with a therapeutic effort, which could compromise (or enhance) the clinician's ability to subsequently engage in intervention with a child. All of these alternative activities allow the child to express his or her thoughts and feelings in reaction to given situations. The clinician should not interpret responses or artistic creations (e.g., Hunsley, Lee, Wood, & Taylor, 2014), as these are primarily used to generate conversation and are prone to clinician biases (see below). In addition, the inclusion of breaks can be useful for regaining/refocusing attention.

The clinician should end the interview with a summary of the main points discussed regarding the presenting problems and other relevant material offered by the interviewee. This is an opportunity for the clinician to ask any final questions or clarify any ambiguous responses. The parent/child should also be given an opportunity to ask any questions or express any concerns not discussed previously.

Unstructured Interviews An *unstructured* interview is conducted as part of most, if not all, evaluations and is commonly the first significant contact the family has with the clinician. The initial interview described above reflected an unstructured interview, and most clinicians begin their assessment with some form of unstructured interview in this manner. A particular strength of the unstructured interview format is the individualized nature, which allows for significant clinician freedom and judgment. Apart from the typically included demographic (e.g., age of child, level of acculturation) and introductory (e.g., "What brings you in today") information, there are no required/standard question sets, which allows for flexibility in pursuing ambiguous responses or gathering greater details. However, in order to collect sufficient information, preparation and organization are required to direct discussion toward topics that are relevant to the problem at hand and that will aid in eventual diagnostic and/or treatment decisions. More experienced clinicians may feel more equipped with the skills necessary for asking the "right" questions (e.g., to elicit useful and relevant information from the child, Sattler & Hoge, 2006); however, less experienced clinicians can become more experienced through practice sessions and supervised unstructured interview administrations. In addition, newer clinicians may benefit from gradually moving from a highly structured to less structured format. For example, becoming familiar with the probe and follow-up questions typically included in more structured interviews, as well as areas of differential diagnosis (e.g., DSM-5, APA, 2013), may help establish a flowing questioning style while remaining comprehensive in the scope of inquiries.

Importantly, unstructured interviews alone are not typically recommended for use in determining clinical diagnoses, given pitfalls and concerns with relying on clinician judgment and experience alone. Detailing the research body surrounding these concerns is beyond the scope of this chapter and has been well-described elsewhere (see Garb & Boyle, 2015; Lilienfeld, Ammirati, & David, 2012; Magnavita & Lilienfeld, 2016); however, it is important to highlight that cognitive errors and biases are commonplace among even the most experienced clinicians and can "compromise the ability of clinicians to use optimal decision-making strategies" (Garb & Boyle, 2015, p. 28). Given the potential for harm that could derive from misdiagnosis (e.g., improper interventions, medications, stigma), it is imperative that clinicians understand these issues and employ best practices (e.g., psychometrically sound measures; multi-informant, multi-measure procedures) to ensure proper diagnosis.

Structured Interviews Many clinicians do not often use standardized interviews due to time constraints (Frick et al., 2010). However, there are a number of benefits to structured interviews. In particular, structured diagnostic interviews were designed to increase the reliability of diagnoses by standardizing the method used to elicit responses. This, in turn, is expected to have the effect of increasing the reliability of the responses and eliminating potential biases (e.g., making decisions prior to the collection of all the information, only collecting confirming or disconfirming evidence) associated with clinical judgment (Angold, 2002; Leffler et al., 2015).

Structured interviews formally examine particular problem areas with several expectations, including that the interviews (1) are internally consistent, (2) have specific rules regarding the content and order of the questions asked (e.g., asking whether depressed mood is present prior to asking the possible effects of the depressed mood) as well as the manner of recording responses, and (3) have some degree of guidance provided for arriving at final diagnostic decisions (Weiss, 1993). Structured interviews are generally geared toward gathering information about specific DSM criteria and are therefore typically ideal for assessing psychiatric symptoms and formulating diagnoses. Furthermore, structured interviews are commonly used because they include a standard set of questions designed to cover the range of topics necessary for obtaining relevant information about the interviewee's presenting problems. The degree to which the interview fits with these expectations and the amount of latitude allotted to the examiner result in classifications of semi-structured or highly structured (also sometimes referred to as respondent- or interview-based; Leffler et al., 2015).

For the most part, the format of (semi-/highly) structured parent and child companion interviews is similar. The typical layout is (1) an introductory section designed to help build rapport with the informant (e.g., demographics, school, psychological history) and elicit initial information regarding presenting problems and history; (2) disorder-specific sections targeting symptom presence, frequency, intensity, duration, and interference; and (3) diagnostic formulations based on pre-set algorithms and/or clinical judgments. All of the interviews can be used in either research or clinical settings and typically require 1–3 h to complete. In addition, for most interview sets, the parent version contains additional diagnostic categories (e.g., the child version of the ADIS-IV does not contain the enuresis section, while the parent version does) and can be used alone when the child is too young to complete his/her respective version. Further, most structured interviews are comprised of questions that are asked in a branching manner. For each diagnostic category, there are screener or core questions that must be administered. Secondary questions are then asked only if the child/parent endorsed the initial screener questions. However, if the initial questions are *not* endorsed, the interview proceeds to the next diagnostic category. Specific descriptions and examples of highly and semi-structured interviews are presented below. However, it is important to highlight that the recent publishing of DSM-5 has resulted in the need for modification to these interviews (e.g., to realign with altered or new diagnostic criteria), and, at present, the majority of these have not yet been released. Therefore, in the descriptions below, specific indication is made as to whether the interview corresponds with DSM-IV or DSM-5.

Highly Structured Interviews Overall, highly structured interviews are more restrictive in the amount of freedom allotted to the interviewer. With these interviews, it is generally expected that examiners ask all questions in the same manner and order, as well as record all responses in a prespecified manner. Given the rigid format, clinical judgment is reduced, and specific and/or extensive training is usually not required. In fact, highly structured interviews are commonly administered by laypersons (e.g., individuals without a formal degree in psychology, psychiatry, or social work), and several have been converted to computer-based formats which have been noted to reduce time and potential recording errors (Leffler et al., 2015). Although these strengths allow for more confidence in the exactness of the interview's administration, the rigidity of the interview may also make it seem impersonal, hinder the establishment of rapport, and limit opportunity to report all difficulties or to explore them fully (Breton et al., 1995; LaGreca & Stone, 1992). As a result, the use of highly structured interviews may result in unanswered questions for the clinician (e.g., potential precipitants, etiological factors, responses by others in the child's environment, developmental context) that may need to be further assessed in a less structured format.

The Diagnostic Interview Schedule for Children (*DISC*; Shaffer, Fisher, Lucas, Dulcan, & Schwab-Stone, 2000) was designed to assess psychiatric disorders that can be identified in children and adolescents. The DISC-IV (for DSM-IV/ICD-10) evaluates symptoms from the past year, as well as recent (last month) symptoms for any areas endorsed. The DISC utilizes "gate" questions that allow the interviewer to skip sections of the interview that are irrelevant to the individual without hindering the reliability of the examination. Given the highly structured format, little training is required for administration. Indeed, lay interviewers and computer administration (C-DISC-4.0) are common given questions are read verbatim following a specified order and diagnoses are computer generated. The DISC has been extensively researched, and several additional versions (e.g., Spanish, Teacher) have been developed (Shaffer et al., 2000).

The *Children's Interview for Psychiatric Syndromes* (*ChIPS*; Weller, Weller, Fristad, Rooney, & Schecter, 2000; Weller, Weller, Teare, & Fristad, 1999) is also considered a highly structured interview and was designed to allow for reports from younger children as well as their parents (both versions for ages 6–18). It is shorter than other structured interviews, and it incorporates concise sentence structure and simple language to ensure comprehension. The ChIPS for DSM-IV includes 20 sections that assess Axis I diagnoses and two sections that examine psychosocial stressors. Lay interviewers can be trained in the administration of the ChIPS, with a scoring manual used to record and summarize responses (Weller et al., 2000). Extensive studies have been conducted and published on the development of the ChIPS (Fristad, Cummins, et al., 1998; Fristad, Glickman, et al., 1998; Fristad, Teare, Weller, Weller, & Salmon, 1998; Teare, Fristad, Weller, Weller, & Salmon, 1998a, 1998b).

The *Mini-International Neuropsychiatric Interview for Children and Adolescents* (*MINI-KID*; Sheehan, Shytle, Milo, Janavs, & Lecrubier, 2009) is a structured interview intended for children ages 6–17 years of age. Recently, the MINI-KID for DSM-5 has been released (Version 7.0.2). The MINI-KID assesses several common psychiatric disorders affecting youth using "branching tree logic" and was designed for efficient administration (15–50 min). Two to four screening questions (yes/no format) are asked for each disorder, and follow-up questions are only asked when symptoms of a disorder are endorsed. The MINI-KID is widely used among diverse groups across the globe (e.g., Uganda; Kinyanda, Kizza, Abbo, Ndyanabangi, & Levin, 2013) and has been translated into many different languages (e.g., Polish, Portuguese, Spanish).

Semi-Structured Interviews Semi-structured interviews represent a combination of structured and unstructured interview formats. These interviews typically include a suggested order and configuration like that of highly structured interviews while also allowing greater opportunity to follow up on questions and flexibility on the phrasing and recording of questions and responses. Emphasis is placed on obtaining consistent and reliable information, and as such extensive training is generally required for administration of semi-structured interviews to ensure that clinical discretion will be applied judiciously.

The *Schedule for Affective Disorders and Schizophrenia for School-Age Children* (*K-SADS*) for DSM-IV has a primary focus on affective disorders; however, several additional psychiatric disorders are also examined. The three most current and widely used versions of the K-SADS are Present State (Ambrosini & Dixon, 1996), Epidemiological (Orvaschel, 1995), and Present/Lifetime (Kaufman et al., 1997). Each of these interviews has child and parent companion versions that differ primarily in regard to the diagnostic time frame examined. For example, the Present State Version examines disorders from the past 12 months and most recent episode, whereas the Epidemiological and Present/Lifetime Versions focus on current and lifetime disorders. Typically, the K-SADS parent version is administered before the child version, with discrepancies addressed in a subsequent joint interview. Following the interviews and consideration of all reports (e.g., parent, child, school, clinicians), the clinician determines summary severity scores, and diagnoses are made based on criteria checklists of symptom severity (i.e., Research Diagnostic Criteria). Other K-SADS sections include behavioral observations, global impressions, and reliability and completeness of the interview. Clinically trained interviewers familiar with K-SADS are required for administering this semi-structured interview, and training costs are noted to vary by version (Ambrosini, 2000).

The *Child and Adolescent Psychiatric Assessment* (CAPA; Angold & Costello, 2000; Angold, Prendergast, Cox, & Harrington, 1995) is a semi-structured interview designed to generate DSM-IV diagnoses. The CAPA has been referred to as "glossary based" because it includes an interview glossary that has detailed definitions of each symptom, which then provides the basis for client response interpretation (Angold & Fisher, 1999). The diagnostic section of the interview is given first and includes evaluation of symptoms and functional impairment followed by the assessment of family structure, functioning, and resources. Each diagnostic section includes a brief description of the symptom being assessed, as well as screening questions, which must be asked verbatim unless modified wording is required for child comprehension. Optional follow-up questions are also provided for the clinician to use if clarification of previous responses is necessary. Additionally, coding rules are applied for rating symptoms in terms of intensity, setting, and timing, as applicable. After the interview, the examiner completes a series of questions based on behavioral observations (i.e., motor behavior, level of activity, apparent mood, and social interaction). Interviewers must have at least a bachelor's degree and receive extensive training in CAPA administration by a qualified CAPA trainer over the course of approximately 1 month.

The *Diagnostic Interview for Children and Adolescents* (*DICA*; Reich, 1998, 2000) is a semi-structured interview designed to examine a wide range of DSM-IV psychiatric disorders. There are two separate youth versions (for ages 6–12 and 13–17 years) and a corresponding parent version. The DICA begins with a joint parent/child interview of demographics, school, and psychiatric and medical histories. This is followed by separately conducted diagnostic sections of the parent and youth interviews. In addition, the parent version also includes inquiries of psychosocial stressors, risk/protective factors, perinatal, delivery, and early child development. The DICA includes structured probes to allow the clinician to clarify interviewee responses when warranted (Silverman, 1994). Following completion of the interview, the interviewer pursues problematic areas which are then resolved by consultation with the DICA manual and/or discussion with more experienced clinicians. A highly structured computerized version of the DICA is also available for administration by trained interviewers or the informant alone. Interviewers must hold at least a bachelor's degree and require approximately 2–4 weeks of training in the DICA. The focus of the interviewer is on rating each symptom and not ruling upon the presence or absence of diagnoses (Reich, 2000).

The *Interview Schedule for Children and Adolescents* (*ISCA*; Kovacs, 1997; Sherrill & Kovacs, 2000) is a semi-structured, symptom-oriented interview that allows for the generation of several diagnoses by mapping symptoms onto the DSM-IV disorders. The ISCA contains five sections: signs and symptoms (e.g., anxiety, dysregulated behavior), mental status (i.e., orientation), behavioral observations (i.e., nonverbal expression), clinical impressions (i.e., social maturity), and developmental milestones (i.e., dating). There is also one item that examines the child's global functioning and social impairment. The ISCA assesses current symptoms; however, separate current/lifetime and current/interim (i.e., since last assessment) versions are also available. The ISCA is usually administered by the same clinician to the parent(s) first and then the child separately. Although all questions are asked of each informant, the interviewer can decide upon the order of administration. At the end of the assessment, the interviewer combines the ratings from both the parent and child to establish an overall symptom rating. A diagnosis is made based on correspondence between established criteria (e.g., DSM) and the clinical significance and temporal sequence of the overall symptom ratings. Clinically relevant experience with semi-structured interviews and diagnostic system(s) is requisite for ISCA administration.

The *Anxiety Disorders Interview Schedule for DSM-IV, Child and Parent Versions* (ADIS-IV:C/P; Silverman & Albano, 1996) is a semi-structured interview that permits diagnoses of all anxiety disorders, as well as several other disorders of childhood and adolescence (e.g., attention deficit hyperactivity disorder, dysthymia) from the DSM-IV. The parent and child versions overlap considerably; however, the parent version contains several additional disorders (e.g., conduct disorder, oppositional defiant disorder, enuresis) as well as requires greater detail regarding the history and consequences of problems. The child version probes for more in-depth descriptions of symptoms and phenomenology while providing a simpler format and wordings (Silverman & Nelles, 1988). During the interview, respondents are first asked to answer "yes" or "no" to several screener questions. If the child or parent responds affirmatively to the screener, the clinician continues to assess symptoms within that section as well as obtains frequency, intensity, and interference ratings as appropriate. These ratings (e.g., symptom count and interference rating) assist the clinician in identifying which diagnostic criteria are met for the child. Following the interview, clinicians assign severity ratings for each diagnosis met based on their subjective interpretation from the child and parent reports. ADIS training is required prior to administration, and it is recommended that the same clinician interview the child and subsequently the parent(s) (Albano & Silverman, 1996).

Psychometrics of Structured Interviews
Psychometric studies have been conducted for each of the above described structured (highly and semi) interviews. In general, researchers have been concerned with demonstrating the reliability (i.e., consistency of measurement), validity (i.e., degree it assesses what it purports to measure), and clinical utility of these interviews. Overall, consistent findings have been reported across the various structured interviews for which reliability data is available (cf, ADIS-Albano & Silverman, 1996; Weems, Silverman, Saavedra, Pina, & Lumpkin, 1999; Wood, Piacentini, Bergman, McCracken, & Barrios, 2002; CAPA-Angold & Costello, 2000; ChIPS-Weller et al., 2000; DICA-Reich, 1998, 2000; DISC-Costello, Edelbrock, & Costello, 1985; Shaffer et al., 2000; ISCA-Sherrill & Kovacs, 2000; K-SADS-Ambrosini, 2000; MINI-KID, Sheehan et al., 2010). Acceptable test-retest and interrater reliability estimates have been documented for each of the structured interviews (Angold, 2002; Grills & Ollendick, 2002, 2008). In contrast, findings for multiple-informant reliability (e.g., parent-child agreement) have been more varied (Angold, 2002; De Los Reyes & Kazdin, 2005; Grills & Ollendick, 2002, 2008), a result also commonly reported for behavior rating scales (Achenbach, Dumenci, & Rescorla, 2002; Achenbach, McConaughy, & Howell, 1987; De Los Reyes & Kazdin, 2005; DiBartolo & Grills, 2006). Attempts to understand informant discordance have been made at the interview (e.g., order effects, length, structure), interviewer (e.g., experience level, site differences, biases), and interviewee (e.g., age, gender, disorder type, motivation) levels with generally inconsistent results (Grills & Ollendick, 2002). Thus, the broad consensus in the youth assessment area is that parent(s) and children should both be involved in the assessment of youth symptoms and diagnoses (Jensen et al., 1999; Silverman & Ollendick, 2005). Varied results have also been presented for the validity of structured interviews. For example, studies have reported positive results regarding construct and/or criterion-related validity (Ambrosini, 2000; Angold & Costello, 2000; Boyle et al., 1996; Cohen, O'Connor, Lewis, Velez, & Malachowski, 1987; Fristad, Cummins, et al., 1998; Fristad, Teare, et al., 1998; Hodges, McKnew, Burbach, & Roebuck, 1987; Kaufman et al., 1997; Piacentini et al., 1993; Reich, 2000; Schwab-Stone et al., 1996; Sheehan et al., 2010; Teare et al., 1998a; Wood et al., 2002). However, concordance for diagnoses generated by structured interviews and "real-world" clinicians have often been poorer (Jensen & Weisz, 2002; Jewell, Handwerk, Almquist, & Lucas, 2004; Lewczyk, Garland, Hurlburt, Gearity, & Hough, 2003).

DSM-5 Considerations As noted previously, the majority of structured interviews described herein were designed to elicit information pertinent to DSM-IV. With the release of the fifth revision of the Diagnostic and Statistical Manual of Mental Disorders (DSM-5; APA, 2013), all of the interviews require modifications. Based on past revisions to these interviews, the structure will likely remain the same, while content will need to be updated to accurately reflect DSM-5 disorders. For example, several diagnoses (i.e., Pervasive Developmental Disorder, Aspergers Disorder) have been subsumed into the Autism Spectrum Disorder category in DSM-5, which will require substantial modification to this section of the structured interviews. Furthermore, certain diagnoses are entirely new to the DSM-5 and are thus absent from previous interview versions. For instance, disruptive mood dysregulation disorder (DMDD) was added to capture acute irritability and explosive behaviors that were previously being attributed to bipolar disorder in children (Baweja, Mayes, Hameed, & Waxmonsky, 2016). These, too, should be considered in the revision process (see Leffler et al., 2015 for review of modifications required for existing interviews to align with DSM-5). While the MINI-KID (described above) has been adapted for DSM-5, as with its previous versions, not all disorders of childhood and adolescence are evaluated. In contrast, the Computer-Assisted Structured Diagnostic Interview (Giannakopoulos, 2017) was specifically designed to align with DSM-5 and appears to be a promising new highly structured interview. The CASDI includes assessment of 37 different disorders that can be diagnosed in youth and has been preliminarily validated with 258 Greek youth ages 8–18 years old and their parents. In summary, structured interviews specifically for DSM-5 are presently limited, with many requiring updates and/or expansion to their present versions and others requiring further evaluation to establish reliability and validity.

Selecting Interview Procedures

In addition to consideration of psychometric issues and alignment with DSM-5, numerous other factors may guide selection among the various structured diagnostic interviews. For example, the structure and rating system used to score responses and compile information, required training for administration, and costs of interviews vary widely. In addition, the setting in which the interview will take place can be influential. For instance, research, epidemiological, or clinical trial settings will likely involve more in-depth and lengthier interview (and overall assessment) processes. Within these settings, a complete structured interview might be given to the parent and child (along with other assessments). Conversely, in a typical practice setting the clinician would be less likely to engage in a complete interview, due to issues such as cost, lengthiness, and relevance. Rather, in these cases, clinicians often select to engage in unstructured interviewing alone, or in combination with the most relevant modules of a structured interview. Not all interviews cover the same diagnostic categories; thus, the primary area of study or presenting problem may also guide the selection of an interview. For example, while all of the structured interviews evaluate for Major Depressive Disorder, only a few (ISCA, CAPA, MINI-KID) assess for Adjustment Disorders.

The child's age may also help determine the type of interview to select. For example, only a subset of the structured interviews are intended to assess younger children (less than 8 years of age). Further, the more structured an interview, the more difficulty younger children may experience, particularly without the benefit of clinician clarifications and/or elaborations. Indeed, some researchers believe the information contained in structured interviews can be too complex or beyond young children's cognitive capabilities (Breton et al., 1995; Brunshaw & Szatmari, 1988; Edelbrock, Costello, Dulcan, Kalas, & Conover, 1985; Ezpeleta, de la Osa, Doménech, Navarro, & Losilla, 1997; Herjanic & Reich, 1982; Welner, Reich, Herjanic, Jung, & Amado, 1987; Young, O'Brien, Gutterman, & Cohen, 1987). The attention spans of younger children are shorter than adolescents and adults, which could also be problematic with lengthier interviews. This is not meant to imply that younger children's input is not valued, but rather that appropriate strategies should be selected based on the developmental level of the child. For instance, the more flexible, semi-structured interviews are often recommended for younger children because multiple examples, visual aids, and explanations can be utilized (Sattler & Hoge, 2006). Furthermore, the use of pictorial aids has been recommended and incorporated into interviews designed for younger children (cf, Scott, Short, Singer, Russ, & Minnes, 2006; Valla, Bergeron, & Smolla, 2000). Nevertheless, given the similarities among interviews, most often the clinician or researcher's discretion or preference guides the final selection. In fact, Hodges (1994) suggested that there is not one "best" interview, but rather, that researchers and clinicians should determine which interview to use based on the sample and focus of their endeavor.

Considerations for Children with Disabilities and Alternative Language Backgrounds

Modifications of Procedures In conducting any kind of an interview with a child who has a disability, modifications may be necessary. For example, if the child has an oral language disorder that interferes with comprehension of speech, it may be necessary to simplify the language of an unstructured or semi-structured interview so that the vocabulary level is appropriate for the child. Furthermore, it may be more difficult to utilize a structured interview with someone who has a comprehension problem because the language is less modifiable. Similarly, reading problems are common in children (and adults). If the highly structured interview is administered on a computer that requires significant reading, this may be frustrating to the child (or to the parent), and it may be necessary to read the items to the interviewee. There are other considerations that may be relevant depending on the presenting problem, and these should always be considered in selecting and administering a semi-structured or highly structured interview. It is always important to ensure that the interview is appropriate for the participant. For example, children with intellectual disabilities or with autism spectrum disorder may not be able to provide adequate self-reports, and, in these cases, it may be important to rely on third-party observers. Similarly, many interviews are only designed for English speakers and are not translated to other languages and/or have little normative data for non-English speakers.

Adaptive Behavior Assessments An important consideration for evaluating children with developmental disabilities is the need to assess adaptive behavior. Adaptive behavior assessments are particularly important for individuals with intellectual disabilities since the definition of an intellectual disability requires evidence of intellectual and adaptive behavior functions that are two standard deviations below average (American Association on Intellectual and Developmental Disabilities; AAIDD, 2017). Given that they rely on third-party informants and address everyday functioning in social and other domains, adaptive behavior assessments can be helpful in evaluating children with autism spectrum disorders as well. In addition, many adaptive behavior scales have separate maladaptive behavior domains that are not computed as part of the adaptive behavior quotient but are very helpful in evaluating children where social function is a major consideration. For instance, while assessments of adaptive behavior are less frequently used for children who have learning disabilities, they can be helpful with other high incidence disabilities when language or attention is a factor (e.g., ADHD), since they are based on the reports of others. For children who have significant language problems, an assessment of adaptive behavior can be helpful in terms of differentiating cognitive problems that interfere with performance on a cognitive test versus the child's capacity for habitual, everyday functioning.

Adaptive behavior is formally defined as "the collection of conceptual, social, and practical skills that have been learned and performed by people in their everyday lives" (AAIDD, 2017). The AAIDD (2017) goes on to indicate that for the diagnosis of intellectual disability, significant limitations in adaptive behavior and intellectual functioning should be established through the use of standardized measures while also thoughtfully considering community environment, linguistic, and cultural differences.

To illustrate the assessment of adaptive behavior, we will briefly summarize three different assessments that vary in their administration characteristics. All three measures share an emphasis on the importance of multiple informants who are familiar with the person being evaluated. This means that adequate assessments of adaptive behavior involve more than just one person. In addition, because of the cognitive limitations of many people who are the subject of adaptive behavior assessments, third-party observers (caretakers, parents, etc.) are critical informants and are often regarded as more reliable than the person themselves. Certainly, it is possible to use adaptive behavior scales to support decisions about vocational abilities, aptitude and judgment, level of independence, etc., particularly in adults. Here it may be more reasonable to complete self-reports based on adaptive behavior scales, but individuals with cognitive impairments are often not reliable informants and may tend to deny their adaptive behavior limitations.

Vineland Adaptive Behavior Scales (Vineland-3; Sparrow, Cicchetti, & Saulnier, 2016). The third edition of the Vineland assesses adaptive behavior in three domains that are comprised of several subdomains (in parentheses), communication (receptive, expressive, written), daily living skills (personal, domestic, community), and socialization (interpersonal relationships, play and leisure, coping skills), as well as includes two optional indices: motor skills (fine motor, gross motor) and maladaptive behavior (internalizing, externalizing, critical items). Vineland-3 items are scored on a 0–2 scale indicating the degree to which a person habitually performs that described item. The domains of the Vineland-3 align with the AAIDD and DSM-5 criteria necessary to diagnose intellectual disability, but the measure is also commonly used to assess adaptive behavior in individuals with other psychiatric disorders (e.g., autism spectrum, ADHD, brain injury, dementia). There are several available forms of the Vineland-3, including an interview form (for all ages), parent/caregiver form (for all ages and available in Spanish), and teacher rating form (for ages 3–21). Each of the forms is available in comprehensive or domain-level (i.e., briefer and for ages 3+) versions. The parent/caregiver and teacher forms use a standard self-report questionnaire format; however, the Vineland-3 is different from other adaptive behavior instruments in that it also includes the option of administration through a semistructured interview with a client's parent/caregiver (i.e., the interview form). All versions of the Vineland-3 are also available in computer-administered format.

The Vineland-3 Interview Form is semistructured, with the interviewer using a starting point in each of the domains to initiate the interview with the parent/caregiver. For example, in discussing language, the interviewer might say "tell me about the kinds of words that Billy uses around the house." From there, additional questions would be asked that would refine the caregiver responses and allow for scoring. Computer administration of the interview form may be particularly beneficial for less experienced clinicians as it includes suggested follow-up prompts and questions based on interviewee responses. The Vineland-3 Comprehensive Interview Form was standardized on a nationally represented sample of 2560 individuals (see Sparrow et al., 2016, for additional standardization information for the other forms) and was aligned with the 2014 US census. The internal consistency reliability for all domains of this form is very high ($\alpha = 0.90$–0.98). Further adequate test-retest (0.73–0.92) and interrater (0.70–0.81) reliabilities, as well as validity, have been reported for all domains (Sparrow et al., 2016).

Adaptive Behavior Assessment System-3 (ABAS-3; Harrison & Oakland, 2015). Like the Vineland-3, the ABAS-3 has been designed to conform with DSM-5 and the AAIDD definitions of adaptive behavior; however, it is typically administered as a rating scale (versus interview). It is typically completed by multiple, third-party informants who are familiar with the individual being assessed. The ABAS-3 includes teacher forms (for ages 2–5 or 5–21), parent forms (for ages 0–5 or 5–21), and adult forms (for ages 16–89). In addition to assessing conceptual, social, and practical domains, it also breaks into 11 specific adaptive skill areas (depending on the client's age) that underline these constructs (communication, community use, functional academics, health and safety, home or school living, leisure, motor, self-care, self-direction, social skills, work). The respondent completes each item using a 0–3 scoring rubric that indicates how often the identified patient correctly performs a behavior without help when behavior is expected to be displayed. The ABAS-3 forms were standardized with 7737 completed forms regarding a sample of 4500 individuals ages 0–89 and is tied to the 2010 census (Rogers, 2015). The ABAS-3 has demonstrated strong psychometric characteristics. The ABAS-3 also has the option of online administration, as well as includes an intervention planner that corresponds with item areas. The internal consistency reliability coefficients for the overall composite and adaptive domains range from 0.85–0.99 to 0.72–0.99 for the skill areas. Adequate test-retest (0.76–0.89 for domains/composite and 0.70–0.80 for skill areas) and interrater (0.77–0.92 for domains/composite and 0.67–0.74 for skill areas) reliabilities, as well as validity, have also been reported (Rogers, 2015).

In addition to the Vineland-3 Interview (and rating forms) and the ABAS-3 rating scales, additional measures of adaptive behavior exist (e.g., Schalock, 1999). For example, the AAIDD has recently developed a semi-structured interview, the Diagnostic Adaptive Behavior Scale, which is designed for individuals aged 4–21 and has already demonstrated strong psychometric properties (Tassé et al., 2016; https://aaidd.org/intellectual-disability/diagnostic-adaptive-behavior-scale). In addition, the Scales of Independent Behavior-Revised (Bruininks, Woodcock, Weatherman, & Hill, 1996) is a highly structured interview that has been a commonly utilized tool for decades, but has not presently been updated to align with current DSM and AAIDD guidelines. Thus, several tools exist for evaluating adaptive behavior skills and incorporating this information into a more extensive assessment. Level of education, the nature of the disability, language dominance factors, and other issues should always be factored into the determination of adaptive behavior level, particularly for a high-stake clinical diagnosis like an intellectual disability. Moreover, the use of multiple responders is critical for adaptive behavior assessments, since they are largely based on third parties.

Report Writing

Many novice clinicians find report writing to be a challenge, likely in part due to inexperience and in part due to differing styles and expectations among supervisors and colleagues. It can be helpful for report writers to develop a standard template, particularly when they are learning to write reports. A standard template that lays out the different parts of the report helps consolidate the data and the different types of interpretations. In addition, it helps the novice report writer deal with the biggest problem in writing reports, which is how to organize the data, which can be voluminous. Organization can also be useful as there is a tendency for report writers to include data that extends beyond the comprehension of non-psychological consumers and too often write reports that are longer than necessary. Oftentimes, addendum tables can be utilized to provide all necessary data and the report can focus on critical data and interpretations. Interviews are often given in the context of other procedures, such as assessments of cognitive function. It is important to integrate the interview information and report it at a construct level, as opposed to individual responses or even detailed discussions of specific scores. A report is always an opinion by a psychologist that utilizes the test data but is tempered by clinical judgment that is informed by the data, behavioral observations, and relevant history.

To help develop a template, consider a report that includes the following (or similar) sections: Referral Information, Procedures Employed, Relevant Background Information, Behavioral Observations, Assessment Results and Interpretations, Clinical Formulation/Conclusions, and Recommendations. The Referral Information section should be a brief summary that provides pertinent demographics, identifying the name, age, and ethnicity of the child. Usually a clinician would include information about the referral source, any specific concerns that led to the referral, and the primary assessment question. Oftentimes this information can be obtained from an intake form or interview

The Procedures section is simply a list of all the instruments, interviews, and other tools used to collect data. The information in the Relevant Background section can come from many sources, including previous evaluations, medical records, unstructured interviews of the child, parent and teacher rating scales, and other sources. Care should be given in revealing personal information, family conflicts, and other information that may need confidentiality if a report is going to a school or at some point could involve a forensic situation. In addition, it is important to apply scrupulous judgment in determining the accuracy of different reports about the child. The clinician does not need to demonstrate their thought processes in summarizing this information but simply provide the most reasonable summary and indicate whether there are consistencies or inconsistencies across different sources. The depth of information summarized in this section may also depend on the referral question or recommendations deriving from the report. For example, a more detailed background of academic testing, services, and supports may be necessary for questions of learning disabilities, whereas greater medical history may be relevant for a case with traumatic brain injury.

The Behavioral Observations section typically entails a brief mental status examination of the child that includes appearance, affect, mood, speech, attention, and any other behaviors that are relevant to understanding the child's presentation and the adequacy of the evaluation. This section should always conclude with a statement about whether the assessor believes the results to appropriately estimate the child's current level of functioning.

Test Results and Interpretations is the data section of the report. The areas covered in this section will vary depending on what measures have been administered. In a typical comprehensive child evaluation, this section is divided into different sections (e.g., Cognitive Assessment, Academic Achievement, Behavioral Adjustment). Information derived from an interview would typically be summarized in the behavioral adjustment section or in a separate diagnostic interview/impressions section that presents parent and/or child interview data. If the interview yields pertinent data, significant elevations may be discussed (as opposed to discussing every single scale). The overall job of the clinician is to integrate the data into a coherent statement (e.g., about the child's intellectual or behavioral level).

The Clinical Formulation/Conclusions section is a precise formulation of the overall results of the assessment. It should be concise, highlighting the essential components of the findings while also tying all relevant pieces of information together. Inclusion of information collected from all informants is imperative for acquiring the most comprehensive and accurate account of the child's presenting problems, particularly given the situation-specific nature of some child behaviors (e.g., inattention at school but not when watching television). Therefore, rather than searching for the "correct" answer among informant reports, it has been recommended that clinicians consider all sources of information and allow discrepancies to be interpreted as informative, not problematic (Boyle et al., 1996; Schwab-Stone et al., 1996). If a diagnostic impression is generated, this will be identified at the end of the Conclusions. Sometimes a justification of differential diagnoses is also provided. Clinicians should be certain to attend to all referral questions in the Conclusions section. Confirming or disconfirming evidence can be provided to specifically address each of the referral questions. Finally, clinicians should attend to client strengths and provide a summation of these in the conclusions section.

Recommendations follow and are often the most important component of a report. It may be helpful to organize the recommendations, for example, by listing them as consecutive numbers that are tied to the formulation. In general, it is important for the recommendations to be flexible and to take into account the resources available to the family. Recommendations should address all the different dimensions covered in the report and should provide detailed suggestions or appropriate referrals whenever possible. Since the purpose of doing an evaluation is often to determine interventions that would be helpful to the child and to the family, the report should be written in a way that supports the recommendations and makes clear the direction recommended by the clinician who conducted the evaluation.

Finally, it is important to write reports that are clear and appropriate for the person who will be a consumer. For example, many physicians are most focused on the conclusion section, whereas school psychologists may be particularly interested in information relevant to an IEP or 504 Plan. Some psychologists may wish to actually see more of the data, in which case a consent form can be signed to release specific data. Importantly, most state rules as well as the rules of publishers prohibit the release of raw data to non-psychologists, and it is up to the clinician to become familiar with the laws and rules governing the distribution of raw data.

Summary

As illustrated throughout this chapter, the interview is a critical element of the psychological assessment of a child, allowing for the evaluation and observation of behavioral and emotional functioning. Unstructured interviews are conducted as part of most clinical evaluations; however structured (i.e., semi or highly) interviews are often preferable for diagnostic and research purposes. The standardization of structured interviews allows for increased diagnostic reliability, and the rigid format permits administration by laypersons or computers, as well as clinicians. On the other hand, the strict format may also interfere with reliability and validity, as it may not provide the interviewee with the opportunity to report all difficulties or explore them in greater depth. As a result, the clinician using the structured interview may have unanswered questions that need to be addressed in a less structured format. Another reason clinicians may choose to use a less structured format, at least initially, is to allow for the establishment of good rapport with the child. As this is one of the most important factors of successful interview administration with children, clinicians should not immediately commence with an inflexible format as the impersonal nature may hinder rapport.

Structured parent-child interviews inquire about disorder-specific information that focuses on symptom presence, frequency, intensity, duration, interference, and diagnostic formulations. Several highly structured (e.g., DISC, ChIPS, MINI-KID) and semi-structured (e.g., K-SADS, CAPA, DICA, ISCA, ADIS) interviews are available; though, at present, only the MINI-KID has been updated to reflect changes in DSM-5. Although structured interviews can be lengthy to deliver, diagnostic disagreement as well as various biases can be minimized through the careful administration of standardized assessments like these (Ely, Graber, & Croskerry, 2011; Frick et al., 2010; Hughes et al., 2000). Clinicians may choose to include only particularly relevant sections of structured interviews to balance time constraints with these benefits. Further, the clinical utility of interviews may be enhanced by incorporating functional assessments/interviews (e.g., Questions About Behavioral Function; Matson, Bamburg, Cherry, & Paclawskyj, 1999) with them. Such interviews can help to establish timelines for presenting problems including the onset, duration, and progress, which can help to guide treatment (Frick et al., 2010).

When interviewing children with disabilities, modifications to the aforementioned interview process and format are usually required. For example, using a structured interview with someone who has a comprehension, reading, or language problem is more difficult because the rigid format does not allow for modification. Therefore, in most cases, semi-structured interviews are preferable for children with disabilities. It is also useful to include assessment of the child's adaptive behaviors in instances when the child has, or is suspected to have, a developmental disability (e.g., autism spectrum disorders). Interviews of adaptive behaviors are typically conducted with individuals who frequently observe the child (e.g., parents/caregivers, teachers) and may be highly or semi-structured (e.g., Vineland-3, ABAS-3).

Finally, the discussion of report writing was included as this is the best way to gather and organize all the data collected during the interview (and any additional assessment measures given). Recommendations for report writing were reviewed in this chapter. In addition, a suggested report template was discussed and included the following sections: Referral Information, Procedures Employed, Relevant Background Information, Behavioral Observations, Assessment Results and Interpretations, Clinical Formulation/

Conclusions, and Recommendations. The recommendations made at the end of the report are crucial as the purpose of doing an evaluation is to determine helpful interventions for the child and family. The inclusion of all of the sections provided will provide a comprehensive report of the child's behavioral and emotional functioning as evidenced from the given assessment.

Appendix: Sample Developmental History Questionnaire

Child's name:		Date of birth:	Age:
Adopted? ☐ Yes ☐ No			
Form completed by:		Date:	
Parent/primary caregiver name:		Parent/primary caregiver name:			
Address:			Address:		
City:	State:	Zip:	City:	State:	Zip:
Phone:			Phone:		
Email:			Email:		

Family Information

Parent/Caregiver

Parent:	Age:			Occupation:
	Years of education:			Highest degree:
	Year married:			If divorced, year:
Parent:	Age:			Occupation:
	Years of education:			Highest degree:
	Year married:			If divorced, year:
Custodial agreement:				

Brothers and Sisters

Name	Sex	Age	Grade	Where living, if out of child's home	Relationship to child (full, half, step)

Family History

	Relationship to child
1. Attention deficit hyperactivity disorder (ADHD)	
2. Learning disability	
3. Speech/language problems	
4. Epilepsy	
5. Slow learner	
6. Anxiety	
7. Depression	
8. Bipolar disorder	
9. Conduct problems/aggression	
10. Alcohol abuse	
11. Substance abuse	
12. Schizophrenia	
13. Intellectual disability	
14. Autism spectrum disorder	
15. Other mental health concerns List:	

Pregnancy Information

Medical Condition

Type	Yes/no	Month of pregnancy	Description
Illness			
Hypertension			
Bleeding			
Diabetes			
Exposure to toxic substance			
Exposure to X-rays			
Medications			

Labor and Delivery

Was labor normal? _____		Labor lasted _____ hours.	
Full term? ☐ Yes ☐ No If no, premature delivery occurred at _____ months of pregnancy.			
Delivery was: _____ Vaginal _____ Head first _____ Breech _____ C-Section			
Birth weight: _____ lbs. _____ ozs.		Length: _____ inches	

Baby

	Yes	No	
Was normal at birth?			
Cried immediately following birth?			
Needed help breathing?			For how long? _____
Needed oxygen?			For how long? _____
Needed blood transfusion?			
Had jaundice during first week?			
Was discharged from newborn nursery at _____ days of life.			

Developmental History

How old (months) was your child when he/she:			
Crawled?	Stood?	Sat?	Walked?
Spoke in simple phrases?		Said first words?	
Did your child ever have difficulty speaking?		☐ No ☐ Yes - Age?	
Completed toilet training?			

Medical History of Child

Illnesses

	Yes/no	Age (yrs.)	Complications
Chickenpox			
Measles			
German measles			
Rheumatic fever			
Pneumonia			
Meningitis			
Encephalitis			
Head injury			
Recurrent strep throat			
Sinus/ear infections			
Asthma			
Allergies			
Other illnesses			
Other injuries			

Operations

Type	Year	Complications/results

Educational History

Current school:		
Address:		
City:	State:	Zip:
Phone:		Fax:
Principal:		Main teacher:
What kinds of grades is your child currently getting in school?		
Has your child's school performance changed from prior years?		

Please complete below, beginning with kindergarten.

Type of class. Please indicate whether your child was in **regular, gifted/talented, special education, 504, or **others** (please explain).

School year	Grade	Age	School name	Pass (Y/N)	Type of class**
	K				
	1				
	2				
	3				
	4				
	5				
	6				
	7				
	8				
	9				
	10				
	11				
	12				

Has your child been diagnosed with:

Diagnosis	Year	Treatment
ADD/ADHD		
Learning disabilities		
Speech or language delay		
Developmental delay		
Fine or gross motor delay		
Intellectual disability		
Autism spectrum disorder		
Tourette's syndrome		
Seizure disorder		
Traumatic brain injury		
Headaches		
Visual problems		
Others please list:		

Has your child had any of these behavioral problems? (Please circle)

Short attention span	Yes	No
Clumsy	Yes	No
Truancy	Yes	No
Overly active	Yes	No
Fighting	Yes	No
Underachieving	Yes	No
Anxiety/fearfulness	Yes	No

Interview and Report Writing

What is your child's current sleeping habits/schedule (e.g., bedtime, time child wakes up in the morning, nightmares/sleep problems)

Abuse history: To your knowledge, has your child ever been physically/sexually abused? Witnessed violence?

Medication History

List prescription medication child has taken on a regular basis (i.e., stimulants, antidepressants, anticonvulsants).

Medication	Dose	Reason for medication	Age

Family Stressors

List any stressors that your child/family has experienced in the past two years (e.g., death of pet, death/illness of family members, school performance issues, financial stresses).

References

Achenbach, T. H. (2001). *Manuals for the child behavior checklist and caregiver/teacher report forms/1½-5, 6–18*. Burlington, VT: ASEBA.

Achenbach, T. M., Dumenci, L., & Rescorla, L. A. (2002). Ten-year comparisons of problems and competencies for national samples of youth: Self, parent and teacher reports. *Journal of Emotional and Behavioral Disorders, 10*, 194–203.

Achenbach, T. M., McConaughy, S. H., & Howell, C. T. (1987). Child/adolescent behavioral and emotional problems: Implications of cross-informant correlations for situational specificity. *Psychological Bulletin, 101*, 213–232.

Albano, A. M., & Silverman, W. K. (1996). *The anxiety disorders interview schedule for children for DSM-IV: Clinician manual (Child and Parent Versions)*. New York, NY: Oxford Press.

Ambrosini, P. J. (2000). Historical development and present status of the Schedule for Affective Disorders and Schizophrenia for school-age children (K-SADS). *Journal of the American Academy of Child and Adolescent Psychiatry, 39*, 49–58.

Ambrosini, P. J., & Dixon, J. F. (1996). *Schedule for affective disorders and schizophrenia for school-age children (K-SADS-IVR)-present state and epidemiological version*. Medical College of Pennsylvania and Hahneman University, Philadelphia, PA.

American Association on Intellectual and Developmental Disabilities. (2017). Definition of intellectual disability. Retrieved from: https://aaidd.org/intellectual-disability/definition#.WSWqcbwrLsE

American Psychiatric Association. (2013). *Diagnostic and statistical manual of mental disorders* (5th ed.). Arlington, VA: American Psychiatric Publishing.

Angold, A. (2002). Diagnostic interviews with parents and children. In M. Rutter & E. Taylor (Eds.), *Child and adolescent psychiatry: Modern approaches* (4th ed., pp. 32–51). Oxford, UK: Blackwell Publishing.

Angold, A., & Costello, E. (2000). The Child and Adolescent Psychiatric Assessment (CAPA). *Journal of the American Academy of Child & Adolescent Psychiatry, 39*, 39–48.

Angold, A., & Fisher, P. (1999). *Interviewer-based interviews. Diagnostic assessment in child and adolescent psychopathology* (pp. 34–64). New York, NY: Guilford Press.

Angold, A., Prendergast, M., Cox, A., & Harrington, R. (1995). The Child and Adolescent Psychiatric Assessment (CAPA). *Psychological Medicine, 25*, 739–753.

Baweja, R., Mayes, S. D., Hameed, U., & Waxmonsky, J. G. (2016). Disruptive mood dysregulation disorder: Current insights. *Neuropsychiatric Disease and Treatment, 12*, 2115–2124. https://doi.org/10.2147/NDT.S100312

Bierman, K., & Schwartz, L. (1986). Clinical child interviews: Approaches and developmental considerations. *Journal of Child & Adolescent Psychotherapy, 3*, 267–278.

Boyle, M. H., Offord, D. R., Racine, Y. A., Szatmari, P., Sanford, M., & Fleming, J. E. (1996). Interviews versus checklists: Adequacy for classifying childhood psychiatric disorder based on adolescent reports. *International Journal of Methods in Psychiatric Research, 6*, 309–319.

Breton, J., Bergeron, L., Valla, J., Lepine, S., Houde, L., & Gaudet, N. (1995). Do children aged 9 through 11 years understand the DISC version 2.25 questions? *Journal of the American Academy of Child and Adolescent Psychiatry, 34*, 946–956.

Bruininks, R., Woodcock, R., Weatherman, R., & Hill, B. (1996). *Scales of independent behavior–revised*. Itasca, IL: Riverside.

Brunshaw, J. M., & Szatmari, P. (1988). The agreement between behaviour checklists and structured psychiatric interviews for children. *Canadian Journal of Psychiatry, 33*, 474–481.

Chambers, W. J., Puig-Antich, J., Hirsch, M., Paez, P., Ambrosini, P. J., Tabrizi, M. A., & Davies, M. (1985). The assessment of affective disorders in children and adolescents by semistructured interview: Test-retest reliability of the schedule for affective disorders and schizophrenia for school-age children, present episode version. *Archives of General Psychiatry, 42*, 696–702.

Cohen, P., O'Connor, P., Lewis, S., Velez, C. N., & Malachowski, B. (1987). Comparison of DISC and K-SADS-P interviews of an epidemiological sample of children. *Journal of the American Academy of Child and Adolescent Psychiatry, 26*, 662–667.

Costello, E., Edelbrock, C., & Costello, A. (1985). Validity of the NIMH diagnostic interview schedule for children: A comparison between psychiatric and pediatric referrals. *Journal of Abnormal Child Psychology, 13*, 579–595.

De Los Reyes, A., & Kazdin, A. E. (2005). Informant discrepancies in the assessment of childhood psychopathology: A critical review, theoretical framework, and recommendations for further study. *Psychological Bulletin, 131*, 483–509.

DiBartolo, P., & Grills, A. (2006). Who is best at predicting children's anxiety in response to a social evaluative task? A comparison of child, parent, and teacher reports. *Journal of Anxiety Disorders, 20*, 630–645.

Edelbrock, C., & Costello, A. J. (1990). Structured interviews for children and adolescents. In G. Goldstein & M. Hersen (Eds.), *Handbook of psychological assessment. Pergamon general psychology series* (Vol. 131, pp. 308–323). New York, NY: Pergamon Press.

Edelbrock, C., Costello, A. J., Dulcan, M. K., Kalas, R., & Conover, N. C. (1985). Age differences in the reliability of the psychiatric interview of the child. *Child Development, 56*, 265–275.

Ely, J. W., Graber, M. L., & Croskerry, P. (2011). Checklists to reduce diagnostic errors. *Academic Medicine, 86*(3), 307–313. https://doi.org/10.1097/ACM.0b013e31820824cd

Ezpeleta, L., de la Osa, N., Doménech, J. M., Navarro, J. B., & Losilla, J. M. (1997). Diagnostic agreement between clinicians and the diagnostic interview for children and adolescents--DICA--R--in an outpatient sample. *Journal of Child Psychology and Psychiatry and Allied Disciplines, 38*, 431–440.

Frick, P. J., Barry, C. T., & Kamphaus, R. W. (2010). *Clinical assessment of child and adolescent personality and behavior* (3rd ed.). New York, NY: Springer Science + Business Media. https://doi.org/10.1007/978-1-4419-0641-0

Fristad, M. A., Cummins, J., Verducci, J. S., Teare, M., Weller, E. B., & Weller, R. A. (1998). Study IV: Concurrent validity of the DSM-IV revised Children's Interview for Psychiatric Syndromes (ChIPS). *Journal of Child and Adolescent Psychopharmacology, 8*, 227–236.

Fristad, M. A., Glickman, A. R., Verducci, J. S., Teare, M., Weller, E. B., & Weller, R. A. (1998). Study V: Children's Interview for Psychiatric Syndromes (ChIPS): Psychometrics in two community samples. *Journal of Child and Adolescent Psychopharmacology, 8*, 237–245.

Fristad, M. A., Teare, M., Weller, E. B., Weller, R. A., & Salmon, P. (1998). Study III: Development and concurrent validity of the Children's Interview for Psychiatric Syndromes (ChIPS). *Journal of Child and Adolescent Psychopharmacology, 8*, 221–226.

Garb, H. N., & Boyle, P. A. (2015). Understanding why some clinicians use pseudoscientific methods: Findings from research on clinical judgment. In S. O. Lilienfeld, S. J. Lynn, & J. M. Lohr (Eds.), *Science and pseudoscience in clinical psychology* (pp. 19–41). New York, NY: Guilford Press.

Giannakopoulos, G. (2017). Concurrent validity of the computer-assisted structured diagnostic interview (CASDI) for children and adolescents aged 8-18 years old. *The Open Psychology Journal, 10*, 1–10.

Greenspan, S., & Greenspan, N. (2003). *The clinical interview of the child* (3rd ed.). Washington, DC: American Psychiatric Publishing, Inc.

Grills, A. E., & Ollendick, T. H. (2008). Diagnostic interviewing. In M. Hersen & A. M. Gross (Eds.), *Handbook of clinical psychology* (Volume 2): Children and Adolescents. New York, NY: Wiley.

Grills, A. E., & Ollendick, T. H. (2002). Issues in parent-child agreement: The case of structured diagnostic interviews. *Clinical Child and Family Psychology Review, 5*, 57–83.

Harrison, P.L., & Oakland, T. (2015). *Adaptive behavior assessment system* (3rd ed.). Torrance, CA : Western Psychological Services

Herba, C., Landau, S., Russell, T., Ecker, C., & Phillips, M. (2006). The development of emotion-processing in children: Effects of age, emotion, and intensity. *Journal of Child Psychology and Psychiatry, 47*, 1098–1106.

Herjanic, B., Herjanic, M., Brown, F., & Wheatt, T. (1975). Are children reliable reporters? *Journal of Abnormal Child Psychology, 3*, 41–48.

Herjanic, B., & Reich, W. (1982). Development of a structured psychiatric interview for children: Agreement between child and parent on individual symptoms. *Journal of Abnormal Child Psychology, 10*, 307–324.

Hodges, K. (1994). Debate and argument: Reply to David Shaffer: Structured interviews for assessing children. *Journal of Child Psychology and Psychiatry and Allied Disciplines, 35*, 785–787.

Hodges, K., McKnew, D., Burbach, D. J., & Roebuck, L. (1987). Diagnostic concordance between the Child Assessment Schedule (CAS) and the Schedule for Affective Disorders and Schizophrenia for school-age children (K-SADS) in an outpatient sample using lay interviewers. *Journal of the American Academy of Child and Adolescent Psychiatry, 26*, 654–661.

Hughes, C. W., Rintelmann, J., Mayes, T., Emslie, G. J., Pearson, G., & Rush, A. J. (2000). Structured interview and uniform assessment improves diagnostic reliability. *Journal of Child and Adolescent Psychopharmacology, 10*, 119–131.

Hunsley, J., Lee, C. M., Wood, J. M., & Taylor, W. (2014). Controversial and questionable assessment techniques. In S. O. Lilienfeld, S. J. Lynn, & J. M. Lohr (Eds.), *Science and pseudoscience in clinical psychology* (pp. 42–82). New York, NY: Guilford.

Jensen, P. S., Rubio-Stipec, M., Canino, G., Bird, H. R., Dulcan, M. K., Schwab-Stone, M. E., & Lahey, B. B. (1999). Parent and child contributions to diagnosis of mental disorder: Are both informants always necessary? *Journal of the American Academy of Child and Adolescent Psychiatry, 38*, 1569–1579.

Jensen, A., & Weisz, J. (2002). Assessing match and mismatch between practitioner-generated and standardized interview-generated diagnoses for clinic-referred children and adolescents. *Journal of Consulting and Clinical Psychology, 70*, 158–168.

Jewell, J., Handwerk, M., Almquist, J., & Lucas, C. (2004). Comparing the validity of clinician-generated diagnosis of conduct disorder to the diagnostic interview schedule for children. *Journal of Clinical Child and Adolescent Psychology, 33*, 536–546.

Karver, M. S. (2006). Determinants of multiple\informant agreement on child and adolescent behavior. *Journal of Abnormal Child Psychology, 34*, 251–262.

Kaufman, J., Birmaher, B., Brent, D., Rao, U., Flynn, C., Moreci, P., … Ryan, N. (1997). Schedule for Affective Disorders and Schizophrenia for School-Age Children-Present and Lifetime version (K-SADS-PL): Initial reliability and validity data. *Journal of the American Academy of Child and Adolescent Psychiatry, 36*, 980–988.

Kinyanda, E., Kizza, R., Abbo, C., Ndyanabangi, S., & Levin, J. (2013). Prevalence and risk factors of depression in childhood and adolescence as seen in 4 districts of northeastern Uganda. *BMC International Health and Human Rights, 13*(19), 1–10.

Kovacs, M. (1997). *The Interview Schedule for Children and Adolescents (ISCA); Current and Lifetime (ISCA-C & L) and Current and Interim (ISCA-C & I) versions*. Pittsburgh, PA: Western Psychiatric Institute and Clinic.

LaGreca, A. M. (1990). *Through the eyes of the child: Obtaining self-reports from children and adolescents*. Needham Heights, MA: Allyn & Bacon.

LaGreca, A. M., & Stone, W. L. (1992). Assessing children through interviews and behavioral observations. In C. E. Walker & M. C. Roberts (Eds.), *Handbook of clinical child psychology* (2nd ed., pp. 63–83). New York: Wiley Interscience.

Lapouse, R., & Monk, M. A. (1958). An epidemiologic study of behavior characteristics of children. *American Journal of Public Health, 48*, 1134–1144.

Leffler, J. M., Riebel, J., & Hughes, H. M. (2015). A review of child and adolescent diagnostic interviews for clinical practitioners. *Assessment, 22*(6), 690–703.

Lewczyk, C., Garland, A., Hurlburt, M., Gearity, J., & Hough, R. (2003). Comparing DISC-IV and clinician diagnoses among youths receiving public mental health services. *Journal of the American Academy of Child & Adolescent Psychiatry, 42*, 349–356.

Lilienfeld, S. O., Ammirati, R., & David, M. (2012). Distinguishing science from pseudoscience in school psychology: Science and scientific thinking as safeguards against human error. *Journal of School Psychology, 50*, 7–36.

MacLeod, E., Woolford, J., Hobbs, L., Gross, J., Hayne, H., & Patterson, T. (2017). Interviews with children about their mental health problems: The congruence and validity of information that children report. *Clinical Child Psychology and Psychiatry, 22*(2), 229–244.

Magnavita, J. J., & Lilienfeld, S. O. (2016). Clinical expertise and decision making: An overview of bias in clinical practice. In J. J. Magnavita (Ed.), *Clinical decision making in mental health practice* (pp. 23–60). Washington, DC: American Psychological Association.

Marin, C. E., Rey, Y., & Silverman, W. K. (2013). Interviews. In B. D. McLeod, A. Jensen-Doss, & T. Ollendick (Eds.), *Diagnostic and behavioral assessment in children and adolescents* (pp. 103–132). New York, NY: Guilford Press.

Matson, J., Bamburg, J., Cherry, K., & Paclawskyj, T. (1999). A validity study on the Questions About Behavioral Function (QABF) scale: Predicting treatment success for self-injury, aggression, and stereotypies. *Research in Developmental Disabilities, 20*, 163–175.

Moretti, M. M., Fine, S., Haley, G., & Marriage, K. (1985). Childhood and adolescent depression: Child-report versus parent-report information. *Journal of the American Academy of Child Psychiatry, 24*, 298–302.

Ollendick, T. H., & Hersen, M. (1993). *Handbook of child and adolescent assessment*. Boston, MA: Allyn and Bacon.

Orvaschel, H. (1995). *Schedule for Affective Disorders and Schizophrenia for School-Age Children Epidemiologic Version-5*. Ft. Lauderdale, FL: Center for Psychological Studies, Nova Southeastern University.

Piacentini, J., Shaffer, D., Fisher, P., Schwab-Stone, M., Davies, M., & Gioia, P. (1993). The diagnostic interview schedule for children-revised version (DISC-R): III. Concurrent criterion validity. *Journal of the American Academy of Child and Adolescent Psychiatry, 32*, 658–665.

Priestley, G., & Pipe, M. E. (1997). Using toys and models in interviews with young children. *Applied Cognitive Psychology, 11*, 69–87.

Reich, W. (1998). *The Diagnostic Interview for Children and Adolescents (DICA): DSM-IV version*. St. Louis, MO: Washington University School of Medicine.

Reich, W. (2000). Diagnostic interview for children and adolescents (DICA). *Journal of the American Academy of Child and Adolescent Psychiatry, 39*, 59–66.

Reid, G., Grills, A. E., Mian, N. D., Merson, R., & Langer, D. (2017). Using research-informed pedagogical practices to maximize learning in youth cognitive behavioral therapy. *Evidence-Based Practice in Child and Adolescent Mental Health, 2*, 82–95.

Reynolds, C. R., & Kamphaus, R. W. (2015). *Behavior assessment system for children – Third edition (BASC-3)*. Bloomington, MN: Pearson.

Rogers, A. K. (2015). *Adaptive Behavior Assessment System-Third Edition* [pdf document]. Retreived from Illinois Association of School Social Workers 2015 conference web site: https://iassw.org/documents/2015Conference/Session%2041%20Rogers%20handout.pdf

Rutter, M., & Graham, P. (1968). The reliability and validity of the psychiatric assessment of the child: I. Interview with the child. *British Journal of Psychiatry, 114*, 563–579.

Rutter, M., Tizard, J., & Whitmore, K. (1970). *Education, health, and behavior*. London, UK: Longmans.

Rutter, M., Tizard, J., Yule, W., Graham, P., & Whitmore, K. (1976). Isle of Wright studies 1964–1974. *Psychological Medicine, 6*, 313–332.

Rutter, M., Tizard, J., Yule, W., Graham, P., & Whitmore, K. (1977). Isle of Wright studies 1964–1974. In S. Chess & A. Thomas (Eds.), *Annual progress in child psychiatry and child development* (pp. 359–392). New York, NY: Brunner/Mazel, Inc.

Salmon, K. (2006). Toys in clinical interviews with children: Review and implications for practice. *Clinical Psychologist, 10*, 54–59.

Sattler, J. M., & Hoge, R. (2006). *Assessment of children: Behavioral and clinical applications* (5th ed.). San Diego, CA: Author.

Schalock, R. L. (1999). The merging of adaptive behavior and intelligence: Implications for the field of mental retardation. In R. L. Schalock (Ed.), *Adaptive behavior and its measurement: Implications for the field of mental retardation* (pp. 43–60). Washington, DC: American Association on Mental Retardation.

Schwab-Stone, M. E., Shaffer, D., Dulcan, M. K., Jensen, P. S., Fisher, P., Bird, H. R., … Rae, D. S. (1996). Criterion validity of the NIMH Diagnostic Interview Schedule for Children version 2.3 (DISC-2.3). *Journal of the American Academy of Child and Adolescent Psychiatry, 35*, 878–888.

Scott, T., Short, E., Singer, L., Russ, S., & Minnes, S. (2006). Psychometric properties of the Dominic interactive assessment: A computerized self-report for children. *Assessment, 13*, 16–26.

Shaffer, D., Fisher, P., Lucas, C. P., Dulcan, M. K., & Schwab-Stone, M. E. (2000). NIMH Diagnostic Interview Schedule for Children version IV (NIMH DISC-IV): Description, differences from previous versions, and reliability of some common diagnoses. *Journal of the American Academy of Child and Adolescent Psychiatry, 39*, 28–38.

Sheehan, D. V., Sheehan, K. H., Shytle, R. D., Janavs, J., Bannon, Y., Rogers, J. E., … Wilkinson, B. (2010). Reliability and validity of the mini international neuropsychiatric interview for children and adolescents (MINI-KID). *Journal of Clinical Psychiatry, 71*, 313–326. https://doi.org/10.4088/JCP.09m05305whi

Sheehan, D., Shytle, D., Milo, K., Janavs, J., & Lecrubier, Y. (2009). *MINI international neuropsychiatric interview for children and adolescents, English version 6.0.* Tampa, FL: University of South Florida.

Sherrill, J., & Kovacs, M. (2000). Interview Schedule for Children and Adolescents (ISCA). *Journal of the American Academy of Child & Adolescent Psychiatry, 39*, 67–75.

Silverman, W. (1994). Structured diagnostic interviews. In *International handbook of phobic and anxiety disorders in children and adolescents* (pp. 293–315). New York, NY: Plenum Press.

Silverman, W. K., & Albano, A. M. (1996). *Anxiety disorders interview schedule, parent/child version.* New York, NY: Oxford University Press.

Silverman, W. K., & Nelles, W. B. (1988). The anxiety disorders interview schedule for children. *Journal of the American Academy of Child and Adolescent Psychiatry, 27*, 772–778.

Silverman, W. K., & Ollendick, T. H. (2005). Evidence-based assessment of anxiety and its disorders in children and adolescents. *Journal of Clinical Child and Adolescent Psychology, 34*, 380–411.

Sparrow, S. S., Cicchetti, D. V., & Balla, D. A. (2016). *Vineland-III: Vineland adaptive behavior scales* (3rd ed.). San Antonio, TX: Pearson.

Tassé, M. J., Schalock, R. L., Thissen, D., Balboni, G., Bersani, H. A., Borthwick-Duffy, S. A., … Navas, P. (2016). Development and standardization of the diagnostic adaptive behavior scale: Application of item response theory to the assessment of adaptive behavior. *American Journal on Intellectual and Developmental Disabilities, 121*, 79–94.

Teare, M., Fristad, M. A., Weller, E. B., Weller, R. A., & Salmon, P. (1998a). Study I: Development and criterion validity of the Children's interview for psychiatric syndromes. *Journal of Child and Adolescent Psychopharmacology, 8*, 205–211.

Teare, M., Fristad, M. A., Weller, E. B., Weller, R. A., & Salmon, P. (1998b). Study II: Concurrent validity of the DSM-III-R Children's interview for psychiatric syndromes. *Journal of Child and Adolescent Psychopharmacology, 8*, 213–219.

Thompson, C. L., & Rudolph, L. B. (2000). *Counseling children* (5th ed.). Belmont, CA: Wadsworth/Thompson Learning.

Tripp, G., Schaughency, E., & Clarke, B. (2006). Parent and teacher rating scales in the evaluation of attention-deficit hyperactivity disorder: Contribution to diagnosis and differential diagnosis in clinically referred children. *Journal of Developmental & Behavioral Pediatrics, 27*, 209–218.

Valla, J., Bergeron, L., & Smolla, N. (2000). The Dominic-R: A pictorial interview for 6- to 11-year-old children. *Journal of the American Academy of Child & Adolescent Psychiatry, 39*, 85–93.

Wareham, P., & Salmon, K. (2006). Mother-child reminiscing about everyday experiences: Implications for psychological interventions in the preschool years. *Clinical Psychology Review, 26*, 535–554.

Weems, C., Silverman, W., Saavedra, L., Pina, A., & Lumpkin, P. (1999). The discrimination of children's phobias using the revised fear survey schedule for children. *Journal of Child Psychology and Psychiatry, 40*, 941–952.

Weiss, D. S. (1993). Structured clinical interview techniques. In J. P. Wilson & R. Beverley (Eds.), *International handbook of traumatic stress syndromes* (pp. 179–187). New York, NY: Plenum Press.

Weller, E. B., Weller, R. A., Fristad, M. A., Rooney, M. T., & Schecter, J. (2000). Children's interview for psychiatric syndromes (ChIPS). *Journal of the American Academy of Child and Adolescent Psychiatry, 39*, 76–84.

Weller, E. B., Weller, R. A., Teare, M., & Fristad, M. A. (1999). *Children's Interview for Psychiatric Syndromes (ChIPS).* Washington DC: American Psychiatric Press.

Welner, Z., Reich, W., Herjanic, B., Jung, K. G., & Amado, H. (1987). Reliability, validity, and parent child agreement studies of the diagnostic interview for children and adolescents (DICA). *Journal of the American Academy of Child and Adolescent Psychiatry, 26*, 649–653.

Wesson, M., & Salmon, K. (2001). Drawing and showing: Helping children to report emotionally laden events. *Applied Cognitive Psychology, 15*, 301–320.

Wood, J., Piacentini, J., Bergman, R., McCracken, J., & Barrios, V. (2002). Concurrent validity of the anxiety disorders section of the anxiety disorders interview schedule for DSM-IV: Child and parent versions. *Journal of Clinical Child and Adolescent Psychology, 31*, 335–342.

Young, J. G., O'Brien, J. D., Gutterman, E. M., & Cohen, P. (1987). Research on the clinical interview. *Journal of the American Academy of Child and Adolescent Psychiatry, 30*, 613–620.

Intelligence Testing

Abigail Issarraras and Johnny L. Matson

Introduction

Intelligence testing has long been a prominent component of childhood psychological assessment, with a history sustaining over 100 years (Boake, 2002; Kamphaus, 2001; White, 2000). Today, a quick Google search of the term "IQ Test" illuminates just how pervasive the concept of intelligence testing is in the public sphere. With hundreds of websites allegedly offering "fast and accurate" tests of how "smart" an individual is, it's no wonder many people misunderstand how and why psychologists use intelligence tests. Intelligence tests purport to measure something qualitatively different than what individuals can master and learn in educational settings, such as would be measured with an achievement test (Kamphaus, 2001). In fact, intelligence testing instigated a wave of interest in assessing many different aspects of human behavior once thought to be immeasurable (Kamphaus, 2001). Intelligence testing is especially crucial to childhood assessments because often the diagnostic considerations taken from test results have the ability to transform a child's life; per the *Diagnostic and Statistical Manual of Mental Disorders, 5th edition* (DSM-5; APA, 2013), intelligence tests can aid in the diagnosis of intellectual disability (ID), a lifelong neurodevelopmental disability. Therefore, clinicians are indebted to their clients to completely understand the history, theoretical frameworks, and strengths and weaknesses of the intelligence tests they choose in order to administer the most appropriate test to their client.

Interestingly, one of the initial questions in considering the most appropriate intelligence test is, what is intelligence? Though different theories have guided psychologists' views of intelligence, perhaps the most widely accepted theory in the field of childhood intelligence testing is the Cattell-Horn-Carroll (CHC) theory of intelligence (Schneider & McGrew, 2012). The CHC theory of intelligence, a combination of Cattell and Horn's Gf-Gc theory (Horn & Blankson, 2012) and Carroll's three-stratum theory (Carroll, 1993), has the most empirical support and thus shapes many of the intelligence tests used in clinical practice today. Briefly, the CHC theory proposes a three-stratum model; stratum 1 holds a large collection of *narrow* or specific abilities, while stratum 2 includes the primary "broad" CHC abilities (Schneider & McGrew, 2012). These abilities include fluid reasoning or intelligence (Gf), comprehension-knowledge or crystallized intelligence (Gc), visual-spatial ability (Gv), long-term storage and retrieval (Glr), auditory processing (Ga), cognitive processing speed

A. Issarraras (✉) · J. L. Matson
Department of Psychology, Louisiana State University, Baton Rouge, LA, USA
e-mail: aissar1@lsu.edu

(Gs), short-term memory (Gsm), and quantitative reasoning (Gq) (Schneider & McGrew, 2012). The final stratum is an overall marker of general intelligence, or g ability (Schneider & McGrew, 2012). This framework will become increasingly familiar to clinicians assessing children's intellectual functioning, especially those who use a variety of assessment tools. This chapter includes a brief overview of the history of intelligence testing; it also discusses some issues related to intelligence testing that clinicians may consider when selecting tests and describes some of the most widely used intelligence tests in clinical practice.

History of Intelligence Testing

Assessment of a child's intellectual functioning can raise many questions for families. Often parents and teachers are somewhat familiar with the most popular intelligence tests, as they may have encountered older editions of the same tests when they themselves were in school (Kamphaus, 2001). The child being tested may also have a plethora of questions about the assessment process and the tasks clinicians are asking them to do. Understanding the history of intelligence testing prepares clinicians to handle any apprehension clients and/or parents may have regarding the testing process, and building rapport and trust in both the intelligence tests and the assessment is essential for any evaluation (Kamphaus, 2001). Though many people are familiar with the controversies surrounding intelligence tests, few people understand the incredible amount of work and time put into developing the tests. Intelligence testing in the United States can trace its origins to the work of French psychologists Alfred Binet and Theodore Simon (Boake, 2002; Cianciolo & Sternberg, 2004; Zenderland, 1998).

Early in the 1900s, the French government passed new laws mandating that all children attend school (Boake, 2002). Alfred Binet was commissioned by the French government to assist in identifying which students were most likely to experience difficulties in school and thus require special services, so he and his colleague, Theodore Simon, set to work on developing questions designed to measure skills they felt were not explicitly taught in schools (Boake, 2002; Kamphaus, 2001). Some of the skills they attempted to measure included attention, problem solving skills, and memory, and they hoped to use these skills to determine which students were more likely to succeed in a traditional school setting (Boake, 2002; Cianciolo & Sternberg, 2004). Interestingly to Binet, children's scores varied across age levels, with some children scoring much higher than children who were chronologically older than them (Cianciolo & Sternberg, 2004). These observations guided Binet's theory of a "mental age," or an average age when most children performed a task well (Boake, 2002). He would later use the term "mental age" after publishing the first modern intelligence test – the Binet-Simon Intelligence Scale (Binet & Simon, 1905; Boake, 2002). A revision to this test grouped each individual test to a certain age level, such as longer sequences in digit span for use with older children. Though these initial publications of the Binet-Simon intelligence tests were easy to administer, critics felt the test relied too much on verbal ability (Boake, 2002). Regardless, as Boake (2002) states, Binet's legacy was solidified, as his scales provided the framework for future intelligence tests, and would soon be noticed by others, particularly in the United States.

At the same time across the globe, Henry Goddard, an American psychologist, was interested in discovering novel ways to assess children's intellectual functioning as well, and thus, when he heard of the work being done by Alfred Binet, he arranged for the scales to be brought to America and translated into English (Boake, 2002; Zenderland, 1998). Unfortunately, Goddard is a major source of the controversy surrounding intellectual testing, as he was a strong believer in eugenics, arguing for the institutionalization of the "feebleminded," whom he considered a burden on society (Zenderland, 1998). Shortly before World War I, a second revision was made to the Binet-Simon intelligence test by Lewis Terman of Stanford University, though this edition of the test was standardized with an American sample of children (Boake, 2002; White, 2000). Terman also extended the age range of what would then be known as the Stanford-Binet Intelligence Scales (Terman, 1916), into adulthood, as well as replacing Binet's "mental age" with the now popularly known "intelligence quotient," a composite score derived by dividing the test taker's mental age by their chronological age, then multiplying by 10 (Boake, 2002). This new revision would quickly dominate the American intellectual testing field (Boake, 2002).

The final development in the history of American intellectual testing began with the widespread testing done by the United States Army during World War I (Boake, 2002). As Boake (2002) mentions, it became imperative for officials in the Army to determine whether new recruits were fit for military service. The main intelligence tests used were the Army Alpha, which was primarily a verbal test for English speaking recruits, and the Army Beta, a nonverbal measure used for recruits either lacking formal education or knowledge of the English language (Boake, 2002). After the war, an American psychologist by the name of David Wechsler was working at Bellevue Hospital, when he became increasingly dissatisfied with the Stanford-Binet intelligence test (Boake, 2002). Wechsler developed a new intelligence test, largely derived from the Army Alpha and Beta tests, which he would first publish as the Wechsler-Bellevue Intelligence Scale (Boake, 2002; Cianciolo & Sternberg, 2004; Kamphaus, 2001; Wechsler, 1939). The Wechsler scales popularity was strengthened by the familiar subtests, its organization into verbal and performance scales, the use of deviation scores, and the large sample including children and adults (Boake, 2002). Wechsler revised his scale for use with children in 1949, which would become the original Wechsler Intelligence Scale for Children (WISC; Wechsler, 1949), further increasing the popularity of the Wechsler scales among American psychologists. Today, though many tests have been developed to meet needs not met by the Stanford-Binet (Terman, 1916) or the Wechsler scales (Wechsler, 1939), the two remain popular and well-researched tests for assessing intellectual functioning across the lifespan (Boake, 2002).

Intelligence Tests

Clinicians have a wide variety of options available to them when planning psychological assessments. With the rise of intelligence tests such as the Stanford-Binet (SB-5; Roid, 2003) and Wechsler Scales (WISC-V; Wechsler, 2014), several new tests have come forth in the last few decades, each claiming to measure intelligence in the most efficient and optimal way. The following tests were each evaluated based on standards put forth by the American Educational Research Association, American Psychological Association, and National Council on Measurement in Education (1999). Many reviews were retrieved from the Buros Mental Measurements Yearbook, now in its twentieth edition (Carlson, Geisinger, & Johnson, 2017), which serves as a valuable tool for any clinician considering a new assessment tool.

Bayley Scales of Infant and Toddler Development

Dr. Nancy Bayley first developed the Bayley Scales of Infant and Toddler Development, Third Edition (Bayley-III; Bayley, 2006), to not only assess the intellectual and developmental functioning of infants and young children but also to identify those children with developmental delays. This test uses multiple methods of assessment to provide examiners with information across five domains: Cognitive, Language, Motor Development, Social-Emotional, and Adaptive Functioning (Bayley, 2006). Though the test is individually administered, primary caregivers are also asked to provide data through questionnaires to inform the assessment (Bayley, 2006). This test can be used in children from the age of 1 month to 42 months, and depending on the child's age at assessment, test time can run from 30 to 90 min (Bayley, 2006; Tobin & Hoff, 2007). Examiners must provide some materials required for administration of the test, including facial tissue, five small coins, food pellets, safety scissors, and other items (Macha & Petermann, 2007).

A total of 19 scores across the 5 domains can be obtained from full administration of the Bayley-III (Bayley, 2006): Cognitive, Language (Receptive Communication, Expressive Communication, Total Score), Motor (Fine Motor, Gross Motor, Total Score), Social-Emotional, and Adaptive Behavior (Communication, Community Use, Functional Pre-Academics, Home Living, Health and Safety, Leisure, Self-Care, Self-Direction, Social, Motor, Total Score). The Bayley-III has strong internal consistency for the measurement of functioning within its five domains. The large normative sample of 1700 children were stratified by race, age, sex, parental education level, and geographic location (Bayley, 2006; Tobin & Hoff, 2007). Reviewers agree that the psychometrics properties have been improved with this third revision of the test, though the predictive ability may not be as strong as the test author purports (Tobin & Hoff, 2007; Venn, 2007). However, the play-based focus of the Bayley-III (Bayley, 2006) and the extended floors and ceilings offered make this instrument invaluable in assessing very young children with both very low and very high cognitive functioning. Bayley (2006) also provides data regarding the use of these instruments with special populations such as children with Down syndrome, pervasive developmental disorders, cerebral palsy, prenatal alcohol exposure, prematurity, etc. (Tobin & Hoff, 2007). Another strength of the Bayley-III is the addition of charts on which clinicians can graph a child's development across each domain over time (Bayley, 2006). Though as mentioned previously, the implications for intervention planning may not be as direct as the author suggests, the tool is still extremely valuable for progress monitoring a child during a period of rapid development (Tobin & Hoff, 2007).

Differential Ability Scales

Though the Differential Ability Scales-II (DAS-II; Elliott, 1990) were not originally devised as an intelligence test but as a means of measuring "a child's strengths and weaknesses in a wide range of cognitive abilities," the utility of this test in clinical assessments is still valuable. Though not specific to any one theory of intelligence, the DAS-II, the test author provides guidelines for interpreting scores within the CHC theoretical framework (Davis, 2010; Elliott, 1990). The DAS-II (Elliott, 1990) includes two individually administered assessment batteries: the Early Years Battery (for children 2 years 6 months through 6 years 11 months) and the School-Age Battery (for children 7 years through 17 years 11 months). The Early Years Battery is further divided into two levels: Lower Level (children ages 2 years 6 months through 3 years 5 months) and Upper Level (children 3 years 6 months to 6 years 11 months). On average, each battery takes between 20 and 40 min to administer, depending on the age of the child being tested. Reviewers note that extensive review and practice with the items is necessary, as there are many subtests and various materials (from manipulatives to stimulus cards) which make interactions more complex (Davis, 2010; Tindal, 2010).

The DAS-II (Elliott, 1990) produces a variety of scores depending on the battery administered. The Lower-Level Early Years Battery yields eight scores: Verbal Ability (Verbal Comprehension and Naming Vocabulary), Nonverbal Ability (Picture Similarities and Pattern Construction), Diagnostic Subtests (Recall of Digits Forward, Recognition of Pictures, and Early Number Concepts), and a General Conceptual Ability (GCA) score. The Upper-Level Early Years Battery generates 19 scores, including those in the Lower-Level Early Years Battery: Verbal Ability (Verbal Comprehension and Naming Vocabulary), Nonverbal Reasoning Ability (Picture Similarities and Matrices), Spatial Ability (Pattern Construction and Copying), a Special Nonverbal Composite, School Readiness (Early Number Concepts, Matching Letter-Like Forms, and Phonological Processing), Working Memory (Recall of Sequential Order and Recall of Digits Backward), Processing Speed (Speed of Information Processing and Rapid Naming), Recall of Objects-Immediate, Recall of Objects-Delayed, Recall of Digits Forward, Recognition of Pictures, and General Conceptual Ability (GCA) composite score.

The School-Age Battery yields 17 scores after testing: Verbal Ability (Word Definitions, Verbal Similarities), Nonverbal Reasoning Ability (Matrices, Sequential and Quantitative Reasoning), Spatial Ability (Recall of Designs, Pattern Construction), a Special Nonverbal Composite, Working Memory (Recall of Sequential Order, Recall of Digits Backward), Processing Speed (Speed of Information Processing, Rapid Naming), Phonological Processing, Recall of Objects-Immediate, Recall of Objects-Delayed, Recall of Digits Forward, Recognition of Pictures, and a General Conceptual Ability (GCA) composite score (Elliott, 1990). All scores were standardized on a highly representative sample based on the US 2002 census data. Additionally, reviewers note the "well-documented" psychometric properties of the DAS-II (Davis, 2010).

The DAS-II (Elliott, 1990) also has clinical utility for special populations. The scales offer an entire Spanish Supplement for all subtests which do not require verbal responses (Davis, 2010; Tindal, 2010), allowing for easy use in bilingual communities. Although the Early Years Battery is designed for children younger than 7 years, the DAS-II manual defends the use of these subtests in assessing children ages 7 years to 8 years 11 months who are suspected of having cognitive delay (Elliott, 1990). In fact, the DAS-II manual states that the GCA score yielded in each battery can be useful to clinicians determining a child's need for special services; however, it is clearly noted that these scores need "further vindication" from other measures in the assessment process, as the results are "hypotheses" of the child's ability (Elliott, 1990; Tindal, 2010). The DAS-II (Elliott, 1990) also defends its use with children with much lower cognitive abilities than other intelligence tests.

Leiter International Performance Scale

The Leiter International Performance Scale, Third Edition (Leiter-3; Rold, Miller, Pomplun, and Koch, 2013), is a completely nonverbal measure of intelligence, for use with individuals from age 3 to 75 and older. Due to the nonverbal nature of the test, administration can be complicated, requiring the use of pantomimed instructions, facial expressions, hand and head movements, and demonstrations to the individual (Rold et al., 2013; Ward, 2017). The training DVD provided as well as the test manual aid first-time examiners in familiarizing themselves with the various instructions (Ward, 2017). Software is also provided to facilitate scoring of the test (Rold et al., 2013). The test author intended this test to be used with individuals that would benefit most from nonverbal assessment methods, including, but not limited to, those with autism spectrum disorder, cognitive delay, English as a second language, and traumatic brain injury (Rold et al., 2013; Ward, 2017). As such, the test manual includes an entire chapter dedicated to administering the test to special populations (Rold et al., 2013).

Building off the CHC theory of intelligence, the domains selected for use include fluid reasoning, visual processing, memory, and attention, though IQ is based solely off performance on the fluid reasoning and visual processing subtests (Ward, 2017). The Leiter-3 (Rold et al., 2013) produces 19 scores overall, which includes 11 subtests (Figure Ground, Form Completion, Classification/Analogies, Sequential Order, Visual Patterns, Attention Sustained, Forward Memory, Reverse Memory, Nonverbal Stroop Incongruent Correct, Nonverbal Stroop Congruent Correct, and Nonverbal Stroop Effect), 3 composite scores (Nonverbal IQ, Nonverbal Memory, and Processing Speed), and 5 supplemental scores (Attention Sustained Errors, Attention Divided Correct, Attention Divided Incorrect, Nonverbal Stroop Congruent Incorrect, and Nonverbal Stroop Incongruent Incorrect). Generally, reviewers found the psychometrics adequate, though they do note the gender differences across age, as females are underrepresented in the lower age ranges of the standardization sample (Ward, 2017). As Ward (2017) also notes, data suggests that performance may vary over time with this measure, so clinicians are cautioned in their interpretation of results across administrations.

Kaufman Brief Intelligence Test

The Kaufman Brief Intelligence Test, Second Edition (KBIT-2), is a brief measure of verbal and nonverbal intelligence, typically used as a screening measure or in periodic reevaluations (Kaufman & Kaufman, 2004; Madle, 2007). This measure can be used with individuals aged 4–90 and usually takes 15–30 min to complete. Based on the Cattell-Horn-Carroll (CHC) theory of intelligence, the KBIT-2 manual discusses how to interpret the three scores yielded (Verbal, Nonverbal, and IQ Composite) within the framework of this theory (Kaufman & Kaufman, 2004; Shaw, 2007). The Verbal score is composed of two subtests (i.e., Verbal Knowledge and Riddles), while the Nonverbal score relies on one subtest (i.e., Matrices); no subtest is given a time constraint. This test requires the child to give a one-word answer or point to the best response, allowing for easy interpretation of instructions. Examiners will also appreciate that due to the limited responses, little querying is necessary.

Reviews of the KBIT-2 emphasize the improvements made in this revision of the measure. As Madle (2007) reports, norms have been updated using a standardization sample of 2120 individuals stratified using the US 2001 Current Population Survey. Additionally, the Matrices subtest was updated, and the Verbal scale was completely novel to the second edition. Because the test now uses the same tasks across the life span, it can easily be used to monitor progress or change in individual performance (Madle, 2007). Another strength of this test is the wide range of populations that examiners can administer the test to. The KBIT-2 manual not only presents variations on administration instructions for individuals with limited English proficiency and severe visual or hearing impairments but also provides instructions and response options in Spanish (Kaufman & Kaufman, 2004; Madle, 2007). The KBIT-2 also establishes strong psychometrics for each subtest, with the exception of the Nonverbal scale in the youngest children (Madle, 2007).

Mullen Scales of Early Learning

Dr. Eileen Mullen, a developmental psychologist, constructed the Mullen Scales of Early Learning: AGS Edition (MSEL:AGS; Mullen, 1995) as a comprehensive test of cognitive functioning in infants and very young children. Accordingly, the age range of this scale is birth to 68 months, and thus the completion time ranges from 15 min to 1 h. The test yields six scores for examiners to interpret: the Gross Motor Scale, the Cognitive Scales (including Visual Reception, Fine Motor, Receptive Language, and Expressive Language), and the Early Learning Composite. As Dumont, Cruse, Alfonso, and Levine (2000) mention in their review, individual items on each scale are scored based on the child's performance, and because items vary in the number of points awarded, examiners should ensure they log the skills the child was able to accomplish on each task. It is also important to note that examiners are expected to bring a variety of items to the test administration, including crayons, cereal, and numerous toys not provided in the testing kit.

Using her extensive experience working with children of differing ability levels, Dr. Mullen designed an interactive test which claims to discriminate between children with and without developmental delays (Mullen, 1995). This is important because as Chittooran (2001) mentions in a review of the MSEL:AGS, this test may be used in determining a child's eligibility for early intervention services, as per federal mandates on infant and preschool assessment. The Early Learning Composite combines the four cognitive scales and thus can be interpreted as a measure of general intelligence (Mullen, 1995). If a child scores 2 standard deviations below the mean on any cognitive subscale of the MSEL:AGS (i.e., a t score less than 30), then early intervention services are deemed necessary (Chittooran, 2001; Mullen, 1995).

The clinical utility of such a test is apparent; however, the MSEL:AGS is not without its critics. Most notably, reviewers draw attention to the inadequacy of the standardization sample, which lacked variability in representation of different ethnicities, community size, and socioeconomic status as compared to the United States 1990 Census data (Dumont et al., 2000). In addition to this, Dumont and colleagues (2000) also note that the standardization sample was combined from data collected across two different time periods, the first from 1981 to 1986 and the second from 1987 to 1989. Because items were dropped from the previous editions of the MSEL over these 8 years of data collection, it is unclear how many individuals received the same assessment instrument (Dumont et al., 2000; Mullen, 1995). Reviewers also mention the strengths of the MSEL:AGS as a clinical tool. First, it is relatively easy for examiners to learn to administer, as the manual is well-organized (Chittooran, 2001; Dumont et al., 2000). The MSEL:AGS also contains colorful and interesting manipulatives that children can easily engage with, such as a red rubber ball. Overall, the test is an efficient and simple tool that examiners can easily engage a variety of children with, including those with special needs; conversely, concerns with psychometric properties may warrant cautious interpretation of results.

Peabody Picture Vocabulary Test

The Peabody Picture Vocabulary Test, Fourth Edition (PPVT-4), developed by Dunn and Dunn (2007), assesses an individual's receptive language skills. Items on the PPVT-4 (Dunn & Dunn, 2007) require the individual to point to one of four pictures arranged on a page that best describes the meaning of the word verbally spoken by the examiner. Examiners can administer one of two parallel forms (Form A and Form B), each consisting of 228 items, to children from the age of 2 years 6 months and to adults over the age of 90. The typical administration time for the PPVT-4 runs from 10 to 15 min, which adds to the simplicity of this assessment tool.

The examiner's manual provides information regarding the standardization sample, which in addition to included children receiving special education services for attention deficit/hyperactivity disorder, emotional/behavioral disturbance, specific learning disability, developmental delays, autism, intellectual disability, and speech language impairment (Dunn & Dunn, 2007). As Kush (2010) notes in his review of this test, the stability of scores in these special populations as well as the straightforward nature of the instructions makes the PPVT-4 a valuable tool for assessing very young children and children with special needs. However, as Dunn and Dunn (2007) note in the PPVT-4 technical manual, though achievement on receptive vocabulary tests has strong empirical relations to cognitive ability, "it is conceptually distinct from them," meaning the PPVT-4 cannot be used as the sole indicator of an individual's intelligence (Kush, 2010). This test can be used and interpreted in conjunction with other measures of the child's psychological evaluation.

Stanford-Binet Intelligence Scales

The Stanford-Binet Intelligence Scales, Fifth Edition (SB-5; Roid, 2003), were designed to assess intelligence in individuals ages 2 years to 89 years 9 months. Based on the CHC theory of intelligence, the SB-5's hierarchical model uses five broad abilities to measure general intelligence (g): Fluid Reasoning (Gf), Knowledge (Gc), Quantitative Reasoning(Gq), Visual-Spatial Reasoning (Gv), and Working Memory (Gsm) (Roid, 2003). These five factor index scores are used in addition to two domain scores (Nonverbal IQ and Verbal IQ) and the full-scale intelligence quotient (FSIQ) score to diagnose children and adults with developmental disabilities (Johnson, 2005; Roid, 2003). The time taken to administer the full battery ranges from 45 to 75 min, while the abbreviated battery may only take 15–20 min.

The psychometric properties of the SB-5 are well-designed and technically sound (Johnson, 2005). The standardization sample used in this revision of the test closely matched the US Census data from 2001, including a total sample of 4800 participants stratified by sex, age, race, socioeconomic level, and geographic region. The SB-5 and its predecessors, as the original methods of childhood intellectual assessment, have withstood the test of time due to the rigorous development process which closely follow recommendations put forth in the Standards for Educational and Psychological Testing (AERA, APA, & NCME, 1999). The SB-5 manual (Roid, 2003) also states that the Nonverbal IQ score is appropriate for assessing special populations such as those with hearing impairments, autism, limited English proficiency, and related areas. Examiners need not purchase a separate instrument for assessing individuals with these needs. However, the SB-5's organization is somewhat complex and thus requires training and practice for examiners to master the test materials in order to accurately assess any individual (Johnson, 2005; Roid, 2003).

Stanford-Binet Intelligence Scales for Early Childhood

Similar to the SB-5, the Stanford-Binet Intelligence Scales for Early Childhood (Early SB-5; Roid, 2005) is an excellent clinical tool for assessing intelligence and cognitive ability. This edition of the SB-5 was specifically designed for identifying the youngest children (ages 2 years to 7 years 3 months) with developmental disabilities or exceptionalities (Roid, 2003; Sink & Eppler, 2007). The Early SB-5 includes modifications such as a test observation checklist, a single-volume test manual, and condensed format which increase the efficiency of the tool (Sink & Eppler, 2007). Like the SB-5, the Early SB-5 includes an abbreviated battery which takes about 15 min to administer, while the full battery can take upwards of 50 min to administer. All items require children to respond either verbally, nonverbally, or through performance of a task (Roid, 2005).

The Early SB-5 (Roid, 2005) yields similar scores to the SB-5: a Nonverbal IQ score, Verbal IQ score, and Full-Scale IQ score. The factor indexes also remain the same in this younger scale (Fluid Reasoning, Knowledge, Quantitative Reasoning, Visual-Spatial Reasoning, and Working Memory). Throughout development of the Early SB-5, special consideration was given to limiting sources of bias due to gender, race, culture, socioeconomic disparities, etc., as well as to increase the validity of the test for its intended use (Sink & Eppler, 2007). As is expected of such a widely used scale, the battery is well supported by strong theoretical foundations and sound psychometric properties (Sink & Eppler, 2007). Reviewers such as Sink and Eppler (2007) also note that criterion-related validity was demonstrated in special populations such as young children with autism, developmental delays, intellectual disability, and other such conditions. Taken together, the Early SB-5 battery has numerous strengths and wide utility for very young children of varying ability levels.

Universal Nonverbal Intelligence Test

As its name suggests, the Universal Nonverbal Intelligence Test (UNIT; Bracken & McCallum, 1998) is a completely nonverbal instrument designed for children age 5 years through 17 years "who may be disadvantaged by traditional verbal and language-loaded measures" (Bracken & McCallum, 1998). There are three batteries an examiner may choose from: the Extended Battery, the Standard Battery, and the Abbreviated Battery (Bracken & McCallum, 1998). Examiners are encouraged to use the Standard Battery, and the UNIT manual suggests only using the Abbreviated Battery as an initial screener (Bracken & McCallum, 1998). Depending on which battery is administered, test time could take between 15 and 45 min.

Bracken and McCallum (1998) developed the UNIT around the theoretical foundation, for the UNIT is based on the conceptualization of intelligence as a general ability factor (g) that encompasses two lower factors of memory and reasoning. This is evident in the design and selection of subtests which include: Symbolic Memory, Cube Design, Spatial Memory, Analogic Reasoning, Object Memory, Mazes, Memory Quotient, Reasoning Quotient, Symbolic Quotient, Nonsymbolic Quotient (Bracken & McCallum, 1998). The test relies heavily on the individual's memory as a measure of their intelligence, and the memory items are notably more difficult than those found on other instruments (Bandalos, 2001). Psychometrically, the UNIT (Bracken & McCallum, 1998) is quite sound. The standardization sample of 2100 children was carefully chosen and was stratified on many variables including gender, race, region, and classroom placement (regular or special education) (Bandalos, 2001). Additionally, the standardization sample included children receiving special education services for learning disabilities, speech and language impairments, serious emotional disturbance, and intellectual disability, as well as children learning English as a second language (Bandalos, 2001). The UNIT also shares concurrent validity with the Wechsler Intelligence Scale for Children, Third Edition (WISC-III), the Woodcock-Johnson Psycho-Educational Battery-Revised (WJ-R), and the Kaufman Brief Intelligence Test (KBIT), but it is important to note that these are not the current editions of any of the reported scales (Bandalos, 2001). Additionally, Bandalos (2001) suggests that more studies on the predictive validity of the UNIT on classroom achievement would strengthen the psychometrics of the test.

Wechsler Intelligence Scale for Children

The Wechsler Intelligence Scale for Children, Fifth Edition (WISC-V; Wechsler, 2014), has significantly progressed from the original scale published by Wechsler in 1949. This clinical instrument is designed to assess intellectual functioning in children from the age of 6 years to 16 years 11 months (Wechsler, 2014). With the most recent update, the WISC-V now consists of 21 subtests and has been revised to improve user friendliness for the examiner and developmental appropriateness for the child being tested (Benson, 2017; Wechsler, 2014). The WISC-V test kit provides the examiner with almost everything needed to administer the test, with the exception of a pencil for the child to use on certain subtests and a stopwatch for the examiner to use throughout the test (Wechsler, 2014). Administration of the WISC-V usually takes around 45 min to a little over an hour, depending on the needs of the child (Wechsler, 2014).

The WISC-V (Wechsler, 2014) consists of 21 subtests: 10 primary subtests (Block Design, Coding, Digit Span, Figure Weights, Matrix Reasoning, Picture Span, Similarities, Symbol Search, Visual Puzzles, and Vocabulary), 6 secondary subtests (Arithmetic, Cancellation, Comprehension, Information, Letter-Number Sequencing, and Picture Concepts), and 5 complementary subtests (Delayed Symbol Translation, Immediate Symbol Translation, Naming Speed Literacy, Naming Speed Quantity, and Recognition Symbol Translation). Interpretation of the WISC-V occurs at several levels, though the test manual asserts various models of intelligence can be applied within the WISC-V interpretative framework (Benson, 2017). At the first level of interpretation is the estimate of general intelligence (g), or the Full-Scale IQ, which is derived from selected primary subtests (Wechsler, 2014). The second level of interpretation is the primary index scale level, which consists of index scores derived from the primary subtests for the following five scales: Fluid Reasoning, Processing Speed, Verbal Comprehension, Visual-Spatial, and Working Memory (Benson, 2017; Wechsler, 2014). This is followed by the third level of interpretation, or the ancillary index scale level, consisting of index scores derived from both primary and secondary subtests for the following five scales: Auditory Working Memory, Cognitive Proficiency, General Ability, Nonverbal, and Quantitative Reasoning (Benson, 2017; Wechsler, 2014). Lastly, the final level of interpretation is the complementary index scale level, which consists of index scores for the following three scales: Naming Speed, Symbol Translation, and Storage and Retrieval (Benson, 2017; Wechsler, 2014).

As with its predecessors, the WISC-V features a large, stratified normative sample of 2200 children (Benson, 2017). In his review of the WISC-V, Benson (2017) emphasizes that evidence is not available to support the absence of bias in this test. Additionally, the WISC-V is of limited utility for children with severe cognitive impairments, as the lowest score a child can receive is a standard score of 40 (Benson, 2017; Wechsler, 2014). Additionally, the test authors note that "disruptive or noncompliant behavior" is likely to have a negative impact on performance (Wechsler, 2014). For many clinicians working with special populations, disruptive behavior is to be expected during an hour-long assessment. Thus, though it is obvious why the WISC-V continues to be a popular tool for intelligence testing in typically developing children, it may be of little utility for clinicians working with children with moderate to severe intellectual disabilities (Benson, 2017).

Wechsler Preschool and Primary Scale of Intelligence

Like the Early SB-5 (Roid, 2005), the Wechsler Preschool and Primary Scale of Intelligence, Fourth Edition (WPPSI-IV; Wechsler, 2012), was designed to provide general intelligence estimates consistent with its "parent" test (i.e., the WISC-V; Wechsler, 2014). However, the WPPSI-IV (Wechsler, 2012) was designed for assessing children much younger than those tested by the WISC-V (Wechsler, 2014). There are two subtest batteries divided by two distinct age groups (from 2 years 6 months to 3 years 11 months and from 4 years to 7 years 7 months) (Wechsler, 2012). Individually administered, this test usually takes 30–60 min to administer.

Consistent with CHC theory, each subtest in the WPPSI-IV measures an overall "global capacity" of intelligence (Canivez, 2014; Wechsler, 2012). Because this test is tailored to toddlers, the stimuli are much more visually engaging, and often the tasks are "game-like" to facilitate child cooperation and easy administration (Canivez, 2014). For example, some of the subtests are quite different from subtests found on the WISC-V (i.e., Animal Coding, Bug Search, Zoo Locations), while others are very familiar to what examiners experienced with other Wechsler scales (i.e., Block Design, Cancellation, Information, Matrix Reasoning, Memory, Picture Naming, etc.). Canivez (2014) mentions the strengths of the WPPSI-IV include these new subtests, geared to early childhood, the ease of administration and scoring, the representative standardization sample, and strong estimates of score reliability (Wechsler, 2012). However, interpretation of WPPSI-IV scores to inform clinical practice lacks specific psychometric evidence and should be considered when using the WPPSI-IV (Canivez, 2014; Wechsler, 2012).

Woodcock-Johnson Test of Cognitive Abilities

The Woodcock-Johnson Test of Cognitive Abilities (WJ-IV COG; Schrank, McGrew, & Mather, 2014) is part of the larger Woodcock-Johnson assessment battery and is a well-known test of cognitive ability for individuals from the age of 2 years to over 90 years. The first seven tests in the Standard Battery take about 35 min to administer, and the WJ-IV testing manual recommends estimating an additional 5 min for each subtest additionally administered (Schrank et al., 2014). Scoring of the WJ-IV COG is now completely done online, further simplifying administration of the test for examiners (Schrank et al., 2014).

The WJ-IV COG (Schrank et al., 2014) yields a variety of scores that can be interpreted hierarchically including 10 Standard Battery test scores (Oral Vocabulary, Number Series, Verbal Attention, Letter-Pattern Matching, Phonological Processing, Story Recall, Visualization, General Information, Concept Formation, Numbers Reversed), 8 Extended Battery test scores (Number-Pattern Matching, Nonword Repetition, Visual-Auditory Learning, Picture Recognition, Analysis-Synthesis, Object-Number Sequencing, Pair Cancellation, Memory for Words), 4 ability scores (General Intellectual Ability, Gf-Gc Composite, Brief Intellectual Ability, and Scholastic Aptitudes in Reading, Math, and Writing), 7 broad ability clusters (Comprehension-Knowledge, Fluid Reasoning, Short-Term Working Memory, Cognitive Processing Speed, Auditory Processing, Long-Term Retrieval, Visual Processing), and

6 narrow ability clusters (Perceptual Speed, Quantitative Reasoning, Auditory Memory Span, Number Facility, Vocabulary, Cognitive Efficiency). Canivez (2017), in his review of the WJ-IV, mentions the strength of the standardization sample, which included 7416 individuals from preschool children to adults. Results taken from the WJ-IV COG, particularly for the general intelligence composite scores, show good reliability estimates (Canivez, 2017). However, though the WJ-IV COG appears to be a good measure of general intelligence, interpreting the scores beyond this should still be done with caution until further research is done with special populations or on the predictive validity of the WJ-IV COG (Canivez, 2017; Schrank et al., 2014). Overall, the WJ-IV assessment battery is an excellent tool that is widely used by many clinicians due its ease of administration and scoring, strong theoretical foundation, and sound psychometric properties (Canivez, 2017; Schrank et al., 2014).

Conclusion

The use of intelligence tests in childhood assessments has increased since the first intelligence tests made by Alfred Binet and David Wechsler. In addition, the variety of intelligence tests now available for clinical practice has also increased. Practitioners must consider a variety of factors when deciding on the most appropriate test for the child. This can include factors related to the intelligence tests themselves (e.g., length of administration, psychometric properties, age norms, etc.) as well as factors related to the child taking the test (e.g., verbal ability, motor skills, presence of a disability, etc.). Having an understanding of the basic properties (e.g., history, theoretical frameworks, strengths, and weaknesses) of the most well-known intelligence tests thus is critical for any clinician. With this knowledge, clinicians are more prepared to administer the most appropriate test to their client and provide the best assessment of the child's intellectual ability at the time.

References

American Educational Research Association (AERA), American Psychological Association (APA), & National Council on Measurement in Education (NCME). (1999). *Standards for educational and psychological testing*. Washington, DC: American Educational Research Association.

American Psychiatric Association. (2013). *Diagnostic and statistical manual of mental disorders* (5th ed.). Arlington, VA: American Psychiatric Publishing.

Bandalos, D. L. (2001). Review of the universal nonverbal intelligence test. In B. S. Plake & J. C. Impara (Eds.), *The fourteenth mental measurements yearbook*. Lincoln, NE: Buros Institute of Mental Measurements.

Bayley, N. (2006). *Bayley scales of infant and toddler development-third edition*. San Antonio, TX: Harcourt Assessment.

Benson, N. F. (2017). Review of the Wechsler intelligence scale for children-fifth edition. In J. F. Carlson, K. F. Geisinger, & J. L. Johnson (Eds.), *The twentieth mental measurements yearbook*. Lincoln, NE: Buros Center for Testing.

Binet, A., & Simon, T. (1905/1916). New methods for the diagnosis of the intellectual level of subnormals. In H. H. Goddard (Ed.), *Development of intelligence in children (the Binet-Simon scale)* (E.S. Kite, Trans., pp. 37–90). Baltimore, MD: Williams & Williams.

Boake, C. (2002). From the Binet-Simon to the Wechsler-Bellevue: Tracing the history of intelligence testing. *Journal of Clinical and Experimental Neuropsychology, 24*(3), 383–405.

Bracken, B. A., & McCallum, R. S. (1998). *Universal nonverbal intelligence test*. Chicago, IL: Riverside.

Canivez, G. L. (2017). Review of the Woodcock-Johnson IV. In J. F. Carlson, K. F. Geisinger, & J. L. Johnson (Eds.), *The twentieth mental measurements yearbook*. Lincoln, NE: Buros Center for Testing.

Canivez, G. L. (2014). Review of the Wechsler preschool and primary scale of intelligence-fourth edition. In J. F. Carlson, K. F. Geisinger, & J. L. Johnson (Eds.), *The nineteenth mental measurements yearbook*. Lincoln, NE: Buros Center for Testing.

Carlson, J. F., Geisinger, K. F., & Johnson, J. L. (Eds.). (2017). *The twentieth mental measurements yearbook*. Lincoln, NE: Buros Center for Testing.

Carroll, J. B. (1993). *Human cognitive abilities*. Cambridge, England: Cambridge University Press.

Chittooran, M. M. (2001). Review of the Mullen scales of early learning: AGS edition. In B. S. Plake & J. C. Impara (Eds.), *The fourteenth mental measurements yearbook*. Lincoln, NE: Buros Institute of Mental Measurements.

Cianciolo, A. T., & Sternberg, R. J. (2004). *Intelligence: A brief history*. Malden, MA: Blackwell Publishing.

Davis, A. S. (2010). Review of the differential ability scales-second edition. In R. A. Spies, J. F. Carlson, & K. F. Geisinger (Eds.), *The eighteenth mental mea-*

surements yearbook. Lincoln, NE: Buros Institute of Mental Measurements.

Dumont, R., Cruse, C. L., Alfonso, V., & Levine, C. (2000). Book review: Mullen scales of early learning: AGS edition. *Journal of Psychoeducational Assessment, 18*(4), 381–389.

Dunn, L. M., & Dunn, D. M. (2007). *Peabody picture vocabulary test, fourth edition*. Minneapolis, MN: Pearson Assessments.

Elliott, C. D. (1990). *Differential ability scales, second edition*. San Antonio, TX: The Psychological Corporation.

Horn, J. L., & Blankson, A. N. (2012). Foundations for better understanding of cognitive abilities. In D. P. Flanagan & P. L. Harrison (Eds.), *Contemporary intellectual assessment: Theories, tests, and issues* (3rd ed., pp. 73–98). New York, NY: Guilford.

Johnson, J. A. (2005). Review of the Stanford-Binet intelligence scales, fifth edition. In R. A. Spies & B. S. Plake (Eds.), *The sixteenth mental measurements yearbook*. Lincoln, NE: Buros Institute of Mental Measurements.

Kamphaus, R. W. (2001). In R. Pascal (Ed.), *Clinical assessment of child and adolescent intelligence* (2nd ed.). Needham Heights, MA: Allyn & Bacon.

Kaufman, A. S., & Kaufman, N. L. (2004). *Kaufman brief intelligence test* (2nd ed.). Bloomington, MN: Pearson, Inc.

Kush, J. C. (2010). Review of the Peabody picture vocabulary test, fourth edition. In R. A. Spies, J. F. Carlson, & K. F. Geisinger (Eds.), *The eighteenth mental measurements yearbook*. Lincoln, NE: Buros Institute of Mental Measurements.

Macha, T., & Petermann, F. (2007). Bayley scales of infant and toddler development, third edition – Deutsche Fassung. *Journal of Psychoeducational Assessment, 25*(2), 139–143.

Madle, R. A. (2007). Review of the Kaufman brief intelligence test, second edition. In K. F. Geisinger, R. A. Spies, J. F. Carlson, & B. S. Plake (Eds.), *The seventeenth mental measurements yearbook*. Lincoln, NE: Buros Institute of Mental Measurements.

Mullen, E. M. (1995). *Mullen scales of early learning*. Circle Pines, MN: American Guidance Service.

Roid, G. H. (2003). *Stanford-Binet intelligence scales, fifth edition*. Itasca, IL: Riverside Publishing.

Roid, G. H. (2005). *Stanford-Binet intelligence scales for early childhood* (5th ed.). Itasca, IL: Riverside Publishing.

Rold, G. H., Miller, L. J., Pomplun, M., & Koch, C. (2013). *Leiter international performance scale-third edition*. Wood Dale, IL: Stoelting Company.

Schneider, W. J., & McGrew, K. S. (2012). The Cattell–Horn–Carroll model of intelligence. In D. P. Flanagan & P. L. Harrison (Eds.), *Contemporary intellectual assessment: Theories, tests, and issues* (3rd ed., pp. 99–144). New York, NY: Guilford.

Schrank, F. A., McGrew, K. S., & Mather, N. (2014). *Woodcock-Johnson IV*. Rolling Meadows, IL: Riverside.

Shaw, S. R. (2007). Review of the Kaufman brief intelligence test, second edition. In K. F. Geisinger, R. A. Spies, J. F. Carlson, & B. S. Plake (Eds.), *The seventeenth mental measurements yearbook*. Lincoln, NE: Buros Institute of Mental Measurements.

Sink, C. A., & Eppler, C. (2007). Review of the Stanford-Binet intelligence scales for early childhood, fifth edition. In K. F. Geisinger, R. A. Spies, J. F. Carlson, & B. S. Plake (Eds.), *The seventeenth mental measurements yearbook*. Lincoln, NE: Buros Institute of Mental Measurements.

Terman, L. M. (1916). *The measurement of intelligence: An explanation of and a complete guide for the use of the Stanford Revision and Extension of the Binet-Simon Intelligence Scale*. Boston, MA: Houghton Mifflin.

Tindal, G. (2010). Review of differential ability scales-second edition. In R. A. Spies, J. F. Carlson, & K. F. Geisinger (Eds.), *The eighteenth mental measurements yearbook*. Lincoln, NE, Buros Institute of Mental Measurements.

Tobin, R. M., & Hoff, K. E. (2007). Review of the Bayley scales of infant and toddler development-third edition. In K. F. Geisinger, R. A. Spies, J. F. Carlson, & B. S. Plake (Eds.), *The seventeenth mental measurements yearbook*. Lincoln, NE: Buros Institute of Mental Measurements.

Venn, J. J. (2007). Review of the Bayley scales of infant and toddler development-third edition. In K. F. Geisinger, R. A. Spies, J. F. Carlson, & B. S. Plake (Eds.), *The seventeenth mental measurements yearbook*. Lincoln, NE: Buros Institute of Mental Measurements.

Ward, S. (2017). Review of the Leiter international performance scale-third edition. In J. F. Carlson, K. F. Geisinger, & J. L. Johnson (Eds.), *The twentieth mental measurements yearbook*. Lincoln, NE: Buros Center for Testing.

Wechsler, D. (1939). *The measurement of adult intelligence*. Baltimore, MD: Williams & Wilkins.

Wechsler, D. (1949). *Wechsler intelligence scale for children. Manual*. New York, NY: Psychological Corporation.

Wechsler, D. (2012). *Wechsler preschool and primary scale of intelligence – Fourth edition*. San Antonio, TX: The Psychological Corporation.

Wechsler, D. (2014). *Wechsler intelligence scale for children—Fifth edition*. San Antonio, TX: The Psychological Corporation.

White, S. H. (2000). Conceptual foundations of IQ testing. *Psychology, Public Policy, and Law, 6*(1), 33–43.

Zenderland, L. (1998). *Measuring minds: Henry Herbert Goddard and the origins of American intelligence testing*. New York, NY: Cambridge University Press.

Adaptive and Developmental Behavior Scales

Jasper A. Estabillo and Johnny L. Matson

Introduction

The purpose of assessment is to integrate information to inform clinical decision-making (Sattler, 2001). Adaptive and developmental behaviors scales are used in assessment for childhood disorders to evaluate the child's level of functioning across various adaptive and developmental domains. These measures may be used in conjunction with developmental history, interviews, rating scales, and clinical observations to assess the child's abilities, make diagnostic decisions, and aid in treatment planning. This chapter reviews a number of widely used adaptive and developmental behavior scales in the assessment of childhood disorders.

Adaptive Behavior Scales

As specified by the American Association on Intellectual and Developmental Disabilities (AAIDD), "for the purpose of making a diagnosis of ruling out Intellectual Disability (ID), a comprehensive standardized measure of adaptive behavior should be used in making the determination of the individual's current adaptive behavior functioning in relation to the general population. The selected measure should provide robust standard scores across the three domains of adaptive behavior: conceptual, social, and practical adaptive behavior" (Schalock et al., 2010). Adaptive behaviors refer to "one's performance of daily activities that are required for personal and social sufficiency" (Bullington, 2011). They may also be defined as how well an individual meets their community's standards for personal independence expected for their age group and sociocultural background (APA, 2013; Bullington, 2011). As such, adaptive behaviors may be understood as the interaction of personal, cognitive, social, and situational variables (Sparrow, Cicchetti, & Balla, 2005). Broadly, areas of adaptive behaviors include communication, community living, self-care, and socialization skills.

Adaptive behaviors may also be referred to as "activities of daily living." Activities of daily living refer to behaviors that are important for self-management of one's health and independent living (Guerra, 2011; Troyer, 2011). These behaviors vary depending on one's developmental level and may be influenced by cognitive functioning (Guerra, 2011). As such, expectations for independent self-care are very different for young children than for adults. Self-care behaviors range from feeding, dressing, and toileting to money management and driving. An individual's ability to engage in these routines independently is central to the assessment of adaptive behaviors.

As defined by the AAIDD, adaptive behaviors are composed of the following:

1. Conceptual skills: memory, communication, reading, and mathematical concepts. These abilities are mostly related to areas of cognitive functioning and intelligence.
2. Social skills: social awareness, interpersonal skills, friendship abilities, and social responsibility. Social skills are related to one's ability to interact with others and function within their community.
3. Practical skills: self-care, activities of daily living, occupational skills, and safety awareness. These skills are related to one's ability to independently care for oneself.

Adaptive behavior assessment is central to the evaluation of intellectual and developmental disabilities. Additionally, it may assist with determining an individual's eligibility for special education programs and social services (Tassé et al., 2012). As current definitions for ID and developmental delays include deficits in adaptive functioning, adaptive behavior assessment may be required by agencies for provision of services. It is important for professionals to note that when assessing adaptive behaviors, scales normed with the general population are appropriate for diagnostic purposes, while scales normed with individuals with ID are appropriate for treatment planning and progress monitoring.

Adaptive behavior scales are also used within this population because individuals with developmental disabilities may require ongoing supports (Sheppard-Jones, Kleinert, Druckenmiller, & Ray, 2015). Identification of one's areas of strengths and weaknesses may be helpful in determining what domains require more support and what services to provide the individual with. Additionally, teaching individuals with disabilities adaptive skills to foster their independence is important. Behavior intervention programs have been found to be effective at teaching individuals with developmental disabilities a range of skills critical to adaptive and developmental behaviors (Alwell & Cobb, 2009; Bouck, 2010; Van Laarhoven & Van Laarhoven-Myers, 2006). These programs provide individuals with living skills that encourage their agency and self-sufficiency and promote their quality of life.

This section reviews some of the most commonly used measures of adaptive behaviors with individuals with ID and developmental delays. These measures assess abilities in a range of domains and are used in a variety of settings.

Vineland Adaptive Behavior Scales, Third Edition (Vineland-III)

The *Vineland Adaptive Behavior Scales, Third Edition* (*Vineland-III*; Sparrow, Cicchetti, & Saulnier, 2016) is a measure designed to assess adaptive behaviors in individuals from birth through 90 years old. The measure was created from the *Vineland Social Maturity Scale* (Doll, 1935) and has since undergone several revisions and re-standardizations. It is the most commonly used adaptive skills measure for assessment of adaptive deficits in individuals with intellectual disabilities and developmental delays (Cicchetti, Carter, & Gray, 2013).

The *Vineland-III* may be administered to parents and other informants familiar with the individual being assessed. There are several forms: interview form, parent/caregiver form, and teacher form. Administration time for the *Vineland-III* is approximately 10–60 min, depending on the form completed. A comprehensive (i.e., full-length) and domain-level (i.e., abbreviated) version of each form is available. In the interview form, the examiner administers questions to the informant in a semi-structured interview. Questions are meant to be open-ended in order to elicit information regarding the examinee's ability to perform various skills. With the parent/caregiver form, the parent/caregiver may rate information themselves. Spanish versions of the parent/caregiver rating forms are available. The teacher form is available for individuals 3–21 years and contains items that are equivalent to domains on the parent report forms.

The *Vineland-III* assesses adaptive behaviors in the domains of communication, daily living, socialization, and motor skills. The communication domain includes expressive and receptive language subdomains, as well as a written domain for older individuals. The daily living skills domain includes behaviors related to self-care (e.g., dressing, health care), domestic, and community living skills. The socialization domain includes skills related to relationships, friendships, and age-appropriate play and leisure. It contains subdomains of interpersonal relationships, play and leisure, and coping skills. The motor domain includes subdomains for both gross and fine motor skills. The motor domain is normed for children through age 9. An Adaptive Behavior Composite is calculated from the communication, daily living, and socialization skills domains to indicate the individual's overall adaptive functioning. In the parent rating form, the *Vineland-III* also contains items pertaining to maladaptive behaviors and includes both internalizing and externalizing subdomains.

Items are rated on a 3-point Likert scale. A "0" indicates that the individual does not perform the behavior, "1" indicates the individual sometimes performs the behavior, and "2" indicates the individuals performs the behavior most of the time. Raw scores yield age-normed standard scores, percentiles, and age equivalents. A broad adaptive behavior composite score is computed to indicate the individual's overall level of adaptive functioning.

Psychometrics for the *Vineland-III* indicate high internal consistency (coefficient alpha ranges 0.90–0.98 across domains). Test-retest reliability is 0.80–0.92 for the adaptive behavior composite. Inter-rater reliability is 0.79 for the adaptive behavior composite and ranges from 0.70 to 0.81 for different domains.

The *Vineland-III* may be used to assist with diagnosis of intellectual and developmental disabilities, as well as intervention planning and progress monitoring. The broad domains computed by the *Vineland-III* correspond to the AAIDD's domains of conceptual, practical, and social domains for adaptive behaviors. The *Vineland-III* may also be used to measure adaptive behaviors in individuals with traumatic brain injury and neurocognitive disorders (e.g., Alzheimer's disease).

Adaptive Behavior Assessment System, Third Edition (ABAS-3)

The *Adaptive Behavior Assessment System, Third Edition (ABAS-3*; Harrison & Oakland, 2015) assesses adaptive behaviors in individuals from birth through 89 years old. There are five forms of the *ABAS-3* available: parent form for ages 0–5 years, teacher/day care form for ages 2–5 years, parent form for ages 5–21 years, teacher form for ages 5–21 years, and adult form for ages 16–89 years. Forms in French-Canadian and Spanish are also available. Administration time is approximately 20 min.

Skills areas of communication, community use, functional academics, health and safety, home or school living, leisure, self-care, self-direction, social, and work skills are assessed. These areas produce standard scores in the domains of conceptual, social, and practical domains, which are aligned with the *DSM-5* and AAIDD models of adaptive behaviors. For young children, motor skills are also assessed. The conceptual domain includes skill areas of communication, functional academics, self-direction, and health and safety skills. The practical domain includes social and leisure skills. Lastly, the social domain includes self-care, home or school living, community use, health and safety, and work skills.

Items are scored on a 4-point Likert scale, where responses indicate if the individual "is not able," "never or almost never when needed," "sometimes when needed," or "always or almost always when needed" performs the behavior. Raw scores are then used to calculate domain composite scores for conceptual, social, and practical skills, as well as a general adaptive composite. The conceptual, social, and practical domains directly align with *DSM-5* and AAIDD domains for adaptive behavior. The general adaptive composite is used to determine the individual's overall level of adaptive functioning.

Psychometrically, the *ABAS-3* has high internal consistency ranging from 0.80 to 0.99 across the general adaptive composite, adaptive behavior domains (i.e., conceptual, practical, social), and skill areas (Burns, 2005). Test-retest reliability ranges from 0.70 to 0.90, and inter-rater reliability ranges from 0.70s to 0.80s depending on the raters and skill areas.

The *ABAS-3* may be used for diagnosis, intervention planning, and monitoring. It may be used to evaluate individuals with developmental delays, autism spectrum disorder (ASD), ID, learning disabilities, and other impairments.

AAMD Adaptive Behavior Scales

The *American Association for Mental Deficiency Adaptive Behavior Scales (AAMD ABS)* has two versions, *Adaptive Behavior Scales-Residential and Community, Second Edition (ABS-RC:2)*, and *Adaptive Behavior Scales-School, Second Edition (ABS-S:2)* (Lyman, 2008). The *ABS-S:2* may be used for individuals aged 3–21 years and the *ABS-RC:2* may be used for individuals aged 18–79 years. These measures are an assessment of adaptive behaviors in terms of personal independence and maladaptive behaviors that are specifically for individuals with intellectual disabilities. Items are rated as yes/no, on a 4-point Likert scale, or by frequency. The *ABS-RC:2* was historically used in institutional settings; however, it is now also used in community settings as well. The *ABS-RC:2* and *ABS-S:2* may be completed by a professional familiar with the individual or administered to an informant.

The *ABS-S:2* was created for use in the school system. Administration time ranges from 20 to 120 min. There are nine adaptive subscales including independent functioning, physical development, economic activity, language development, numbers and time, prevocational/vocational activity, self-direction, responsibility, and socialization. The behavioral domains include social behavior, conformity, trustworthiness, stereotyped and hyperactive behavior, self-abusive behavior, social engagement, and disturbing interpersonal behavior. Raw scores are converted to standard scores, percentiles, and age equivalents for each subdomain. Scores also loaded onto five factors including personal self-sufficiency, community self-sufficiency, personal social responsibility, social adjustment, and personal adjustment. These factor scores also may be converted to percentiles, standard scores, and age equivalents.

The *ABS-RC:2* also has two parts, but a greater number of subscales. Administration time ranges from 15 to 50 min. The adaptive subscales include independent functioning, physical development, economic activity, language development, numbers and time, domestic activity, prevocational/vocational activity, self-direction, responsibility, and socialization. The behavioral subscales include social behavior, conformity, trustworthiness, stereotypes and hyperactive behavior, sexual behavior, self-abusive behavior, social engagement, and disturbing interpersonal behavior.

Both the *ABS-S:2* and *ABS-RC:2* have good psychometrics. The *ABS-S:2* internal consistency ranges from 0.79 to 0.98, and inter-rater reliability ranges from 0.95 to 0.98 for Part I and 0.96 to 0.99 for Part II (Lyman, 2008). For the *ABS-RC:2* internal consistency ranges from 0.81 to 0.97. When examining discriminant validity, the *ABS-RC:2* Part II was not found to be related to the Vineland Adaptive Behavior Scales or Adaptive Behavior Inventory. The *ABS-S:2* was normed on students with and without intellectual disabilities, but the *ABS-RC:2* was not.

Adaptive Behavior Inventory (ABI)

The *Adaptive Behavior Inventory (ABI*; Brown & Leigh, 1986) assesses functional adaptive behaviors in children aged 6 years to 18 years, 11 months. It was designed to identify children who may have intellectual disability. This measure takes approximately 30 min to administer. A short form of the ABI is also available. It is typically completed by the child's classroom teacher.

The measure has five subtests: self-care skills, communication skills, social skills, academic skills, and occupational skills. Items are rated on a 4-point Likert scale. Responses of "0" indicate that the student does not perform the behavior, "1" indicate that the student is beginning to perform the behavior, "2" indicate that the student performs the behavior most of the time, and "3" indicate that the student has mastered the behavior. Raw scores are used to calculate standard scores and percentiles. Scores can be compared to two different sets of norms. One set of norms are used to compare the student with individuals with normal intelligence, while the other set is representative of students with ID.

The *ABI* has good psychometrics, with good internal consistency and test-retest reliability (Brown & Leigh, 1986). Coefficient alpha was found to range from 0.86 to 0.97 depending on age group. Internal consistency was above 0.90 for each age group. For test-retest reliability, the subtests, composite score, and short-form composite were all above 0.90.

Scales of Independent Behavior – Revised (SIB-R)

The *Scales of Independent Behavior – Revised* (*SIB-R*; Bruininks, Woodcock, Weatherman, & Hill, 1996) is a standardized measure of adaptive behaviors for individuals 3 months to 80 years old. There are three forms: early development form for children 3 months to 8 years, full-scale form for individuals 3 months to 80 years, and short form for individuals 3 months to 80 years. Both the early development and short forms are abbreviated versions of the full-scale *SIB-R*. The full-scale *SIB-R* takes 45–60 min for administration, and the early development form and short form each take approximately 15–20 min.

The *SIB-R* may be administered via either a structured interview or checklist procedure. Raw scores are used to calculate standard scores, percentile ranks, age equivalents, and instructional and developmental ranges. The measure has 14 subscales that are organized into four adaptive domains: motor skills, personal living skills, social interaction and communication skills, and community living skills. The maladaptive indices include general, internalized, asocial, and externalized behaviors. The *SIB-R* also has a functional limitations index, which provides details on the presence and severity of limitations of one's adaptive behavior. Support scores are also provided, which may assist in determining the level of support the individual needs (e.g., pervasive, extensive, frequent, limited, intermittent, or infrequent/no support). The measure also includes an individual plan recommendation form that may be used by professionals to plan and monitor the individual's needs and progress.

Adaptive Behavior Diagnostic Scale (ABDS)

The *Adaptive Behavior Diagnostic Scale* (*ABDS*; Pearson, Patton, & Mruzek, 2016) is an interview-based measure that assesses adaptive behaviors in individuals ages 2 through 21 years. Administration takes approximately 30 min. The *ABDS* is one of the newest standardized adaptive behavior scales available for use.

Items on the *ABDS* yield scores across the domains of conceptual, social, and practical. There are 50 items in each domain. Raw scores are used to calculate standard scores for each domain and an overall adaptive behavior index. These standard scores may be interpreted for diagnostic purposes, as well as determining target areas for treatment planning.

Psychometrics for the *ABDS* have been found to be good; internal consistency was at least 0.90 for all domain and composite scores. Additionally, sensitivity was found to be 0.85, specificity was 0.99, and classification accuracy was 0.98. However, because the *ABDS* is a newer measure, outside validation studies have not yet been conducted. Additional research on this scale with individuals with and without intellectual and developmental disabilities is needed.

Diagnostic Adaptive Behavior Scale (DABS)

The *Diagnostic Adaptive Behavior Scale* (*DABS*; Tassé et al., 2016) is another new standardized measure for adaptive behaviors. It was specifically designed to aid in diagnosis for ID individuals aged 4–21 years. The *DABS* is administered via a semi-structured interview which takes approximately 30 min to complete. It contains a total of 75 items that were tailored to adhere to the tripartite definition of adaptive behavior (i.e., conceptual, social, practical). A unique component of the *DABS* is that the measure was developed based on item response theory rather than classical test theory.

Items are administered to an informant who answers based on the individual's performance of certain behaviors. Responses of "0" indicate "no, does not do," "1" indicates "does it with reminders," "2" is "does it sometimes independently," and "3" is "yes, does it." Raw scores are converted to standard scores for the domains of conceptual skills, social skills, practical skills, and a *DABS* total score.

The *DABS* was normed on the general population for the purpose of being used as a diagnostic measure. Its sensitivity ranges from 81% to 98% depending on the age group, and specificity ranges from 89% to 91%, also depending on age group (Balboni et al., 2014). The measure also has good convergent and divergent validity with the *VABS-II* (Balboni et al., 2014).

Developmental Behavior Scales

When conducting evaluations for developmental disabilities, assessing across several developmental domains provides information on the individual's functioning overall, as well as within specific domains. Evaluating abilities in cognitive, motor, social, and communication domains provides a picture of the child's functioning within each area, and such measures allow for comparison with same-aged peers and a better understanding of the individual's strengths and weaknesses. Assessing developmental milestones in children is particularly helpful due to the instability of IQ tests at young ages (Rapin, 2003). Because assessing IQ in young children is not reliable, evaluation of capabilities in various domains may provide professionals with a broader assessment of the child's functioning.

In addition to full developmental scales, abbreviated screening measures have been created for use in clinical settings. These measures allow for quick assessment of a child's development, and if their scores meet established cutoffs, they are typically referred for further evaluation. The purpose of screening is to identify individuals who may be at risk for disorders (American Academy of Pediatrics, 2001; Baird et al., 2001). Various screening measures for specific disorders (e.g., ASD) are available; however, this chapter will review some broader developmental screening measures for overall delays rather than specific disorders. Screening measures are appropriate for use in settings where full evaluations are not necessary or feasible. They are cost effective and allow for greater numbers of children to be screened for possible delays. Ultimately, screening allows for the early identification of disorders in order to facilitate earlier diagnosis and intervention (American Academy of Pediatrics, 2001). This section reviews some of the most commonly used developmental behavior scales and abbreviated screening measures for the assessment of developmental delays in children.

Battelle Developmental Inventory, Second Edition (BDI-2)

The *Battelle Developmental Inventory, Second Edition* (*BDI-2*; Newborg, 2005), is a widely used developmental measure that assesses a child's skills in the domains of personal/social, adaptive, motor, communication, and cognitive skills. It is valid for children from birth through 7 years, 11 months old. Administration time ranges from 60 to 90 min. Examiners rate the quality of the child's development on a scale of 0–2 based on direct observation of the child's behavior or per informant report. A score of "0" indicates "no ability," "1" indicates an "emerging ability," and "2" indicates "ability present." Raw scores are converted to standard scores, age equivalents, percentile ranks, and developmental quotients, which all provide information on the child's developmental level. The developmental quotient is based on a mean of 100 and standard deviation of 15; it can be understood as the child's general functioning level. The *BDI-2* has acceptable test-retest reliability of $\alpha = 0.80$ and excellent internal consistency of 0.98–0.99 (Bliss, 2007; Newborg, 2005).

Skills are assessed through interaction and observation with the child, as well as interview with parents/caregivers. Domains may be administered in any order. The adaptive domain assesses skills related to self-care and personal responsibility and includes items pertaining to eating/feeding, dressing, toileting, and safety awareness. It is divided into the subdomains of adult interaction, peer interaction, and self-concept and social role. The personal/social domain assesses the child's capacity for self-concept and ability to interact with peers and adults. Communication is divided into receptive (i.e., comprehension) and expressive skills (i.e., ability to communicate with others through use of vocalizations and gestures). The motor domain assesses the child's gross motor, fine motor, and perceptual motor skills, where perceptual motor requires integration of perceptual and fine motor abilities (e.g., stacking blocks). The cognitive domain is divided into attention and memory, reasoning and academic skills, and perception and concepts. It assesses skills related to attention, perception, thinking, and information processing.

Concurrent validity studies of the *BDI-2* and *Bayley Scales of Infant Development, Second Edition* (*BSID-II*; Bayley, 1993) showed moderate to moderately high correlations between corresponding domains on each measure. Studies with special populations including children with autism and various developmental delays indicated very good specificity in correctly identifying children across diagnoses (Hilton-Mounger, 2011).

The *BDI-2* is also useful in assessing areas for intervention. Because of the various domains assessed, the *BDI-2* provides a profile of development that may be used by providers to determine broad areas for treatment.

Bayley Scales of Infant and Toddler Development – Third Edition (Bayley-III)

The *Bayley Scales of Infant and Toddler Development – Third Edition* (*Bayley-III*; Bayley, 2006a, 2006b) is another widely used developmental measure that is designed for identification of children with developmental delays across domains of cognitive, language, motor, social-emotional, and adaptive skills. It is valid for administration with children 16 days to 42 months, 15 days old, and administration time is typically 30–90 min.

Examiners administer items to the child through playful activities which aid in assessing the child's level of functioning in the cognitive, language, and motor domains. Start points are based on the child's chronological age, and once a basal is established, items are administered until the ceiling is achieved. Items are scored as "1" if the behavior is observed/child receives credit for their performance and "0" if the behavior is not observed/no credit given. Subtests may be administered in any order, with the exception of the Receptive Communication subtest, which must be given prior to the Expressive Communication subtest. The cognitive domain evaluates abilities such as the child's sensorimotor development, concept formation, memory, visual acuity, and visual preference. Tasks include age-appropriate skills including object assembly, puzzle completion, and pattern discrimination. The language domain assesses both expressive and receptive language. Expressive skills include babbling, gesturing, and vocabulary development, while receptive skills include the child's ability to identify objects and understanding of pronouns and prepositions. In the motor domain, examiners assess fine motor skills (e.g., grasping, reaching, functional hand

and finger skills) and gross motor skills (e.g., locomotion, balance, motor planning).

To assess the child's social-emotional and adaptive development, parents/caregivers provide ratings for the child's abilities. To assess social-emotional development, parents/caregivers answer questions related to the child's social-emotional growth and functioning to determine if deficits or problems are present (Greenspan, 2004). All questions in the social-emotional scale must be completed until the informant reaches the child's age-appropriate stop point. Lastly, adaptive behaviors assessed by parent ratings include communication skills, functional pre-academic skills, home and community skills, self-care skills, social skills, and motor skills. All questions on the adaptive behavior scale are completed by parents/caregivers.

Scores obtained from the *Bayley-III* provide information on the child's developmental level. Raw scores are converted to standard scores, age equivalents, percentiles, and T-scores to allow for comparison with peers. The *Bayley-III* may be used in intervention settings to calculate growth scores and monitor the child's progress. While other measures of adaptive and developmental behavior may not be appropriate for individuals with severe delays, a strength of the *Bayley-III* is that it may also be used for individuals over 42 months who experience significant delays. Additionally, a screening measure is available. The *Bayley-III Screening Test* contains selected items from the *Bayley-III* full assessment battery and takes approximately 15–25 min to administer. The abbreviated measure allows for quick assessment of the child's developmental functioning and aids in determining if comprehensive evaluation is needed.

Mullen Scales of Early Learning: American Guidance Service Edition (MSEL:AGS)

The *Mullen Scales of Early Learning: American Guidance Service Edition* (*MSEL:AGS*; Mullen, 1995) is an assessment measure for young children's cognitive and motor abilities. It is appropriate for use with children from birth to 68 months old. Administration time ranges from 15 to 60 min, depending on the age of the child being assessed.

The measure comprises of 124 items which assess abilities pertaining to gross motor, visual reception, fine motor, expressive language, and receptive language abilities. The gross motor scale is only administered to children up to 33 months. Items are scored based on the child's completion of various tasks or through interview with an informant. Items may be scored as "1" to indicate that the child exhibited a correct response or "0" to indicate an incorrect response. Scores on the visual reception, fine motor, receptive language, and expressive language scales are combined to compose an Early Learning Composite (ELC), which may be interpreted as a measure of the child's overall cognitive functioning. Raw scores are used to calculate T-scores, percentile ranks, age equivalents, and standard scores.

Studies on the measure's psychometrics have shown good internal consistency and reliability (Mullen, 1995). Internal consistency coefficients ranged from 0.75 to 0.83 for the four scales and 0.91 for the ELC. Test-retest reliability was 0.96 for the gross motor scale and 0.82–0.85 (younger children) or 0.71–0.79 (older children) for the cognitive scales. Inter-rater reliability was also found to be high, ranging from 0.91 to 0.99.

The *MSEL:AGS* may be used to aid in identifying strengths and weaknesses and is recommended for use in early intervention programs and assessing for school readiness. As recommended by the creator, the *MSEL:AGS* may be used to determine eligibility for services (e.g., early intervention, special education), evaluation for developmental delays, and individualized program planning (Mullen, 1995). As such, the measure is useful in a variety of clinical and educational settings.

Ages and Stages Questionnaires (ASQ-3)

The *Ages and Stages Questionnaires (ASQ-3): A Parent-Completed Child Monitoring System, Third edition* (*ASQ-3*; Squires et al., 2009), is a screening measure designed for early identification of delays in infants and young children. The *ASQ-3* has 21 separate questionnaires for ages 2, 3, 6, 8, 9, 10, 12, 14, 16, 18, 20, 22, 24, 27, 30, 33, 36, 42, 48, 54, and 60 months, which are intended to be completed at each age for monitoring. The *ASQ:SE* (social-emotional) is also available for the child's social-emotional development. Completion of both components of the *ASQ* provides information regarding the child's functioning across a number of domains. The questionnaires are completed by parents/caregivers, and completion time is approximately 15 min. Scoring may be completed in 2–3 min. Questionnaires are available in English, Spanish, and French.

Each questionnaire is comprised of 30 items pertaining to communication, gross motor, fine motor, problem solving, and personal-social skills. Items are answered as "yes" (i.e., child performs behavior), "sometimes" (i.e., emerging behavior), or "not yet" (i.e., child does not perform behavior). Items are scored and total scores are compared to established cutoff points.

Standardization studies have indicated good psychometrics on the *ASQ-3* (Squires et al., 2009). Test-retest reliability was high (0.92), as was inter-rater reliability (0.93). The *ASQ-3* also has a sensitivity of 0.86 and specificity of 0.85.

As a screening measure, the *ASQ-3* provides valuable information regarding a child's development starting at very young ages. Because of its various forms, parents/caregivers and professionals may monitor a child's progress over time. This may be particularly useful for intervention purposes, as the *ASQ-3* may identify difficulties at very early ages. Scores that are found to be in the "monitoring zone" are useful to aid in treatment planning and progress monitoring.

Denver Developmental Screening Test II (DDST-II)

The *Denver Developmental Screening Test* (*DDST*; Frankenburg & Dodds, 1967) was the first widely used screening measure designed for identification of young children at risk for developmental delays. The subsequent *Denver II* (Frankenburg, Dodds, Archers, Shapiro, & Bresnick, 1992) was created as an update to the *DDST*. The instrument was created for children 0–6 years and assesses skills in personal-social, fine motor-adaptive, language, and gross motor domains. An examiner administers the measure through various standardized items (e.g., blocks, pictures). Administration time is approximately 10–20 min. Items are rated based on if the child's response falls within or outside of the expected range for the child's age. The child's scores are compared to same-aged peers on bar graphs which indicate the ages that 25%, 50%, 75%, and 90% of typically developing children were able to complete each task. Items which the child could not complete but 90% of typically developing children could are considered to be delays. Items that the child could not complete but 75–90% of typically developing children could are marked as "cautions." The graphs provide a visual to depict where the child is developmentally compared to same-aged peers.

Standardized on over 1000 children, the *DDST* showed high specificity (>0.87) but very low sensitivity (0.13–0.46). Thus, the *DDST* was not good at detecting children with delays, which is a major concern given the purpose of the measure was to screen children. With the *Denver II*'s re-standardization, sensitivity improved to 0.83 but specificity decreased to 0.43 (Glascoe et al., 1992). As such, this led to concerns regarding high numbers of typically developing children being screened as needing further evaluation for delays. Test-retest and inter-rater reliability were both reported to be 0.90 or greater (Frankenburg et al., 1992).

At present, the *Denver II* is no longer widely used for screening for developmental delays. However, as the first developmental screening tool widely used in the health field, it is important to note. There are currently a number of other screening tools and comprehensive developmental measures available to aid in the assessment of developmental delays and disabilities in children.

Conclusion

This chapter discussed a number of adaptive and developmental behavior scales available to aid in the assessment of developmental delays. Adaptive behavior scales are designed to assess skills across domains relevant to an individual's ability to care for oneself. Delays are determined by the social and cultural expectations at each age. Changes in the conceptualization of ID have led to many of these measures to evaluate behaviors in conceptual, social, and practical domains, which reflect the current *DSM-5* and AAIDD definitions for ID. Similarly, developmental behavior scales are designed to assess skills across a variety of domains; however, these measures tend to be broader in the areas assessed and are primarily for use in the assessment of developmental disabilities in children. Because of the broad domains assessed in these measures, they may also be used for intervention planning and progress monitoring. Both adaptive and developmental behavior scales are widely used in the field of child psychopathology and developmental disabilities, and their use is central to the assessment and treatment of these disorders.

References

Alwell, M., & Cobb, B. (2009). Functional life skills curricular interventions for youth with disabilities: A systematic review. *Career Development for Exceptional Individuals, 32*(2), 82–93.

American Academy of Pediatrics. (2001). Developmental surveillance and screening of infants and young children. *Pediatrics, 108*(1), 192–195.

American Psychiatric Association (APA). (2013). Diagnostic and statistical manual of mental disorders (5th ed.). Arlington, VA: American Psychiatric Publishing.

Baird, G., Charman, A., Cox, S., Baron-Cohen, S., Swettenham, J., Wheelwright, S., & Drew, A. (2001). Screening and surveillance for autism and pervasive developmental disorders. *Archives of Disease in Childhood, 84*, 468–475.

Balboni, G., Tassé, M. J., Schalock, R. L., Borthwick-Duffy, S. A., Spreat, S., Thissen, D., … Navas, P. (2014). The diagnostic adaptive behavior scale: Evaluating its diagnostic sensitivity and specificity. *Research in Developmental Disabilities, 35*(11), 2884–2893.

Bayley, N. (1993). *Bayley scales of infant and development-second edition*. San Antonio, TX: The Psychological Corporation.

Bayley, N. (2006a). *Bayley scales of infant and toddler development, third edition: Administration manual*. San Antonio, TX: Harcourt Assessment.

Bayley, N. (2006b). *Bayley scales of infant and toddler development, third edition: Technical manual*. San Antonio, TX: Harcourt Assessment.

Bouck, E. C. (2010). Reports of life skills training for students with intellectual disabilities in and out of school. *Journal of Intellectual Disability Research, 54*(12), 1093–1103.

Bliss, S. L. (2007). Test reviews: Newborg, J. (2005). Battelle developmental inventory-second edition. Itasca, IL: Riverside. *Journal of Psychoeducational Assessment, 25*(4), 409–415.

Bruininks, R., Woodcock, R., Weatherman, R., & Hill, B. (1996). *Scales of independent behavior – Revised*. Rolling Meadows, IL: Riverside Publishing.

Brown, L., & Leigh, J. E. (1986). Adaptive behavior inventory. Austin, TX: PRO-ED.

Bullington, E. A. (2011). Adaptive behavior. In S. Goldstein & J. A. Naglieri (Eds.), *Encyclopedia of child behavior and development*. New York, NY: Springer.

Burns, M. K. (2005). Review of the adaptive behavior assessment system – Second edition. In R. Spies & B. Plake (Eds.), *The sixteenth mental measurements yearbook*. Lincoln, NE: Buros Institute of Mental Measurements.

Cicchetti, D. V., Carter, A. S., & Gray, S. A. O. (2013). Vineland adaptive behavior scales. In F. R. Volkmar (Ed.), *Encyclopedia of autism Spectrum disorders*. New York, NY: Springer.

Doll, E. A. (1935). *Vineland social maturity scale: Manual of directions*. Minneapolis, MN: Educational Test Bureau.

Frankenburg, W. K., & Dodds, J. (1967). The Denver developmental screening test. *Journal of Pediatrics, 71*, 181–191.

Frankenburg, W. K., Dodds, J., Archer, P., Shapiro, H., & Bresnick, B. (1992). The Denver II: A major revision and restandardization of the Denver developmental screening test. *Pediatrics, 89*, 91–97.

Glascoe, F. P., Byrne, K. E., Ashford, L. G., Johnson, K. L., Chang, B., & Strickland, B. (1992). Accuracy of the Denver II in developmental screening. *Pediatrics, 89*, 1221–1225.

Greenspan, S. I. (2004). *Greenspan social-emotional growth chart: A screening questionnaire for infants and young children*. San Antonio, TX: Harcourt.

Guerra, N. S. (2011). Activity of daily living. In S. Goldstein & J. A. Naglieri (Eds.), *Encyclopedia of child behavior and development*. New York, NY: Springer.

Harrison, P., & Oakland, T. (2015). *Adaptive behavior assessment system* (3rd ed.). San Antonio, TX: Harcourt Assessment.

Hilton-Mounger, A. (2011). Batelle developmental inventory: Second edition. In S. Goldstein & J. A. Naglieri (Eds.), *Encyclopedia of child behavior and development*. New York, NY: Springer.

Lyman, W. (2008). Test review. In N. Lambert, K. Nihira, & H. Lel (1993). AAMR Adaptive behavior scales: school. *Assessment for Affective Intervention, 33*, 55–57.

Mullen, E. M. (1995). *Mullen scales of early learning: AGS education*. Circle Pines, MN: American Guidance Service.

Newborg, J. (2005). *Battelle developmental inventory* (2nd ed.). Itasca, IL: Riverside Publishing.

Pearson, N. A., Patton, J. R., & Mruzek, D. W. (2016). *Adaptive behavior diagnostic scale: Examiner's manual*. Austin, TX: PRO-ED.

Rapin, I. (2003). Value and limitations of preschool cognitive tests, with an emphasis on longitudinal study of children on the autistic spectrum. *Brain and Development, 25*, 546–548.

Sattler, J. M. (2001). *Assessment of children, cognitive applications* (4th ed.). San Diego, CA: Jerome Sattler Publishing.

Schalock, R. L., Borthwick-Duffy, S. A., Bradley, V. J., Buntinx, W. H. E., Coulter, D. L., Craig, E. M., ... Yeager, M. H. (2010). *Intellectual disability: Diagnosis, classification, and systems of supports* (11th ed.). Washington, DC: American Association on Intellectual and Developmental Disabilities.

Sheppard-Jones, K., Kleinert, H. L., Druckemiller, W., Ray, M. K. (2015). Students with intellectual disability in higher education: Adult service provider perspectives. *Intellectual and Developmental Disabilities, 53*(2), 120–128.

Sparrow, S., Cicchetti, D., & Balla, D. (2005). *Vineland adaptive behavior scales* (2nd ed.). Circle Pines, MN: American Guidance Service.

Sparrow, S. S., Cicchetti, D. V., & Saulnier, C. A. (2016). *Vineland adaptive behavior scales, (Vineland-3)* (3rd ed.). Bloomington, MN: Pearson.

Squires, J., Bricker, D., Twombly, E., Nickel, R., Clifford, J., Murphy, K., ... Farrell, J. (2009). *Ages & stages questionnaires, (ASQ-3)* (3rd ed.). Baltimore, MD: Paul H. Brookes.

Tassé, M. J., Schalock, R. L., Balboni, G., Bersani, H., Borthwick-Duffy, S. A., Spreat, S., ... Zhang, D. (2012). The construct of adaptive behavior: Its conceptualization, measurement, and use in the field of intellectual disability. *American Journal on Intellectual and Developmental Disabilities, 117*(4), 291–303.

Tassé, M. J., Schalock, R. L., Thissen, D., Balboni, G., Bersani, H. H., Borthwick-Duffy, S. A., ... Navas, P. (2016). Development and standardization of the diagnostic adaptive behavior scale: Application of item response theory to the assessment of adaptive behavior. *American Journal on Intellectual and Developmental Disabilities, 121*(2), 79–94.

Troyer, A. K. (2011). Activities of daily living. In J. S. Kreutzer, J. DeLuca, & B. Caplan (Eds.), *Encyclopedia of clinical neuropsychology*. New York, NY: Springer.

Van Laarhoven, T., & Van Laarhoven-Myers, T. (2006). Comparison of three video-based instructional procedures for teaching daily living skills to persons with developmental disabilities. *Education and Training in Developmental Disabilities, 41*(4), 365–381.

Academic Assessment

George H. Noell, Scott P. Ardoin, and Kristin A. Gansle

Academic Assessment

Children growing up in information-age societies are immersed in educational contexts in which academic demands are pervasive. These educational contexts are the gateways into adult life, work, independence, and relative self-sufficiency. Poor academic attainment is associated with a host of negative life outcomes including earnings, social engagement, and mental health (Hu & Wolniak, 2013; Jhang, 2017). Poor academic achievement is a common trigger event for children's referrals for assessment to both within-school (Smeets & Roeleveld, 2016) and out-of-school resources. A complex interaction exists between children's academic and social-emotional functioning in which academic attainment can affect mental health outcomes and mental health problems can adversely impact children's educational success (Johnson, McGue, & Iacono, 2006). Children who suffer from depression, anxiety, or attention-deficit/hyperactivity disorder (ADHD) are at an apparent disadvantage in attending to, completing, and profiting from instruction. Children who exhibit substantial conduct problems are also at increased risk for poor academic achievement that may be the result of the interaction of diverse factors (Montague, Enders, & Castro, 2005). The academic attainment mental health synergy may also emerge from the opposite perspective, with children who experience poor educational outcomes being more likely to exhibit anxiety, depression, negative self-esteem, and conduct problems (Weidman, Augustine, Murayama, & Elliot, 2015).

Co-occurring phenomena naturally raise the question of causality. Are academic difficulties the result of psychopathology, is psychopathology the result of chronic stress due to school failure, or are both concerns the result of a third factor? A strong causal determination is likely not possible due both the limitations of epidemiological correlational research and the practical reality that the emergence of these concerns may be substantively idiographic. Psychopathology may create substantive barriers to academic achievement for some children, while for others, chronic negative life events resulting from academic failure may drive psychopathological symptoms. The inescapable nature of school stressors in an age of mandatory school attendance may further exacerbate these stressors. Although it may be common

G. H. Noell (✉)
Department of Psychology, Louisiana State University, Baton Rouge, LA, USA
e-mail: gnoell@lsu.edu

S. P. Ardoin
Department of Educational Psychology, University of Georgia, Athens, GA, USA

K. A. Gansle
School of Education, Louisiana State University, Baton Rouge, LA, USA

to think in terms of psychopathology as causing academic concerns, for some children the reverse relationship may hold (Weidman et al., 2015).

Given the central nature of education in the lives of children, comprehensive psychological assessment for them should include assessment of the client's educational context and achievement; thus, the inclusion of this chapter in a volume devoted to the assessment of psychopathology. It is organized around the assumption that assessments will be designed to answer the same broad questions relevant to diagnosis and treatment that drive assessment for nonacademic concerns. First, is there a problem, and if so, what is the nature of that problem (diagnosis)? Second, if academic performance is a part of the presenting problem, what can be done to ameliorate that problem (treatment specification)? Although these two questions generally provide a simple, powerful organizing heuristic for psychological assessment, the challenge is in specifying the details to develop an assessment that is valid and has treatment utility. The selection of measurement tools and the integration of assessment data that vary in their direct relevance to treatment planning and in their technical quality create substantial challenges for the design, execution, and interpretation of the assessment.

This chapter is organized into three sections. The first section discusses diagnostic considerations relevant to academic concerns with primary consideration devoted to the Individuals with Disabilities Education Improvement Act of 2004 (IDEA). IDEA is central to the treatment of academic concerns in schools and is likely to be less familiar to readers of this volume as compared to the Diagnostic and Statistical Manual of Mental Disorders (DSM-5, American Psychiatric Association, 2013). The second section describes the types of assessments that are commonly deployed in school systems with a multitiered system of supports and direct assessments of academic skills that have commonly been described as curriculum-based measures (CBM). The types of measures used in these systems potentially can be used for universal screening, treatment selection, progress monitoring, and ultimately entitlement decisions provided they are appropriately implemented. The final section describes critical considerations in the design of interventions for academic concerns. The authors wish to acknowledge at the outset that space limitations preclude a comprehensive treatment of the issues surrounding academic assessment relevant to psychopathology and developmental disabilities. Each year many journals and complete volumes are devoted to the topics reviewed herein. This chapter provides an overview of selected topics relevant to academic concerns in the assessment of childhood psychopathology and developmental disabilities.

Diagnostic Considerations

The *Diagnostic and Statistical Manual of Mental Disorders* (DSM-5, American Psychiatric Association [APA], 2013) and Public Law 108–446, or IDEA, are the primary diagnostic sources used for the identification of academic concerns of children in the United States. Poor achievement may be accounted for either by within-child factors, poor instruction and/or environmental disadvantage, or an interaction of the two (Fuchs, Fuchs, & Hollenbeck, 2007; Gresham & Gansle, 1992). Despite the reality that both within-child and environmental factors are well documented, both diagnostic schemes conceptualize the cause of poor achievement as contained within the child rather than in an interaction between the child and the classroom environment. Although IDEA does explicitly state that environmental disadvantage must not be the reason for diagnosis of a learning disability, the extent to which this is commonly assessed or integrated into assessment in practice is uncertain. Further, despite the requirement of a disability diagnosis to allow a student to receive services in schools and community settings, the needs of the student, rather than the disability, should determine the treatment or intervention for academic concerns (Yell, 2016). A diagnosis from either DSM-5 or IDEA has little if any treatment utility for academic concerns; the diagnoses are nosological rather than functional. It is also worth acknowledging that a diagnosis under either system may be needed to allow a client to access services they need or to trigger civil rights protections in the schools (Yell, 2016).

Academic problems or their early childhood equivalents, social and communication problems, are features common to many of the diagnoses first identified in infancy, childhood, adolescence, or in school settings. The Neurodevelopmental Disorders include Intellectual Disabilities, Communication Disorders, Autism Spectrum Disorder, and Specific Learning Disorder, all of which contain deficits either in intellectual functioning or social communication and social interaction as primary criteria (DSM-5, 2013). Further, children diagnosed with many of the other DSM-5 diagnoses including post-traumatic stress disorder, schizophrenia spectrum and other psychotic disorders, or disruptive, impulse-control, and conduct disorders are likely to demonstrate problems with academic achievement. In the latter cases, however, it is probable that academic concerns will be secondary to problems with social-emotional functioning. This chapter's focus is on matters for which academic performance is the central issue.

Although they may be used for different purposes in different settings, DSM-5 and IDEA diagnoses share features that contribute to efficient and effective communication among practitioners in clinical and educational settings. Each seeks to address intellectual functioning and its relationship to achievement in reading, mathematics, and written expression. However, DSM-5 and educational diagnoses differ with respect to the diagnoses that may be made as well as specificity of their features. Traditionally, children who struggle with academics in the general curriculum have been assessed using standardized, norm-referenced tests in clinical and school settings. These instruments generally have technical properties appropriate to and adequate for diagnostic use.

Diagnostic and Statistical Manual of Mental Disorders, 5th Edition (DSM-5)

Intellectual Disability (Intellectual Developmental Disorder, ID) Depending on the extent to which the impairments resulting from an intellectual disability are pervasive, academic concerns may take a more central or a more secondary focus. Given the increasing emphasis on integrating all students into the general curriculum to the maximum extent possible (IDEA, 2004), the general education curriculum is likely to be a more central concern for students whose ID is milder than those whose impairment is more severe. For many individuals functioning in the mild range of intellectual disability, academic concerns are likely to be of central importance. Common diagnostic requirements for ID include *intellectual functioning* that is approximately two standard deviations (or more) below the population mean (DSM-5, APA, 2013). IDEA (2004) cites "significantly subaverage intellectual functioning" as a diagnostic requirement; this is interpreted by many, but not all, states as two standard deviations below the mean. Given that measurement error is inherent in assessment, the DSM-5 cautions that individuals with scores somewhat above 70 may still qualify for the diagnosis if additional indicators are significantly impaired. Similarly, individuals with scores more than two standard deviations below the mean may *not* qualify for the diagnosis if other diagnostic indicators do not confirm the diagnosis (APA, 2013).

Second, individuals who qualify for an ID diagnosis must have concurrent deficits in *adaptive functioning*. DSM-5 defines adaptive functioning as "how well a person meets community standards of personal independence and social responsibility, in comparison to others of similar age and sociocultural background" (APA, 2013, p. 37). Deficits in adaptive functioning must be observed in either the conceptual, social, or practical domains. At least one domain must be sufficiently impaired that the person needs support to function. Adaptive functioning skills include all areas relevant to social independence, such as communication and social skills, work and community involvement, academic skills, and health and safety (APA, 2013). The deficits in adaptive functioning must be related to the deficits in intellectual functioning (APA, 2013). Third, the *onset of the disorder* must be before the age of

18 years. An initial ID diagnosis may be made after the age of 18, but there must be evidence of onset prior to that age.

Specific Learning Disorders In DSM-5, when an individual's achievement in reading, written expression, or mathematics on individually administered standardized tests is *substantially and quantifiably below* what is expected given the individual's age and it causes *significant interference* with achievement, work performance, or activities of daily living, a specific learning disorder may be diagnosed. The DSM-5 does not provide a standard regarding what scores qualify for the diagnosis but does suggest low achievement within an academic domain as "at least 1.5 standard deviations [SD] below the population mean for age…are needed for the greatest diagnostic certainty" (p. 69), but that "a more lenient threshold may be used…when learning difficulties are supported by converging evidence from clinical assessment, academic history, school reports, or test scores" (p. 69). Specific learning disorder is assumed to have a biological etiology residing within the central nervous system. For a diagnosis to be made, the disorder must have an important negative impact on academic achievement or daily living skills. One important feature of this disorder is persistent problems learning critical academic skills that begins during years of formal academic instruction and may be associated with delays in attention or language skills.

Attention-Deficit/Hyperactivity Disorder A DSM-5 diagnosis of attention-deficit/hyperactivity disorder (ADHD) may be used when a child displays a pattern of inattention and/or impulsivity/hyperactivity that is persistent and interferes with functioning or development. Several of the symptoms must have been present prior to the child's 12th birthday, and they must manifest in two or more settings. There is quantitative standard for qualification for the diagnosis. The word "often" is common to all 18 specific behavioral diagnostic criteria for ADHD (e.g., "often fails to give close attention to details," APA, p. 59–60). Individuals with ADHD may be diagnosed as predominantly hyperactive/impulsive, predominantly inattentive, or combined. When the individual has major symptoms of ADHD but specific criteria for ADHD subtypes are not met, ADHD Not Otherwise Specified may be diagnosed. Mild delays in language development, social development, or motor development may occur with ADHD as well as low frustration tolerance, irritability, or mood swings (APA, p. 61).

Individuals with Disabilities Education Improvement Act of 2004 (IDEA)

Children in the United States are entitled to a free and appropriate public education in the least restrictive environment that is appropriate to their individual needs (IDEA, 2004). Children with disabilities must receive a diagnosis of those disabilities within the due process provisions of IDEA and applicable case law, using nondiscriminatory, multifactored evaluation in order to receive special services under IDEA (Yell, 2016). Diagnostic evaluations are completed with the express purpose of ascertaining eligibility for and providing services to children with disabilities. Eligibility must be determined based on the presence of a disability defined in IDEA and by state law and the documentation of need for special services to remediate the educational deficits caused by the disability. Once eligibility has been established and a service plan designed and implemented, schools receive supplemental federal and state funding to partially offset the increased cost of providing educational services to students with disabilities.

Under IDEA, disabilities for which special education services may be provided are identified in 13 categories. The diagnoses available for use by multidisciplinary teams (MDTs) in schools address concerns about children that have an impact on their educational achievement; however, many of them require planning for issues in addition to academic achievement (e.g., deaf-blindness, other health impairment, or emotional disturbance). For this chapter, assessment for diagnoses whose primary focus is academic will be addressed. Although the educational diagnostic categories are broadly delineated in federal legislation (IDEA, 2004), each state determines the specific operational diagnostic criteria for use in their jurisdiction. It is also worth noting that states vary widely in terms of the qualifications of the examiners that are required in order for data to contribute to a MDT determination. Typically, assessor qualifications focus on educational licenses or certifications.

Intellectual Disability In 2010, "Rosa's Law" was signed by President Obama, changing the name of the previously designated IDEA diagnosis of "Mental Retardation" to "Intellectual Disability" (Pub L. 111–256). It applies to all federal health, education and labor laws including IDEA (Friedman, 2016). The criteria for the diagnosis are the same as they had been under IDEA (2004). In IDEA, intellectual disability is defined as "significantly subaverage general intellectual functioning, existing concurrently with deficits in adaptive behavior and manifested during the developmental period, that adversely affects a child's educational performance" (IDEA, 2004). Although IDEA does not define "significantly subaverage intellectual functioning," leaving that determination to the states, an IQ score approximately two standard deviations below the mean is considered such by the American Association on Intellectual and Developmental Disabilities (AAIDD, Schalock, Borthwick-Duffy, Buntinx, Coulter, & Craig, 2010), a leader in advocacy, policy, and research for individuals with ID. It is the most common standard adopted by states. Not all education agencies, however, choose to use two standard deviations as the IQ criterion for the diagnosis, and the degree to which a child's intellectual functioning must deviate from the mean differs according to the agency setting the policy.

Adaptive behavior is "the collection of conceptual, social, and practical skills that are learned and performed by people in their everyday lives" (AAIDD, Schalock et al., 2010). Adequate adaptive behavior may be inferred from the degree to which individuals function independently, taking expectations of age and culture into account. Although DSM-5 further classifies ID by severity, IDEA does not provide similar categories. Services are made available to students according to need, and those needs are established using descriptions of current levels of educational performance and goals for future performance (Yell, 2016).

Specific Learning Disabilities IDEA (2004) describes specific learning disability (SLD) as "a disorder in one or more of the basic psychological processes involved in understanding or in using language, spoken or written, that may manifest itself in the imperfect ability to listen, think, speak, read, write, spell, or to do mathematical calculations." It may include disorders such as dyslexia, brain injury, and developmental aphasia. The seven areas that may be affected by the disability are a much broader application of SLD than the three areas of specific learning disorders (reading impairment, written expression impairment, and mathematics impairment) used by DSM-5, despite the lack of clear empirical support for all seven areas as distinct SLDs (Fletcher et al., 1998). Exclusionary criteria for the diagnosis indicate that other factors such as visual, hearing, motor problems, intellectual disabilities, emotional disturbance, and environmental, cultural, or economic disadvantage may *not* be responsible for the learning problem (IDEA, 2004). Although this is spelled out in the federal definition, research on identification practices demonstrates that in the face of criteria that exclude students from receiving special services for some of the very reasons they need assistance in the first place, MDTs identify large numbers of students who fail to meet eligibility criteria as exhibiting SLD (Lyon, 1996; MacMillan, Gresham, & Bocian, 1998; Shaywitz, Shaywitz, Fletcher, & Escobar, 1990).

Whereas DSM-5 defines the disorder concretely as a discrepancy between ability and achievement, IDEA describes SLD as a disorder in psychological processes. Therefore, the resulting diagnosis for SLD focuses on those processes which cannot be observed directly and in some instances are logically incoherent (Gresham, 2002). The original IDEA indicated that children labeled as SLD must have a "severe discrepancy" between ability and achievement (U. S. Office of Education, 1977, p. 65083). The US Department of Education has proposed a number of formulas for determining discrepancy and all have been challenged (Heward, 2006). This is likely due to a number of documented problems with these formulas (Fletcher, Francis, Morris, & Lyon, 2005; Fletcher et al., 1998; Kavale, 2002).

Given the problems associated with discrepancy formulas, a burgeoning literature describes a range of alternatives including different discrepancy formulas and response to intervention models (RTI, see Gresham, 2002; Kavale, 2002); however, none has gained widespread acceptance in the policy, research, and practice communities. The current IDEA mentions neither discrepancy nor specific criteria for determining the diagnosis but does describe RTI as a possibility for determining a specific learning disorder. The states, then, are left to operationalize the definition. This, in turn, has led to *substantial* heterogeneity between states in the criteria and procedures for classifying children with learning disabilities (Kavale, 2002; MacMillan & Siperstein, 2002). Despite these differences, however, the most common practice for identifying SLD is to determine whether a severe discrepancy exists between achievement predicted by individually administered measures of intellectual ability and actual achievement (Heward, 2006), that severe discrepancy, of course, being defined at the state or local level.

Attention-Deficit/Hyperactivity Disorder Despite the well-documented relationship between ADHD and achievement problems (e.g., O'Neill, Thornton, Marks, Rajendran, & Halperin, 2016; Rabiner, Carrig, & Dodge, 2016), IDEA does not include ADHD as a diagnosis. Modifications and accommodations for ADHD may be made on the child's Individual Education Program (IEP) if the child has been determined eligible for and receives special services for another disability. Some students have received a diagnosis of Other Health Impaired (OHI) under IDEA as a result of ADHD symptoms that are sufficiently severe that they require an individualized program of special education; however, the applicability of OHI to ADHD varies based on the specific operational definition employed in each state. The key issue from the federal definition of OHI in IDEA is the possibility that a chronic medical condition can cause problems with alertness which has been interpreted by some to include the attention problems that are part of the core of ADHD. Accommodations and modifications for students with ADHD may also be provided through Section 504 of the Rehabilitation Act of 1973, provided the student is not covered by IDEA.

Traditional Diagnostic Assessment Tools

The poor treatment utility of the instruments and procedures traditionally used to make diagnostic determinations for academic concerns have been discussed at length (Gresham, 2002; Shinn, 1989). Academic assessment that leads to diagnosis typically lacks an empirical basis for guiding treatment recommendations. Assessment practices that were developed primarily for treatment selection and progress monitoring are discussed later in the chapter. Diagnostic assessments under both DSM-5 and IDEA have emphasized the use of individually administered standardized tests of intelligence and achievement. Although group tests of intelligence and achievement are less expensive, the magnitude of the implications of assessment outcomes has argued for using instruments that generally are regarded as producing the most accurate assessment results.

Tests of Intelligence Standardized tests of intelligence commonly are used for diagnoses of ID and for SLD, as, in most cases, the child's level of intellectual functioning must be established before a diagnosis may be assigned and/or educational services provided. Tests of intelligence are norm-referenced; they are designed to convey information about the individual's performance as compared to a large representative sample of other children (with and without disabilities) of the same age. They are standardized, or given in the same way to every person to whom the test is administered as an effort to control for variations in test scores due to testers. Although there are other quality tests available, the Wechsler Intelligence Scale for Children (5th ed., Wechsler, 2014) and the Stanford-Binet (5th ed., Roid, 2003) are the two intelligence tests in widest use (Heward, 2006).

Measures of Adaptive Behavior Systematic assessment of adaptive behavior is important for determining supports needed for success in the person's environment (Simões, Santos, Biscaia, & Thompson, 2016) as well as establishing deficits concomitant with those in intellectual functioning for diagnosing ID (AAIDD, Shalock et al., 2010; DSM-V, APA, 2013; IDEA, 2004). In most cases, an informant who is familiar with the client answers questions in the form of an interview or a questionnaire. The AAMR Adaptive Behavior Scale: 2 has different forms that describe behavior either in school (ABS-S:2, Lambert, Nihira, & Leland, 1993) or in residential and community settings (ABS-RC:2, Nihira, Leland, & Lambert, 1993). The Vineland Adaptive Behavior Scales, 2nd edition (Vineland-II, Sparrow, Cicchetti, & Balla, 2008), measures a wide range of adaptive behaviors in the communication, daily living skills, socialization, and motor skill domains, using either interviews or a questionnaire for classroom teachers. The Scales of Independent Behavior—Revised (SIB-R, Bruininks, Woodcock, Weatherman, & Hill, 1997) is a norm-referenced assessment of 14 areas of adaptive behavior and eight areas of problem behavior and is designed to be used with individuals of all ages.

Measures of Achievement Standardized tests of achievement are routinely given to children to determine SLD and, in educational contexts, may be given to children with ID to determine their present levels of functioning in specific academic areas. For diagnostic purposes, standardized tests of achievement are used in order to establish a discrepancy between IQ and achievement but may also be used to document educational impairment for other disorders such as OHI or severe emotional disturbance. These tests of educational achievement appear to be the most ubiquitous element of diagnostic assessment under IDEA. Some achievement tests are designed to measure achievement in one area of academic functioning, such as the KeyMath-3 (Connolly, 2007), which provides scores for Basic Concepts, Operations, and Applications; the Test of Written Language, 4th ed. (TOWL-4, Hammill & Larsen, 2009), which has 10 subtest scores in a variety of areas from Vocabulary to Conventions to Story Composition; and the Gates-MacGinitie Reading Tests (4th ed., MacGinitie, MacGinitie, Maria, & Dreyer, 2000), which measures a variety of skills from letter-sound correspondence to vocabulary to comprehension. Others measure overall achievement and may take the form of group achievement tests administered to a group of students in a classroom, such as the Iowa Tests of Basic Skills (ITBS, Hoover et al., 2003), or individual achievement tests that are administered to one student at a time, such as the Woodcock-Johnson IV Tests of Achievement (Schrank, McGrew, Mather, Wendling, & Dailey, 2014).

Rating Scales Additional measures may be used to gather information from individuals familiar with children's behavior in home and school settings. Rating scales provide norm-referenced comparisons of children's behavior relative to that of same-aged peers. These instruments ask teachers, parents, the child, or other individuals who spend time with the child to rate the frequency with which he or she engages in specific behaviors. Some rating scales are directed at specific diagnoses, such as the Conners 3 (Conners, 2008), which focuses on behaviors relevant to ADHD diagnosis. Rating scales that most commonly are used in schools, however, sample a wide range of behaviors, such as the Achenbach System of Empirically Based Assessment (2015 Update, Achenbach et al., 1980/2015) and the Behavior Assessment System for Children-3 (Reynolds & Kamphaus, 2015).

Summary Diagnostic Assessment Standardized norm-referenced tests provide clinicians with estimates of students' skills relative to a national normative sample. Although these tests have established utility for making diagnostic determinations, generally they are inadequate for academic intervention planning or monitoring. Tests typically contain very few items specific to any skill due to the broad nature of the assessment they provide. They generally fail to provide information regarding clients' proficiency in particular skills and as a result are substantially deficient for treatment planning (Deno, 1985). Additionally, norm-referenced assessments do not consider variables that are well established as critical to educational attainment such as the quality of instruction. They appear to assume a normative or generic school experience that may be irrelevant to the education of the client. Comparing an individual's skills to others who have received the same instruction provides a better indication of whether the student may be having difficulty with *learning* rather than terminal achievement. Furthermore, norm-referenced tests are poor choices for monitoring intervention effects because of the cost of administration, practice effects, and insensitivity to small changes in student performance (Shinn, 1989). Given the limitations of norm-referenced tests, it is important that alternative measures are used when evaluating student skills, developing intervention plans, and monitoring the effects of intervention.

Direct Academic Assessment

Since the passage of the IDEA (2004), an increasing number of schools are employing response to intervention (RtI) within multitiered systems of supports (MTSS) as their process for identifying students with special education needs. RtI is an assessment and intervention model in which the need and potentially the eligibility for specialized supports are determined based on the student's response to an evidence-based intervention matched to their needs (Jimerson, Burns & VanDerHeyden, 2016). MTSS models are designed to provide systematic and layered levels of support to students such that the intensity of intervention can be matched to the student's needs. Typically these tiered systems include three levels with universal services, standardized protocol intervention services, and intensive individualized interventions for students with more intensive needs (Jimerson et al., 2016).

Core features of both RtI and MTSS models include the collection of data on all students within schools in order to identify students with academic concerns (i.e., universal screening), evaluation of the instructional environment, and determination of the instructional supports a child needs (Jimerson et al., 2016; Sugai & Horner, 2009). Although determining students' special education eligibility is often viewed as the primary purpose of these models, the data collected for these purposes have great potential treatment utility both for (a) practitioners within a school and (b) clinicians outside of the school with access to the data.

Schools successfully implementing RtI/MTSS typically administer universal screeners to students three times annually, beginning in the first year of formal schooling (i.e., kindergarten). The resulting data have the potential to serve multiple purposes, with a primary purpose being the identification of students whose level of performance is significantly discrepant from peers receiving similar/identical instruction (Ardoin, Wagner, & Bangs, 2016). Administration of universal screeners multiple times per year beginning in students' kindergarten year of schooling also allows for the evaluation of individual students growth. These data allow schools to attend to whether students who are behind or ahead of their peers are making growth that will allow them to catch up to the average performing student or maintain their high level of achievement (Jimerson et al., 2016). Universal screening data can also be used to evaluate the quality of instruction provided to students at the district/school/classroom/ instructional program levels. Data can be collapsed across students who are receiving similar or identical instruction, and the rate of growth of those data can be compared to national normative rates of growth or to the rates of growth of students from other schools, in other classrooms, or receiving different instructional programs within the same or different classrooms (Hosp, Hosp, & Howell, 2016; Hosp & Ardoin, 2008). Given that these data are generally collected as early as a child' kindergarten year of school, universal screening data can also be used to assess when students' academic difficulties commence.

There are two primary genres of universal screeners administered by schools to assess students' academic achievement and academic growth: computer-adaptive tests (CATs) and curriculum-based measurement (CBM). These two genres of universal screening measures are described below, followed by a description of how resulting data might be used to inform the diagnoses and recommendations made by clinicians.

Computer-Adaptive Tests (CATs)

CATs are administered individually to students via a computer, are designed to require minimal administration time (15–30 min), and allow for both the comparison of student achievement to national norms and local norms and the evaluation of the rates of growth made by individuals and groups of students within and across grade levels. Unlike standard norm-referenced tests, CATs personalize the set of items administered to a student. The difficulty of each item administered to a student is known based upon data collected during test development, and the difficulty of each item administered is based upon a student's response accuracy to previously administered items (Davey, Pitoniak, & Slater, 2016). This adaptive nature of CATs to student responding allows for the administration of items that are restricted to the assessment of skills within a tighter range of difficulty. Thus, a student achieving below grade level will be administered items that assess skills at that grade level but will not be forced to answer questions he/she has no chance of answering correctly. Likewise, students achieving above grade level are not presented with items that are too easy. Such personalization of items administered allows for the delivery of fewer items and thus shorter administration time.

Furthermore, resulting data have greater treatment utility in that information can be provided regarding what specific skills a student has mastered, needs additional practice with, and has yet to develop (Davey et al., 2016).

Curriculum-Based Measurement (CBM)

CBM is a set of procedures that assesses students' performance in the areas of reading, mathematics, and writing and allows for both the comparison of students' achievement to local and national norms and the measuring of individual students' progress across time. A common element of all CBM procedures is that student performance is timed, thus providing information regarding response accuracy and rate of responding. Measuring students' rate of accurate responding allows for the evaluation of not only whether a student has the knowledge to perform the skill(s) being measured but whether the student has developed sufficient fluency in the skill to allow for the generalization and adaptation of the skill to other situations (Hosp et al., 2016).

Originally, CBM procedures were developed to be used by special education to establish meaningful individual education plan goals and to monitor students' progress toward achieving those established goals. Based upon an extensive base of empirical evidence demonstrating its sensitivity to instruction and its technical adequacy for identifying struggling students, along with the fact that it is cheap and quick to administer, elementary schools have widely adopted CBM procedures as part of their RtI and MTSS models (Mellard, McKnight, & Woods, 2009; Reschly, Busch, Betts, Deno & Long, 2009). Generally, schools administer CBM-Pre-reading measures to students beginning in kindergarten, and in first grade, they administer CBM-Reading (CBM-R), CBM-Mathematics (CBM-M), and CBM-Writing (CBM-W) assessments to students (Hosp et al., 2016). Although multiple companies exist that provide schools with the necessary materials and computer software to employ CBM as part of their RtI/MTSS model, it is important to know that CBM is a set of evidence-based standardized procedures for assessing student performance not a specific set of materials (Ardoin & Christ, 2009).

Due to the popularity, wide use, and marketing of CBM measures, educators do not always refer to the CBM procedures they are engaging in as CBM but rather will associate the procedures and materials with the product name provided by the publisher. For instance, educators might state that they are "Dibeling" students when in fact they are employing CBM materials developed by DIBELS (Diagnostic Indicators of Basic Early Literacy Skills) to assess students' skills in a specified area. Although the probes/materials published by these companies differ and thus the specific items to which students are responding differ, the associated procedures and research on which it relies are largely consistent. With that said, not all probes are created equal, and thus reliability and validity estimates are not consistent across publishers of CBM materials (Ardoin & Christ, 2009). Some of the companies that produce CBM materials include DIBELS, AimsWeb, FastBridge, and EasyCBM.

Basic descriptions of the primary CBM administration and scoring procedures employed by schools are provided below. It is important that clinicians understand these procedures for two reasons. First, it is essential that clinicians are able to understand the data provided to them by schools (see *Uses of Universal Screening Data*, below). Second clinicians might employ the procedures on their own to assess a client in a given skill either by obtaining the materials from a publisher or through a website such as www.interventioncentral.com that allows for the development of some basic CBM materials.

CBM-Pre-reading Most publishers of CBM-Pre-reading measures provide schools with probes for assessing students' letter naming and letter sound fluency as substantial evidence demonstrating the validity of these two measures in predicting future reading outcomes exists (Catts, Nielsen, Bridges, Liu, & Bontempo. 2015; Ritchey, 2008; Sáez, Nese, Alonzo, & Tindal, 2016). Administration of these measures requires a probe (worksheet) with letters placed in random order. The student is provided with the probe and the directive to either provide the letter name or sound associated with each letter, depending on the skill being assessed, or to proceed across and down the page. When the student begins providing responses, the examiner starts a countdown timer set for 1 min. During this minute, the examiner records accurate responses as well as any errors made by the student and asks the student to stop at the conclusion of the minute. Considering the focus of CBM assessment is on accurate and fluent responding, error correction is never provided during the administration of CBM probes as it would interfere with a student's production of responses. Correct responses are, however, provided to students when they hesitate on an item/word for 3 s (Hosp et al., 2016).

Another common CBM-Pre-reading measure is nonsense word fluency (NWF). NWF probes generally consist of single syllable three letter nonsense words (e.g., nug, cag). Students are asked to respond to each nonword by either saying the word as a whole or sounding out each letter. Given the novelty of this task, administrators should provide modeling of these two response options and allow the student to practice reading a nonword with corrective feedback prior to the NWF probe being presented to the student. After providing the student with the opportunity to practice, the NWF probe is presented to the student, and the student is again informed of the option to read the "fake" words as whole words or individual sounds and told to read across and then down. Once the student provides the first sound/nonword, the examiner starts the timer and allows the student to respond to the nonwords until 1 min elapses. In an identical fashion to other CBM probes, error correction is not provided, but sounds/words are provided to students when they hesitate on a sound/word for 3 s. The dependent measure for NWF is the number of sounds provided correctly in a minute. Thus, regardless of whether a student correctly reads a nonword as a whole word or provides the sounds of each letter, the student would gain the same score. Likewise, if a student blends the three sounds of a nonword but provides two correct and one incorrect sound, the student would score two letter sounds correct just as if the student were to say the sounds individually and say only two of the three letter sounds correctly (January, Ardoin, Christ, Eckert & White, 2016).

Publishers of CBM materials also provide measures that can be used to assess students' phonemic awareness skills, such as probes that assess students' rhyming, blending, and segmenting of words. There is greater variability in the format of the materials employed for measuring these skills as well as the administration and scoring procedures associated with these assessments as compared to other standardized CBM procedures. Given the variability of these assessment procedures, they will not be discussed.

CBM-Reading There exist a large literature base demonstrating the relationship between CBM-Reading, a measure of students' oral reading fluency, and students' word reading skills, reading comprehension, and global reading achievement (Reschly et al., 2009). Although there are those who believe that CBM-Reading is simply a measure of students' ability to read words quickly and thus CBM-Reading fails to identify students who can read words but lack comprehension skills (word callers), research suggests otherwise. Students identified by teachers as "word callers" in fact have poor reading fluency and lack sufficient comprehension (Hamilton & Shinn, 2003). Researchers have also provided evidence to indicate that comprehension skills facilitate students' reading of text, with students being able to read words within connected text at a much faster rate than they can read the same words presented outside of connected text (Ardoin et al., 2013; Jenkins, Fuchs, van den Broek, Espin, & Deno, 2003).

CBM-Reading universal screening procedures require individual administration of three grade level CBM-Reading passages to each student. Students are directed to start at the beginning of the passage and to read from left to right and down the page. Consistent with the procedures for administering pre-reading measures, students are provided with 1 min to read the passage, reading errors are not corrected, and the examiner only provides the correct word on occasions when a student hesitates on a word for 3 s. Errors are counted for any word skipped, word read incorrectly, word pronounced incorrectly given the context of the sentence, and word substitutions (e.g., student reads mom instead of mother) or which the student drops or adds a suffix (e.g., -s, -ing). Inserted words are ignored and thus not counted toward the number of correct or incorrectly words read by the student. Examiners calculate the number of words read correctly per minute (WRCM) for each passage by subtracting the number of errors made from the total number of words read. After administered three passages, students' median WRCM is used to examine each student's performance relative to local and national norms (Hosp et al., 2016)

In addition to CBM-Reading probes, some schools also administer CBM-Maze probes. Maze probes are reading passages with the first sentence intact and every seventh word thereafter removed. For each missing word, three word choices are provided, and students are asked to circle the word choice which best fits into the space. Three minutes is given to the student to circle as many words that fill in the blanks as they can. It is occasionally suggested that maze probes allow for better measurement of students' reading comprehension skills; however, research contradicts this perception. Numerous studies have provided clear evidence suggesting that CBM-R is a better predictor of both reading comprehension and global reading achievement and that in fact students do not have to understand the text they are reading to accurately select the words which best fits into the space. It is therefore not recommended that maze probes be used as a means of assessing students' comprehension skills (Ardoin et al., 2004; January & Ardoin, 2012).

CBM-Mathematics Concepts and Applications The ability to accurately and rapidly complete basic math facts is an essential skill for students to achieve, and it also forms the basis of essentially all mathematical work. When conducting universal screening procedures as part of their RtI process, schools, therefore, frequently employ CBM-Mathematics probes to assess students' basic math fluency. When conducting universal screening in mathematics, the probes should generally consist of 3–5 skills that will be assessed across the academic year. Although single-skilled probes can be useful for identifying whether a student has or has not mastered a specific skill, multiskilled probes are best for universal screening purpose (Hosp et al., 2016).

CBM-Mathematics probes can be administered to students in groups, with students being provided with 2–5 min to complete the probes, with the time depending on the skills being assessed. Probes are scored for the number of digits correct per minute (DCPM) as opposed to number of problems correct per minute. For example, the product of five times five would be scored as 2 digits correct if the students provided the response of 25, but the student would earn 1 digit correct if only the number in the ones (i.e., 5) or tens (i.e., 2) column was correct. Students also earn digits correct for the multiple steps in a multiplication or division problems that include multiple levels (Hosp et al., 2016). Example of how to score such probes can be found in the math worksheet generator of www.interventioncentral.com.

Similar to the assessment of phonemic awareness skills, the publishers of CBM materials vary in the format and procedures that they provide to schools for measuring students' math application and problem solving skills. Students are often provided with more time to complete these measures than other types of CBM given that each problem can require from several seconds to minutes. Scoring procedures might also vary depending on the specific problem types measured (Hosp et al., 2016; Jitendra, Dupuis, & Zaslofsky, 2014).

CBM-Writing Administration of CBM-Writing probes can also be conducted with groups of students. A story starter (e.g., My best day at school was when…) is provided to students on the sheet that they will write their story on, 1 min is allowed for students to think about what they will write, and then 3 min is provided for students to write their story. At the conclusion of the 3 min, students must immediately stop writing, and the examiner retrieves the worksheets (Hosp et al., 2016). Unlike other CBM procedures for which only one standard scoring procedure exists, there are multiple technically adequate methods for scoring CBM-Writing probes (total words written, correct word sequences, and words spelled correctly). For total words written, the number of words written by a student is counted without consideration of correct spelling or grammar. In contrast when scoring writing probes for correct word sequences, each word pair is evaluated for spelling and grammar. For a correct sequence to be scored, both words must be spelled correctly and be grammatically correct. For the first word in a sentence, capitalization is considered, and for the last word, punctuation is considered in evaluating the sequence. Finally, when using words spelled correctly as the dependent measure, one simply counts the total number of words the student spelled correctly (Furey, Marcotte, Hintze, & Shackett, 2016; Gansle, Noell, VanDerHeyden, Naquin, & Slider, 2002).

Utility of Universal Screeners Universal screening data provides clinicians with a unique means of examining the quality of instruction being provided to a client, a means of identifying how a client compares to that of peers receiving similar instruction, as well as a potential mechanism for determining when a client's academic difficulties commenced. The only other possible sources of such objective information would be data from state-mandated tests, but universal screening data have many advantages over results from state-mandated tests. For instance, whereas at the school level, state-mandated tests generally provide only information regarding the percent of students in a school who exceeded, met, and failed to meet state standards, the criteria set by universal screening data are generally based upon national norms. In contrast, schools can provide clinicians with universal screening data regarding how specific groups of students (e.g., students with specific learning disabilities, gifted students) performed on the measure as compared to other groups of students within the school as well as compared to national norm-referenced data. The school may also be able to provide the clinician with information regarding how a client performed relative to peers within the same classroom or grade level. Thus, if provided with the appropriate universal screening data, clinicians can determine the extent to which a client differs from other students with similar educational experiences.

A second advantage of universal screening data is that whereas state-mandated tests provide a static view of students' achievement, universal screening measures are administered to students triannually, allowing for analyses of students' rates of growth. Such data are useful as they allow for a determination of not simply whether a client is discrepant from peers academically but also whether that discrepancy has increased with time. Knowledge that a student's level of discrepancy is continuing to increase over time provides evidence of the need to act immediately so as to prevent the problem from worsening.

Universal screening data also differ from state-mandated tests in that schools generally begin administering universal screening measures to students in kindergarten, whereas state-mandated tests are not typically administered until students are in third grade. Access to a client's universal screening data across their academic career provides clinicians with the opportunity to evaluate when the client's achievement began to become discrepant from peers within the same school as well as nationally. Knowledge of when a client's achievement began to decline could be especially useful in matching the information with other historical data from the client's life (e.g., change in school, parental relationships, health issues).

A final potential benefit of universal screening data is that if a client has been provided with intervention services within the school system, the clinician can examine the data to determine whether during that time period the client's rate of academic growth improved as compared to the client's prior rates of growth and rates of growth relative to peers. Clinicians might also continue to attend to universal screening data in order to examine whether the treatment they are providing to a client is improving the client's rates of growth by comparing growth rates prior to the beginning of treatment with that collected posttreatment.

In addition to employing universal screening data provided to them by a client's school, clinicians should also consider adopting CBM procedures as a means of evaluating their suggested treatments. Administering CBM is relatively quick and easy and in addition to being useful as a universal screening measure and for monitoring individual students' academic growth; research suggests that it is sensitive to medication effects (Ardoin & Martens, 2000). Clinicians might therefore wish to administer CBM probes or train parents to administer the measures to their child when the child is on and off medication as a means of evaluated the effects of medication on a client's academic performance.

Intervention: Moving from Identifying Problems to Acting on Them

Assessments that end with diagnostic or nomothetic outcomes may have limited utility in improving clients' life outcomes (Nelson-Gray, 2003). To the extent that diagnostic assessments result in clients being placed in effective intervention programs, they may have considerable benefit. However, substantial evidence exists that individualized educational interventions programs are uneven in their efficacy (Morgan, Frisco, Farkas, & Hibel, 2017). Interestingly, even when assessments of psychopathology do result in clients gaining access to effective educational treatment programs, those treatment programs often need to include additional assessments that are more focused on the interaction of skills and environmental supports to devise an effective program for an individual student. The range of potential assessments, interventions, and client needs is sufficiently broad that a comprehensive treatment of assessment for academic intervention is beyond the scope of this chapter. Interested readers might choose to consult one of the following resources (Jimerson et al., 2016; Little & Akin-Little, 2014).

This section of the chapter is designed to outline some of the core considerations that clinicians should be aware of regarding assessment for academic intervention design. The organizing heuristic to guide assessment is reduced to four core tasks. First, define the problem operationally. Second, identify environmental supports that lead to learning gains. Third, devise supports that lead to implementation of the support plan. Fourth, devise and implement a strategy for monitoring progress and adjusting the plan. The balance of this section considers each of these tasks in turn.

Define the task operationally The initial task in supporting parents and educators in devising an intervention to accelerate a child's academic development is to define the problem in a way that is measurable and captures the mismatch between expectations and current performance (Noell & Gansle, 2014). For example, broad reading concerns might be operationalized as poor reading fluency which can be measured through CBM-Reading. Alternatively, a homework completion problem might be defined as the percentage of homework assignments turned in per week with at least 90% accuracy (assuming homework is being used primarily for reinforcement and review). A critical challenge at this stage is moving from diverse and numerous concerns to specific, actionable, and measurable concerns.

Completing this process typically will require prioritizing among multiple competing concerns. Many clients will have deficits across reading, writing, mathematics, and task completion. In prioritizing concerns, it is typically most important to prioritize those that have the broadest impact on the client's functioning and those that have the highest risk for triggering adverse consequences (Barnett, Bauer, Ehrhardt, Lentz, & Stollar, 1996). The broad importance of reading for success across all academic domains partially explains how frequently it emerges as the focus for intervention. It is critical at the operational definition stage that clinicians help educators and parents prioritize and identify a manageable initial set of actions that will begin the ameliorative process. A critical step in helping clients take ownership of the challenges confronting them is to help them simplify and focus their diverse concerns to a set they can act on and begin to experience success with (Beck, 2011). If they can achieve success with one or a few initial targets, they will be much better positioned to circle back to other issues that were initially deferred.

Identify environmental supports that lead to learning gains Academic concerns, like most human behaviors, emerge as an expression of the complex interplay between biological endowments and environmental experience. This reality may initially appear to be paralyzing, as it may suggest the need for assessments that are impossibly complex in the comprehensiveness of their coverage. However, nature and the available scientific evidence have conspired to provide clinicians, educators, and parents a more manageable path. An overwhelming body of evidence exists demonstrating that environmentally based interventions are effective for academic difficulties whose etiology maybe biological, at least in part, environmental, or are largely unknown (Linstead et al., 2017; O'Reilly, 1997; Vereenooghe, & Langdon, 2013). Although it may ultimately prove useful in some cases, we typically do not have to know the etiology of an academic concern to correct it.

The details of academic interventions that have been developed by educators and psychologists can be overwhelming in their number and variety and are beyond the scope of this chapter. However, a smaller set of first principles underlie much of this work, and it is possible to summarize these principles herein. First, establishing an appropriate context for academic instruction is a critical principle. Attempting to teach students in classrooms that are chaotic or asking clients to complete homework assignments in environments that are distracting can be futile

(Day, Connor, & McClelland, 2015; Xu, 2010). Generally speaking, effective educational contexts arrange stimuli such that attention is drawn to the instructional task or materials, and distracting stimuli or contingencies for off task behavior are minimized. A second fundamental principle underlying effective instruction is the importance and availability of effective models. The actual models can vary widely such as listening to a competent reader read a passage fluently prior to the student attempting the passage (e.g., Begeny, Krouse, Ross, & Mitchell, 2009) to providing models of correct mathematics problem completion when using the cover-copy-compare procedure (Poncy, & Skinner, 2011). Although models can serve a range of instructional functions, a core purpose is to help the learner begin producing correct responses quickly so that they, rather than error responses, can be reinforced.

A third critical principle underlying effective instruction is appropriately paced opportunities to practice. An overwhelming and long-standing research literature has demonstrated that learning is better facilitated by active responding than passive receipt of information or observations of models. For example, outlining material you have read is more effective than simply reading that material. Interestingly, active practice is routinely integral to learning in some domains, mathematics, or playing musical instruments but can be strangely absent in others such as studying history or science. A critical challenge is designing interventions such that the students are active participants who are responding rather than passively reviewing information.

An effective intervention plan that sets an appropriate context, provides helpful models, and occasions relevant responses by students establishes the foundation for two additional core principles of effective instruction. The fourth critical principle in the current heuristic is the importance of timely accuracy feedback. Students learn more effectively when they receive accuracy feedback about their responses in a timely fashion (Carroll, Kodak, & Adolf, 2016). Delayed feedback is notoriously problematic. A student who completes an essay or paper and only receives feedback on their performance a month later may not connect their work, the feedback, and their future writing in a way that leads to skill acquisition. It is equally important that feedback be sufficiently specific and clear to occasion learning. For example, it may be helpful to tell a student they solved a multiplication problem incorrectly, but it would be more helpful to also show them the correct answer. Even more critically, vague global feedback has very limited instructional value. If the essay was "good," what was good about it and what is necessary to move to great writing?

A final core principle of effective academic intervention should be broadly familiar to clinicians: reinforcement. Behavior change is effortful whether it is exercise targeting weight reduction or outlining chapters in social studies to improve reading comprehension. Although both behaviors may ultimately lead to positive consequences that might be considered reinforcing, in both cases, the consequences may be too delayed, too incremental, and too cumulative to actually be reinforcing (e.g., Malott, 1989). Behavior change is most effectively reinforced by consequences that are proximal to the behavior (Carroll et al., 2016). A range of studies have demonstrated the power of planned reinforcement in supporting academic behavior change (e.g., Dolezal, Weber, Evavold, Wylie, & McLaughlin, 2007).

Support implementation Assuring treatment plan implementation is often more challenging than identifying a beneficial intervention. For academic interventions, this reality is often exacerbated by the fact that the consulting mental health-care provider is not providing the academic intervention. Implementation of intervention in schools as well as parent-implemented interventions can often be extremely problematic in the absence of systematic programming to support implementation (Noell, Volz, Henderson, & Williams, 2017). The school-based literature examining treatment plan implementation has repeatedly demonstrated poor and deteriorating implementation in the absence of systematic follow-up (Noell et al., 2014). Follow-up support that has been effective in sustaining implementation has included objective assessment of intervention implementation (often through permanent products), graphing implementation as well as student outcomes, and feedback to the treatment agent on implementation (see Noell & Gansle, 2013, for a review). This general approach has been found to be effective across a number of studies (Noell et al., 2014) and appears to be practical in many contexts treating psychopathology. The intervention agent can be asked to bring the work products in for a weekly review and consultation regarding the academic intervention as well as other pertinent issues that can be provided.

Monitor progress Extensive and varied research supports the assumption that monitoring patient or student performance through time and making treatment decisions based upon those data result in improved outcomes (National Center on Student Progress Monitoring, 2006). Although a number of strategies are viable for monitoring academic progress, it is worth noting that progress monitoring is one of the key purposes for which CBM was developed. Commonly, CBM probes are administered twice a week, which is facilitated by their brevity. Data are commonly plotted against a goal line that expresses desired gain over time. The origin of the goal line is often the median of three initial data points with the terminus being the target terminal rate based on a published criterion, local norm, or research-based norms (see Hosp et al. 2016 for research-based norms). Typically, if four consecutive data points over 2 weeks fall below the goal line, intervention modification is suggested (Marston & Tindal, 1996). An alternative approach to evaluating intervention effectiveness is to evaluate the slope of client gain for obtained data through a process such as least squares estimation. The obtained slope is then compared to the target slope. Although early recommendations suggested that 10 data points were sufficient to evaluate intervention effectiveness, subsequent research suggests that more data are needed in order to accurately predict a client's growth rate (Christ & Silberglitt, 2007).

Summary and Conclusion

The same core questions, what is the problem and what can be done about it, drive the assessment of both psychopathology and academic concerns. Specifying the problem will often include molar assessments that are typically norm-referenced as well as more molecular assessment of specific skills and response to instruction that may be evaluated against normative or criterion-based standards. Diagnosis will frequently be the referral sources' initial concern and also may be necessary to obtain services for the client. However, current diagnostic systems lack the degree of detail necessary to provide specific treatment planning for academic concerns. Additionally, the instruments most commonly useful for making diagnostic determinations have very limited treatment utility due to the limited coverage of specific skills at any given level (Marston & Tindal, 1996). An additional barrier is presented by the reality that achievement tests typically assess academic skill as broad constructs (e.g., mathematics) rather than specific skills (e.g., 20 digits correct per minute on addition facts). Under IDEA, newer approaches to diagnosis in schools based on RtI within MTSS have the potential to provide diagnostic information that also has treatment utility (Jimerson et al., 2016).

Although RtI/MTSS approaches can provide data for treatment planning and diagnosis (Jimerson et al., 2016), current common practice for academic treatment specification often requires additional assessment that is more direct and skill based and examines RtI. Additionally, this assessment should consider classroom expectations and broader environmental factors that may be critical to placing the academic deficit into a sufficiently comprehensive context that a useful case formulation and treatment plan is possible. Perhaps the most important and most challenging aspects of assuring effective educational services for children exhibiting academic concerns and psychopathology are assuring that services are delivered as designed (Noell et al., 2017) and that progress monitoring data are collected to guide ongoing program modification.

References

Achenbach, T. M., Rescorla, L. A., McConaughey, S. H., Pecora, P. J., Wetherbee, K. M., Ruffle, T. M., & Ivanova, M. Y. (1980). *Achenbach system of empirically based assessment* [2015 update]. Burlington, VT: University of Vermont Research Center for Children, Youth, & Families.

American Psychiatric Association. (2013). *Diagnostic and statistical manual of mental disorders* (5th ed.). Washington, DC: Author.

Ardoin, S. P., & Christ, T. J. (2009). Curriculum based measurement of oral reading: Standard errors associated with progress monitoring outcomes from DIBELS, AIMSweb, and an experimental passage set. *School Psychology Review, 38*, 266–283.

Ardoin, S. P., Eckert, T. L., Christ, T. J., White, M. J., Morena, L., Baxter, S. A., & Hine, J. (2013). Examining variance in reading comprehension among developing readers: Words in context (CBM-R) versus words out of context (word list). *School Psychology Review, 42*, 243–261.

Ardoin, S. P., & Martens, B. K. (2000). Testing the ability of children with ADHD to accurately report the effects of medication on their behavior. *Journal of Applied Behavior Analysis, 33*, 593–610.

Ardoin, S. P., Wagner, L., & Bangs, K. E. (2016). Applied behavior analysis: A foundation for RtI. In S. R. Jimerson, M. K. Burns, & A. M. VanDerHeyden (Eds.), *Handbook of response to intervention: The science and practice of multi tiered systems of support* (2nd ed., pp. 29–42). New York, NY: Springer.

Ardoin, S. P., Witt, J. C., Suldo, S. M., Connell, J. E., Koenig, J. L., Resetar, J. L., & Slider, N. J. (2004). Examining the incremental benefits of administering a maze and three versus one curriculum-based measurement reading probe when conducting universal screening. *School Psychology Review, 33*, 218–233.

Barnett, D. W., Bauer, A. M., Ehrhardt, K. E., Lentz, F. E., & Stollar, S. A. (1996). Keystone targets for change: Planning for widespread positive consequences. *School Psychology Quarterly, 11*, 95–117. https://doi.org/10.1037/h0088923

Beck, J. S. (2011). *Cognitive behavior therapy: Basics and beyond* (2nd ed.). New York, NY: Guilford Press.

Begeny, J. C., Krouse, H. E., Ross, S. G., & Mitchell, R. C. (2009). Increasing elementary-aged students' reading fluency with small-group interventions: A comparison of repeated reading, listening passage preview, and listening only strategies. *Journal of Behavioral Education, 18*(3), 211–228. https://doi.org/10.1007/s10864-009-9090-9

Bruininks, R. H., Woodcock, R. W., Weatherman, R. F., & Hill, B. K. (1997). Scales of independent behavior-revised. Itasca, IL: Riverside Publishing.

Carroll, R. A., Kodak, T., & Adolf, K. J. (2016). Effect of delayed reinforcement on skill acquisition during discrete-trial instruction: Implications for treatment-integrity errors in academic settings. *Journal of Applied Behavior Analysis, 49*(1), 176–181. https://doi.org/10.1002/jaba.268

Catts, H. W., Nielsen, D. C., Bridges, M. S., Liu, Y. S., & Bontempo, D. E. (2015). Early identification of reading disabilities within an RTI framework. *Journal of Learning Disabilities, 48*, 281–297. https://doi.org/10.1177/0022219413498115

Christ, T. J., & Silberglitt, B. (2007). Estimates of the standard error of measurement for curriculum-based measures of oral reading fluency. *School Psychology Review, 36*(1), 130–146.

Conners, C. K. (2008). *Conners* (3rd ed.). North Tonawanda, NY: Multi-Health Systems.

Connolly, A. J. (2007). *KeyMath-3 diagnostic assessment*. San Antonio, TX: Pearson Assessments.

Davey, T., Pitoniak, M. J., & Slater, S. C. (2016). Designing computerized adaptive tests. In S. Lane, M. R. Raymond, T. M. Haladyna, S. Lane, M. R. Raymond, & T. M. Haladyna (Eds.), *Handbook of test development* (2nd ed., pp. 467–484). New York, NY: Routledge/Taylor & Francis Group.

Day, S. L., Connor, C. M., & McClelland, M. M. (2015). Children's behavioral regulation and literacy: The impact of the first grade classroom environment. *Journal of School Psychology, 53*, 409–428. https://doi.org/10.1016/j.jsp.2015.07.004

Deno, S. L. (1985). Curriculum-based measurement: The emerging alternative. *Exceptional Children, 52*, 219–232.

Dolezal, D. N., Weber, K. P., Evavold, J. J., Wylie, J., & McLaughlin, T. F. (2007). The effects of a reinforcement package for on-task and reading behavior with at-risk and middle school students with disabilities. *Child & Family Behavior Therapy, 29*, 9–25. https://doi.org/10.1300/J019v29n02_02

Fletcher, J. M., Francis, D. J., Morris, R. D., & Lyon, G. R. (2005). Evidence-based assessment of learning disabilities in children and adolescents. *Journal of Clinical Child and Adolescent Psychology, 34*, 506–522.

Fletcher, J. M., Francis, D. J., Shaywitz, S. E., Lyon, G. R., Foorman, B. R., Stuebing, K. K., & Shaywitz, B. A. (1998). Intelligent testing and the discrepancy model for children with learning disabilities. *Learning Disabilities Research and Practice, 13*, 186–203.

Friedman, C. (2016). Outdated language: Use of "mental retardation" in Medicaid HCBS waivers post-Rosa's law. *Intellectual and Developmental Disabilities, 54*, 342–353. https://doi.org/10.1352/1934-9556-54.5.342

Fuchs, L. S., Fuchs, D., & Hollenbeck, K. N. (2007). Extending responsiveness to intervention to mathematics at first and third grades. *Learning Disabilities Research & Practice, 22*, 13–24. https://doi.org/10.1111/j.1540-5826.2007.00227.x

Furey, W. M., Marcotte, A. M., Hintze, J. M., & Shackett, C. M. (2016). Concurrent validity and classification accuracy of curriculum-based measurement for written expression. *School Psychology Quarterly, 31*, 369–382. https://doi.org/10.1037/spq0000138

Gansle, K. A., Noell, G. H., VanDerHeyden, A. M., Naquin, G. M., & Slider, N. J. (2002). Moving beyond total words written: The reliability, criterion validity, and time cost of alternate measures for curriculum-based measurement in writing. *School Psychology Review, 31,* 477–497.

Gresham, F. M. (2002). Responsiveness to intervention: An alternative approach to the identification of learning disabilities. In R. Bradley, L. Danielson, & D. P. Hallahan (Eds.), *Identification of learning disabilities: Research to practice* (pp. 467–519). Mahwah, NJ: Lawrence Erlbaum Associates.

Gresham, F. M., & Gansle, K. A. (1992). Misguided assumptions of DSM-III-R: Implications for school psychological practice. *School Psychology Quarterly, 7,* 79–95.

Hamilton, C., & Shinn, M. R. (2003). Characteristics of word callers: An investigation of the accuracy of teachers' judgments of reading comprehension and oral reading skills. *School Psychology Review, 32,* 228–240.

Hammill, D. D., & Larsen, S. C. (2009). *Test of written language–fourth edition.* Austin, TX: Pro-Ed.

Heward, W. L. (Ed.). (2006). *Exceptional children: An introduction to special education* (8th ed.). Upper Saddle River, NJ: Pearson Education, Inc.

Hoover, H. D., Dunbar, S. B., Frisbie, D. A., Oberley, K. R., Ordman, V. L., Naylor, R. J., & Qualls, A. L. (2003). *Iowa tests of basic skills(r), Forms A and B.* Itasca, IL: Houghton Mifflin Harcourt.

Hosp, J. L., & Ardoin, S. P. (2008). Assessment for instructional planning. *Assessment for Effective Intervention, 33,* 69–77.

Hosp, M. K., Hosp, J. L., & Howell, K. W. (2016). *The ABCs of CBM: A practical guide to curriculum-based measurement.* New York: Guilford Publications.

Hu, S., & Wolniak, G. C. (2013). College student engagement and early career earnings: Differences by gender, race/ethnicity, and academic preparation. *Review of Higher Education: Journal of The Association for the Study of Higher Education, 36,* 211–233. https://doi.org/10.1353/rhe.2013.0002

Individuals with Disabilities Education Improvement Act, 20 U.S.C 1400 et seq. (2004).

January, S.-A. A., & Ardoin, S. P. (2012). The impact of context and word type on students' maze task accuracy. *School Psychology Review, 41,* 262–271.

January, S.-A. A., Ardoin, S. P., Christ, T. J., Eckert, T. L., & White, M. J. (2016). Evaluating the interpretations and use of curriculum-based measurement in reading and word lists for universal screening in first and second grade. *School Psychology Review, 45,* 310–326.

Jenkins, J. R., Fuchs, L. S., van den Broek, P., Espin, C., & Deno, S. L. (2003). Accuracy and fluency in list and context reading of skilled and RD groups: Absolute and relative performance levels. *Learning Disabilities Research & Practice, 18,* 237–245.

Jhang, F. (2017). Economically disadvantaged adolescents' self-concept and academic achievement as mediators between family cohesion and mental health in Taiwan. *International Journal of Mental Health and Addiction, 15,* 407. https://doi.org/10.1007/s11469-017-9737-z

Jimerson, S. R., Burns, M. K., & VanDerHeyden, A. M. (2016). *Handbook of response to intervention: The science and practice of multi tiered Systems of Support.* New York, NY: Springer.

Jitendra, A. K., Dupuis, D. N., & Zaslofsky, A. F. (2014). Curriculum-based measurement and standards-based mathematics: Monitoring the arithmetic word problem-solving performance of third-grade students at risk for mathematics difficulties. *Learning Disability Quarterly, 37,* 241–251. https://doi.org/10.1177/0731948713516766

Johnson, W., McGue, M., & Iacono, W. G. (2006). Genetic and environmental influences on academic achievement trajectories during adolescence. *Developmental Psychology, 42,* 514–532.

Kavale, K. A. (2002). Discrepancy models in the identification of learning disability. In R. Bradley, L. Danielson, & D. P. Hallahan (Eds.), *Identification of learning disabilities: Research to practice* (pp. 369–426). Mahwah, NJ: Lawrence Erlbaum Associates.

Lambert, N., Nihira, K., & Leland, H. (1993). *AAMR adaptive behavior scale – school* (2nd ed.). Austin, TX: Pro-Ed.

Linstead, E., Dixon, D. R., French, R., Granpeesheh, D., Adams, H., German, R., … Kornack, J. (2017). Intensity and learning outcomes in the treatment of children with autism spectrum disorder. *Behavior Modification, 41,* 229–252. https://doi.org/10.1177/0145445516667059

Little, S. G., & Akin-Little, A. (2014). *Academic assessment and intervention.* New York, NY: Routledge/Taylor & Francis Group.

Lyon, G. R. (1996). Learning disabilities. *The Future of Children: Special Education for Students with Disabilities, 6,* 56–76.

MacGinitie, W., MacGinitie, R., Maria, R. K., & Dreyer, L. G. (2000). *Gates-MacGinitie reading tests* (4th ed.). Itasca, IL: Riverside.

MacMillan, D. L., & Siperstein, G. N. (2002). Learning disabilities as operationally defined by schools. In R. Bradley, L. Danielson, & D. P. Hallahan (Eds.), *Identification of learning disabilities: Research to practice* (pp. 287–333). Mahwah, NJ: Lawrence Erlbaum Associates.

MacMillan, D. L., Gresham, F. M., & Bocian, K. M. (1998). Discrepancy between definitions of learning disabilities and school practices: An empirical investigation. *Journal of Learning Disabilities, 31,* 314–326.

Malott, R. (1989). The achievement of evasive goals. In S. C. Hayes (Ed.), *Rule-governed behavior: Cognition, contingencies, and instructional control.* New York, NY: Springer.

Marston, D., & Tindal, G. (1996). Best practices in performance monitoring. In A. Thomas & J. Grimes (Eds.), *Best practices in school psychology III*. Bethesda, MD: NASP Publications.

Mellard, D. F., McKnight, M., & Woods, K. (2009). Response to intervention screening and progress-monitoring practices in 41 local schools. *Learning Disabilities Research & Practice, 24*, 186–195.

Montague, M., Enders, C., & Castro, M. (2005). Academic and behavioral outcomes for students at risk for emotional and behavioral disorders. *Behavioral Disorders, 31*, 84–94.

Morgan, P. L., Frisco, M. L., Farkas, G., & Hibel, J. (2017). Republication of 'A propensity score matching analysis of the effects of special education services'. *The Journal of Special Education, 50*, 197–214.

National Center on Student Progress Monitoring. (2006). What are the benefits of progress monitoring? Retrieved October 02, 2006, from www.studentprogress.org.

Nelson-Gray, R. O. (2003). Treatment utility of psychological assessment. *Psychological Assessment, 15*, 521–531. https://doi.org/10.1037/1040-3590.15.4.521

Nihira, K., Leland, H., & Lambert, N. (1993). *AAMR adaptive behavior scale – residential and community* (2nd ed.). Austin, TX: Pro-Ed.

Noell, G. H., & Gansle, K. A. (2013). The use of performance feedback to improve intervention implementation in schools. In L. M. H. Sanetti & T. R. Kratochwill (Eds.), *Treatment integrity: A foundation for evidence-based practice in applied psychology* (pp. 161–185). Washington, D.C.: American Psychological Association.

Noell, G. H., & Gansle, K. A. (2014). A general case framework for academic intervention. In S. G. Little & A. Akin-Little (Eds.), *Academic assessment and intervention* (pp. 7–26). New York, NY: Routledge.

Noell, G. H., Gansle, K. A., Mevers, J. L., Knox, R. M., Mintz, J. C., & Dahir, A. (2014). Improving treatment plan implementation in schools: A meta-analysis of single subject design studies. *Journal of Behavioral Education, 23*, 168–191. https://doi.org/10.1007/s10864-013-9177-1

Noell, G. H., Volz, J. R., Henderson, M. Y., & Williams, K. L. (2017). Evaluating an integrated support model for increasing treatment plan implementation following consultation in schools. *School Psychology Quarterly, 32*, 525. https://doi.org/10.1037/spq0000195

O'Neill, S., Thornton, V., Marks, D. J., Rajendran, K., & Halperin, J. M. (2016). Early language mediates the relations between preschool inattention and school-age reading achievement. *Neuropsychology, 30*, 398–404. https://doi.org/10.1037/neu0000247

O'Reilly, M. F. (1997). Functional analysis of episodic self-injury correlated with recurrent otitis media. *Journal of Applied Behavior Analysis, 30*, 165–167. https://doi.org/10.1901/jaba.1997.30-165

Poncy, B. C., & Skinner, C. H. (2011). Enhancing first-grade students' addition-fact fluency using class-wide cover, copy, and compare, a sprint, and group rewards. *Journal of Applied School Psychology, 27*, 1–20. https://doi.org/10.1080/15377903.2011.540499

Rabiner, D. L., Carrig, M. M., & Dodge, K. A. (2016). Attention problems and academic achievement: Do persistent and earlier-emerging problems have more adverse long-term effects? *Journal of Attention Disorders, 20*, 946–957. https://doi.org/10.1177/1087054713507974

Reschly, A. L., Busch, T. W., Betts, J., Deno, S. L., & Long, J. D. (2009). Curriculum-based measurement oral reading as an indicator of reading achievement: A meta-analysis of the correlational evidence. *Journal of School Psychology, 47*, 427–469. https://doi.org/10.1016/j.jsp.2009.07.001

Reynolds, C. R., & Kamphaus, R. W. (2015). *Behavior assessment system for children* (3rd ed.). San Antonio, TX: Pearson Assessment.

Ritchey, K. D. (2008). Assessing letter sound knowledge: A comparison of letter sound fluency and nonsense word fluency. *Exceptional Children, 74*, 487–506.

Roid, G. H. (2003). *Stanford-Binet intelligence scales* (5th ed.). Austin, TX: Pro-Ed.

Rosa's Law, Pub. L. No. 111-256 (2010).

Sáez, L., Nese, J. T., Alonzo, J., & Tindal, G. (2016). Individual differences in kindergarten through grade 2 fluency relations. *Learning and Individual Differences, 49*, 100–109. https://doi.org/10.1016/j.lindif.2016.05.020

Schalock, R. L., Borthwick-Duffy, S. A., Buntinx, W. H. E., Coulter, D. L., & Craig, E. M. (2010). *Intellectual disability: Definition, classification, and systems of supports* (11th ed.). Washington, DC: AAIDD.

Schrank, F. A., McGrew, K. S., Mather, N., Wendling, B. J., & Dailey, D. (2014). *Woodcock-Johnson® IV*. Itasca, IL: Houghton Mifflin Harcourt.

Shaywitz, S. E., Shaywitz, B. A., Fletcher, J. M., & Escobar, M. D. (1990). Prevalence of reading disability in boys and girls: Results of the Connecticut Longitudinal Study. *Journal of the American Medical Association, 264*, 998–1002.

Shinn, M. R. (1989). *Curriculum-based measurement: Assessing special children*. New York, NY: Guilford.

Simões, C., Santos, S., Biscaia, R., & Thompson, J. R. (2016). Understanding the relationship between quality of life, adaptive behavior and support needs. *Journal of Developmental and Physical Disabilities, 28*, 849–870. https://doi.org/10.1007/s10882-016-9514-0

Smeets, E., & Roeleveld, J. (2016). The identification by teachers of special educational needs in primary school pupils and factors associated with referral to special education. *European Journal of Special Needs Education, 31*, 423–439. https://doi.org/10.1080/08856257.2016.1187879

Sparrow, S. S., Cicchetti, D. V., & Balla, D. A. (2008). *Vineland adaptive behavior scales* (2nd ed.). San Antonio, TX: Pearson Assessments.

Sugai, G., & Horner, R. H. (2009). Responsiveness-to-intervention and school-wide positive behavior supports: Integration of multi-tiered system approaches. *Exceptionality, 17*, 223–237.

U. S. Office of Education. (1977). Procedures for evaluating specific learning disabilities. *Federal Register, 42*, 65082–65085.

Vereenooghe, L., & Langdon, P. E. (2013). Psychological therapies for people with intellectual disabilities: A systematic review and meta-analysis. *Research in Developmental Disabilities, 34*, 4085–4102. https://doi.org/10.1016/j.ridd.2013.08.030

Wechsler, D. (2014). *Wechsler intelligence scale for children* (5th ed.). San Antonio, TX: NCS Pearson.

Weidman, A. C., Augustine, A. A., Murayama, K., & Elliot, A. J. (2015). Internalizing symptomatology and academic achievement: Bi-directional prospective relations in adolescence. *Journal of Research in Personality, 58*, 106–114. https://doi.org/10.1016/j.jrp.2015.07.005

Xu, J. (2010). Predicting homework distraction at the secondary school level: A multilevel analysis. *Teachers College Record, 112*, 1937–1970.

Yell, M. L. (2016). *The law and special education* (4th ed.). Boston, MA: Pearson.

Neuropsychological Testing

Peter J. Castagna and Matthew Calamia

Neuropsychology is "dedicated to enhancing the understanding of brain-behavior relationships and the applications of such knowledge to human problems" (American Psychological Association, 2003). The process of conducting a neuropsychological assessment assumes (1) there are established brain-behavior relationships, (2) we can identify dysfunction that occurs in those relationships, and (3) we can describe the consequences that occur due to that dysfunction. Originally, neuropsychology was focused mostly on identifying the presence and location of brain damage ("Period of Neuropsychological Localization"; Ruff, 2003). As neuroimaging has improved, neuropsychology now focuses less on identifying the presence of brain damage and more on describing the consequences of neural dysfunction in terms of a patient's current level of cognitive and emotional functioning ("Period of Neurocognitive Evaluations"; Ruff, 2003). A comprehensive neuropsychological assessment battery typically includes measures of a number of different cognitive functions including verbal and visuospatial reasoning, attention, memory, processing speed, learning, memory, and motor functioning (Larrabee, 2014). Because the results of a neuropsychological assessment include a patient's cognitive strengths and weaknesses, those results can also be used to suggest interventions. For example, patients with impairments in some types of memory can be put in rehabilitation programs that teach skills that rely on their other domains of intact cognitive functioning (e.g., Greenaway, Hanna, Lepore, & Smith, 2008).

Neuropsychological assessment is used diagnostically for several neurodevelopmental disorders, for example, impairments in intellectual and language functioning are diagnostic specifiers for autism spectrum disorder (American Psychiatric Association, 2013). The conditions most often assessed by pediatric neuropsychologists include attention-deficit/hyperactivity disorder, seizure disorder, traumatic brain injury, brain tumors, pervasive developmental disorder, and other medical and neurological conditions (Sweet, Benson, Nelson, & Moberg, 2015). However, neuropsychological assessment can yield information on cognitive functioning across many types of childhood psychopathology. For example, children with major depressive disorder have been found to have reductions in executive functioning, verbal memory, and sustained attention (Wagner, Müller, Helmreich, Huss, & Tadić, 2015), and children with obsessive-compulsive

P. J. Castagna (✉)
Department of Psychology, Louisiana State University, Baton Rouge, LA, USA
e-mail: pcasta1@lsu.edu

M. Calamia
Department of Psychology, Louisiana State University, Baton Rouge, LA, USA

disorder have specific executive functioning problems that parallel with those found in adults with obsessive-compulsive disorder (Shin et al., 2008). Although many childhood disorders are associated with neuropsychological deficits in studies comparing groups of children with and without a disorder, the clinical utility of a comprehensive individual neuropsychological assessment in evaluating neurodevelopmental disorders such as ADHD and specific learning disorder has been debated (Barkley, 2014; Fletcher & Miciak , 2017; Schneider & Kaufman, 2017). Given the costs, both in time and money, required for a neuropsychological assessment, some recommend that it only be conducted when the results of such an assessment would aid in answering a specific referral question and guide treatment or educational planning (Klin, Saulnier, Tsatsanis, & Volkmar, 2005). This chapter describes popular measures used in the neuropsychological assessment of children.

Neuropsychological Assessment of Noncredible Responding

The assessment of noncredible responding, which occurs "when individuals present themselves in an inaccurate way during an assessment by behaving in a manner inconsistent with their actual abilities or concerns" (Suhr, 2015), has historically not been as large a focus of attention in child and adolescent assessment compared to adult assessment (Kirkwood, 2015a). However, a growing body of research has identified the extent to which measures of noncredible responding used in adult assessment can successfully be used in the assessment of children and adolescents (Kirkwood, 2015a). Additionally, measures have been developed specifically for the assessment of noncredible responding in children and adolescents, for example, the Memory Validity Profile (Sherman & Brooks, 2015b). The presence of noncredible responding can significantly distort the scores obtained in an evaluation and, despite beliefs of some clinicians to the contrary, clinical judgment alone is not sufficient to identify noncredible responding in the absence of specific measures designed to detect it (Kirkwood, 2015a).

The inclusion of these measures in a neuropsychological assessment battery can be important as research has shown that noncredible responding can occur across many different clinical populations and settings (Kirkwood, 2015a). Young children are capable of deception (Peterson & Peterson, 2015) and may provide poor effort on testing or deliberately answer items incorrectly to obtain low scores for a host of reasons, including financial reasons, an interest in obtaining academic accommodations such as extra time to complete standardized tests, a desire to avoid attending school, or as a "cry for help" due to being overwhelmed and wanting to make it clear to the examiner that they are in need of assistance (Baker & Kirkwood, 2015). Of note, noncredible responding is not limited to performance on cognitive or achievement measures; children or adolescents, or their parents or caregivers, may also overreport or underreport psychological symptoms during an evaluation. Unfortunately, this is an understudied area, even though some measures do include scales designed for this purpose, such as the F Index on the Behavior Assessment System for Children – Second Edition (BASC-2) or the Negativity scale on the Behavior Rating Inventory of Executive Functioning (BRIEF) (Kirkwood, 2015b).

Neuropsychological Assessment of Intellectual Functioning

Neuropsychologists frequently administer measures of intellectual functioning as part of their evaluations with the Wechsler intelligence batteries ranking among the most widely used neuropsychology measures (Rabin, Paolillo, & Barr, 2016). The assessment of intellectual functioning is critical for several developmental disorders, most notably intellectual disability (American Psychiatric Association, 2013). Given the importance of intellectual functioning to both diagnosis and functional outcomes, special normative studies are often conducted when developing intellectual functioning measures; for example, development of the Wechsler Intelligence Scale for Children – Fifth Edition (WISC-V; Wechsler, 2014) included data collection from children and adolescents with intellectual disability, autism spectrum disorder, ADHD, and traumatic brain injury. Although conditions such as ADHD do not require an assessment of intellectual functioning for the purposes of diagnosis, weaknesses or deficits identified on aspects of intellectual functioning commonly affected in ADHD, such as working memory (Mayes & Calhoun, 2006), may be useful to assess given the association of poor working memory with academic underachievement (Gathercole, Pickering, Knight, & Stegmann, 2004) and psychopathology (Huang-Pollock, Shapiro, Galloway-Long, & Weigard, 2016).

Numerous batteries exist for the assessment of intellectual functioning in children and adolescents including the WISC-V (Wechsler, 2014), Woodcock-Johnson IV Tests of Cognitive Abilities (WJ-IV COG; Schrank, Mather, & McGrew, 2014), and *Stanford-Binet Intelligence Scales, Fifth Edition* (SB5; Roid, 2003). The WISC-V is used only with children and adolescents (ages 6–16) with other Wechsler batteries used at both younger and older ages, while the WJ-IV COG and SB5 are used throughout the lifespan (ages 2 to 90+ and 2 to 85+, respectively). An in-depth description of the subtests included on each of these batteries is beyond the scope of this chapter, but for the three batteries noted, there is a high degree of overlap in the intellectual abilities they assess, and they have been examined in relation to Cattell-Horn-Carroll theory (e.g., Roid, 2003; Schrank et al., 2014), a hierarchical model of cognitive abilities that is popular areas of clinical practice and research such as school psychology (Sotelo-Dynega & Dixon, 2014).

Among the domains assessed by these batteries are fluid intelligence, or novel problem-solving and reasoning; crystallized intelligence, or the ability to use access and deploy prior knowledge or experience; working memory, or the ability to temporarily store and manipulate information; processing speed, or the ability to quickly process and perform simple tasks; and visual or visual-spatial processing, or the ability to process visual information, including identifying relationships based on visual features (McGrew, 2009). It is important to note that although measures may assess the same domains to some degree, the designs of the specific subtests on these measures can vary widely and, in addition, differences do exist in the specific abilities included on specific test batteries. For example, unlike the WISC-V, the WJ-IV COG includes composites for auditory processing and long-term memory (Schrank et al., 2014).

On the WISC-V, the primary index scores are derived from the administration of ten subtests in approximately 65 min (Wechsler, 2014). The Fluid Reasoning Index is measured using Matrix Reasoning, a subtest in which the examinee must detect patterns and use reasoning to choose the response which best completes a matrix, and Figure Weights, a subtest involving both fluid and quantitative reasoning in which an examinee must choose a response that will balance a scale given other examples of balanced scales. The Verbal Comprehension Index, a measure of crystallized verbal intelligence, is measured using Similarities, a subtest in which the examinee must apply previously acquired knowledge to determine in what way two presented words are similar, and Vocabulary, a subtest in which the examinee is asked to recall previously acquired knowledge concerning the definition of words. The Working Memory Index is measured using Digit Span, a task in which the examinee has to store and manipulate auditory presented numbers (e.g., by saying the list of numbers backwards) and Picture Span, a measure in which the examinee has to recall the serial order of visual stimuli. The Processing Speed Index is measured using Coding, a task in which the examinee has to quickly fill in missing symbols below numbered boxes using a key which matches numbers to specific symbols, and Symbol Search, a task in which the examinee has to quickly scan a row of visual figures to determine whether one of two figures in a key is present. The Visual-Spatial Index is measured using Block Design, a subtest in which the examinee must physically manipulate three-dimensional blocks with block faces which are white, red, or half white and half red such that the design created by the tops of those blocks matches a two-dimensional image, and Visual Puzzles, a subtest in which the examinee must mentally determine how to create various designs from a selection of images of different shaped pieces. An abbreviated list of subtests taking only 48 min to administer can be given if the goal of the evaluation is to obtain the Full-Scale Intelligence Quotient (FSIQ) only rather than individual primary index scores. A number of ancillary index scores are also available which require the administration of additional subtests.

Neuropsychological Assessment of Academic Achievement

The neuropsychological assessment of academic achievement is essential to evaluating skills that are required to be a successful student. Typically, three primary areas, reading, mathematics, and writing, are evaluated within this domain. The assessment of academic achievement is often used to assess whether an individual meets Criterion B for a specific learning disability (SLD), as outlined by the *Diagnostic and Statistical Manual of Mental Disorders, Fifth Edition* (*DSM-5*; American Psychiatric Association, 2013). Specifically, Criterion B establishes that an individual's performance of a certain academic skill (i.e., reading, writing, or mathematics) is well below average for their age. Children low academic achievement within a particular domain causes significant interference in school performance (e.g., school reports, teacher's grades/ratings). Moreover, Criterion B "requires psychometric evidence from an individually administered, psychometrically, sound and culturally appropriate test of academic achievement that is norm- or criterion-referenced" (*DSM-5*, pg. 69). Although academic achievement is distributed along a continuum, any threshold is largely arbitrary; nevertheless, the *DSM-5* suggests using a cutoff of 1.5 standard deviations below the population mean for age (i.e., standard score of 78 or less, 7th percentile) for "greatest diagnostic certainty" (pg. 69). However, it is worth noting that the *DSM-5* does allow a more lenient threshold to be used (e.g., 1.0–2.5 standard deviations) on the basis of clinical judgment (e.g., converging evidence of learning difficulties from clinical assessment, academic history, school reports, and/or test scores). Other criteria, as outlined by the *DSM-5*, indicate that the individual must also have persistent difficulties learning a certain keystone academic skill (i.e., Criterion A), with onset during early school years (i.e., Criterion C); learning difficulties are considered persistent when they restrict progress in learning for at least 6 months despite home- or school-based interventions. The final diagnostic feature of a SLD is that it is indeed specific to a certain academic domain (i.e., Criterion D). Criterion D is necessary to ensure that an individual's academic difficulties are not attributed to intellectual disabilities, global developmental delay, hearing or vision disorder, and neurological or motor disorders. Overall, the neuropsychological assessment of academic achievement is a crucial in determining whether an individual meets Criterion B of a SLD as outlined by the *DSM-5*, which aligns with three federal laws (i.e., the Individuals with Disabilities Education Act [IDEA], Title II of the Americans with Disabilities Act of 1990 [ADA; Title II], and Section 504 of the Rehabilitation Act of 1973 [Section 504]) that outline the obligations of public schools to meet the communication needs of students with disabilities.

Overview of Academic Achievement Assessments

Overall, the WIAT-III is normed for youth aged 4–19 years, 11 months, and includes 16 subtests to measure the 8 areas of achievement specified by US federal legislation (i.e., IDEA) to identify and classify learning disabilities. The subtests include Listening Comprehension, Oral Expression, Early Reading Skills, Word Reading, Pseudoword Decoding, Reading Comprehension, Oral Reading Fluency, Alphabet Writing Fluency, Spelling, Sentence Composition, Essay Composition, Math Problem-Solving, Numerical Operations, Math Fluency-Addition, Math Fluency-Subtraction, and Math Fluency-Multiplication. These 16 subtests measure eight areas (i.e., composites) of academic achievement: Oral Language (i.e., Listening Comprehension and Oral Expression subtests), Total Reading (i.e., Early Reading Skills, Reading Comprehension, Word Reading, Pseudoword Reading, and Oral Reading Fluency subtests), Basic Reading (i.e., Word Reading, Pseudoword Decoding), Reading Comprehension and Fluency (i.e., Reading Comprehension and Oral Reading Fluency subtests), Written Expression (i.e., Sentence Composition, Essay Composition, Spelling subtests), Mathematics (i.e., Math Problem-Solving and Numerical Operations subtests), Math Fluency (i.e., Math Fluency-Addition, Math Fluency-Subtraction, and Math Fluency-Multiplication subtests), and Total Achievement.

The WJ-IV ACH is normed in individuals aged 3 to 90+ and includes 11 standard, and 20 extended, subtests to measure 14 domain-specific clusters across three broad areas of achievement: Reading (i.e., Reading, Broad Reading, Basic Reading Skills, Reading Comprehension, Reading Fluency, and Reading Rate), Writing (i.e., Written Language, Broad Written Language, and Written Expression), and Math (i.e., Mathematics, Broad Mathematics, and Math Calculation Skills), along with six cross-domain clusters (i.e., Academic Skills, Academic Fluency, Academic Applications, Academic Knowledge, Phoneme-Grapheme Knowledge, and Brief/Broad Achievement). The 11 standard subtests that comprise the 14 domain-specific and cross-domain clusters include Letter-Word Identification, Applied Problems, Spelling, Passage Comprehension, Calculation, Writing Samples, Word Attack, Oral Reading, Sentence Reading Fluency, Math Facts Fluency, and Sentence Writing Fluency.

Reading

Reading is a central academic skill that young children learn during the early elementary school years and is basic to success in school. Consequently, teachers have ranked student motivation and creating an interest in reading as their first priority in teaching reading (O'Flahavan et al., 1992). Assessing a child's reading abilities can be broken down into two main components: phonemic coding, reading comprehension, and reading rate or fluency. Decoding refers to the ability to sound out the words, presented in a list or in the context of a story. The second component, comprehension, is a child's ability to understand written material, such as a written story. Finally, reading rate or fluency is a child's capacity to read smoothly and with relative speed. These three components are directly in line with the SLD with impairment in reading specifiers outlined by the *DSM-5* (i.e., word reading accuracy, reading rate or fluency, and/or reading comprehension).

Assessment of Reading: The Wechsler Individual Achievement Test – Third Edition (WIAT-III)

The WIAT-III assesses reading abilities through children's scores on the Early Reading Skills, Word Reading, Pseudoword Decoding, Reading Comprehension, and Oral Reading Fluency subtests. The Early Reading Skills subtest is administered to children currently in prekindergarten to 3rd grade. The subtest requires children to name letters of the alphabet, identify and generate rhyming words, identify words with the same beginning and ending sounds, blend sounds, match sounds with letters and letter blends, and match written words with pictures that illustrate their meaning, thus providing a measure of young children's understanding of essential prerequisite skills to both phonemic coding and reading comprehension. Youth in grades 1 through 12+ are administered the Word Reading, Pseudoword Decoding, Reading Comprehension, and Oral Reading Fluency subtests. Word Reading measures the speed and accuracy of word recognition without the aid of context. This task requires youth to reads aloud from a list of words that increase in difficulty, providing a measure of an examinees' ability to apply phonemic coding to words they may or may not be familiar with. Similarly, Pseudoword Decoding assesses youth's ability to decode nonsense words, where the examinee reads aloud from a list of pseudowords that increase in difficulty. Therefore, the Pseudoword Decoding subtest measures youth's ability to apply phonemic coding to words they are not familiar with, providing an assessment of phonemic coding irrespective of previous word knowledge. The Reading Comprehension subtest requires the examinee read passages, aloud or silently, and, after each passage, orally respond to literal and inferential comprehension questions read aloud by the examiner, where the examinee is allowed to refer to passage to answer questions. The Reading Comprehension subtest, therefore, measures reading comprehension of various types of text in an untimed format (i.e., fictional stories, informational text, advertisements, and how-to passages). Finally, the Oral Reading Fluency subtest requires youth to read passages aloud and then orally respond to comprehension questions, as a measure of speed, fluency, accuracy, and prosody of contextualized oral reading.

Assessment of Reading: The Woodcock-Johnson Tests of Achievement – Fourth Edition (WJ-IV ACH)

The WJ-IV ACH utilizes the Letter-Word Identification, Passage Comprehension, Word Attack, Oral Reading, and Sentence Reading Fluency subtests as measures of youth's reading abilities. These five subtests are used to create six reading clusters: Reading (i.e., Letter-Word Identification and Passage Comprehension subtests), Broad Reading (i.e. Letter-Word Identification, Passage Comprehension, and Sentence Reading Fluency subtests), Basic Reading Skills (i.e., Letter-Word Identification and Word Attack subtests), Reading Fluency (i.e., Oral Reading and Sentence Reading Fluency subtests), Reading Comprehension (i.e., Reading Comprehension subtest), and Reading Rate (Sentence Reading Fluency subtest). Letter-Word Identification, similar to the Word Reading subtest on the WIAT-III, requires the examinee to identify printed letters and words to assess their ability to recognize visual word forms from a phonological lexicon and their pronunciations associated with visual word forms. Conversely, the Passage Comprehension subtest asks an individual to identify a missing key word that is logical given the context of a written passage. Together, the Reading cluster measures youth's phonemic coding (i.e., Letter-Word Identification) and reading comprehension (i.e., Passage Comprehension) abilities. The Broad Reading cluster also includes these subtests, with the addition of the Sentence Reading Fluency subtest, which assesses timed semantic decision-making, requiring reading ability by having youth read printed statements and responding "yes" or "no." The Basic Reading Skills cluster includes the aforementioned Letter-Word Identification subtest, as well as the Word Attack subtest. Word Attack is comparable to the Pseudoword Decoding subtest of the WIAT-III, and asks youth to read phonically regular non-words to assess grapheme-to-phoneme translation by accessing pronunciations of pseudowords not contained in the lexicon. Taken together, the Basic Reading Skills cluster measures youth's capacity to phonemically decode words they may be familiar with (i.e., Letter-Word Identification) or non-words (i.e., Word Attack). The Reading Fluency cluster is comprised of the Oral Reading and Sentence Reading Fluency subtests; Oral Reading asks the examinee to read sentences orally with accuracy and fluency as a measure of orthographic, phonological, and semantic processes. The final two clusters are comprised of single subtests previously discussed: Reading Comprehension cluster (i.e., Passage Comprehension subtest) and Reading Rate cluster (i.e., Sentence Reading Fluency subtest).

Writing

Writing is a complex academic skill that young children begin learning during the early elementary school years and is essential for high academic achievement. The multifaceted nature of writing requires this domain to be examined from a number of subcomponents: grammatical rules, spelling, and ability to organize and convey a message in written form. Additionally, aspects of writing such as the quality of the letters and how they are formed can be important when measuring a child's writing abilities. However, the latter components, though salient on measures of writing achievement, are often indicative of visuomotor and fine motor abilities and therefore better assessed with neuropsychological assessments specific these constructs. A child's writing abilities can be broken down into three main components: essay writing, grammar/punctuation, and spelling. Notably, these three components directly map on to the SLD with impairment in written expression specifiers outlined by the *DSM-5* (i.e., clarity or organization of written expression, grammar and punctuation accuracy, and/or spelling accuracy, reading rate or fluency, and/or reading comprehension).

Assessment of Writing: The Wechsler Individual Achievement Test – Third Edition (WIAT-III)

The WIAT-III assesses written expression through children's scores on the Alphabet Writing Fluency, Sentence Composition, Essay Composition, and Spelling subtests, which comprise the Written Expression composite. The Alphabet Writing Fluency subtest is administered to children in prekindergarten through 3rd grade. The subtest requires children to write letters in any order, in upper- or lowercase, in 30 s as a measure of written letter knowledge, formation, and sequencing. Thus, this assessment provides a measure of young children's understanding of essential prerequisite skills to both letter knowledge, formation, and sequencing. Youth in grades 1 through 12+ are administered the Sentence Composition subtest to measure sentence formulation skills and written semantics, grammar, and mechanics. These constructs are assessed by having children combine (i.e., Sentence Combination) and build sentences (i.e., Sentence Building), where they are scored on their syntax, grammar, and mechanics. Sentence Combination involves children being presented with two independent clauses and having them create single sentence that preserves the meaning using correct spelling, grammar, and punctuation. Sentence Building presents children with a single word (e.g., "and"), and requires them to create a single sentence that includes the word, again, using correct spelling, grammar, and punctuation. The Essay Composition subtest is administered to youth in grades 3 through 12+ and requires the examinee to construct an essay in response to a prompt (i.e., write a single page about their favorite game, providing at least three reasons why), therefore, providing a measure of youth's spontaneous compositional writing abilities within a 10-min time limit. The essay is scored on six features: the inclusion of five paragraphs, an introduction, transitions, three or more reasons of support, one or more elaborations to support each reason, and a conclusion. Moreover, the essay is assessed for number of words used, correct, and incorrect, word sequences. Finally, the Spelling subtest measures written spelling of letter sounds and single words by orally presenting the child with each letter sound within the context of a word, and each word within the context of a sentence, and then the child writes the target letter sound or word. The Spelling subtest is administered to youth in grades kindergarten through 12 + .

Assessment of Writing: The Woodcock–Johnson Tests of Achievement – Fourth Edition (WJ–IV ACH)

The WJ-IV ACH utilizes the Spelling, Writing Samples, and Sentence Writing Fluency subtests as measures of youth's writing abilities. These subtests comprise four writing clusters: Written Language (i.e., Spelling and Writing Samples subtests), Broad Written Language (i.e., Spelling,

Writing Samples, and Sentence Writing Fluency subtests), Basic Writing Skills (i.e., Spelling subtest), and Written Expression (i.e., Writing Samples and Sentence Writing Fluency). The Spelling subtest asks children to spell orally presented words to assess their ability to translate phonological segments into graphemic units or by activating spellings of words from the semantic lexicon. Writing Samples requires youth to write meaningful sentences for a given purpose. In doing so, the Writing Sample subtest assess children's retrieval of word meanings, application of psycholinguistic rules of case, grammar, and syntax, as well as planning and construction of bridging inferences in immediate awareness. Finally, the Sentence Writing Fluency subtest asks the examinee to formulate and write simple sentences rapidly as a measure of their ability to form constituent sentence structures that require fluent access to semantic and syntactic knowledge.

Mathematics

Strong math skills are important for admission to most colleges and are critical for many career and job opportunities. However, many students discontinue their mathematical training early in high school due to their rigor (National Center for Educational Statistics, 1984). Mathematics is an extremely broad domain, and therefore abilities are evaluated in multiple ways. First, a child's ability to solve number problems is examined to provide an assessment of their general functioning in terms of knowledge of the basic mathematical procedures. Second, it is important to assess youth's ability to apply mathematical skills to practical tasks, such as telling time, counting money, word problems, and reading graphs.

Assessment of Mathematics: The Wechsler Individual Achievement Test – Third Edition (WIAT–III)

The WIAT-III assesses mathematic abilities through children's scores on the Math Problem-Solving and Numerical Operations subtests, which comprise the Mathematics composite. Additionally, the Math Fluency-Addition, Math Fluency-Subtraction, and Math Fluency-Multiplication subtests make up the Math Fluency composite. The Math Problem-Solving and Numerical Operation subtest is administered to children in prekindergarten, kindergarten through 12th + grade, respectively. Math Problem-Solving requires children to provide oral, and at times pointing responses, in response to questions presented orally, which often include visual cues, requiring the application of math reasoning skills. This subtest assesses children's untimed math problem-solving skills in terms of basic concepts, real-world applications, geometry, and algebra. During the Numerical Operations subtest, the examinee completes mathematic calculation problems presented in a worksheet format. The Numerical Operations subtest measures untimed, written math calculation skills in terms of basic skills, basic operations with integers, geometry, algebra, and calculus. The three Math Fluency subtests (i.e., Addition, Subtraction, and Multiplication) are administered to youth in grades 1 through 12+, and all follow the same format: the examinee solves written math problems using the specified operation (i.e., addition, subtraction, or multiplication) within a 60-s time limit, where their score reflects the number of correct answers. Children's scores are thought to reflect the speed and accuracy of their math (either addition, subtraction, or multiplication) calculations. *Assessment of Mathematics: The Woodcock-Johnson Tests of Achievement – Fourth Edition (WJ-IV ACH).*

The WJ-IV ACH utilizes the Applied Problems, Calculation, and Math Facts Fluency subtests as measures of youth's mathematic abilities. These subtests comprise four mathematic clusters: Mathematics (i.e., Applied Problems and Calculation subtests), Broad Mathematics (i.e., Applied Problems, Calculation, and Math Facts Fluency subtests), Math Calculation Skills (i.e., Calculation and Math Facts Fluency subtests), and Math Problem-Solving (i.e., Applied Problems subtest). The Applied Problems subtest has children performing math calculations in response to orally presented problems as a measure of their application of calculation and/or quantitative reasoning, as well as formation of insight. During the Calculation subtest, the examinee is required to performing various mathematical calculations in response to written problems. The Calculation subtest assesses the application of knowledge of numbers and calculation procedures to written mathematic problems. The final subtest, Math Facts Fluency, instructs children to complete as many simple mathematic problems (i.e., either addition, subtraction, or multiplication) as they can in 3 min. This subtest measures children's access to and application of digit-symbol arithmetic procedures in a timed format.

Neuropsychological Assessment of Learning and Memory

It has been posited that there are over 100 different types of memory (Tulving, 2002); therefore, it may be unsurprising that the assessment of learning and memory is complex. Although once conceptualized as a unitary construct, memory is multidimensional with a plethora of subsystems and processes. The assessment of memory hinges on properly defining and understanding learning. Learning has been defined as the process of acquiring new information, conversely, memory refers to the persistence of learned material that can be later retrieved (Squire, 1987). Thus, the assessment of memory functioning cannot be fully assessed without knowledge that the information has been properly learned.

There are numerous theories regarding the types of memory systems that exist; however two of the most empirically supported approaches to understanding memory are the systems approach and process approach (Lezak, Howieson, Loring, Hannay, & Fischer, 2004) that are seen as complimentary, though distinct (Schacter, Wagner, & Buckner, 2000). The systems approach suggests that each interrelated system is independent, producing a distinction between procedural and declarative memory systems (Tulving, 2000). Declarative memory refers to knowing that some information was learned, whereas the procedural memory system consists of knowing how to perform a specific skill outside of conscious awareness of the procedural steps necessary to accomplish the particular skill.

Nearly all assessments of memory are measuring children's episodic memory, likely because this system is most vulnerable to dysfunction or damage. The quantitative assessment of learning and memory measures children's ability to learn and remember information that is compared to a normative, same-age group to determine whether the child is demonstrating impairment. As previously mentioned, memory cannot be adequately assessed without first knowing whether the target information has been learned. However, most neuropsychological assessments of memory do not assess learning directly or in a comprehensive manner. A thorough clinical assessment of memory and learning should look to determine where in the memory process (i.e., encoding, consolidation, and/or retrieval) a child is experiencing dysfunction.

Learning and memory assessment in children can be broken down into verbal and visual learning and memory. Furthermore, a child can be assessed whether the type of information (i.e., verbal or visual) can be recalled immediately (i.e., within the first several minutes) or after an extended period of time (i.e., delayed recall). Finally, children's abilities can be assessed for whether they can recall the information without a prompt (i.e., free recall) or recognize the information among other distractor items (i.e., recognition). Recognition trials are essential as they provide information on whether subpar performances are due to learning impairment or retrieval problems. Overall, learning and memory for verbal and visual information can be assessed for immediate and delayed recall as well as recognition.

California Verbal Learning Test for Children (CVLT–C)

Neuropsychological assessments of verbal memory and learning are defined by requiring the child to learn and remember verbal information such as words, sentences, and/or stories. One of the most widely used measures of verbal memory and learning in children is the California Verbal Learning Test for Children (CVLT-C; Delis, Kramer, Kaplan, & Ober, 1994). The CVLT-C is normed on children aged 5–16 and can be used to assess mild to severe learning disabilities, attention-deficit/hyperactivity disorder, intellectual disability, and other neurological disorders and can be administered in 20 min, plus a 20-min delay. The CVLT-C presents the child with a list of 15 words that can be organized into three semantic categories. The list of words is presented over five trials to assess a child's ability to learn verbal information of a series of trials (i.e., list A) as well as whether the child is utilizing learning strategies. Following learning trials, the child is presented with an interference list of 15 different words (i.e., list B), followed by a short free recall for both list A and B. Afterward, the child is assessed for their short cued recall of list A. Finally, the examinee's ability to free and cued recall, as well as recognition, is assessed following a long delay (i.e., 20 min).

The CVLT-C assesses a multitude of memory and learning domains, and importantly, it allows for differentiation between learning and retrieval, as well as an examination of the learning process through a variety of procedures. For instance, the CVLT-C quantifies the rate of learning, recall consistency, and learning strategy employed (e.g., serial or semantic clustering). The CVLT-C also generates traditional measures of immediate and delayed free recall and cued recall, as well as delayed recognition. As well, the CVLT-C allows for the assessment of interference through the presentation of a second list of words that is only assessed once for immediate recall.

Children's Memory Scale (CMS)

The Children's Memory Scale (CMS; Cohen, 1997) is an individually administered comprehensive assessment of learning and memory functioning in children aged 5–16; two record forms are provided for students of 5–8 and 9–16 years old. The immediate portion of the CMS takes approximately 30–40 min to administer, with an additional 10–20 min required for administration of the delayed recognition sections. The CMS measures ability to learn and remember information presented verbally and visually, utilizing three domains: Auditory/Verbal, Visual/Nonverbal, and Attention/Concentration (i.e., working memory). Therefore, the current section will focus on the verbal and visual portions of the CMS, with the following section on attention containing information on the attention/concentration components of the CMS. Each domain assessed (i.e., Auditory/Verbal, Visual/Nonverbal, and Attention/Concentration) contains two core subtests and one supplemental subtest, with each subtest in the Auditory/Verbal and Visual/Nonverbal domains containing both an immediate memory and a delayed memory portion. The Auditory/Verbal memory subtests produces four index scores: Verbal Immediate (VI), Verbal Delayed (VD), Delayed Recognition (DR), and Learning calculated from two Auditory/Verbal and one Visual/Nonverbal subtests (i.e., Stories, Word Pairs, and Dot Locations, respectively). VI provides a neuropsychological assessment of children's immediate recall, whereas VD measures children's delayed recall. Starting with the former, the VI subtest orally presents children with two, age-dependent, short stories, and the child is then asked to retell each story immediately following hearing it. Conversely, the VD subtest contains the delayed condition that assesses children's long-term memory for the story from the immediate recall condition (i.e., VI), in a free recall trial, and then with a recognition task for certain details of the story. The recognition task asks the child to respond yes/no to questions about both stories. To provide an assessment of youth's learning, the Learning subtest assesses verbal memory for word pairs; the examiner reads 10–14 word pairs and then reads the first word of each pair, asking the child to provide the corresponding word. The same list of word pairs is presented over three trials. Following, the Learning subtest quantifies children's free and cued recall of the verbally paired information; during which, children are orally presented with the first word of each word pair learned in the immediate condition and asked to provide the corresponding word freely. As well, the examinee is read a list of word pairs and asked to identify whether each word pair was from the immediate recall condition or a new word pair (i.e., recognition).

As mentioned above, the Visual/Nonverbal domain contains two core subtests and one supplemental subtest, containing both an immediate memory and a delayed memory portion. The Visual/Nonverbal domain consists of three indices: Learning, Visual Immediate (ViI), and Visual Delayed (ViD) calculated from two subtests (i.e., Dot Location and Faces). During the administration of the Dot Location subtest, the child is shown an array of blue dots located within a rectangle. Following, the page is removed, and the child is asked to replicate the spatial location of the dots by placing chips on a rectangular grid. The task includes three learning trials, which is combined with the Verbal Learning subtest to form the Learning Index, followed by a distractor array of red dots. After, the child is assessed for their immediate (i.e., ViI) and delayed recall (i.e., ViD) of the original blue dot array. In addition, the Faces subtest consists of a series of 12 (5–8-year-olds) or 16 (9–16-year-olds) pictured human faces one at a time. The child is then asked to recall the faces immediately (i.e., ViI) and following a delay (i.e., ViD), where they must identify the stimulus faces from a different set of distractor items (36 or 48 colored photos).

Child and Adolescent Memory Profile (ChAMP)

The Child and Adolescent Memory Profile (ChAMP; Sherman & Brooks, 2015a, b) assesses visual and verbal memory in children, adolescents, and young adults. The ChAMP is an individually administered comprehensive assessment of learning and memory functioning in individuals aged 5–21 and takes approximately 35 min to administer with a potential 10-min screening index consisting of two subtests. The full assessment measures two domains, consisting of a total of 10 subtests: Verbal Memory (i.e., Lists Immediate Recall, Instructions Immediate Recall, Lists Delayed Recall, Instructions Delayed Recall, Lists Recognition, and Instructions Recognition) and Visual Memory (i.e., Objects Immediate Recall, Places Immediate Recall, Objects Delayed Recall, and Places Delayed Recall). The Lists subtest is a typical list learning tasks consisting of 16 nouns. The children are assessed for their ability to immediately recall the list (i.e., Lists Immediate Recall), recite the list following a long delay (i.e., Lists Delayed Recall), and recognize the nouns among distractors (i.e., Lists Recognition). Similarly, the ChAMP also incorporates the Instructions subtests, in which youth are read a paragraph to assess contextual auditory and verbal memory. Children's abilities to recall the instructions immediately (i.e., Instructions Immediate Recall) and after a delay (i.e., Instructions Delay Recall).

The ChAMP also includes a Visual Memory domain that consists of two subtests (i.e., Objects and Places), which creates four indices (i.e., Objects Immediate Recall, Places Immediate Recall, Objects Delayed Recall, and Places Delayed Recall). The Objects subtest visually presents children with shapes, textures, and three-dimensional characteristics, which they are asked to look at, two at a time, for 2 s. Children aged 5 are presented with 16 items, whereas children 6 years or older are shown 32 items. Following their presentation, children are asked to identify the objects among three choices (i.e., two distractors and one target), which is administered twice immediate recall (i.e., Objects Immediate Recall) and once for delayed recall (i.e., Objects Delayed Recall). Finally, on the Places subtest, youth are shown a visual scene (e.g., a bedroom or public place). Next, they are asked to recognize the spatial configurations and contextual visual details of the visual scene, which administration very similar to the Objects subtest; children choose among three choices (i.e., two distractors and one target; Places Immediate Recall). Following a delay children are administered a forced choice recognition section (i.e., Places Delayed Recall). Notably, both visual memory tasks contain delayed recall tasks; however, they function as forced choice recognition tasks.

All tasks provide scaled scores and base rates for verbal memory, visual memory, immediate memory, delayed memory, total memory, and screening index indices. All indices can be administered in isolation or scored as part of the overall testing profile.

Wide Range Assessment of Memory and Learning, 2nd Edition (WRAML2)

The Wide Range Assessment of Memory and Learning, 2nd Edition (WRAML2; Sheslow & Adams, 2003), is a standardized assessment of verbal memory, visual memory, learning, and attention/concentration in individuals aged 5–90. The WRAML2 takes approximately 75–90 min to administer and consists of six core tests: two verbal, two visual, and two attention/concentration, which yield three index scores (i.e., Verbal Memory [VeM], Visual Memory [ViM], and Attention/Concentration [AC]), as well as a General Memory Index (GMI). In addition, clinicians can choose to administer up to 11 optional subtests that produce additional clinical index scores, though these indices are not included in the WRAML2 structural validation studies reported in the *Administration and Technical Manual* (Sheslow & Adams, 2003). The current section will focus on the verbal and visual portions of the WRAML2, with the following section on attention containing information on the attention/concentration components of the WRAML2. The VeM index is comprised of the Story Memory and Verbal Learning subtests. Story Memory involves the clinician reading two short stories to the child, where the child is asked to orally recall as many parts of the story as possible. Of note, the VeM also includes the two optional Story Memory subtests that may be particularly helpful to test administrators: Story Memory Delayed Recall and Story Memory Delayed Recognition subtests. The latter measures a child's ability to recall the story after a long delay, whereas the former asks the child to recognize certain components of the story utilizing contextual cues. The Verbal Learning subtest requires the evaluator to orally present a list of common single-syllable words to a child followed by an immediate free recall; this same procedure is repeated over three identical trials. Individuals 8 years and younger are administered a 13-word list, whereas youth aged 9 and up are presented with 16-word list. Additionally, the optional Verbal Recognition subtest can be administered to test youth's ability to recognize the words following a delay.

The ViM index includes the Design Memory and Picture Memory subtests. The Design Memory subtest is a measure of youth's short-term visual memory of quasi-meaningful visual stimuli. During the task, five 4x6 cards with multiple, simple geometric figures are presented, one at a time, for 10 s of exposure. Following each card, there is a 10-s delay where the participant is then asked to draw the content she/he remembers. The Picture Memory subtest evaluates visual memory using skills to detect changes in specific features or details within meaning visual arrays in four different scenes. The task evaluates a child's ability to remember new, context-related visual information. The Picture Memory subtest involves briefly showing the child a scene which they are asked to scan for 10 s prior to it being removed. Afterward, a similar, alternate scene is immediately presented, and the participant is asked to identify elements of the scene that have been moved, changed, or added. Optionally, the clinician can administer the Design Recognition and Picture Recognition subtests where the child is assessed visual recognition recall following a delay. The WRAML2 also includes an optional Working Memory Index that is comprised of two subtests: Verbal Working Memory and Visual Working Memory.

Neuropsychological Assessment of Attention

Attention is defined as the process of selecting for active processing specific aspects of the environment or information stored in memory (Raz, 2004). Whereas early theories conceptualized attention as a unitary process (e.g., Broadbent, 1958), it is now understood that attention comprises a system of networks that include alerting, orienting, and selection (Fan et al., 2002). Alerting refers to the process of changes in internal states in preparation for perceiving a particular stimulus, sometimes termed vigilance. Orienting, in contrast, involves the selection of information from sensory systems that is either triggered by external stimulus or through voluntary control (Fernandez-Duque & Posner, 1997). Therefore, orienting can be a reflexive behavior when a stimulus directs an individual's attention to its location or voluntary when an individual is instructed to search a visual field for a particular stimulus, for example. Selection describes the process of selecting from among a multitude of often conflicting actions or responses (Lamar & Raz, 2007). Although these processes are thought to be largely independent, the neuropsychological assessment of attention often involves their interaction due to a lack of specificity with our current methods of measuring attention. Overall, visual attention is guided by a combination of bottom-up processes grounded on spatiotemporal differences in visual input (Itti & Koch, 2001), as well as top-down networks based on prior knowledge of a particular stimuli (Wolfe, Horowitz, Kenner, Hyle, & Vasan, 2004).

The theorized orthogonal components of attention (i.e., altering, orienting, and selection) are typically not reflecting in the neuropsychological assessment of attention. Rather, a youth's simple and sustained auditory and visual attention is often assessed when attentional difficulties are reported. This disconnect may reflect the fact that neuropsychological measures typically involve the interaction of alerting, orienting, and selection, making it difficult to tease apart these related, yet theoretically independent, constructs.

Simple attention tasks involve visual-motor processing demands, mostly on speeded measures, with a short duration. In contrast, sustained attention requires goal-oriented attention over a longer period of time. Both simple and sustained attention can be assessed in the visual and auditory domains.

Simple Attention

The Trail Making Test – Part A (TMT-A; Army Individual Test Battery, 1944) is one of the most widely used neuropsychological measures of children's simple attention. The intermediate version of the TMT-A can be administered to children aged 9–14, whereas the adult version is administered to individuals 15 years or older. The TMT-A takes approximately 5 min to administer, where the examiner instructs the child to connect a series of numbered circles randomly distributed in a spatial array. The intermediate version (i.e., for ages 9–14) requires the child to connect the dots, in order starting at circle 1 and ending at circle 18, as fast as he or she can without lifting the pencil from the paper. Both time-to-completion in seconds and number of errors, when compared to readily available norms, provide an indication of youth's level of simple attention. The Trail Making Test – Part B (TMT-B) is often given following Part A and will be described in detail below (see Neuropsychological Assessment of Executive Functioning) as it assesses various aspects of executive functioning. Worth noting, there are a number of variants of the Trail Making Test such as the Children's Color Trails Test (CCTT; D'Elia, Satz, Uchiyama, & White, 1996; Llorente, Williams, Satz, & D'Elia, 2003) and the Delis-Kaplan Executive Function System's Trail Making Test (D-KEFS TMT; Delis, Kaplan, & Kramer, 2001). The CCTT was designed to minimize the influence of language to allow for it to be used cross-culturally and can be administered to youth aged 8–16. Part one of the CCTT is similar to TMT-A, except all odd-numbered circles are pink and even-numbered circles are yellow. Although the colors of the circles are irrelevant for part one, they are used for part two, which is analogous to TMT-B. Similarly, D-KEFS TMT can be administered to individuals aged 8–89 and includes five variants of the TMT, with condition two being analogous to TMT-A, with the exception that the D-KEFS TMT condition two also includes distractor items (i.e., letters) that are to be ignored by the examinee. More detail regarding the D-KEFS will be provided in the section below (i.e., Neuropsychological Assessment of Executive Functioning).

The Test of Everyday Attention for Children (TEA-Ch; Manly, Robertson, Anderson, Nimmo-Smith, 2001) is a neuropsychological measure of various attentional capacities in youth between the ages of 6 and 15.11 and takes about an hour to administer. The TEA-Ch assesses youth's simple attention, sustained attention, as well as executive functioning (i.e., switching and inhibition). Therefore, the current section will focus on subtests measuring simple and sustained attention, whereas the following section on the assessment of executive functioning will describe subtests of switching and/or inhibition. The TEA-Ch includes seven subtests: Sky Search, Score!, Creature Counting, Sky Search DT, Map Mission, Score DT, and Walk, Don't Walk, with three primarily measuring simple or sustained attention (i.e., Sky Search, Score!, and Map Mission). Sky Search is a brief, timed subtest. This is a brief, timed subtest. Children have to find as many spaceship targets as possible on a sheet filled with similar distractor spaceships. The second portion of the task is the same format, but there are no distractors. Subtracting part two from part one gives a measure of a child's ability to make this selection that is relatively free from the influence of processing or motor speed. Similar to Sky Search, Score! examines sustained auditory, as opposed to visual, attention. Score! asks children to count of the number of scoring sounds they hear across a number of trials on a standardized recording. Finally, Map Mission assesses children's simple visual attention by asking the examinee to search a map to find as many target symbols as they can in 1 min.

Sustained Attention

The Conners' Continuous Performance Test 3 (CPT 3; Conners & Staff, 2015a) is a neuropsychological measure of various attention-related problems in youth older than 8 years and includes successive 360 trials over the course of 14 min. Youth are instructed to press the space bar for all letters presented, except for "X." Various letters are presented, one at a time, at various time intervals. The CPT 3 utilizes four dimensions: Inattentiveness, Impulsivity, Sustained Attention, and Vigilance. Dimensions are assessed through on three to six standardized performance scores. The Inattentiveness dimension is comprised of Detectability, Omissions, Commissions, Hit Reaction Time (HRT), HRT Standard Deviation (SD), and Variability. Briefly, detectability is a score that reflects youth's ability to discriminate between targets (X) and nontargets (non-X); omissions reflect missed targets; commissions are incorrect responses to nontargets; HRT is youth's reaction time; HRT SD is their response speed consistency; and variability scores are indicative of youth's variability in response speed consistency. Thus, high scores on these constructs may reflect a young person's inattention. Similarly, the Impulsivity dimension is made up of a number of the same performance scores within the Inattention domain (i.e., HRT and Commissions), as well as perseverations – random or anticipatory responses (i.e., responses with HRT < 100 ms). Scores on the HRT block change, omissions by block, and commissions by block comprise the Sustained Attention domain. HRT block change documents an examinee's change in response speed across blocks of trials; omissions by block are missed targets by block; commissions by block are incorrect responses to nontargets by block. Finally, the Vigilance dimension is reflected by scores on the HRT interstimulus interval (ISI) change (i.e., change in response speed at various ISI), omissions by ISI (i.e., missed targets by ISI), and commissions by ISI (i.e., incorrect responses to nontargets by ISI).

Conners' Continuous Auditory Test of Attention (CATA; Conners & Staff, 2015a) assesses auditory processing and attention-related problems in individuals 8 years or older. The CATA consists of 200 trials that are divided into types and sounds: warned trials (i.e., low tone, followed by a high tone) and unwarned trials (i.e., high-tone by itself with no warning), taking approximately 14 min to complete. During the test, examinees are presented with high-tone sounds that are either preceded by a low-tone warning sound (i.e., warned trials) or played alone (i.e., unwarned trials). The individual is instructed to respond only to high-tone sounds on warned trials and to ignore those on unwarned trials. Typically, the low-tone and the high-tone sounds are played in the same ear (non-switch trials). However, there are also switch trials; the low-tone warning sound and the high-tone target sound are played in different ears. The CATA includes three dimensions: Inattentiveness (i.e., Detectability, Omissions, Commissions, Hit Reaction Time [HRT], HRT Standard Deviation [SD]), Impulsivity (i.e., HRT, Commissions, Perseverative Commissions), and Sustained Attention (i.e., HRT Block Change, Omissions by Block, Commissions by Block), as well as descriptive information regarding respondent's Auditory Laterality and Auditory Mobility is also provided. Auditory Laterality is comprised of respondents' HRT and percentage of hits in the right versus left ear, measuring youth's preference for right versus left targets. Similarly, Auditory Mobility utilizes HRT and percentage of hits in the switch versus non-switch trials, measuring individuals' ability to switch attention from one ear to the other. Moreover, results can be broken down into blocks to track an examinees performance over the entirety of the test.

Neuropsychological Assessment of Executive Functioning

Executive functioning (EF) is a broad term that is comprised of a number of higher-order cognitive domains that aid in processes such as judgment, decision-making, and planning (Baron, 2004; Lezak, Howieson, & Loring, 2004). Moreover, EFs are high-level cognitive processes that enable individuals to regulate their thoughts and actions during goal-directed behavior through their influence on lower-level processes (Friedman and Miyake, 2016). EFs are critical to assess as strengths and weaknesses can represent protective- and risk-factors for developmental psychopathology (Pennington & Ozonoff, 1996). As such, the transition from adolescence to adulthood is a particularly important time for EF development, as it is a period during which performance matures. Some studies have suggested more unity of EF at young ages (Brydges, Fox, Reid, and Anderson, 2014; Wiebe et al., 2011); however, studies tend to find evidence that shifting is separable from updating or working memory in older children and adults, with inconsistencies involving the inhibition factor. Functional neuroimaging studies of EF tasks suggest that children and adolescents use the same circuitry as adults, just less efficiently (Luna, Garver, Urban, Lazar, & Sweeney, 2004; Luna et al., 2001; Scherf, Sweeney, & Luna, 2006). These findings in youth fit nicely with the bifactor model of EF proposed by Friedman and colleagues (2008) where updating and shifting are independent, and a common EF latent variable relates to both updating and shifting, as well as subsumes the inhibition factor. Notably, the field of neuropsychology typically utilizes the three-factor model of EF that includes inhibition, updating, and shifting (Miyake et al., 2000). Inhibition is defined as the cognitive ability to inhibit a proponent response; updating is an individual's ability to update working memory given new information; shifting is the ability to shift cognitive resources between task-sets. Although working memory itself is separable from updating working memory, and there are other aspects of working memory (i.e., maintenance and manipulation), these domains are beyond the scope of the current section.

Inhibition

Delis-Kaplan Executive Function System (D-KEFS; Delis et al., 2001) includes nine tasks designed to assess various components of EF: Trail Making Test, Verbal Fluency Test, Design Fluency Test, Color-Word Interference Test, Sorting Test, Twenty Questions Test, Word Context Test, Tower Test, and Proverb Test. The D-KEFS can be administered to individuals from the ages of 8 to 89 and takes approximately 90 min to administer in its entirety. A recent factor structure of the D-KEFS in 8- to 19-year-olds indicated that the Trail Making Test-B, Color-Word Interference (Inhibition), and Color-Word Interference (Inhibition/Switching) most strongly relate to inhibition; the Verbal Fluency Test (i.e., Letter Fluency, Category Fluency, Category Switching total, and Category Switching Accuracy) maps on to updating; and shifting is best captured by the Sorting Test (i.e., Sorting Condition 1, Free Sort; Sorting Condition 2, Free Sort Description; and Sorting Condition 3, Sort Recognition; Latzman & Markon, 2010). As well, Crawford, Sutherland, and Garthwaite (2008) demonstrated that the reliability of the contrast measures is low, with a few tests reliably assessing current conceptualizations of EF. Therefore, only a select number of tests from the D-KEFS will be discussed (i.e., Trail Making Test, Verbal Fluency Test, Color-Word Interference Test, and Sorting Test).

The Color-Word Interference Test is a Stroop task that is comprised of four trials: Color Naming, Color-Word Reading, Inhibition, and Inhibition/Switching. The latter two are typically used to assess baseline processing ability for contrast scores. The inhibition test presents youth a series of color names in different colored ink, and the child is required to name the ink color in which color words are printed, and not read the word. Total time to complete in seconds, corrected errors, and uncorrected errors are assessed as a measure of inhibition. Conversely, the Inhibition/Switching condition requires the individual to switch back and forth between naming the ink color the word is printed and reading the color name, depending on whether the word is within a black box. Again, total time to complete in seconds, corrected errors, and uncorrected errors area assessed to provide information on youths' ability to inhibit a proponent response, as well as shift task-set in an efficient manner.

The Trail Making Test (TMT) of the D-KEFS has five different conditions. As previously mentioned, condition one is Visual Scanning, where the child is instructed to rapidly locate a number of letter among an array of distractors; condition two is comparable to the aforementioned TMT-A, with the exception that it also includes distractors (i.e., letters) that are to be ignored; condition three is also comparable to TMT-A, but the child is asked to connect the letters in order while ignoring distractors (i.e., numbers); condition four is the most related to inhibition and shifting, equivalent to TMT-B. During this test, the child is instructed to connect the circles containing number and letters in order, alternating between numbers and letters (i.e., 1-A-2-B-3-C, etc.).

Test of Everyday Attention for Children (TEA-Ch; Manly et al., 2001) has a number of subtests that assess youths' inhibition abilities. For example, the Walk, Don't Walk task asks children to take a "step" on a paper path, using a pen, after each tone they hear on a tape. Unpredictably one tone ends differently than the rest, which signals the child to stop. The test measures whether or not the child is able to stop responding when the signal occurs and is thus a measure of inhibition.

Overall, these neuropsychological measures reflect multidimensional clinical assessments; however, it is worth noting that cognitive psychology tends to use computer-based measures such as the antisaccade task as a measure of inhibition.

Updating

The Verbal Fluency Test (VFT) of the D-KEFS has been found to most closely relate to updating working memory and is comprised of three conditions: Letter Fluency, Category Fluency, and Category Switching. During Letter Fluency, the examiner asks the child to list all words they can think of that begin with a certain letter in 60 s, with three trials consisting of different letters. The words cannot be people, places, or numbers; they are also instructed to not say the same words with different endings (i.e., if they say "make," they should not also say "makes" or "making"). The child's score is based on the number of correct words said in 60 s over the three trials, as well as number of intrusions (i.e., words that do not start with the instructed letter) and repetitions. Number of words can be grouped in 15-s groups and collapsed across letter trials (i.e., words said from 0–15 s, 15–30 s, etc.). The second subtest in VFT is Category Fluency, which includes two trials, where the child is told to name as many animal and boy names as they can in 60 s, respectively. The youth's score is garnered from the number of correct category words said over the two 60-s trials, number of intrusions, and repetitions. As with Letter Fluency, Category Fluency also quantifies individuals' responses grouped across trials in 15-s groups. Finally, Category Switching is similar to Category Fluency but requires the examinee to switch back and forth between saying as many fruits and as many pieces of furniture as they can in one 60-s trial. Youth are scored on the number of total correct switching (i.e., total number of correct fruits and furniture stated in 60 s) and their switching accuracy (i.e., total number of correct switches from fruit to furniture). Again, total number of fruits and furniture stated can be grouped in 15-s groups and collapsed across the single trials (i.e., words said from 0 to 15 s, 15 to 30 s, etc.). In sum, these subtests of the VFT have been found to be indicative of a child's ability to update their working memory.

The Children's Paced Auditory Serial Addition Task (CHIPASAT; Dyche & Johnson, 1991) has norms for children aged 8–14.5 years and is a measure of youth's updating ability. During the task, the child is orally presented with a random series of numbers from 1 to 9, and the child is instructed to consecutively add pairs of numbers (i.e., each number is added to the one that immediately preceded: the second number is added to the first, the third number to the second, etc.). In youth, the sum never exceeds 10. This response requirement is sustained over numerous items until the end of the trial. The interstimulus interval is then decreased, and the same process is repeated. The interstimulus intervals are 2.8 (practice), 2.4, 2.0, 1.6, and 1.2 s. Thus, the CHIPASAT incrementally increases demands over trials by increasing the speed of stimulus input and decreasing the available response time. There are 61 items per trial, with scores available for each interstimulus interval (i.e., 2.4, 2.0, 1.6, and 1.2 s), as well as a total score.

The Brown-Peterson Task (BPT; Brown, 1958; Peterson & Peterson, 1959) is a measure of youth's updating of working memory and can be administered to individuals aged 9–84 years, taking approximately 10 min to complete. Notably, the task is sometimes called the Auditory Consonant Trigrams, which is abbreviated as CCC (i.e., Paniak, Millar, Murphy, and Keizer, 1997; ages 9–15 years). The BPT and CCC require children to recall a series of items (i.e., three consonants) after a variable delay, during which they are asked to complete an interference task (i.e., mental addition or subtraction for BPT; count backwards by one for CCC). Three-letter trigrams with retention intervals ranging from 0 to 18 s are used. The CCC includes 5 trials (without an interference task, delay of 0 s) and 15 trials that have a random delay (i.e., either 3, 9, or 18 s), as well as a random starting point for the child to count backward from. The CCC provides a total score and scores for each of the 0-, 3-, 9-, and 18-s delays.

Shifting

The Sorting Test of the D-KEFS has found to most closely relate to shifting, or cognitive flexibility, and is comprised of two conditions: Free Sorting and Sort Recognition. During, condition one (i.e., Free Sorting), the child asked to sort six cards into two groups, with three cards in each group, according to as many different possible sorting categories as possible (e.g., grouped by shape, grouped by color, grouped by semantic relationship, etc.). Free Sorting includes two trials that utilize different stimuli. Free Sorting scores are generated based on the correct number of sorts and a description score for each of the two trials. During condition two (i.e., Sort Recognition), the examinee has to identify and describe the correct rules the examiner used to generate a particular sort. Sort Recognition includes two trials, using the same cards from the Free Sorting condition. Sort Recognition provides a single description score for each trial. Scores on the Free Sorting and Sort Recognition subtest of the Sorting Test have been shown to relate to a child's ability to think flexibly (Latzman & Markon, 2010).

The Wisconsin Card Sorting Test (WCST; Heaton, Chelune, Talley, Kay, and Curtis, 1993) can be used in individuals aged 6:5 to 89 years as a measure of ability to form abstract concepts, to shift and maintain set, and to utilize feedback. The test consists of four stimulus cards, placed in front of the examinee (i.e., the first with a red triangle, the second with two green stars, the third with three yellow crosses, and the fourth with four blue circles). The youth is then given two packs each containing 64 response cards, which have designs similar to those on the stimulus cards (i.e., varying in color, geometric form, and number). The examiner instructs the child to match each of the cards in the decks to one of the four key cards. Following the examiner provides feedback each time whether he or she is right or wrong. The child continues until he or she provides ten consecutive correct answers. After, with no warning provided, the sorting rule changes (e.g., rule changes from matching based on color to matching based on geometric form). This procedure continues until the subject has successfully completed six sorting categories (color, geometric form, number, color, geometric form, number) or until all 128 cards have been placed. Seven scores can be generated from the WCST: number of categories completed (i.e., number of sequences of ten consecutive correct matches; maximum = 6), trials to complete the first category (i.e., total number of trials to complete first category), perseveration responses/perseveration errors (i.e., number of items in which the patient persists in responding to a stimulus characteristic that is incorrect), percent perseveration errors (i.e., concentration of perseverative errors in relation to overall test performance), failure to maintain set (i.e., examinee makes five or more consecutive correct matches but then makes an error before successfully completing the category), percent conceptual level responses (i.e., consecutive correct responses occurring in runs of three), and learning to learn (i.e., average change in conceptual efficiency across the successive stages or categories, based on percent error difference scores for each consecutive pair of adjacent categories).

The Test of Everyday Attention for Children (TEA-Ch; Manly et al., 2001) also has a number of subtests that measure youths' shifting abilities. The subtests include Creature Counting and Opposite Worlds. During Creature Counting, the children is required to repeatedly switch between two simple activities (i.e., of counting upwards and counting downwards). Specifically, they are asked to count aliens in their burrow, with occasional arrows that indicate to change the direction in which they are counting. Time taken and accuracy are used as an assessment of shifting abilities. The Opposite Worlds subtest is similar; children follow a path naming the digits one and two that are scattered along the path. Then, in the "opposite world," the same type of task is presented except the child must now say "one" when they see a two and "two" when they see a one. The speed in seconds with which the child can perform the cognitive reversal is indicative of their shifting abilities and attentional control.

Neuropsychological Assessment of Visuospatial and Visuoconstruction Functioning

Visuospatial (VS) and visuoconstruction (VC) abilities play an important role in every day functioning, though they are often automatic processes. VS is a broad term that involves the identification of a stimulus and its location.

Generally speaking, VC is the ability to integrate, organize, and manipulate spatial information to achieve a desired goal (e.g., a certain design), typically through a motor response. In sum, neuropsychological tests of VS functioning would include identifying, and possibly mentally manipulating, stimulus and its location. In contrast, the neuropsychological assessment of VC comprises integrating visual information (i.e., a certain design) with motor responses (e.g., orienting blocks) to achieve a particular outcome. In addition to the tests described below, subtests from measures of intellectual functioning are also used to measure these abilities (e.g., WISC-V Block Design and Visual Puzzles; Wechsler, 2014).

The Beery-Buktenica Developmental Test of Visual-Motor Integration, Sixth Edition (VMI; Beery, Buktenica, & Beery, 2010), can be administered to individuals aged 2 to 99:11 as a neuropsychological measure of visual-motor integration. Overall, the VMI includes three subtests (i.e., Visual-Motor Integration [VI], Visual Perception [VP], and Motor Coordination [MC]) and takes approximately 10–15 min to administer. The VI portion requires the child to copy a series of developmentally staged geometric forms using paper and pencil. The following section, VP, instructs the examinee to look at a series of pictures and select the geometric figure that matches a target figure from a series of choices. Finally, the MC subtest instructs the child draw lines with a pencil through narrow paths without crossing over or drawing outside the path. When scoring the VMI, children receive one point for each correctly drawn (i.e., VI and MC) and selected figure (i.e., VP), until three consecutive failures.

The Judgment of Line Orientation (JOL; Benton, Varney, and Hamsher, 1978) can be administered to individuals aged 7–96 years and is a measure of spatial perception and orientation. The JOL takes approximately 15–20 min to administer. The test utilizes a single spiral-bound booklet that consists of 35 stimuli in the upper part of the booklet, with the bottom portion including a multiple-choice card that stays the same for all stimuli. The multiple-choice response card has an array of lines, labeled "1" through "11," drawn at 18-degree intervals. The test begins with five practice items, and generally speaking, items are presented in ascending difficulty. During the test, the youth is required to identify which two lines, utilizing the multiple-choice array, match the directions of the lines on the stimulus card. Scoring the JOL includes summing the examinees' total number of correct responses.

The Rey-Osterrieth Complex Figure Test-Copy (ROCFT-C; Osterrieth, 1944) has available norms for individuals aged 6–93 years as a measure of both visual-spatial constructional ability and visual memory. The ROCFT presents the youth with a complex figure consisting of a number of smaller geometric figures. The test includes a copy trial, followed by a 3-min, 30-min recall trials, as well as a recognition trial. Recall and recognition trials serve as a measure of an individual's visual memory abilities. In contrast, the copy trial can provide valuable information on youth's visuoconstruction and planning abilities. During the copy trial, the child is presented with the complex figure and is timed as they copy the figure to a blank piece of paper. The copy trial is scored by providing the examinee 0, 1, or 2 points for each of the smaller geometric figures that comprise the larger, complex figure depending on whether they are directly drawn and/or in the correct location.

Concluding a Neuropsychological Evaluation: Providing Feedback and Recommendations

Following a neuropsychological evaluation, which involves the administration of measures such as the ones detailed in this chapter, the neuropsychologist may provide feedback on both the neuropsychologist's impressions about a patient's diagnosis and prognosis, as well as specific recommendations related to the patient's everyday functioning. For example, parents may receive feedback that their child's symptoms and neuropsychological test performance are consistent with a diagnosis of attention-deficit/hyperactivity disorder and then be given recommendations for helpful behavioral techniques in managing symptoms as well as referral options for additional psychological or pharmacological treatment. Unfortunately, compared to the large research literatures for other areas of clinical intervention, the scientific study of how best to provide neuropsychological feedback is underwhelming.

A handful of experimental studies have demonstrated the utility of certain techniques, for example, the provision of written feedback in addition to oral feedback (Fallows and Hilsabeck, 2013; Meth, Calamia, & Tranel, 2016) and the provision of individualized fables to children to explain test results and recommendations (Tharinger & Pilgrim, 2012). Research has shown that although patients report a high level of satisfaction with being provided with feedback (Westervelt, Brown, Tremont, Javorsky, & Stern, 2007), their recall of specific recommendations can be quite poor (Fallows and Hilsabeck, 2013; Meth et al., 2016). Therefore, the provision of written feedback, in addition to oral feedback, should be provided to increase the likelihood that patients and their families will be able to implement the recommendations given after a neuropsychological evaluation.

References

American Psychiatric Association. (2013). *Diagnostic and statistical manual of mental disorders* (5th ed.). Arlington, VA: American Psychiatric Publishing.

American Psychological Association Council of Representatives (1996, reapproved. 2003). *Archival Description of Clinical Neuropsychology*. Retrieved from https://www.scn40.org/

Baker, D. A., & Kirkwood, M. W. (2015). Motivations behind noncredible presentations: Why children feign and how to make this determination. In M. W. Kirkwood (Ed.), *Validity testing in child and adolescent assessment evaluating exaggeration, feigning, and noncredible effort*. New York, NY: The Guilford Press.

Barkley, R. (2014). Psychological assessment of children with ADHD. In R. A. Barkley (Ed.), *Attention-deficit hyperactivity disorder: A handbook for diagnosis and treatment*. New York, NY: The Guilford Press.

Baron, I. S. (2004). *Neuropsychological evaluation of the child*. New York, NY: Oxford University Press.

Army Individual Test Battery. (1944). *Manual of directions and scoring*. Washington, DC: War Department, Adjutant General's Office.

Beery, K. E., Buktenica, N. A., & Beery, N. A. (2010). *The beery-Buktenica developmental test of visual motor integration* (6th ed.). Bloomington, MN: Pearson.

Benton, A. L., Varney, N. R., & Hamsher, K. D. (1978). Visuospatial judgment: A clinical test. *Archives of Neurology, 35*, 364–367.

Broadbent, D. E. (1958). *Perception and communication*. New York, NY: Oxford University Press.

Brown, J. (1958). Some tests of the decay of immediate memory. *Quarterly Journal of Experimental Psychology, 10*, 12–21.

Brydges, C. R., Fox, A. M., Reid, C. L., & Anderson, M. (2014). The differentiation of executive functions in middle and late childhood: A longitudinal latent-variable analysis. *Intelligence, 47*, 34–43. https://doi.org/10.1016/j.intell.2014.08.010

Cohen, M. J. (1997). *Children's memory scale*. San Antonio, TX: The Psychological Corporation.

Conners, C. K., & Staff, M. H. S. (Eds.). (2015a). *Conners' continuous auditory test of attention III: Computer program for windows technical guide and software manual*. North Tonawanda, NY: Multi-Health Systems.

Conners, C. K., & Staff, M. H. S. (Eds.). (2015b). *Conners' continuous performance test III: Computer program for windows technical guide and software manual*. North Tonawanda, NY: Multi-Health Systems.

Crawford, J. R., Sutherland, D., & Garthwaite, P. H. (2008). On the reliability and standard errors of measurement of contrast measures from the D-KEFS. *Journal of the International Neuropsychological Society, 14*, 1069–1073. https://doi.org/10.1017/S1355617708081228

D'Elia, L. F., Satz, P., Uchiyama, C. L., & White, T. (1996). *Color trails test*. Odessa, FL: PAR.

Delis, D. C., Kaplan, E., & Kramer, J. H. (2001). *Delis-Kaplan executive function system (D-KEFS)*. New York, NY: Psychological Corporation.

Delis, D. C., Kramer, J. H., Kaplan, E., & Ober, B. A. (1994). *Manual for the California verbal learning test for children*. New York, NY: Psychological Corporation.

Dyche, G. M., & Johnson, D. A. (1991). Development and evaluation of CHIPASAT, an attention test for children: II. Test-retest reliability and practice effect for a normal sample. *Perceptual and Motor Skills, 72*, 563–572.

Fallows, R. R., & Hilsabeck, R. C. (2013). Comparing two methods of delivering neuropsychological feedback. *Archives of Clinical Neuropsychology, 28*, 180–188. https://doi.org/10.1093/arclin/acs142

Fan, J., McCandliss, B. D., Sommer, T., Raz, A., & Posner, M. I. (2002). Testing the efficiency and independence of attentional networks. *Journal of Cognitive Neuroscience, 14*(3), 340–347.

Fernandez-Duque, D., & Posner, M. I. (1997). Relating the mechanisms of orienting and alerting. *Neuropsychologia, 35*, 477–486.

Fletcher, J. M., & Miciak, J. (2017). Comprehensive cognitive assessments are not necessary for the identification and treatment of learning disabilities. *Archives of Clinical Neuropsychology, 32*, 2–7. https://doi.org/10.1093/arclin/acw103

Friedman, N. P., Miyake, A., Young, S. E., DeFries, J. C., Corley, R. P., & Hewitt, J. K. (2008). Individual differences in executive functions are almost entirely genetic in origin. *Journal of Experimental Psychology: General, 137*(2), 201.

Friedman, N. P., & Miyake, A. (2016). Unity and diversity of executive functions: Individual differences as a window on cognitive structure. *Cortex, 86*, 186–204. https://doi.org/10.1016/j.cortex.2016.04.023

Gathercole, S. E., Pickering, S. J., Knight, C., & Stegmann, Z. (2004). Working memory skills and educational attainment: Evidence from national curriculum assessments at 7 and 14 years of age. *Applied Cognitive Psychology, 18*, 1–16. https://doi.org/10.1002/acp.934

Greenaway, M. C., Hanna, S. M., Lepore, S. W., & Smith, G. E. (2008). A behavioral rehabilitation intervention for amnestic mild cognitive impairment. *American Journal of Alzheimer's Disease and Other Dementias, 23*, 451–461. https://doi.org/10.1177/1533317508320352

Heaton, R. K., Chelune, G. J., Talley, J. L., Kay, G. G., & Curtis, G. (1993). *Wisconsin card sorting test (WCST) manual, revised and expanded*. Odessa, FL: Psychological Assessment Resources.

Huang-Pollock, C., Shapiro, Z., Galloway-Long, H., & Weigard, A. (2016). Is poor working memory a Transdiagnostic risk factor for psychopathology? *Journal of Abnormal Child Psychology*. https://doi.org/10.1007/s10802-016-0219-8 Advance Online Publication.

Itti, L., & Koch, C. (2001). Computational modelling of visual attention. *Nature Reviews Neuroscience, 2*, 194–203.

Kirkwood, M. W. (2015a). A rationale for performance validity testing in child and adolescent assessment. In M. W. Kirkwood (Ed.), *Validity testing in child and adolescent assessment evaluating exaggeration, feigning, and noncredible effort*. New York, NY: The Guilford Press.

Kirkwood, M. W. (2015b). Review of pediatric performance and symptom validity tests. In M. W. Kirkwood (Ed.), *Validity testing in child and adolescent assessment evaluating exaggeration, feigning, and noncredible effort*. New York, NY: The Guilford Press.

Klin, A., Saulnier, C., Tsatsanis, K., & Volkmar, F. R. (2005). Clinical evaluation in autism Spectrum disorders: Psychological assessment within a transdisciplinary framework. In F. R. Volkmar, R. Paul, A. Klin, & D. Cohen (Eds.), *Handbook of autism and pervasive developmental disorders* (Vol. 2, 3rd ed.). Hoboken, NJ: John Wiley & Sons, Inc.

Lamar, M., & Raz, A. (2007). Neuropsychological assessment of attention and executive functioning. *Cambridge handbook of psychology, health, and medicine*. 2nd ed, 290–294.

Larrabee, G. J. (2014). Test Validity and Performance Validity: Considerations in Providing a Framework for Development of an Ability-Focused Neuropsychological Test Battery. *Archives of Clinical Neuropsychology, 29*(7), 695–714.

Latzman, R. D., & Markon, K. E. (2010). The factor structure and age-related factorial invariance of the delis–Kaplan executive function system (D-KEFS). *Assessment, 17*, 172–184. https://doi.org/10.1177/1073191109356254

Lezak, M. D., Howieson, D. B., & Loring, D. W. (2004). The behavioral geography of the brain. *Neuropsychological Assessment, 4*, 39–85.

Lezak, M. D., Howieson, D. B., Loring, D. W., Hannay, H. J., & Fischer, J. S. (2004). Neuropsychological Assessment 4th edition Oxford University Press. New York.

Llorente, A. M., Williams, J., Satz, P., & D'Elia, L. F. (2003). *Children's color trails test (CCTT)*. Odessa, FL: PAR.

Luna, B., Garver, K. E., Urban, T. A., Lazar, N. A., & Sweeney, J. A. (2004). Maturation of cognitive processes from late childhood to adulthood. *Child Development, 75*, 1357–1372.

Luna, B., Thulborn, K. R., Munoz, D. P., Merriam, E. P., Garver, K. E., Minshew, N. J., … Sweeney, J. A. (2001). Maturation of widely distributed brain function subserves cognitive development. *NeuroImage, 13*, 786–793.

Manly, T., Robertson, I. H., Anderson, V., & Nimmo-Smith, I. (2001). *TEA-Ch: The test of everyday attention for children*. Bury St. Edmunds, UK: Thames Valley Test Company.

Mayes, S. D., & Calhoun, S. L. (2006). WISC-IV and WISC-III profiles in children with ADHD. *Journal of Attention Disorders, 9*, 486–493. https://doi.org/10.1177/1087054705283616

McGrew, K. S. (2009). CHC theory and the human cognitive abilities project: Standing on the shoulders of the giants of psychometric intelligence research. *Intelligence, 37*, 1–10. https://doi.org/10.1016/j.intell.2008.08.004

Meth, M., Calamia, M., & Tranel, D. (2016). Does a simple intervention enhance memory and adherence for neuropsychological recommendations? *Applied Neuropsychology: Adult*. https://doi.org/10.1080/23279095.2014.996881

Miyake, A., Friedman, N. P., Emerson, M. J., Witzki, A. H., Howerter, A., & Wager, T. D. (2000). The unity and diversity of executive functions and their

contributions to complex "frontal lobe" tasks: A latent variable analysis. *Cognitive Psychology, 41*(1), 49–100.
National Center for Education Statistics. (1984). Quality of responses of high school students to questionnaire items. Washington, DC: U.S. Government Printing Office.
O'Flahavan, J., Gambrell, L. B., Guthrie, J., Stahl, S., Baumann, J., & Alvermann, D. (1992). Poll results guide activities of research center. *Reading Today, 10*, 12.
Osterrieth, P. A. (1944). The test of copying a complex figure: A contribution to the study of perception and memory. *Archives de Psychologie, 30*, 286–356.
Paniak, C. E., Millar, H. B., Murphy, D., & Keizer, J. (1997). A consonant trigrams test for children: Development and norms. *The Clinical Neuropsychologist, 11*, 198–200. https://doi.org/10.1093/arclin/11.5.431a
Pennington, B. F., & Ozonoff, S. (1996). Executive functions and developmental psychopathology. *Journal of Child Psychology and Psychiatry, 37*, 51–87.
Peterson, E., & Peterson, R. L. (2015). A understanding deception from a developmental perspective. In M. W. Kirkwood (Ed.), *Validity testing in child and adolescent assessment evaluating exaggeration, feigning, and noncredible effort*. New York, NY: The Guilford Press.
Peterson, L., & Peterson, M. J. (1959). Short-term retention of individual verbal items. *Journal of Experimental Psychology, 58*, 193.
Rabin, L. A., Paolillo, E., & Barr, W. B. (2016). Stability in test-usage practices of clinical neuropsychologists in the United States and Canada over a 10-year period: A follow-up survey of INS and NAN members. *Archives of Clinical Neuropsychology, 31*, 206–230. https://doi.org/10.1093/arclin/acw007
Raz, A. (2004). Anatomy of attentional networks. In *The anatomical record part B: The new anatomist* (Vol. 281, pp. 21–36).
Roid, G. H. (2003). *Stanford-Binet intelligence scales, fifth edition*. Itasca, IL: Riverside Publishing.
Ruff, R. M. (2003). A friendly critique of neuropsychology: Facing the challenges of our future. *Archives of Clinical Neuropsychology, 18*, 847–864. https://doi.org/10.1016/j.acn.2003.07.002
Schacter, D. L., Wagner, A. D., & Buckner, R. L. (2000). Memory systems of 1999. In E. Tulving & F. I. M. Craik (Eds.), *The Oxford handbook of memory*. New York, NY: Oxford University Press.
Scherf, K. S., Sweeney, J. A., & Luna, B. (2006). Brain basis of developmental change in visuospatial working memory. *Journal of Cognitive Neuroscience, 18*, 1045–1058.
Schneider, J. W., & Kaufman, A. S. (2017). Let's not do away with comprehensive cognitive assessments just yet. *Archives of Clinical Neuropsychology, 32*, 8–20. https://doi.org/10.1093/arclin/acw104

Schrank, F. A., Mather, N., & McGrew, K. S. (2014). *Woodcock-Johnson IV tests of achievement*. Rolling Meadows, IL: Riverside.
Sherman, E. M. S., & Brooks, B. L. (2015a). *Child and adolescent memory profile (ChAMP)*. Lutz, FL: Psychological Assessment Resources.
Sherman, E. M. S., & Brooks, B. L. (2015b). *Memory validity profile*. Lutz, FL: Psychological Assessment Resources.
Sheslow, D., & Adams, W. (2003). *Wide range assessment of memory and learning, second edition*. Lutz, FL: Psychological Assessment Resources.
Shin, M. S., Choi, H., Kim, H., Hwang, J. W., Kim, B. N., & Cho, S. C. (2008). A study of neuropsychological deficit in children with obsessive-compulsive disorder. *European Psychiatry, 23*, 512–520. https://doi.org/10.1016/j.eurpsy.2008.03.010
Sotelo-Dynega, M., & Dixon, S. G. (2014). Cognitive assessment practices: A survey of school psychologists. *Psychology in the Schools, 51*, 1031–1045. https://doi.org/10.1002/pits.21802
Squire, L. R. (1987). *Memory and brain*. New York, NY: Oxford University Press.
Suhr, J. (2015). *Psychological assessment: A problem solving approach*. New York, NY: The Guilford Press.
Sweet, J. J., Benson, L. M., Nelson, N. W., & Moberg, P. J. (2015). The American Academy of Clinical Neuropsychology, National Academy of Neuropsychology, and Society for Clinical Neuropsychology (APA Division 40) 2015 TCN professional practice and 'salary survey': Professional practices, beliefs, and incomes of US neuropsychologists. *The Clinical Neuropsychologist, 29*, 1069–1162. https://doi.org/10.1080/13854046.2016.1140228
Tharinger, D. J., & Pilgrim, S. (2012). Parent and child experiences of neuropsychological assessment as a function of child feedback by individualized fable. *Child Neuropsychology, 18*, 228–241. https://doi.org/10.1080/09297049.2011.595708
Tulving, E. (2000). Concepts of memory. The Oxford handbook of memory, 33–43.
Tulving, E. (2002). Episodic memory: From mind to brain. *Annual Review of Psychology, 53*, 1–25. https://doi.org/10.1146/annurev.psych.53.100901.135114
Wagner, S., Müller, C., Helmreich, I., Huss, M., & Tadić, A. (2015). A meta-analysis of cognitive functions in children and adolescents with major depressive disorder. *European Child & Adolescent Psychiatry, 24*, 5–19. https://doi.org/10.1007/s00787-014-0559-2
Wechsler, D. (2014). *Wechsler intelligence scale for children* (5th ed.). San Antonio, TX: Pearson.
Westervelt, H. J., Brown, L. B., Tremont, G., Javorsky, D. J., & Stern, R. A. (2007). Patient and family perceptions of the neuropsychological evaluation:

How are we doing? *The Clinical Neuropsychologist, 21*, 263–273. https://doi.org/10.1080/13854040500519745

Wiebe, S. A., Sheffield, T., Nelson, J. M., Clark, C. A., Chevalier, N., & Espy, K. A. (2011). The structure of executive function in 3-year-olds. *Journal of Experimental Child Psychology, 108*, 436–452. https://doi.org/10.1016/j.jecp.2010.08.008

Wolfe, J. M., Horowitz, T. S., Kenner, N., Hyle, M., & Vasan, N. (2004). How fast can you change your mind? The speed of top-down guidance in visual search. *Vision Research, 44*, 1411–1426.

The Assessment of ADHD in Persons with Developmental Disabilities

Pamela McPherson, Michelle Yetman, Claire O. Burns, and Bob Wynn

Vignette

Anthony is an 11-year-old boy with intellectual disability (ID) receiving special education services. His teacher has documented that he is unable to focus, even with direct one-on-one instruction. He is very impulsive compared to the other students in the class. In fact, his impulsivity has become a safety concern. On two occasions, Anthony ran from the classroom. He has had trouble waiting his turn and listening to his teacher. He constantly blurts out comments or makes noises during work time. Weekly conduct notes home indicate that he frequently disrupts the class. Anthony's parents have observed that he cannot sit still to complete homework and is distracted from simple tasks. Even with accommodations for ID, Anthony's behavior is impairing his progress. His teacher has tracked his lack of progress in the classroom under the school district's response to intervention (RtI) protocol (see education section below). When tier interventions did not provide the help he needed, his teacher and parents questioned the possibility of ADHD. Anthony's parents sought the advice of his pediatrician.

Reviewing Anthony's history, his pediatrician recalled referring the family to the local zero-to-three early intervention program to address Anthony's developmental delays. The home-based program provided physical therapy to help Anthony learn to walk and later speech therapy. When Anthony entered second grade, the school psychologist tested Anthony and explained that his delays were due to an intellectual disability. She explained that it was mild and that Anthony would benefit from receiving special education services. The school has conducted annual meetings to review Anthony's progress and update his individualized educational program (IEP). The pediatrician asked the parents and teacher to complete behavior screening forms. When the results indicated possible ADHD, a psychological referral was made for a full assessment.

P. McPherson (✉)
Northwest Louisiana Human Services District, Shreveport, LA, USA
e-mail: Pamela.McPherson@LA.GOV

B. Wynn · M. Yetman
Louisiana State University Health Sciences Center, Shreveport, LA, USA

C. O. Burns
Louisiana State University, Department of Psychology, Baton Rouge, LA, USA

Overview of ADHD in Children with Developmental Disabilities

Attention deficit hyperactivity disorder (ADHD) is the most common neurodevelopmental disorder diagnosed in childhood. A recent meta-analysis of 175 studies reported a prevalence rate of 7.2% (Thomas, Sanders, Doust, Beller, &

Glasziou, 2015). Significant educational, psychological, and medical resources are expended in the assessment and treatment of persons with ADHD, with estimates in excess of $100 billion annually (Doshi et al., 2012). The National Survey of Children's Health (NSCH) indicates that 11%, approximately 6.4 million children, received treatment for ADHD in 2011 (Visser et al., 2014). This represents a significant increase from the 9.4% reported by the NSCH in 2003 (Visser et al., 2014; Bramlett & Blumberg, 2007). Treatment rates may be greater than prevalence rates because children with developmental disabilities are often excluded from ADHD research. In fact, until 2013 the Diagnostic and Statistical Manual of the American Psychiatric Association did not allow the diagnosis of ADHD in children with intellectual disability.

The NSCH documented that among children with ADHD, comorbid conditions are the rule rather than the exception; 67% of children with ADHD had a comorbid condition, including 46% with a learning disability, 12% with speech issues, and 6% with autism (Larson, Russ, Kahn, & Halfon, 2011). ADHD is comorbid in approximately 50% of youth with fragile X syndrome (Vortsman & Ophoff, 2013). ADHD is estimated to be present in 22.5% of children with cerebral palsy (Gabis, Tsubary, Leon, Ashkenasi, & Shefer, 2015). Recent meta-analysis reported a 51.2% prevalence of ADHD among youth with fetal alcohol syndrome disorder (FASD) (Han et al., 2015; Millichap, 2008; Popova et al., 2016). Tobacco use can result in intrauterine growth retardation (Milnerowicz-Nabzdyk & Bizon, 2014). This in turn causes low birth weight and developmental complications. Maternal smoking and maternal nicotine replacement use during pregnancy are associated with increased risk of ADHD (Joelsson et al., 2016; Zhu et al., 2014). The use of illicit substances during fetal development is associated with birth defects which contribute to developmental disorders, including ADHD (Hagan et al., 2016; Konijnenberg, 2015). Postnatal lead exposure has been linked to higher risk of clinical ADHD (Kim, Lee, Lee, & Hong, 2014). See Table 1.

Table 1 Frequency of ADHD in selected developmental disabilities

Developmental disability	Frequency of co-occurring ADHD
Preterm children	10–30.6%
Intellectual disability	18–40%
Cerebral palsy	22.5%
Autism spectrum disorders	22–83%
Fetal alcohol spectrum disorders	49.4–94%
Fragile X syndrome	49.3%
Velocardial facial syndrome	35–55%

Approximately 3% of the population is estimated to have intellectual disability with an intelligence quotient <70; and within this population, ADHD is the most common comorbid mental health diagnosis (Ageranioti-Bélanger et al., 2012; Hastings, Beck, Daley, & Hill, 2005; La Malfa, Lassi, Bertelli, Pallanti, & Albertini, 2008; Neece, Baker, & Lee, 2013). The impact of ADHD on intellectual function and the inverse, the impact of intellectual function on ADHD, have been matters of psychometric and broader clinical debate. Until recently it was generally accepted that ADHD did not significantly lower IQ. A meta-analysis found that children with ADHD (without ID), scored approximately 9 IQ points lower than peers without ADHD (Frazier, Demaree, & Youngstrom, 2004). A study by Bridgett and Walker (2006) replicated this finding in adults but cautioned that the difference was small and likely reflects only a subset of individuals with ADHD. The greater controversy has been the relationship between ID and ADHD. Historically, ADHD symptoms among an ID population were considered to be part of the ID diagnosis, as such ADHD symptoms were considered to be common features in this population (Einfeld & Aman, 1995; Gjaerum & Bjornerem, 2003; Hurley, 1996). The widely held belief that ADHD symptoms were inherent in an ID population discouraged comorbid diagnosis and curtailed ADHD research among youth with ID (Antschel, Phillips, Gordon, Barkley & Faraone, 2006).

More recently, numerous large-scale studies have examined the association between children who have ID and ADHD. Approximately 18–40% of children with an intellectual disability (ID) meet criteria for ADHD (Epstein, Cullinan, & Polloway; 1986; Koller, Richardson, Katz, & McLaren, 1983; Pearson & Aman, 1994; Stromme & Diseth, 2000). Emerson (2003) conducted a population-based study examining the prevalence of psychiatric disorders among children and adolescents with and without ID. Using a clinical interview, Emerson compared ICD-10 diagnoses, including hyperkinesis. The ID population presented with the diagnosis of hyperkinesis at a rate of 8.7%, in contrast to the non-ID population, rate of 0.9%. The youth with ID showed a tenfold greater risk for hyperkinesis. These studies have concluded that the prevalence of ADHD symptoms cannot be explained by rater bias or by co-occurring psychiatric conditions separate from ADHD (Hastings et al., 2005; Simonoff, Pickles, Wood, Gringras, & Chadwick, 2007). The ADHD symptoms met criteria for comorbid ADHD (Pliszka, 2009). Subsequent research has supported findings that children with ID are at an increased risk for ADHD. Risk increases in relation to the severity of intellectual disability (Voigt, Barbaresi, Colligan, Weaver, & Katusic, 2006). The association of lower IQ with increased ADHD risk has been documented in the normal range of intellectual functioning and the mild to moderate ID range (Simonoff et al., 2007).

Studies have shown that a relationship exists between lower IQ and increased disability due to ADHD (Kuntsi et al., 2004). For persons with ADHD, disability is common and occurs in multiple settings. Longitudinal studies have demonstrated that ADHD symptoms remain clinically significant in most ADHD patients into adulthood (Weiss and Weiss, 2004). Impairment may become significant when structure and social supports provided by family and school decrease. Once out of high school, young adults may face a less scheduled or routine environment or a change of living situations or start a job (Wagner, Newman, & Javitz, 2014). Stresses such as vocational training or emotional stress from changing relationships, having children, handling finances, and other factors may lead to increased impairment due to ADHD symptoms.

Abbreviated History of the ADHD Diagnosis

Symptoms that we now associate with ADHD first appeared in the medical literature over 200 years ago (Lange, Reichl, Lange, Tucha, & Tucha, 2010). Over time, the etiology of ADHD has been explained as moral deficiency, poor parenting, nerve disturbances, encephalitis, catecholamine imbalance, cortical inhibition, and lesions of the brain stem (Baumeister, Henderson, Pow, & Advokat, 2012). Multiple risk factors for ADHD including genetic markers, prenatal toxin exposure, and early environmental experiences have been identified and suggest an early and stable etiology (Arnett, MacDonald, & Pennington, 2013). Some risk factors for intellectual disability such as low birth weight or preterm birth are also shared with ADHD (Morales, Polizzi, Sulliotti, Mascolino, & Perricone, 2013).

Baumeister et al. (2012) outlined the evolution of theories regarding the etiology of ADHD over the last 200 years. Baumeister linked the first account of ADHD to Crichton in 1798, who associated this disorder with nerve disturbances, although some accounts posit that Weikard described similar features (e.g., inattentive, overactive impulse) 20 years earlier (Niggs & Barkley, 2014). Following these early accounts, several other clinical descriptions were recorded (see Niggs & Barkley, 2014, for specific accounts). In the early 1900s, encephalitis, with basal ganglia and brain stem involvement, was implicated in ADHD symptoms such as impulsivity and overactivity. The children surviving the epidemic were some of the first to be treated with stimulant medication for symptoms of hyperactivity (Baumeister et al., 2012, Bradley, 1937; Niggs & Barkley, 2014).

The role of the brain stem was further supported by Kahn and Cohen's theory of "organic drivenness," which they believed caused hyperkinesis (Kahn & Cohen, 1934, cited from Baumeister et al., 2012). They expanded on previous research by suggesting that organicity was not caused solely by encephalitis but could have many etiologies (Baumeister et al., 2012). These findings contributed to the prevailing theory of the time that neurodevelopmental disorders such as intellectual disability were "brain-injured child syndromes." Children who displayed behavioral concerns associated with hyperactivity were considered to have "minimal brain dysfunction" (Nigg & Barkley, 2014). Minimal brain damage or dysfunction (MBD) represented the prominent theory of ADHD at the time, highlighting a neurological etiology and focus on cognitive abilities (Taylor, 2011).

The advent of EEGs provided additional evidence for the role of neurological differences in children with behavioral symptoms characteristic of ADHD. Early studies found abnormalities in EEGs for children with hyperactive symptoms, which researchers hypothesized were due to differences in cortical systems (Knobel, Wolman, & Mason, 1959). Research on ADHD shifted toward neuropsychological testing around the 1950s with research focused on using neuropsychological measures to assess and diagnose disorders that were considered organic brain disorders (Baumeister et al., 2012). This trend has continued, as assessment of ADHD currently typically includes psychological measures. However, there is continued debate over whether ADHD has a primarily neurological or behavioral/psychosocial basis. Cultural differences in such viewpoints have been reported, as many North American countries view ADHD as a neurodevelopmental disorder, while European countries historically perceived the disorder as a behavioral one related to conduct disorder (Niggs & Barkley, 2014).

Burks (1960) first used the term "hyperactive child syndrome," hypothesizing that ADHD symptoms were related to cortical overstimulation (Niggs & Barkley, 2014). These findings reinforced the hypothesis that hyperactive symptoms had an organic origin, providing further support for the use of pharmacological interventions (Baumeister et al., 2012). In 1970, Kornetsky (cited in Baumeister et al., 2012) proposed the "catecholamine hypothesis" based on observations of the effect of amphetamine on individuals with hyperactivity. He hypothesized that hyperkinetic activity was caused by an excess of norepinephrine and that amphetamines inhibit this monoamine. More recently scientific advances have shown that stimulant medications actually do the opposite; however, his hypothesis set the stage for further research in to the role of catecholamines in ADHD (Baumeister et al., 2012). Although the DSM-5 states that no specific biological markers can be used solely for diagnosis (APA, 2013), there is substantial evidence of neurological and genetic contributions (Niggs & Barkley, 2014). Magnetic resonance imaging (MRI) is exploring the neural signatures of ADHD subtypes (Fair et al., 2012). Whole-genome sequencing is providing evidence of the genetic and epigenetic influences in the etiology of "neurodevelopmental spectrum disorders" including ADHD, ID, and ASD (Kiser, Rivero, & Lesch, 2015).

Official Classification of ADHD

Over time neuropsychological advances have informed our understanding of ADHD. This is reflected in shifting terminology that can be confusing. Tracking the name changes through the editions of the Diagnostic and Statistical Manual helps explain the variety of terms in the literature and the "Does he have ADD or ADHD?" questions from parents. What is now called ADHD was first formally recognized as a diagnosis in the DSM-II (APA, 1968) as "hyperkinetic reaction of childhood." This name reflects psychologist's observations and measurements of behavior leading to a shift from the idea of brain damage as a cause for ADHD symptoms.

As neuropsychological advances expanded, our understanding of brain function focus shifted to the inattention symptom domain. Douglas (1972) emphasized the role of core difficulties that included ability to sustain attention, ability to inhibit impulsivity, and organized planning. Douglas highlighted the importance of integrating information from multiple sources (e.g., teacher report, parent report, behavioral observations, and clinical tests) in making a diagnosis. This conceptualization gave rise to performance-based measures, such as the Conners' Continuous Performance Test, third edition (CPT-3; Conners, 2008), which assesses difficulties with attention. The pattern of responses can indicate symptoms such as inattention, impulsivity, vigilance issues, or difficulties with arousal (Conners & Sitarenios, 2011). This is reflected in the DSM-III (American Psychiatric Association, 1980) shift to "attention deficit disorder."

The DSM-III was the first version to use the terminology "attention deficit disorder" allowing for the specifier "with or without hyperactivity." This marked an important shift, as it acknowledged that children may meet criteria if they were inattentive but lacked hyperactive behaviors (Niggs & Barkley, 2014). The DSM-III specifically precluded the diagnosis of ADHD in children with ID or PDD (Mallett, Natarajan, & Hoy, 2014). The name "attention-deficit/hyperactivity disorder" was first used in DSM-III-R in 1987, though subtypes related to inattention and hyperactivity were not included until DSM-IV in 1994 (American Psychiatric Association, 2000). The DSM-III-R allowed the diagnosis of ADD in children with ID but not pervasive developmental disorders (Mallet et al., 2014). Under DSM-IV criteria, ADHD was diagnosed in children with "mental retardation" only when the symptoms of inattention or hyperactivity are excessive for the child's mental age (p. 82, APA, 1994). While acknowledging the co-occurrence of ADHD and ID, the DSM-IV did not provide guidance to clinicians as to how to best determine when symptoms are excessive (Antschel et al. 2006).

The *Diagnostic and Statistical Manual, Fifth Edition* (DSM-5) states ADHD is a neurodevelopmental disorder (American Psychiatric Association, 2013). A major shift in the DSM-5 is that ASD is no longer considered an exclusionary diagnosis for ADHD (American Psychiatric Association, 2013). Prior to DSM-5, individuals with ASD could not receive a comorbid diagnosis of ADHD, as symptoms of hyperactivity and inattention were thought to be better explained by autism symptomology. However, recent research has indicated that the etiological and developmental mechanisms associated with these two disorders are distinct (May, Sciberras, Hiscock, & Rinehart, 2016). This shift raises additional considerations in the assessment of comorbid ASD and ADHD. For individuals with an existing ASD diagnosis, Mahajan et al. (2012) recommend that the individual receive a comprehensive ADHD evaluation if they display ADHD symptoms that do not improve through the intervention plan to target difficulties associated with ASD. Although intervention approaches may overlap, there are often different recommended treatment approaches for ASD and ADHD (May et al., 2016).

In parallel to the DSM, the International Classification of Diseases (ICD) has evolved from a descriptive to etiologically based diagnostic approach. The ICD system of classification dates to the early 1900s. The early versions were called the *International List of Causes of Death*. By the 1940s, the World Health Organization assumed major responsibilities for the ICD with a major shift toward disease classification. At the time of the 9th revision of the ICD in the mid-1970s, a standard international terminology for mental disorders did not exist. The process of integrating DSM and ICD classification systems was initiated with a major shift in the ICD which included a new section "Mental and Behavioral Disorders." Since October 2015 the United States has used the ICD-10-CM for federal billing purposes. The ICD 11 is scheduled for release in 2018 (French, 2015). Despite the changes in terminology, research has supported the stable description of core symptoms of ADHD across revisions of the DSM and ICD (Moriyama, Loy, Robb-Smith, Rosenberg, & Hoyert, 2011).

Overview of the Assessment of ADHD

Although ADHD is a common diagnosis, the assessment is not simple. There is no single test or checklist to diagnose ADHD. First, the clinician is faced with the task of verifying the presence of hyperactivity, inattention, and impulsivity in excess of the level expected for mental age (American Psychiatric Association, 2013). This requires knowledge of typical development as well as the developmental trajectories of persons

Table 2 Conditions mistaken for ADHD in children with developmental disabilities

Psychological	Medical	Social
Anxiety disorder	Seizures	Inappropriate expectations
Oppositional defiant disorder	Infections	Stressors
Disruptive mood dysregulation disorder	Sleep apnea	Bullying
PTSD	Metabolic disorders	
Substance use	Lead/toxin exposures	
Reactive attachment disorder	Sensory impairment	
Intermittent explosive disorder	Diabetes	
Depressive disorder	Tourette's syndrome	
	Head trauma	
	Allergies	
	Medication side effect	
	Illicit substances	

with intellectual disability, autism, and other developmental disabilities. Next, symptoms must be documented in more than one setting. Caregivers at home, school, day care, and/or work environments must be queried with sensitivity to familial and cultural expectations. Finally, the clinician's skill is tested by the third task – ruling out social, environmental, psychological, or medical issues as causes for the symptoms. The diagnosis of ADHD can only be made when there is no other explanation for the symptoms of hyperactivity, inattention, and impulsivity (see Table 2). The assessment for ADHD requires clinical expertise to obtain developmental, social, and medical histories and well-honed professional judgment to integrate this history with skilled observation and information from collateral sources.

The assessment of ADHD may require several office visits to review medical history, social history, educational history, and family history and conduct clinical interviews and observations (Taylor et al., 2004). Assessment for co-occurring behavioral disturbances must be completed as well. Reassessment should be conducted annually or with changes in symptoms. The level of impairment must be continually evaluated to inform therapeutic and educational interventions (Pliszka, 2009).

The DSM-5 encourages comparing the severity of ADHD symptoms to peers of comparable mental age. To assist the diagnostician, the DSM-5 (APA, 2013) includes age-appropriate examples of symptoms. When assessing children with developmental disabilities for ADHD, it is important to make the differentiation between normative levels of hyperactivity and inattention for the individual's chronological vs. mental age. In fact, the individual's developmental level and intellectual function should be a primary consideration in the assessment of ADHD symptoms (May et al., 2016). The assessment of ADHD in persons with developmental disabilities is challenging, requiring psychologists, teachers, physicians, and families to work in unison.

Current Diagnostic Criteria

The DSM-5 classifies attention deficit hyperactivity disorder as neurodevelopmental disorder with the onset of symptoms before the age of 12. The 18 symptoms of ADHD are divided into two symptom domains, inattention and hyperactivity/impulsivity. See Table 3. To meet criteria for the diagnosis, 6 symptoms in persons under 17 years, and 5 over 17, must be present for at least 6 months with a severity inappropriate for the person's developmental level. Symptoms must impair function in two or more settings (APA, 2013). Based on the symptoms present, ADHD may be characterized as combined presentation, predominantly inattentive presentation, or predominantly hyperactive-impulsive presentation. This characterization does not capture the diverse presentations of individuals with ADHD. Not only do the 18 core symptoms of ADHD combine in thousands of ways to yield the diagnosis, comorbidity is common. Thorough assessment is critical to formulate individualized patient interventions.

Table 3 Attention deficit hyperactivity disorder symptoms (Present in two settings at an incidence inappropriate for developmental level)

Inattention	Hyperactivity/impulsivity
1. Often fails to give close attention to details or makes careless mistakes in schoolwork, at work, or with other activities	1. Often fidgets with or taps hands or feet or squirms in seat
2. Often has trouble holding attention on tasks or play activities	2. Often leaves seat in situations when remaining seated is expected
3. Often does not seem to listen when spoken to directly	3. Often runs about or climbs in situations where it is not appropriate (adolescents or adults may be limited to feeling restless)
4. Often does not follow through on instructions and fails to finish schoolwork, chores, or duties in the workplace (e.g., loses focus, side-tracked)	4. Often unable to play or take part in leisure activities quietly
5. Often has trouble organizing tasks and activities	5. Is often "on the go" acting as if "driven by a motor"
6. Often avoids, dislikes, or is reluctant to do tasks that require mental effort over a long period of time (such as schoolwork or homework)	6. Often talks excessively
7. Often loses things necessary for tasks and activities (e.g., school materials, pencils, books, tools, wallets, keys, paperwork, eyeglasses, mobile telephones)	7. Often blurts out an answer before a question has been completed
8. Is often easily distracted	8. Often has trouble waiting his/her turn
9. Is often forgetful in daily activities	9. Often interrupts or intrudes on others (e.g., butts into conversations or games)

Professional Guidelines for the Assessment of ADHD

The American Academy of Pediatrics, American Academy of Child and Adolescent Psychiatry, American Academy of Family Practitioners, the American Academy of Neurologists, and Autism Speaks are among the organizations with guidelines on ADHD. The American Academy of Pediatrics (AAP) clinical practice guideline for ADHD is endorsed by the American Psychological Association and warrants review.

In 2011, the American Academy of Pediatrics released new guidelines for diagnosis and treatment of ADHD titled *ADHD: Clinical Practice Guideline for the Diagnosis, Evaluation, and Treatment of Attention-Deficit/Hyperactivity Disorder in Children and Adolescents*. The Guideline recognizes ADHD as a chronic condition requiring special care. The clinician is advised to assess for comorbid conditions and rule out alternative causes for inattention, hyperactivity, and impulsivity. Age-specific treatment recommendations are noted (Fiks et al., 2016). The AAP website provides additional guidance and tools for the assessment, monitoring and treatment of ADHD.

The American Academy of Child and Adolescent Psychiatry (AACAP) released practice parameters in 2007. AACAP practice parameters recommend that the clinician carefully distinguish both symptoms and impairment with the reminder to document impairment in more than one setting. If a patient's symptoms are observed only at school but an inordinate amount of time is spent finishing schoolwork at home, the multiple setting requirement would be met (Pliszka, 2009). The importance of assessing familial issues is also noted. ADHD is highly heritable, necessitating family history and family function inquiry during the clinical assessment.

Screening Versus Assessment

The American Psychological Association defines screening as brief queries to determine the need for a full diagnostic assessment. Screening instruments are designed to identify persons with symptoms of a specific disorder but are not sufficient to diagnose a specific disorder (American Psychological Association, 2017). For the purposes of this chapter, screening and assessment for ADHD include observations and questions that may be obtained in person or through the completion of standardized instruments. Screening for ADHD alerts the clinician to selected symptoms of ADHD. Assessment for ADHD contains queries for all 18 DSM-5 ADHD symptoms and comprehensive evaluation.

Screening

Educational Screening

Vignette
Anthony is an 11-year-old boy with intellectual disability (ID) receiving special education services. His teacher has tracked his lack of progress in the classroom under the school district's response to intervention (RtI) protocol. When tier interventions did not provide the help he needed, his teacher and parents questioned the possibility of ADHD.

The academic, behavioral, and social demands of the school setting often present challenges to children with ADHD. Federal law provides for students with challenges under the Individuals with Disability Education Act (IDEA). The IDEA was enacted in 1975 to ensure a free and appropriate public education (FAPE) for children with disabilities. The IDEA details the requirements for individualized educational plans (IEPs) for students who do not benefit from routine instruction. The first step toward an IEP is tier interventions as part of response to intervention (RtI). RtI does not qualify as special education under IDEA. Federal law encourages intervention without labeling students; therefore tier interventions occur without an educational assessment or assignment of an exceptionality (Preston, Wood, & Stecker, 2015). In order to promote the early identification and prompt intervention for struggling students, educators have implemented response to intervention (RtI) (Haraway, 2012).

RtI addresses the academic and behavioral needs of students. Academic progress is monitored with reading and math achievement screening many times each school year. Behavioral needs are monitored via school-wide Positive Behavioral Supports and Interventions (Haraway, 2012). RtI typically includes three tiers. Tier one is considered a "core instructional intervention" and offered to all students. Tier two interventions are offered to at-risk students, and tier three interventions are individualized interventions (Berkeley, Bender, Peaster, & Saunders, 2009). Anthony's teacher started the school year introducing a tier one behavioral RtI in the form of a classroom behavior management program with rewards and consequences and daily conduct grades. When positive behavioral supports of tier one did not provide the supports Anthony needed, his teacher referred him to a tier two behavior skills group. When Anthony continued to struggle, she requested a tier three functional behavioral assessment. Tier two and three interventions vary by school and state but may include small group interventions, check-ins with the school counselor, functional behavioral assessment, and/or teaching self-monitoring and regulation skills (Smith, Cumming, Merrill, Pitts, & Daunic, 2015). The Individuals with Disabilities Education Improvement Act (IDEIA) and No Child Left Behind (NCLB) require schools to document tier interventions. If tier interventions prove insufficient to address challenges, a full assessment for special services should be requested by the parent in writing.

While grounded in decades of research, RtI was catapulted into schools following the mandates of the 2004 IDEIA and the 2001 NCLB (Fuchs & Fuchs, 2006). It is critical to understand that federal mandates promote RtI as a method of "early intervention and assessment." Federal mandates allow for schools to designate the exceptionality of specific learning disability and other health impairment without intellectual testing (Reynolds & Shaywitz, 2009).

Medical Screening

Vignette
Anthony's parents sought the advice of his pediatrician. After reviewing Anthony's history, his pediatrician asked the parents and teacher to complete behavior screening forms. When the results indicated possible ADHD, a psychological referral was made for a full assessment.

The AAP recommends developmental screening as a routine part of well-child medical visits (2014 Recommendations for Pediatric Preventive Health Care, 2014). This early screening allowed Anthony's pediatrician to identify motor and speech delays leading to an early intervention referral. Pediatricians and primary care providers are advised to initiate an ADHD assessment for children between 4 and 18 years old presenting with academic or behavioral problems due to symptoms including inattention, hyperactivity, or impulsiveness (AAP, 2011). As in Anthony's case, many parents seek the advice of their family physicians or pediatricians when a teacher raises concern about a possible ADHD diagnosis. In fact, the pediatrician or family practitioner diagnoses ADHD in 53% of cases involving children between 4 and 17 years of age as compared to 18% and 14% diagnosed by psychiatrists and psychologists, respectively (Visser, Danielson, & Wolraich, 2016). In complex cases involving developmental disability and ADHD symptoms, pediatricians often refer children to a psychologist for assessment after screening for medical etiologies for the symptoms of inattention, hyperactivity, and impulsivity.

The symptoms of ADHD may be due to a medical condition or psychological condition other than ADHD (French, 2015). Medical disorders such as sleep apnea, sensory impairment, thyroid disorders, lead poisoning, and metabolic disorders should be considered (Kolar et al., 2008). In addition, comorbid medical and psychological disorders are common. Common medical comorbidities include headache, seizure disorders, and chronic pain (Jameson, et al., 2016). Persons with ID are diagnosed with epilepsy at a rate three to four times higher than compared to the general population (Robertson et al., 2015). Children with autism experience numerous medical conditions at high rates (Kohane et al., 2012). The pediatrician may order laboratory studies, an EEG, genetic studies, or other diagnostic tests to fully explore medical conditions. If indicated by the history and medical evaluation, the pediatrician might consider referral to a medical specialist such as a neurologist, geneticist, endocrinologist, gastroenterologist, ENT/sleep specialist, or child and adolescent psychiatrist.

Psychological Screening

Vignette
On receiving the pediatrician's request for psychological assessment of Anthony's ADHD symptoms, the psychologist requested all medical and school records. In addition, the parents and teacher were asked to complete a detailed history form and complete a symptom checklist.

A cornerstone of any mental health assessment should include screening for signs and symptoms of ADHD (AACAP, 2007). In addition to specifically inquiring about symptoms of ADHD, clinicians should attempt to gather all pertinent documentation that could shed light onto how the child functions within the classroom. Documentation should include report cards, previous standardized testing, former evaluation reports (through the school system or privately), special education reports, IEPs, and medical records. After carefully reviewing the documentation and interviewing the parent for details of developmental disability and the presence of symptoms indicating possible ADHD or other mental disorders, the clinician can determine if a full psychological assessment is necessary (AACAP, 2007).

ADHD Screening and Assessment Instruments

ADHD symptoms have been found to occur at higher rates among children with intellectual disabilities when examined in large-scale population studies using rating questionnaires (Linna, Piha, Kumpulainen, Tamminen, & Almqvist, 1999). Computerized or pencil and paper instruments and checklists, such as the Vanderbilt and the Conners' Rating Scale (Conners, 2008), are often used in the screening process. These instruments are available in parent and teacher versions and have been shown to be useful screening tools

(Wolraich et al., 2003; DuPaul, Power, Anastopoulos, & Reid, 1998). Such instruments are easy to administer and score, fast, and economical and provide the clinician with immediate feedback regarding the need for a full assessment (Biederman et al., 1995). Few screening tools have been adapted for use in young children. Those that exist have limited evidence in prediction of later ADHD (Arnett et al., 2013). It is important to note that the diagnosis of ADHD should never be made from a rating scale alone (AACAP, 2007). A rating scale is merely one piece of a puzzle requiring clinical judgment to assemble the full diagnostic picture.

Common instruments used to assess and monitor ADHD are summarized in Table 4. The majority of these instruments have not been normed in an ID population. The Child Behavior Checklist is an exception (CBCL; Achenbach and Rescorla 2001). Einfeld and Tonge (1996) used a modified version of the CBCL (96 items) in one of the largest epidemiological studies of psychopathology in children with ID. Among the 507 children surveyed in the study, 40.7% qualified for ID with a comorbid severe emotional and behavior disorder. The Conners' Teachers Rating Scale (CTRS) has also been normed for children with ID. Fee, Matson, and Benavidez (1994)

Table 4 Common ADHD rating scales. The Conner's short or long versions may be scored by the parent, teacher, or child to screen for ADHD and comorbid issues in youth 6 to 18 years

Name of scale	Description
ADHD Rating Scale-IV (ADHD RS-IV)	An 18-item scale corresponding to the 18 items in the DSM criteria that is divided into 2 subscales: Hyperactivity/impulsivity and inattentiveness. Items are scored on a 4-point frequency scale ranging from 0 = never/rarely to 3 = very often. It has both a parent and teacher form. There is also a self-report version that is used less frequently due to individuals' general lack of insight. Contains 108 items divided into subscales that aligns with DSM-5 criteria for ADHD, oppositional defiant disorder, and conduct disorder. The instrument also provides ratings on the following scales: Inattention, hyperactivity/impulsivity, learning problems, executive functioning, defiance/aggression, peer relations, ADHD inattentive, ADHD hyperactive-impulsive, and ADHD Combined
Brown Rating Scales for Children and Adolescents	These scales come in two age versions, ages 3–7 years and 8–12 years. Self-report adolescent and adult versions also exist. These measures assess a wide range of symptoms of executive function impairments associated with ADHD
Conners' Rating Scale	
Child Behavior Checklist (CBCL/6-18)	The CBCL is a widely used measure for identifying problem behavior in youths ages 6–18 years. Consists of 120-question checklist with items scored On a 3-point scale from 0 = not true to 2 = very true or often true. Scoring provides information about the presence of possible syndromes and internalizing/externalizing problems
Home Situation Questionnaire-Revised (HSQ-R) School Situation Questionnaire-Revised (SSQ-R)	The HSQ-R is a 14-item scale designed to assess attention and concentration across home and public situations. This instrument uses a 9-point scale ranging from mild to severe. The SSQ-R examines the child's behavior across a range of school settings, e.g., classroom, recess, field trips, etc.
NICHQ Vanderbilt ADHD Teacher Rating Scale Parent Rating Scale	Available in the public domain, both scales are commonly used by health-care providers to evaluate ADHD symptoms. The teacher version assesses symptoms and performance within the school setting; parent version assesses perception of school performance and social functioning. Higher score indicates more severe symptoms, except for the performance section, where higher score indicates greater performance in academics and classroom behavior
SNAP-IV Teacher & Parent Rating Scale	This instrument is available in the public domain and allows parents or teachers to rate a child using DSM-IV criteria for ADHD symptoms. Informants rate each item on a 4-point Likert scale. 26 of the 90 items specifically address ADHD; the remaining items address other possible conditions contained in the DSM, including ODD, conduct disorder, OCD, anxiety, and numerous other conditions

used the CTRS to assess children with ADHD and children with ID and co-occurring ADHD. The authors had teachers rate 100 boys between the ages of 6 and 8 using the CTRS. The study divided 100 boys into 4 groups – children with ADHD without ID, children with ID, children with ADHD and ID, and a control group of typically developing children. The study found that the clinical profiles of children with ADHD and with ID/ADHD did not have significant differences with the exception of increased anxiety in ID youth. The CTRS is a useful instrument of screening and monitoring of ADHD symptoms in youth with ID.

The Conners' Parent Rating Scale (CPRS) does not need to be modified for use with children with ID. A small study conducted by Handen et al. (1997) compared mental versus chronological age norms in order to assess ADHD symptoms in children with intellectual disabilities. Using the CPRS, children were scored using both sets of norms, and results were statistically similar on the majority of the scales. The authors concluded that it is acceptable to use norms based on a child's chronological age when examining ADHD in an ID population. Other studies have supported this finding (Pearson & Aman, 1994).

The NICHQ Vanderbilt Assessment Scales are in the public domain. In addition to ADHD, the Vanderbilt screens for oppositional defiant disorder, conduct disorder, anxiety, and depression. The teacher version includes queries regarding academic progress and peer interactions to gauge impairment. Figure 1 shows a sample Vanderbilt questions.

The Aberrant Behavior Checklist (ABC; Aman & Singh, 1986) is one of the few scales specifically designed for use with an ID population. The ABC consists of a 58-item checklist that rates inappropriate and maladaptive behaviors in either children or adults with intellectual disability. The ABC has five subscales: disruptive behavior, social withdrawal, stereotypic behavior, hyperactivity/noncompliance, and inappropriate speech. While not designed specifically for ADHD, the ABC is one of the most psychometrically validated instruments for determining ADHD in persons with ID (Miller, Fee, & Jones, 2004, Miller, Fee, & Netterville, 2004). Perhaps the focus on aberrant behavior rather than ADHD specifically explains why the ABC is not used more broadly (Antshel et al. 2006).

Rating scales are not the only instruments psychologists have at their disposal. Continuous performance tests (CPTs) have proven valuable in assessing inattentiveness, impulsivity, sustained attention, and vigilance. CPTs measure the ability to maintain focused attention over a period of time (5–20 min depending on program used) as the child responds to a target stimuli (letter, number, or picture) and inhibits responses to nontarget stimuli. Several different versions of CPTs are commercially available including the Gordon Diagnostic System (Gordon, 1983), the Conners' CPT (Conners, 1994), and the Integrated Variables of Attention, 2nd Edition (Sanford & Turner, 1994). Although CPTs are commonly used to assess symptoms of ADHD, these instruments have not been normed on an ID population. If used, results should be interpreted with caution in persons with IQ < 70. Likewise, caution is indicated in interpreting CPT results in persons with ASD. The CPT performance of persons with ASD has indicated deficits in sustained attention tasks in individuals with and without comorbid ADHD (Chien et al., 2014; Lundervold

Symptom	Never	Occasionally	Often	Very Often
1. Does not pay attention to details or makes careless mistakes with, for example, homework	0	1	2	3
2. Has difficulty keeping attention to what needs to be done.	0	1	2	3
3. Does not seem to listen when spoken to directly	0	1	2	3

Fig. 1 Sample of Vanderbilt questions, three of the thirty-five symptom questions

et al., 2012; Murphy et al., 2014). Lundervold et al. (2012) caution that low IQ may impair CPT performance in youth with ASD rendering a false indication of ADHD. Some additional measures include the Brown Rating Scales for Children and Adolescents (Brown, 2001) and the Swanson, Nolan, and Pelham Rating Scale (SNAP) (Swanson, 1992), which are described in Table 4.

Assessment

Vignette

The psychologist reviewed psychological testing from the school psychologist documenting ID. During screening, the psychologist observed Anthony staring blankly and making a chewing motion with his mouth. His parents hadn't noticed this behavior and were asked to make notes if it was observed at home. The psychologist also noticed that Anthony had a long face and large ears. The psychologist sent a note to the pediatrician describing these concerns and asking the pediatrician to consider referrals to a neurologist to rule out a seizure disorder and a geneticist to screen for fragile X or other genetic condition.

Medical Specialty Assessments

If psychological or medical screening raises concerns of medical illness, a referral to a neurologist, geneticist, ENT (ear, nose, and throat specialist/otolaryngologist), or other medical specialist may be necessary. Many insurances require the pediatrician to make medical specialty referrals; therefore, it is helpful to provide the parent with a detailed written description of observations or historical factors suggesting the need for additional medical assessment. The note should also request a copy of the medical specialist report.

Neurologist

Neurological disorders, including seizures, are common among children with intellectual disabilities (Corbett, 2000). The clinician should ask for records of any past neurological assessments. In addition, the clinician should inquire about staring spells, tics, headaches, and head trauma. If a child has brief staring spells lasting 10–15 s and has no memory for that time, absence seizures may be the reason for inattention. If seizures are suspected or there is a history of seizures, it is helpful to keep a seizure log describing the seizure, how long it lasts, and behaviors immediately before and after the seizure. When Anthony saw the neurologist, he was referred for an EEG. His parents were asked to keep him up very late the night before the EEG so he would fall asleep during the test. This increases the possibility of seizure activity. Anthony's EEG showed diffuse slowing consistent with ID but no seizure activity or focal deficits. Knowing that Tourette's syndrome may mimic ADHD, the neurologist considered the possibility of a tic disorder and asked Anthony's parents and teacher to complete a tic checklist for a week. Stimulant medications used to treat ADHD may increase tics in children with tic disorders.

Neurologists may refer children with cerebral palsy (CP) for psychological assessment. CP is a disorder of poor muscle control due to an abnormality of brain development which occurs before, during, or after delivery. As a result of CP, children may have poor balance, stiffness, poor coordination, or uncontrollable movements. The CDC has reported that approximately 1 in 323 children is diagnosed with CP (Christensen et al., 2014). Children with CP are at increased risk for ID, ASD, epilepsy, communication disorders and ADHD (Bjorgaas, Elgen, Boe, & Hysing, 2013). CP encompasses a broad array of cognitive and motor impairments. The specific area of brain dysfunction and the etiology of the abnormality should be considered by the clinician assessing the child with CP for ADHD. For example, orofacial motor cortex involvement may result in an expressive language disorder that will impact choice of psychological test to determine mental age (Ballester-Plané et al., 2016). An expressive language disorder may result in a child attempting to speak less. This may confound the assessment of hyperactivity/impulsivity symptoms of playing loudly, talking excessively, blurting out, and interrupting. If the child also has restricted movement, the assessment of attention may be the primary focus of the ADHD assessment. The clinician will need to take into account that children with CP often demonstrate executive function impairment across all domains (Bodimeade, Whittingham, Lloyd, & Boyd, 2013; Whittingham, Bodimeade, Lloyd, & Boyd, 2014).

Geneticist

Genetic testing may inform the ADHD assessment of children with developmental disabilities. Due to recent advances in genetic testing, it is becoming increasingly common for pediatricians to order genetic testing for children with developmental disabilities. When the karyotype or microassay reveals an abnormality, genetic consultation may be sought. The clinician should request genetic reports and consider requesting testing if not previously done.

Specific genetic causes can be identified in over half of patients with intellectual disability referred for genetic testing (Moeschler, 2008). Chromosomal aberrations are the most common known cause of intellectual disability (Kaufman, Ayub, & Vincent, 2010). In a review of genetic anomalies associated with ADHD, several had greater than 50% prevalence, including fragile X syndrome, Klinefelter syndrome, velocardiofacial syndrome, and Williams syndrome (Vorstman & Ophoff, 2013). The behavioral phenotype of a genetic disorder may predict behavioral challenges and prognosis. For example, velocardiofacial syndrome is associated with inattention more commonly than hyperactivity (Antshel et al., 2007; Niklasson, Rasmussen, Oskarsdottir, & Gillberg, 2009). The behavioral phenotype may complicate the assessment of ADHD (Vorstman & Ophoff, 2013). For example, the social and communication skills of children with Williams syndrome may lead to inflated estimates of mental age. This may lead to expectations that frustrate the child, causing the child to appear inattentive or hyperactive (Deutsch, Dube, & McIlvane, 2008). Children with intellectual disability should be referred for genetic testing as a specific genetic cause can be identified in over 50% of cases and inform treatment and care planning (Moeschler, 2008).

ENT/Otolaryngologist

The pediatrician may consider referral to an otolaryngologist (ENT) if a child has an abnormal sleep study. The CDC has deemed insufficient sleep an epidemic (CDC, 2013). The clinician should consider signs that a child is not getting enough sleep including difficulty getting out of bed in the morning, daytime sleepiness, dark circles under the eyes, inattention and concentration problems, and behavioral difficulties such as irritability, hyperactivity, depression, impatience, impulse control problems, aggression, moodiness, and temper tantrums (Bonuck, Chervin, Cole, et al., 2011). Sleep disturbance may be the etiology of inattention, impulsivity, and hyperactivity. Dahl and colleagues noted the similarities between chronic sleep deprivation and ADHD over 25 years ago. More recently, the Avon Longitudinal Study of Parents and Children found that sleep disorders clearly mimic numerous symptoms of ADHD. In this study of over 2400 children, high rates of inattention, hyperactivity, and impulsivity were common in youth with sleep-disordered breathing and sleep difficulties. At 4 years of age, these children were 40% more likely to have behavioral problems, and at 7 years of age, they were 60% more likely to suffer from behavioral problems in comparison to a group of children who did not have sleep-disordered breathing (Perfect, Archbold, Goodwin, Levine-Donnerstein, & Quan, 2013). Among children with ADHD, 1 h of sleep disruption has been shown to decrease the ability to perform cognitive tasks and exacerbate ADHD symptoms (Gruber et al., 2011). The seriousness of sleep deprivation in children cannot be understated. Research indicates that untreated sleep disorders are often chronic and result in academic underachievement or failure, depression, conflict with peers, and a variety of health problems including obesity (Aldabal and Bahammam 2011).

Sleep disorders are found comorbid with ADHD in approximately 25–55% of patients (Corkum, Moldofsky, Hogg-Johnson, Humphries, & Tannock, n.d.; Hodgkins et al., 2013; Owens, 2005; Sung, Hiscock, Sciberras, & Efron, 2008). Children with developmental disabilities are at increased risk for sleep disorders. Sleep difficulties in children with ASD are well documented (Richdale & Baglin, 2015; Richdale & Schreck, 2009). Developmental disabilities, including fragile X, Down's syndrome, FAS/FAE, cerebral palsy, and Williams syndrome, are associated with disordered sleep (Breslin et al., 2014; Maris, Verhulst, Wojciechowski, Van de Heyning, & Boudewyns, 2016; Goril, Zalai, Scott, & Shapiro, 2016; Koyuncu, Türkkani, Sarikaya, & Özgirgin, 2017; Curran, Debbarma and Sedky, 2017; Santoro, Giacheti, Rossi, Campos, & Pinato, 2016).

Sleep disorders associated with ADHD typically present as breathing problems, peripheral limb movements, or activity on somnography. Breathing concerns can range from obstructive sleep apnea to primary snoring (Owens et al., 2012). Recent reviews indicate that obstructive sleep apnea may be more prevalent in the ADHD population (25–30%) than the general population (approx 3%) (Youssef, Ege, Angly, Strauss, & Marx, 2011). The American Academy of Pediatrics recommends screening for sleep apnea in children with ADHD symptoms (AAP, 2011). Following screening, a referral for a sleep study may be made with subsequent consultation with an ENT if indicated. Surgical treatment of obstructive sleep apnea with adenotonsillectomy can lead to substantial improvement of ADHD symptoms in many patients (Huang et al., 2007).

Children described as "restless sleepers," those who throw covers and pillows from the bed during sleep and wake askew, may experience excessive peripheral limb movements. Movements are tracked during sleep studies and correlated with EEG readings to rule out seizure activity. Up to 44% of patients with ADHD have symptoms of restless legs syndrome or periodic limb movement disorder. In children with limb movements, pain or discomfort may be mistaken for ADHD or ODD (Cortese et al., 2005). Treatment of sleep disturbances with subsequent improved sleep efficiency may eliminate the need for ADHD assessment.

There are several confounders in evaluating sleep with ADHD and developmental disabilities. Sleep deficit in children is known to have neurocognitive effects that overlap with core features of ADHD (Owens et al., 2012). Also, stimulant medications used for ADHD are known to impair sleep in some patients (Spruyt & Gozal, 2011). However, stimulants can also have the opposite effect and cause paradoxical calming in some patients (Hvolby, 2015). A thorough sleep history should be part of all assessments (see Table 5). Clinicians suspecting that a sleep disorder may be complicating the assessment of ADHD should discuss good sleep hygiene practices and have parents complete a sleep diary.

Psychological Assessment

Vignette

After pediatric and specialty medical assessments were completed, the psychologist met with Anthony's parents to gather detailed developmental, medical, social, educational, and family history. His teacher provided RtI tracking forms, functional behavioral assessment results, and copies of behavioral reports which were valuable in documenting symptoms and the resulting impairment in the school setting.

The psychological assessment of ADHD symptoms in children with developmental disabilities will require more time, preparation, and clinical decision-making than typically budgeted for routine evaluations. Given the complexity of ADHD and the numerous possible ADHD presentations, it is not surprising that there is no single test that can diagnose ADHD

Table 5 A sleep history should be included in all assessments

Sleep history
Evening routine, including electronic/TV use
Desired bedtime
Difficulty getting the child to bed
Difficulty keeping the child in bed
Sleep onset latency
Sleep disruptions including snoring
Nocturnal enuresis
Wake time and mood
Daytime sleepiness/napping

(National Institute of Mental Health, 2012). Instead, one must approach the assessment like a puzzle with many pieces that may not be completed in a single sitting. Multiple sessions will be required to explore the complex history and evaluate the child. Children with developmental disorders may find lengthy sessions overstimulating. An initial parent meeting without the child may be helpful as the parent interview is very likely the most important source of data. Parent interviews provide valuable information that could not be obtained from child. Interviewing children is critical to learn how they understand symptoms and to observe how they express themselves but will not yield the wealth of information parents and teachers can provide (Mitis, McKay, Schulz, Newcorn, & Halperin, 2000). The parent interview gathers data to fully understand symptoms of inattention, hyperactivity, and impulsivity and to rule out comorbid conditions. The symptoms explored should include queries regarding anxiety, depression, and behavior disorders. Higher rates of oppositional defiant disorder and conduct disorder in children with ID have been suggested (Lindblad, Gillberg, & Fernell, 2011; Ahuja, Martin, Langley, & Thapar, 2013). A full description of each symptom including age of onset, course over time, and impact on function at home and school should be obtained. In addition, the clinician can screen for conditions, such as prenatal exposure to drugs and/or alcohol, head trauma, prematurity, sleep disturbances, or a seizure disorder, which could explain or exacerbate ADHD symptoms.

Psychological testing results will often be available for children with developmental disability presenting for ADHD assessment. Because the diagnostic criteria for ADHD stipulate consideration the child's developmental level in assessing ADHD symptoms, retesting may be necessary to understand the degree and nature of discrepancies between chronological age and cognitive/developmental age (APA, 2013; Tannock, 2002). It is critical to review disability specific assessments including autism, speech/language, occupational therapy, and physical therapy evaluations.

Intellectual Disability

In order to accommodate the unique needs of each youth, collateral information should be reviewed before the assessment. The clinician should consider how the assessment will accommodate the child's mental age, physical requirements, and speech/language development.

In addition to individual needs, the assessment of ADHD symptoms in youth with ID requires special attention a broad range of diagnoses and situations. Pearson and colleagues concluded that children with ID/ADHD have more symptoms of depression, family conflict, noncompliance, anxiety, hyperactivity, inadequate social skills, and academic problems compared to children with only ADHD. The authors clearly demonstrated that the clinical picture is more complicated when there is the dual diagnosis of ID and ADHD (Pearson et al., 2000). Using a structured clinical interview process to apply the DSM-IV diagnostic criteria to an ID population, Dekker and Koot (2003) found that 14.8% of their recruited sample met criteria for ADHD and 44% had co-occurring oppositional defiant disorder. Obviously these rates are significantly higher than what would be predicted among the general population.

The parent's understanding of her child's intellectual abilities and challenges is critical to clinical judgment regarding symptoms of inattention, hyperactivity, and impulsivity. The parent's expectations should conform to the child's mental age just as clinician's assessment of ADHD symptoms should be in accord with the child's mental age. Reviewing functional assessments or asking about the child's ability to complete self-care tasks will provide a baseline for ability level and assist the clinician in ruling out an expectation-ability discrepancy as a cause for ADHD concern. Aligning parental expectations with the child's ability is critical for successful treatment.

Autism Spectrum Disorder

The DSM-5 highlights the presentation of ASD as a spectrum of symptoms (APA, 2013). Given the variability in the clinical presentation of persons with ASD and the high rate and wide range of comorbidities, the clinician must fully assess ASD symptoms and comorbid conditions before rendering an ADHD diagnosis (Kohane et al., 2012). Intellectual disability (ID) and autism spectrum disorders (ASD) co-occur at high rates with the severity of one disorder impacting the other (Matson & Shoemaker, 2009). Children with both ID and ASD have different needs, and often a different prognosis, than children who have either condition alone (Carminati, Gerber, Baud, & Baud, 2007; Gilchrist et al., 2001). Therefore, it is important that the clinician distinguish symptoms due to each condition.

In addition to comorbid disorders, the symptoms of ASD may confound the diagnosis of ADHD. For example, children with ASD and hyperreactivity to sensory stimuli may be fidgety or overactive; others may shut down when overstimulated and appear inattentive. Careful inquiry into antecedents to periods of overactivity and inattention is critical. Detailed descriptions of specific behaviors and modulating factors should be obtained. In order to obtain detail, parents may be asked to describe behaviors as if they are describing a movie of their child. Social impairment in children with ASD must be distinguished from that of ADHD. The lack of social reciprocity which is a core symptom of ASD may be mimicked or exacerbated by the impulsivity of ADHD. While children with ADHD may form friendships with greater ease than children with ASD, difficulty sustaining friendships is characteristic of both. Descriptions of social interactions from the perspectives of caregivers and the child provide the clinician with clues to understanding the contributions of ASD and ADHD to challenges (Leitner, 2014). In addition, the brain maturation of individuals with ASD differs from those with ADHD but not ASD and has implications for prognosis and the need for treatment into adulthood (Murphy et al., 2014).

Fetal Alcohol Syndrome Disorder

Fetal alcohol syndrome disorder (FASD) is the leading preventable cause of developmental delay. The American Academy of Pediatrics describes with diagnosis of FASD as a constellation of physical, behavioral, and intellectual impairments resulting from prenatal alcohol exposure (Williams and Smith, 2015). The AAP has published an extensive Fetal Alcohol Spectrum Disorders Toolkit on their Healthy Initiative website (American Academy of Pediatrics, 2017). The DSM-5 section for further study has included the FASD-related condition, Neurobehavioral Disorder Associated with Prenatal Alcohol Exposure (ND-PAE). ND-PAE proposed diagnostic criteria include impairments of neurocognitive functioning (intellect, executive functioning, learning, memory, and/or visual-spatial reasoning), self-regulation (mood/behavior, attention, or impulse control), and adaptive functioning (language, social communication/interaction, daily living skills, and/or motor skills) (APA, 2013). Doyle and Mattson (2015) have published guidelines for the assessment of ND-PAE. Young et al. (2016) have published *Guidelines for the identification and treatment of individuals with AD/HD and associated fetal alcohol spectrum disorders based upon expert consensus.*

Distinguishing between behavioral symptoms due to FASD and ADHD presents unique challenges. ADHD and FASD represent distinct entities. The expert consensus guidelines note youth with ADHD and FASD-ADHD differ on tests of executive function, response to stimulant medication, and adaptive functioning (Young et al., 2016). On psychometric testing youth with FASD tend to have difficulties with encoding information and shifting attention, whereas children with ADHD have problems with focus and sustaining attention (Peadon & Elliott, 2010; Doyle and Mattson, 2015). Children with FASD often present with early-onset ADHD with predominant inattentive symptoms (O'Malley & Nanson, 2002; Kingdon, Cardoso, & McGrath, 2015). In fact, ADHD diagnosis often precedes FASD diagnosis. FASD should be considered when children have poor response to treatment for ADHD and history of PAE (Young et al., 2016). In addition, children with FASD have greater impairment of activities of daily living than children with ADHD (Crocker, Vaurio, Riley, & Mattson, 2009).

The clinical assessment of youth should always include detailed inquiry regarding prenatal alcohol exposure (PAE). Obtaining PAE history may be difficult. The clinician must take care to be nonjudgmental. The mother should not be questioned in front of her child or others. Asking about alcohol use "before you knew you were pregnant" may encourage more open disclosure. Youth in foster care and adopted children are 10–15 times more likely to suffer FASD than youth who have not been in placement (Astley, Stachowiak, Clarren, & Clausen, 2002). PAE history may not be available for these youth. In addition, these populations are more likely to have experienced abuse and/or neglect with resulting behaviors that may complicate the diagnosis and treatment of ADHD.

Educational Assessment

Vignette

After the psychologist diagnosed Anthony with ADHD, an IEP team meeting was scheduled. The exceptionality of "other health impaired" was added to Anthony's IEP. A behavior intervention plan (BIP) was created to address challenging behaviors.

The increased incidence of academic challenges and disciplinary interventions for students with ADHD is well documented (Cuffe et al., 2015; Reed, Jakubovski, Johnson, & Bloch, 2017; Martin & Burns, 2014). When RtI is not successful, further assessment is indicated. IDEA, state departments of education, and local school districts detail the procedures for assessment, exceptionality assignment, and implementation of accommodations via an individualized accommodation plan (IAP) or individualized educational plan (IEP). IDEA defines educational disabilities or exceptionalities. IDEA designates 14 exceptionalities including autism, intellectual disability, specific learning disability, developmental delay, emotional disturbance, speech or language impairment, traumatic brain injury, hearing impairment, deafness, visual impairment, deaf-blindness, multiple disabilities, orthopedic impairment, and other health impairment. While exceptionality terminology may appear congruent with behavioral health/medical diagnoses, exceptionalities are defined by state and federal governments, not the DSM. Under IDEA, ADHD is classified under the exceptionality "Other Health Impairment." Within IDEA parameters, the states are allowed to define "developmental delay," "autism," and "intellectual disability." States may assign the exceptionality of developmental delay to children between the ages of 3 and 9 who display delays in physical, cognitive, social/emotional, communication, or adaptive development. The exceptionalities of autism and intellectual disability are similar to behavioral health/medical diagnoses but state specific exceptionality definitions should be referenced for specific details (Fisher & Rhodes, 2017).

Although students with ADHD often qualify for assessment and services under IDEA, the number of students receiving services for ADHD is unclear because the "other health impairment" exceptionality includes health problems such as asthma, epilepsy, and diabetes. During the 2013–2014 school year, US Department of Education data indicates 6.5 million students qualified for special education services. The greatest number qualified for special learning disability (2,275,000), followed by other health impairment (845,000), autism (520,000), and intellectual disability (455,000). Comorbidity is common for students with ADHD; however only 0.3% of youth, 132,000, receiving special services during the 2013–2014 school year were qualified under the multiple disabilities exceptionality (U. S. Department of Education, 2016).

The other health impairment (OHI) exceptionality requires a diagnosis of a chronic illness. Educational assessments identify symptoms consistent with ADHD through classroom observations, parent and teacher interviews, and rating scales. Educational assessments do not render diagnoses; therefore, the school will refer to a psychologist, pediatrician, psychiatrist, or other professional for the assessment and diagnosis of ADHD (Gordon, 2015).

Summary and Future Directions

Even the most seasoned clinician will face challenges when assessing ADHD in children with developmental disabilities. The core symptoms of ADHD combine in thousands of ways to render the diagnosis and comorbid conditions abound. Likewise, specific developmental disabilities may vary in presentation. Symptoms of ADHD and developmental disabilities may wax and wane over time due to development, environment, stressors, or other factors. The clinician must understand a child's unique experience with the identified developmental disability before attempting to assess for ADHD. The child's intellectual age and functional abilities must be fully determined.

Before making the diagnosis of ADHD, the clinician must exclude other possible etiologies for the symptoms, of inattention, hyperactivity, and impulsivity. Diagnosing specific sleep disorders is of particular importance because of the pervasiveness of the sleep disturbances and the persistence and severity of the sleep disorders that tend to be present in children with DD (Wiggs, 2001). Accurate diagnosis and successful treatment depend on the accurate identification of impairments due to ADHD and those due to comorbid conditions, taking into account the child's mental age and familial and cultural behavioral expectations. The assessment depends on a high degree of clinical skill to gather information from multiple informants and collateral sources and rally the cooperation of parents, teachers, behavioral health, and medical professionals. In persons with developmental disabilities, impairment due to ADHD will require reassessment as the child matures or symptoms change and accommodations extending to the adult years.

The twenty-first century holds the promise of astounding advances in neuroscience.

The assessment and treatment of ADHD will be informed by advances in genetics, neurochemistry, cell biology, and technology. Recent advances in genetics, epigenetics, neurochemistry, and cell biology foreshadow the ability to increase our understanding of ADHD and developmental disabilities (Hamza, et al., 2017; Fair, et al., 2012; Franke, Neale, & Faraone, 2009; Thapar et al., 2016; Williams et al., 2010). "Synaptopathy," synaptic dysfunction as the source of brain disorders, will open new avenues in our understanding of ADHD and DD (Torres, Vallejo, & Inestrosa, 2017). Technological advances, including the use of virtual reality, dysmorphological analysis using facial recognition technology, and social media, will inform our assessment and treatment of ADHD and developmental disabilities (Rodriquez, Garcia & Areces, 2017; Veldhuizen & Cairney, 2017). As scientific progress refines our understanding of ADHD, the clinical assessment will evolve and provide new challenges to clinician.

References

Achenbach, T. M., & Rescorla, L. A. (2001). *Manual for the ASEBA school age forms & profiles*. Burlington, VT: University of Vermont.

Ageranioti-Bélanger, S., Brunet, S., D'Anjou, G., Tellier, G., Boivin, J., & Gauthier, M. (2012). Behaviour disorders in children with an intellectual disability. *Paediatrics & Child Health, 17*(2), 84–88.

Ahuja, A., Martin, J., Langley, K., & Thapar, A. (2013). Intellectual disability in children with attention deficit hyperactivity disorder. *The Journal of Pediatrics, 163*, 890–895.

Aldabal, L., & Bahammam, A. S. (2011). Metabolic, endocrine, and immune consequences of sleep deprivation. *Open Respiratory Medicine Journal, 5*, 31–43.

Aman, M. G., & Singh, N. N. (1986). *Aberrant behavior checklist manual*. East Aurora, NY: Slosson Educational Publications.

American Academy of Child and Adolescent Psychiatry. (2007). Practice parameter for the assessment and treatment of children and adolescents with attention deficit hyperactivity disorder. *Journal of the American Academy of Child and Adolescent Psychiatry, 46*, 894–921.

American Academy of Pediatrics. (2017). Fetal alcohol spectrum disorders toolkit. Retrieved 15 May 2017, from https://www.aap.org/en-us/advocacy-and-policy/aap-health-initiatives/fetal-alcohol-spectrum-disorders-toolkit/Pages/default.aspx

American Psychiatric Association. (1968). *Diagnostic and statistical manual of mental diseases (DSM-II)*. Washington, DC: American Psychiatric Association.

American Psychiatric Association. (1980). *Diagnostic and statistical manual (DSM-III)*. Washington, DC: American Psychiatric Association.

American Psychiatric Association. (1994). *Diagnostic and statistical manual of mental disorders: DSM-IV.* Washington, DC: American Psychiatric Association.

American Psychiatric Association. (2000). *Diagnostic and statistical manual-text revision.* Washington, DC: American Psychiatric Association.

American Psychiatric Association. (2013). *Diagnostic and statistical manual of mental disorders (DSM-5)* (5th ed.). Washington, DC: American Psychiatric Association.

American Psychological Association. (2017). *Distinguishing between screening and assessment for mental and behavioral health problems.* Retrieved from APA Practice Organization: http://www.apapracticecentral.org/reimbursement/billing/assessment-screening.aspx

Antshel, K. M., Phillips, M. H., Gordon, M., Barkley, R., & Faraone, S. V. (2006). Is ADHD a valid disorder in children with intellectual delays? *Clinical Psychology Review, 26*(5), 555–572.

Antshel, K. M., Aneja, A., Strunge, L., Peebles, J., Fremont, W. P., Stallone, K., et al. (2007). Autistic spectrum disorders in velo-cardio facial syndrome (22q11.2 deletion). *Journal of Autism and Developmental Disorders, 37,* 1776–1786.

Arnett, A. B., MacDonald, B., & Pennington, B. F. (2013). Cognitive and behavioral indicators of ADHD symptoms prior to school age. *Journal of Child Psychology and Psychiatry, 54*(12), 1284–1294.

Astley, S. J., Stachowiak, J., Clarren, S. K., & Clausen, C. (2002). Application of the fetal alcohol syndrome facial photographic screening tool in a foster care population. *The Journal of Pediatrics, 141*(5), 712–717.

Ballester-Plané, J., Laporta-Hoyos, O., Macaya, A., Póo, P., Meléndez-Plumed, M., Vázquez, É., … Pueyo, R. (2016). Measuring intellectual ability in cerebral palsy: The comparison of three tests and their neuroimaging correlates. *Research in Developmental Disabilities, 56,* 83–98.

Baumeister, A. A., Henderson, K., Pow, J. L., & Advokat, C. (2012). The early history of the neuroscience of attention-deficit/hyperactivity disorder. *Journal of the History of the Neurosciences, 21*(3), 263–279. https://doi.org/10.1080/0964704X.2011.595649

Berkeley, S., Bender, W. N., Peaster, L. G., & Saunders, L. (2009). Implementation of response to intervention: A snapshot of progress. *Journal of Learning Disabilities, 42*(1), 85–95.

Biederman, J., Wozniak, J., Kiely, K., Ablon, S., Faraone, S., Mick, E., … Kraus, I. (1995). CBCL clinical scales discriminate prepubertal children with structured interview – Derived diagnosis of mania from those with ADHD. *Journal of the American Academy of Child & Adolescent Psychiatry, 34,* 464–471.

Bjorgaas, H. M., Elgen, I., Boe, T., & Hysing, M. (2013). Mental health in children with cerebral palsy: Does screening capture the complexity? *The Scientific World Journal, 2013,* 468402.

Bodimeade, H. L., Whittingham, K., Lloyd, O., & Boyd, R. N. (2013). Executive functioning in children and adolescents with unilateral cerebral palsy. *Developmental Medicine and Child Neurology, 55*(10), 926–933.

Bonuck, K. A., Chervin, R. D., Cole, T. J., et al. (2011). Prevalence and persistence of sleep disordered breathing symptoms in young children: A 6-year population based cohort study. *Sleep, 34*(7), 875–884.

Bradley, C. (1937). The behavior of children receiving Benzedrine. *American Journal of Psychiatry, 94,* 577–585.

Bramlett, M. D., & Blumberg, S. J. (2007). Family structure and children's physical and mental health. *Health Affairs, 26*(2), 549–558.

Breslin, J., Spanò, G., Bootzin, R., Anand, P., Nadel, L., & Edgin, J. (2014). Obstructive sleep apnea syndrome and cognition in down syndrome. *Developmental Medicine and Child Neurology, 56*(7), 657–664.

Bridgett, D. J., & Walker, M. E. (2006). Intellectual functioning in adults with ADHD: A meta-analytic examination of full scale IQ differences between adults with and without ADHD.

Brown, T. E. (2001). *The Brown attention deficit disorder scales.* San Antonio, TX: Psychological Corporation.

Burks, H. F. (1960). The hyperkinetic child. *Exceptional Children, 27*(1), 18–26.

Carminati, G. G., Gerber, F., Baud, M. A., & Baud, O. (2007). Evaluating the effects of a structured program for adults with autism spectrum disorders and intellectual disabilities. *Research in Autism Spectrum Disorders, 1,* 256–265.

Centers for Disease Control and Prevention. (2013). Insufficient sleep is a public health epidemic. http://cdc.gov/Features/dsSleep

Chien, Y.-L., Gau, S. S.-F., Chiu, Y.-N., Tsai, W.-C., Shang, C.-Y., & Wu, Y.-Y. (2014). Impaired sustained attention, focused attention, and vigilance in youths with autistic disorder and Asperger's disorder. *Research in Autism Spectrum Disorders, 8*(7), 881–889.

Christensen, D., Van Naarden Braun, K., Doernberg, N. S., Maenner, M. J., Arneson, C. L., Durkin, M. S., … Yeargin-Allsopp, M. (2014). Prevalence of cerebral palsy, co-occurring autism spectrum disorders, and motor functioning – Autism and developmental disabilities monitoring network, USA, 2008. *Developmental Medicine and Child Neurology, 56*(1), 59–65.

Conners, C. K. (1994). *The Conners continuous performance test.* Toronto, Canada: Multi-Health Systems.

Conners, C. K. (2008). *Conners (Conners 3)* (3rd ed.). North Tonawanda, NY: Multi-Health Systems.

Conners, C. K., & Sitarenios, G. (2011). Conners' continuous performance test (CPT). In *Encyclopedia of clinical neuropsychology* (pp. 681–683). New York: Springer.

Corbett, J. A. (2000). Epilepsy and mental retardation. *The British Journal of Psychiatry, 177*(5), 473. https://doi.org/10.1192/bjp.177.5.473-a

Corkum, P., Moldofsky, H., Hogg-Johnson, S., Humphries, T., & Tannock, R. (n.d.). Sleep problems in children with attention-deficit/hyperactivity disorder: Impact of subtype, comorbidity, and stimulant medication. *Journal of the American Academy of*

Child & Adolescent Psychiatry, 38(10), 1285–1293. https://doi.org/10.1097/00004583-199910000-00018

Cortese, S., Konofal, E., Lecendreux, M., Arnulf, I., Mouren, M.-C., Darra, F., & Dalla Bernardina, B. (2005). Restless legs syndrome and attention-deficit/hyperactivity disorder: A review of the literature. Sleep, 28(8), 1007–1013.

Crocker, N., Vaurio, L., Riley, E. P., & Mattson, S. N. (2009). Comparison of adaptive behavior in children with heavy prenatal alcohol exposure or attention-deficit/hyperactivity disorder. Alcoholism, Clinical and Experimental Research, 33(11), 2015–2023.

Cuffe, S. P., Visser, S. N., Holbrook, J. R., Danielson, M. L., Geryk, L. L., Wolraich, M. L., & McKeown, R. E. (2015). ADHD and psychiatric comorbidity: Functional outcomes in a school-based sample of children. Journal of Attention Disorders. https://doi.org/10.1177/1087054715613437

Curran, C., Debbarma, S., & Sedky, K. (2017). Fragile X and obstructive sleep apnea syndrome: Case presentation and management challenges. Journal of Clinical Sleep Medicine, 13(1), 137–138.

Dekker, M. C., & Koot, H. M. (2003). DSM-IV disorders in children with borderline to moderate intellectual disability I: Prevalence and impact. Journal of the American Academy of Child & Adolescent Psychiatry, 42, 915–922.

Deutsch, C. K., Dube, W. V., & McIlvane, W. J. (2008). Attention deficits, attention-deficit hyperactivity disorder, and intellectual disabilities. Developmental Disabilities Research Reviews, 14(4), 285–292. http://doi.org/10.1002/ddrr.42.

Doshi, J. A., Hodgkins, P., Kahle, J., Sikirica, V., Cangelosi, M. J., Setyawan, J., ... Neumann, P. J. (2012). Economic impact of childhood and adult attention-deficit/hyperactivity disorder in the United States. Journal of the American Academy of Child and Adolescent Psychiatry, 51(10), 990–1002.e2.

Douglas, V. I. (1972). Stop, look and listen: The problem of sustained attention and impulse control in hyperactive and normal children. Canadian Journal of Behavioural Science, 4(4), 259–282. Canada: University of Toronto Press. doi:10.1037/h0082313. ISSN 1879-2669. Retrieved 10 Nov 2014.

Doyle, L. R., & Mattson, S. N. (2015). Neurobehavioral disorder associated with prenatal alcohol exposure (ND-PAE): Review of evidence and guidelines for assessment. Current Developmental Disorders Reports, 2(3), 175–186.

DuPaul, G. J., Power, T. J., Anastopoulos, A. D., & Reid, R. (1998). ADHD rating scale-IV: Checklists, norms, and clinical interpretations. Journal of Psychoeducational Assessment, 10, 172–178.

Einfeld, S. L., & Aman, M. (1995). Issues in the taxonomy of psychopathology in mental retardation. Journal of Autism and Developmental Disorders, 25(2), 143–167.

Einfeld, S. L., & Tonge, B. J. (1996). Population prevalence of psychopathology in children and adolescents with intellectual disability: II epidemiological findings. Journal of Intellectual Disability Research, 40, 99–109.

Emerson, E. (2003). Prevalence of psychiatric disorders in children and adolescents with and without intellectual disability. Journal of Intellectual Disability Research, 47, 51–58.

Epstein, M. H., Cullinan, D., & Polloway, E. D. (1986). Patterns of maladjustment among mentally retarded children and youth. American Journal of Mental Deficiency, 91, 127–134.

Fair, D. A., Nigg, J. T., Iyer, S., Bathula, D., Mills, K. L., Dosenbach, N. U. F., ... Milham, M. P. (2012). Distinct neural signatures detected for ADHD subtypes after controlling for micro- movements in resting state functional connectivity MRI data. Frontiers in Systems Neuroscience, 6, 80.

Fee, V. E., Matson, J. L., & Benavidez, D. A. (1994). Attention deficit-hyperactivity disorder among mentally retarded children. Research in Developmental Disabilities, 15(1), 67–79.

Fiks, A. G., Ross, M. E., Mayne, S. L., Song, L., Liu, W., Steffes, J., ... Wasserman, R. (2016). Preschool ADHD diagnosis and stimulant use before and after the 2011 AAP practice guideline. Pediatrics, 138(6). https://doi.org/10.1542/peds.2016-2025.

Fisher, O., & Rhodes, G. (2017). "Office of Special Education Programs (OSEP) – Home page," March. http://www.ed.gov/about/offices/list/osers/osep/index.html

Franke, B., Neale, B. M., & Faraone, S. V. (2009). Genome-wide association studies in ADHD. Human Genetics, 126(1), 13–50. http://doi.org/10.1007/s00439-009-0663-4.

Frazier, T. W., Demaree, H. A., & Youngstrom, E. A. (2004). Meta-analysis of intellectual and neuropsychological test performance in attention deficit hyperactivity disorder. Neuropsychology, 18, 543–555.

French, W. P. (2015). Assessment and treatment of attention-deficit/hyperactivity disorder: Part 1. Pediatric Annals, 44(3), 114–120.

Fuchs, D., & Fuchs, L. S. (2006). Introduction to response to intervention: What, why, and how valid is it? Reading Research Quarterly, 41(1), 93–99.

Gabis, L. V., Tsubary, N. M., Leon, O., Ashkenasi, A., & Shefer, S. (2015). Assessment of abilities and comorbidities in children with cerebral palsy. Journal of Child Neurology, 30(12), 1640–1645. https://doi.org/10.1177/0883073815576792

Gilchrist, A., Green, J., Cox, A., Burton, D., Rutter, M., & LeCouteur, A. (2001). Development and current functioning in adolescents with Asperger syndrome: A comparative study. Journal of Child Psychology and Psychiatry, 42, 227–240.

Gjaerum, B., & Bjornerem, H. (2003). Psychosocial impairment is significant in young referred children with and without psychiatric diagnoses and cognitive delays. European Child & Adolescent Psychiatry, 12(5), 239–248.

Gordon, M. (1983). The gordon diagnostic system. DeWitt, NY: Gordon Systems.

Gordon, M. (2015). Challenges surrounding the education of children with chronic diseases. IGI Global.

Goril, S., Zalai, D., Scott, L., & Shapiro, C. M. (2016). Sleep and melatonin secretion abnormalities in children and adolescents with fetal alcohol spectrum disorders. *Sleep Medicine, 23*, 59–64. https://doi.org/10.1016/j.sleep.2016.06.002

Gruber, R., Wiebe, S., Montecalvo, L., Brunetti, B., Amsel, R., & Carrier, J. (2011). Impact of sleep restriction on neurobehavioral functioning of children with attention deficit hyperactivity disorder. *Sleep, 34*(3), 315–323.

Hagan, J. F., Balachova, T., Bertrand, J., Chasnoff, I., Dang, E., Fernandez-Baca, D., ... Zubler, J. (2016). Neurobehavioral disorder associated with prenatal alcohol exposure., *138*(6).

Hamza, M., Halayem, S., Bourgou, S., Daoud, M., Charfi, F., & Belhadj, A. (2017). Epigenetics and ADHD. *Journal of Attention Disorders*, 108705471769676.

Han, J. Y., Kwon, H. J., Ha, M., Paik, K. C., Lim, M. H., Lee, S. G., ... Kim, E. J. (2015). The effects of prenatal exposure to alcohol and environmental tobacco smoke on risk for ADHD: A large population-based study. *Psychiatry Research, 225*(1), 164–168.

Handen, B. L., Feldman, H. M., Lurier, A. M., & Murray, P. H. (1997). Efficacy of methylphenidate among preschool children with developmental disabilities and ADHD. *Journal of the American Academy of Child and Adolescent Psychiatry, 38*, 805–812.

Haraway, D. L. (2012). Monitoring students with ADHD within the RTI framework. *The Behavior Analyst Today, 13*(2), 17–21.

Hastings, R. P., Beck, A., Daley, D., & Hill, C. (2005). Symptoms of ADHD and their correlates in children with intellectual disabilities. *Research in Developmental Disabilities, 26*, 456–468.

Hodgkins, P., Setyawan, J., Mitra, D., Davis, K., Quintero, J., Fridman, M., ... Harpin, V. (2013). Management of ADHD in children across Europe: Patient demographics, physician characteristics and treatment patterns. *European Journal of Pediatrics, 172*(7), 895–906. https://doi.org/10.1007/s00431-013-1969-8

Huang, Y.-S., Guilleminault, C., Li, H.-Y., Yang, C.-M., Wu, Y.-Y., & Chen, N.-H. (2007). Attention-deficit/hyperactivity disorder with obstructive sleep apnea: A treatment outcome study. *Sleep Medicine, 8*(1), 18–30. https://doi.org/10.1016/j.sleep.2006.05.016

Hurley, A. D. (1996). Psychiatric disorders in children and adolescents with mental retardation and developmental disabilities. *Current Opinion in Pediatrics, 8*(4), 361–366.

Hvolby, A. (2015). Associations of sleep disturbance with ADHD: Implications for treatment. *Attention Deficit and Hyperactivity Disorders, 7*(1), 1–18. https://doi.org/10.1007/s12402-014-0151-0

Jameson, N. D., Sheppard, B. K., Lateef, T. M., Vande Voort, J. L., He, J.-P., & Merikangas, K. R. (2016). Medical comorbidity of attention-deficit/hyperactivity disorder in US adolescents. *Journal of Child Neurology, 31*(11), 1282–1289.

Joelsson, P., Chudal, R., Talati, A., Suominen, A., Brown, A. S., & Sourander, A. (2016). Prenatal smoking exposure and neuropsychiatric comorbidity of ADHD: A Finnish nationwide population-based cohort study. *BMC Psychiatry, 16*(1), 306.

Kahn, E., & Cohen, L. (1934). Organic drivenness a brainstem syndrome and an experience. *The New England Journal of Medicine, 210*, 748–756.

Kaufman, L., Ayub, M., & Vincent, J. B. (2010). The genetic basis of non-syndromic intellectual disability: A review. *Journal of Neurodevelopmental Disorders, 2*(4), 182–209. https://doi.org/10.1007/s11689-010-9055-2

Kim, J., Lee, S. H., Lee, J. H., & Hong, K. H. (2014). The role of intrinsic defects in methylammonium lead iodide perovskite. *The journal of physical chemistry letters, 5*(8), 1312–1317.

Kingdon, D., Cardoso, C., & McGrath, J. J. (2015). Research review: Executive function deficits in fetal alcohol spectrum disorders and attention-deficit/hyperactivity disorder – A meta-analysis. *Journal of Child Psychology and Psychiatry, and Allied Disciplines, 57*(2), 116–131. https://doi.org/10.1111/jcpp.12451

Kiser, D. P., Rivero, O., & Lesch, K. P. (2015). Annual research review: The (epi) genetics of neurodevelopmental disorders in the era of whole-genome sequencing–unveiling the dark matter. *Journal of Child Psychology and Psychiatry, 56*(3), 278–295.

Knobel, M., Wolman, M. B., & Mason, E. (1959). Hyperkinesis and organicity in children. *AMA archives of general psychiatry, 1*(3), 310–321.

Kohane, I. S., McMurry, A., Weber, G., MacFadden, D., Rappaport, L., Kunkel, L., ... Churchill, S. (2012). The co-morbidity burden of children and young adults with autism spectrum disorders. *PLoS One, 7*(4), e33224.

Kolar, D., Keller, A., Golfinopoulos, M., Cumyn, L., Syer, C., & Hechtman, L. (2008). Treatment of adults with attention-deficit/hyperactivity disorder. *Neuropsychiatric Disease and Treatment, 4*(2), 389–403.

Koller, H., Richardson, S. A., Katz, M., & McLaren, J. (1983). Behavior disturbance since childhood among a 5-year birth cohort of all mentally retarded young adults in a city. *American Journal of Mental Deficiency, 87*, 386–395.

Konijnenberg, C. (2015). Methodological issues in assessing the impact of prenatal drug exposure. *Substance abuse research and treatment, 9*(Suppl 2), 39–44.

Koyuncu, E., Türkkani, M. H., Sarikaya, F. G., & Özgirgin, N. (2017). Sleep disordered breathing in children with cerebral palsy. *Sleep Medicine, 30*, 146–150. https://doi.org/10.1016/j.sleep.2016.01.020

Kuntsi, J., Eley, T. C., Taylor, A., Hughes, C., Asherson, P., Caspi, A., & Moffitt, T. E. (2004). Co-occurrence of ADHD and low IQ has genetic origins. *American Journal of Medical Genetics, 124B*, 41–47.

La Malfa, G., Lassi, S., Bertelli, M., Pallanti, S., & Albertini, G. (2008). Detecting Attention-Deficit/Hyperactivity Disorder (ADHD) in adults with intellectual disability the use of Conners' Adult ADHD Rating Scales (CAARS). *Research in Developmental Disabilities, 29*(2), 158–164. https://doi.org/10.1016/j.ridd.2007.02.002

Lange, K. W., Reichl, S., Lange, K. M., Tucha, L., & Tucha, O. (2010). The history of attention deficit hyperactivity disorder. *Attention Deficit and Hyperactivity Disorders, 2*(4), 241–255. https://doi.org/10.1007/s12402-010-0045-8

Larson, K., Russ, S. A., Kahn, R. S., & Halfon, N. (2011). Patterns of comorbidity, functioning, and service use for US children with ADHD, 2007. *Pediatrics, 127*(3), 462–470.

Leitner, Y. (2014). The co-occurrence of autism and attention deficit hyperactivity disorder in children – What do we know? *Frontiers in Human Neuroscience, 8*, 268.

Lindblad, I., Gillberg, C., & Fernell, E. (2011). ADHD and other associated developmental problems in children with mild mental retardation. The use of the "Five-To-fifteen" questionnaire in a population-based sample. *Research in Developmental Disabilities, 32*, 2805–2809.

Linna, S. L., Moilanen, I., Ebeling, H., Piha, J., Kumpulainen, K., Tamminen, T., & Almqvist, F. (1999). Psychiatric symptoms in children with intellectual disability. *European Child & Adolescent Psychiatry, 8*, 77–82.

Lundervold, A. J., Stickert, M., Hysing, M., Sorensen, L., Gillberg, C., & Posserud, M.-B. (2012). Attention deficits in children with combined autism and ADHD: A CPT study. *Journal of Attention Disorders, 20*(7), 599–609.

Mahajan, R., Bernal, M. P., Panzer, R., Whitaker, A., Roberts, W., Handen, B., … Veenstra-VanderWeele, J. (2012). Clinical practice pathways for evaluation and medication choice for attention-deficit/hyperactivity disorder symptoms in autism spectrum disorders. *Pediatrics, 130*(Supplement 2), S125–S138.

Mallett, C. A., Natarajan, A., & Hoy, J. (2014). Attention deficit/hyperactivity disorder: A DSM timeline review. *International Journal of Mental Health, 43*(4), 36–60. https://doi.org/10.1080/00207411.2015.1009310

Maris, M., Verhulst, S., Wojciechowski, M., Van de Heyning, P., & Boudewyns, A. (2016). Sleep problems and obstructive sleep apnea in children with down syndrome, an overview. *International Journal of Pediatric Otorhinolaryngology, 82*, 12–15. https://doi.org/10.1016/j.ijporl.2015.12.014

Martin, A. J., & Burns, E. C. (2014). Academic buoyancy, resilience, and adaptability in students with ADHD. *The ADHD Report, 22*(6), 1–9.

Matson, J. L., & Shoemaker, M. (2009). Intellectual disability and its relationship to autism spectrum disorders. *Research in Developmental Disabilities, 30*, 1107–1114.

May, T., Sciberras, E., Hiscock, H., & Rinehart, N. (2016). The comorbid diagnosis of ASD and ADHD: Clinical and neuropsychological perspectives. In J. L. Matson (Ed.), *Handbook of assessment and diagnosis of autism spectrum disorder* (pp. 259–284). Springer International Publishing. Retrieved from http://link.springer.com/chapter/10.1007/978-3-319-27171-2_14

Miller, M. L., Fee, V., & Jones, C. J. (2004). Psychometric properties of ADHD rating scales among children with mental retardation I: Validity. *Research in Developmental Disabilities, 25*, 477–492.

Miller, M. L., Fee, V. E., & Netterville, A. K. (2004). Psychometric properties of ADHD rating scales among children with mental retardation I: Reliability. *Research in Developmental Disabilities, 25*(5), 459–476.

Millichap, J. G. (2008). Etiologic classification of attention-deficit/hyperactivity disorder. *Pediatrics, 121*(2), e358–e365.

Milnerowicz-Nabzdyk, E., & Bizoń, A. (2014). Effect of cigarette smoking on vascular flows in pregnancies complicated by intrauterine growth restriction. *Reproductive Toxicology, 50*, 27–35.

Mitis, E. M., McKay, K. E., Schulz, K. P., Newcorn, J. H., & Halperin, J. M. (2000). Parent-teacher concordance for DSM-IV attention deficit hyperactivity disorder in a clinic referred sample. *Journal of the American Academy of Child & Adolescent Psychiatry, 39*, 308–313.

Moeschler, J. B. (2008). Genetic evaluation of intellectual disabilities. *Seminars in Pediatric Neurology, 15*(1), 2–9. https://doi.org/10.1016/j.spen.2008.01.002

Morales, M. R., Polizzi, C., Sulliotti, G., Mascolino, C., & Perricone, G. (2013). Early precursors of low attention and hyperactivity in moderately and very preterm children at preschool age. *Pediatric reports, 5*(4), 18.

Moriyama, I. M., Loy, R. M., Robb-Smith, A. H. T., Rosenberg, H. M., & Hoyert, D. L. (2011). *History of the statistical classification of diseases and causes of death*. Department of Health and Human Services Public Health Service.

Murphy, C. M., Christakou, A., Daly, E. M., Ecker, C., Giampietro, V., Brammer, M., … Rubia, K. (2014). Abnormal functional activation and maturation of fronto-striato-temporal and cerebellar regions during sustained attention in autism spectrum disorder. *The American Journal of Psychiatry, 171*(10), 1107–1116.

National Institute of Mental Health. (2012). *Attention deficit hyperactivity disorder (ADHD)*. Washington, DC: U.S. Department of Health and Human Services. NIH Publication No. 12-3572.

Neece, C. L., Baker, B. L., & Lee, S. S. (2013). ADHD among adolescents with intellectual disabilities: Pre-pathway influences. *Research in Developmental Disabilities, 34*(7), 2268–2279. https://doi.org/10.1016/j.ridd.2013.02.025

Niggs, J. T., & Barkely, R. A. (2014). Attention-deficit/hyperactivity disorder. In *Child psychopathology* (3rd ed.). New York: Guildford Press.

Niklasson, L., Rasmussen, P., Oskarsdottir, S., & Gillberg, C. (2009). Autism, ADHD, mental retardation and behavior problems in 100 individuals with 22q11 deletion syndrome. *Research in Developmental*

Disabilities, 30(4), 763–773. https://doi.org/10.1016/j.ridd.2008.10.007

O'Malley, K. D., & Nanson, J. (2002). Clinical implications of a link between fetal alcohol spectrum disorder and attention-deficit hyperactivity disorder. *Canadian Journal of Psychiatry. Revue Canadienne de Psychiatrie, 47*(4), 349–354.

Owens, J., Gruber, R., Brown, T., Corkum, P., Cortese, S., O'Brien, L., … Weiss, M. (2012). Future research directions in sleep and ADHD. *Journal of Attention Disorders, 17*(7), 550–564. https://doi.org/10.1177/1087054712457799

Owens, J. A. (2005). The ADHD and sleep conundrum redux: Moving forward. *Sleep Medicine Reviews, 10*(6), 377–379. https://doi.org/10.1016/j.smrv.2006.08.002

Peadon, E., & Elliott, E. J. (2010). Distinguishing between attention-deficit hyperactivity and fetal alcohol spectrum disorders in children: Clinical guidelines. *Neuropsychiatric Disease and Treatment, 6*, 509–515.

Pearson, D. A., & Aman, M. G. (1994). Ratings of hyperactivity and developmental indices: Should clinicians correct for developmental level? *Journal of Autism and Developmental Disorders, 24*, 395–411.

Pearson, D. A., Lachar, D., Loveland, K. A., Santos, C. W., Faria, L. P., Azzam, P. N., … Cleveland, L. A. (2000). Patterns of behavioral adjustment and maladjustment in mental retardation: Comparison of children with and without ADHD. *American Journal on Mental Retardation, 105*(4), 236–251.

Perfect, M. M., Archbold, K., Goodwin, J., Levine-Donnerstein, D., & Quan, S. F. (2013). Risk of behavioral and adaptive functioning difficulties in youth with previous and current sleep disordered breathing. *Sleep, 36*(4), 517–525B.

Pliszka, S. R. (2009). *Treating ADHD and comorbid disorders. Psychosocial and psychopharmacological interventions*. New York: Guilford Press.

Popova, S., Lange, S., Shield, K., Mihic, A., Chudley, A. E., Mukherjee, R. A. S., … Rehm, J. (2016). Comorbidity of fetal alcohol spectrum disorder: A systematic review and meta-analysis. *The Lancet, 387*(10022), 978–987.

Preston, A. I., Wood, C. L., & Stecker, P. M. (2015). Response to intervention: Where it came from and where it's going. *Preventing School Failure: Alternative Education for Children and Youth, 60*(3), 173–182.

Reed, M. O., Jakubovski, E., Johnson, J. A., & Bloch, M. H. (2017). Predictors of long-term school-based behavioral outcomes in the multimodal treatment study of children with attention-deficit/hyperactivity disorder. *Journal of Child and Adolescent Psychopharmacology, 27*(4), 296–309.

Reynolds, C. R., & Shaywitz, S. E. (2009). Response to intervention: Prevention and remediation, Perhaps. Diagnosis, No. *Child Development Perspectives, 3*(1), 44.

Richdale, A. L., & Baglin, C. L. (2015). Self-report and caregiver-report of sleep and psychopathology in children with high-functioning autism spectrum disorder: A pilot study. *Developmental Neurorehabilitation, 18*(4), 272–279.

Richdale, A. L., & Schreck, K. A. (2009). Sleep problems in autism spectrum disorders: Prevalence, nature, & possible biopsychosocial aetiologies. *Sleep Medicine Reviews, 13*(6), 403–411. https://doi.org/10.1016/j.smrv.2009.02.003

Robertson, J., Hatton, C., Emerson, E., & Baines, S. (2015). Prevalence of epilepsy among people with intellectual disabilities: A systematic review. *Seizure: The Journal of the British Epilepsy Association, 29*, 46–62.

Rodríguez, C., García, T., & Areces, D. (2017). New and future challenges concerning the use of virtual reality tools for assessing ADHD. *Current Developmental Disorders Reports, 4*(1), 8–10.

Sanford, J. A., & Turner, A. (1994). *Integrated Visual and Auditory continuous performance test (IVA+Plus), interpretation manual*. Brain Train, Inc.

Santoro, S. D., Giacheti, C. M., Rossi, N. F., Campos, L. M. G., & Pinato, L. (2016). Correlations between behavior, memory, sleep-wake and melatonin in Williams-Beuren syndrome. *Physiology & Behavior, 159*, 14–19. https://doi.org/10.1016/j.physbeh.2016.03.010

Simon, G. R., Baker, C., Barden, G. A., Brown, O. W., Hardin, A., Lessin, H. R., … Bright Futures Periodicity Schedule Workgroup. (2014). 2014 recommendations for pediatric preventive health care. *Pediatrics, 133*(3), 568–570.

Simonoff, E., Pickles, A., Wood, N., Gringras, P., & Chadwick, O. (2007). ADHD symptoms in children with mild intellectual disability. *Journal of the American Academy of Child and Adolescent Psychiatry, 46*, 591–600.

Smith, S. W., Cumming, M. M., Merrill, K. L., Pitts, D. L., & Daunic, A. P. (2015). Teaching self-regulation skills to students with behavior problems: Essential instructional components. *Beyond Behavior, 24*(3), 4–13.

Spruyt, K., & Gozal, D. (2011). Sleep disturbances in children with attention-deficit/hyperactivity disorder. *Expert Review of Neurotherapeutics, 11*(4), 565–577. https://doi.org/10.1586/ern.11.7

Stromme, P., & Diseth, T. H. (2000). Prevalence of psychiatric diagnoses in children with mental retardation: Data from a population-based study. *Developmental Medicine and Child Neurology, 42*, 266–270.

Subcommittee on Attention-Deficit/Hyperactivity Disorder, Steering Committee on Quality Improvement and Management, Wolraich, M., Brown, L., Brown, R. T., DuPaul, G., … Visser, S. (2011). ADHD: Clinical practice guideline for the diagnosis, evaluation, and treatment of attention-deficit/hyperactivity disorder in children and adolescents. *Pediatrics, 128*(5), 1007–1022.

Sung, V., Hiscock, H., Sciberras, E., & Efron, D. (2008). Sleep problems in children with attention-deficit/hyperactivity disorder: Prevalence and the effect on the child and family. *Archives of Pediatrics & Adolescent Medicine, 162*(4), 336–342.

Swanson, J. M. (1992). *School based assessments and intervention for ADD students*. Irvine, CA: KC Publishing.

Tannock, R. (2002). Cognitive correlates of ADHD. In P. S. Jensen & J. R. Cooper (Eds.), *Attention deficit hyperactivity disorder: State of the science* (pp. 8–27). Kingston, NJ: Civic Research Institute.

Taylor, E. (2011). Antecedents of ADHD: A historical account of diagnostic concepts. *ADHD Attention Deficit and Hyperactivity Disorders, 3*(2), 69–75. https://doi.org/10.1007/s12402-010-0051-x

Taylor, E., Dopfner, M., Sergeant, J., Asherson, P., Banaschewski, T., Buitelaar, J., … Zuddas, A. (2004). European clinical guidelines for hyperkinetic disorder – First upgrade. *European Child & Adolescent Psychiatry, 13*(Suppl 1), 17–30. https://doi.org/10.1007/s00787-004-1002-x.

Thapar, A., Martin J., Mick E., Arias Vasquez A., Langley K., Scherer S. W., Schachar R., et al. (2016). Psychiatric gene discoveries shape evidence on ADHD's biology. *Molecular Psychiatry, 21*(9),1202–1207. https://doi.org/10.1038/mp.2015.163.

Thomas, R., Sanders, S., Doust, J., Beller, E., & Glasziou, P. (2015). Prevalence of attention-deficit/hyperactivity disorder: A systematic review and meta-analysis. *Pediatrics, 135*(4), e994–e1001.

Torres, V. I., Vallejo, D., & Inestrosa, N. C. (2017). Emerging synaptic molecules as candidates in the etiology of neurological disorders. *Neural Plasticity, 2017*, 8081758.

U. S. Department of Education, National Center for Education Statistics. (2016). *Digest of education statistics, 2015* (NCES 2016-014), Chapter 2.

Veldhuizen, S., & Cairney, J. (2017). Digital technology and screening for developmental concerns in the early years. *Current Developmental Disorders Report, 4*(1), 5–7.

Visser, S., Danielson, M., & Wolraich, M. (2016). Vital signs: National and state-specific patterns of attention deficit/hyperactivity disorder treatment among insured children age 2–5 years. *Morbidity and Mortality Weekly Report*, (65), 443–450. http://dx.doi.org/10.15585/mmwr.mm6517e1.

Visser, S. N., Danielson, M. L., Bitsko, R. H., Holbrook, J. R., Kogan, M. D., Ghandour, R. M., … Blumberg, S. J. (2014). Trends in the parent-report of health care provider-diagnosed and medicated attention-deficit/hyperactivity disorder: United States, 2003–2011. *Journal of the American Academy of Child and Adolescent Psychiatry, 53*(1), 34–46.e2.

Voigt, R. G., Barbaresi, W. J., Colligan, R. C., Weaver, A. L., & Katusic, S. K. (2006). Developmental dissociation, deviance, and delay: Occurrence of attention deficit hyperactivity disorder in individuals with and without borderline to mild intellectual disability. *Developmental Medical Child Neurology, 48*, 831–835.

Vorstman, J. A. S., & Ophoff, R. A. (2013). Genetic causes of developmental disorders. *Current Opinion in Neurology, 26*(2), 128–136. https://doi.org/10.1097/WCO.0b013e32835f1a

Wagner, M. M., Newman, L. A., & Javitz, H. S. (2014). The influence of family socioeconomic status on the post–high school outcomes of youth with disabilities. *Career Development and Transition for Exceptional Individuals, 37*(1), 5–17.

Weiss, M. D., & Weiss, J. R. (2004). A guide to the treatment of adults with ADHD. *The Journal of Clinical Psychiatry, 65*(Suppl 3), 27–37.

Whittingham, K., Bodimeade, H. L., Lloyd, O., & Boyd, R. N. (2014). Everyday psychological functioning in children with unilateral cerebral palsy: Does executive functioning play a role? *Developmental Medicine and Child Neurology, 56*(6), 572–579.

Wiggs, L. (2001). Sleep problems in children with developmental disorders. *Journal of the Royal Society of Medicine, 94*, 177–179.

Williams, J. F., Smith, V. C., & Committee on Substance Abuse. (2015). Fetal alcohol spectrum disorders. *Pediatrics, 136*(5), e1395–e1406.

Williams, N. M., Zaharieva, I., Martin, A., Langley, K., Mantripragada, K., Fossdal, R., et al. (2010). Rare chromosomal deletions and duplications in attention-deficit hyperactivity disorder: A genome-wide analysis. *Lancet, 376*(9750), 1401–1408. https://doi.org/10.1016/S0140-6736(10)61109-9

Wolraich, M. L., Lambert, W., Doffing, M., Bickman, L., Simmons, T., & Worley, K. (2003). Psychometric properties of the Vanderbilt ADHD diagnostic parent rating scale in a referred population. *Journal of Pediatric Psychology, 8*(8), 559–568.

Young, S., Absoud, M., Blackburn, C., Branney, P., Colley, B., Farrag, E., … Mukherjee, R. (2016). Guidelines for identification and treatment of individuals with attention deficit/hyperactivity disorder and associated fetal alcohol spectrum disorders based upon expert consensus. *BMC Psychiatry*, (1), 16. https://doi.org/10.1186/s12888-016-1027-y

Youssef, N. A., Ege, M., Angly, S. S., Strauss, J. L., & Marx, C. E. (2011). Is obstructive sleep apnea associated with ADHD? *Annals of Clinical Psychiatry: Official Journal of the American Academy of Clinical Psychiatrists, 23*(3), 213–224.

Zhu, J. L., Olsen, J., Liew, Z., Li, J., Niclasen, J., & Obel, C. (2014). Parental smoking during pregnancy and ADHD in children: The Danish national birth cohort. *Pediatrics, 134*(2), e382–e388.

Assessment of Autism Spectrum Disorders

Leland T. Farmer, Michelle S. Lemay, and Robert D. Rieske

Autism Assessment

The prevalence of autism spectrum disorder (ASD) has seen a rapid increase in the past 20 years. Since autism was first introduced into the third edition of the *Diagnostic and Statistical Manual of Mental Disorders* (DSM-III, APA 1980), the prevalence has risen to roughly 1 in every 68 children based on a recent study conducted by the Centers for Disease Control and Prevention (CDC, 2014). This rapid change in prevalence strongly contrasts the prior rates of 6 per every 1000 children in the 1990s (Wing & Potter, 2002). Although multiple theories exist regarding the cause of this rise in prevalence, the most hypothesized reason is an increased awareness for it. More pediatricians are screening patients, more parents are aware of ASD symptoms, and it is even becoming more prominent in the media.

Although a greater awareness of ASD symptoms and the need to screen for these symptoms is important, proper assessment of the observed symptoms is the only way to ensure that the symptoms fall within a diagnosis of autism. Unfortunately, many children are often misdiagnosed or are not diagnosed until much later in life, which can negatively affect development and reduces effectiveness of behavioral and developmental interventions. This chapter will discuss the different components to consider when conducting an ASD assessment including the purpose, which assessments have the best validity and reliability, and which areas of functioning should be considered to provide appropriate case conceptualization.

Purpose of ASD Assessment

ASD, which is classified as a neurodevelopmental disorder, can affect multiple aspects of an individual's functioning including language abilities, social skills, adaptive skills, and overall cognitive abilities, to name a few. Due to the complex nature of the presentation for this diagnosis, assessment of ASD becomes quite complex. Specifically, it is important when performing an ASD diagnostic assessment that all the above-mentioned areas are being assessed within the assessment battery. Best clinical practice recommends a multi-method, multi-informant approach to assessment. This is an extensive process that includes administering standardized clinician-administered assessments of cognitive abilities, language skills, adaptive behaviors, as well as informant-report measures with multiple infor-

L. T. Farmer · M. S. Lemay · R. D. Rieske (✉)
Department of Psychology, Idaho State University, Pocatello, ID, USA
e-mail: riesrobe@isu.edu

mants including parents, teachers, or other raters such as speech-language pathologists, occupational therapists, and oftentimes the clinician.

Process of Assessment

Although the source of ASD is still undetermined, test developers have created a wide range of assessment tools and protocols for the use of determining whether or not an individual does in fact have ASD. Diagnosis, especially early diagnosis, can be a determining factor in the outcomes and implementation of services such as applied behavior analysis (ABA) or functional skills training. Several parameters have been set in place by the American Academy of Neurology, the American Academy of Child and Adolescent Psychiatry, and a panel of individuals from multiple professional societies detailing the requirements for an assessment of ASD (Filipek et al., 1999, 2000; Volkmar, Cook, Pomeroy, Realmuto, & Tanguay, 1999). These parameters state that the first level of screening and evaluation should be conducted by professionals such as pediatricians or general practitioners who are meant to monitor the child's developmental milestones for any noticeable abnormalities within their development. The second level of evaluation occurs following a positive screening during the first level of evaluation. These children are typically referred to a psychologist who then receive a more comprehensive psychodiagnostic assessment. However, the first thing that must happen in order for a child to go through the abovementioned steps is for the caregiver and/or pediatrician to be aware of the different symptom presentations associated with ASD.

Autism Spectrum Disorder Symptomology

Symptoms of ASD vary across children as well as age range, especially when rehabilitative services such as occupational therapy, speech-language therapy, or ABA are implemented. For example, some children with ASD may exhibit poor eye contact and have a very strong but limited interest in few activities, whereas other children could present as nonverbal with no interest in social interaction but are willing to play with a wide range of toys. Therefore, it is important to understand the range of symptoms associated with ASD and the high levels of heterogeneity between individuals.

ASD symptoms are not always consistent across age and development. Just like any typically developing child, the challenging behaviors and symptoms of ASD change with development and maturation. Therefore different tools have been developed to assess for symptomology at different age points based on findings from research that characterize the disorder at differing developmental ages.

Infants and Toddlers

Although one of the more difficult age ranges to assess and diagnose ASD is in the infant/toddler age range, this is attributed to the fact that, unless the child is on the severe end of the spectrum, parents and caregivers are less likely to notice any abnormalities in their child's behavior or functioning until they enter school or other social settings. However, the presentation of ASD in toddlers is probably one of the most well-researched developmental stages. Tools designed for assessing ASD begin as young as 12 months of age. Within this age range, children on the spectrum may display developmental delays in behaviors such as joint attention, pointing, and gaze following, which typically develop between 9 and 14 months (Johnson, 2008). In addition to deficits in these behaviors, children with ASD may also have limited verbal ability, little shared interest, poor eye contact, or poor communication skills (Klaiman, Fernandez-Carriba, Hall, & Saulnier, 2015). Frequently, infants or toddlers that are higher functioning will be "missed" in terms of diagnosis at this age level because they are not expected to engage in as complex social interactions as older school-aged children who interact more with same-aged children in a school or daycare setting.

School-Age Children

Most parents or caregivers who have children on the spectrum first begin to notice their child is different when they begin attending daycare, preschool, or kindergarten. This is thought to be due to the fact that parents are able to observe their child's behaviors in comparison to a wider range of other children in a social context, where deviations in their child's behavior are more noticeable. Parents or teachers may notice a child on the spectrum being less interested in joint-play activities or having a preference for solitary play. Within this age group, symptoms such as language delays and behavioral differences become more apparent. For example, school-age children with ASD are more likely to display aggression, tantrums, and "meltdowns" which are often tied to language difficulties and an inability to communicate their wants or needs (Klaiman et al., 2015). Additionally, children in this age range also experience other mental health symptoms such as anxiety, depression, attention deficit hyperactivity disorder (ADHD), and oppositional or defiant behavior at higher rates than typically developing children which causes diagnostic clarification to be even more difficult (Ghanizadeh, 2012; Goldin, Matson, Tureck, Cervantes, & Jang, 2013). When these aggressive behavioral problems begin to occur, caregivers will typically begin the assessment and treatment process in an attempt to abate the behavioral problems. However, if these problems persist into adolescence, they may become more severe or could manifest in other ways.

Adolescence

The adolescent period of development is when we begin to see an increase in comorbid diagnoses and more distress related to social functioning. For example, if an adolescent with ASD is attempting to make friends but is not skilled in appropriately initiating social interaction, he may struggle to form or maintain friendships (Gotham, 2010). This may lead to increased rates of depression or anxiety and decrease the likelihood that this teen may attempt to talk with his peers again. Studies have shown that up to 30% of adolescents with ASD also meet the criteria for major depressive disorders and up to 84% of adolescents with ASD also meet the criteria for an anxiety disorder (Klaiman, Fernandez-Carriba, Hall, & Saulnier, 2015). Additionally, adolescents with ASD are more likely to be teased or bullied because of their social differences. This period in life is important for the implementation of social skills training or continued ABA-based therapies based on the severity of the diagnosis due to the psychosocial effect of bullying on the adolescent. It is possible that adolescents with a diagnosis of ASD will continue to display limited speech abilities, restricted interests, poor social skills, and limited eye contact, but therapeutic interventions continue to be effective within this age range.

Adulthood

Although individuals on the more severe end of the ASD spectrum may continue to be nonverbal, have poor social skills and restricted interests, and make little-to-no eye contact, some adults on the ASD spectrum are able to live their lives with little or no support from others. Some symptoms that are prominent in adults with ASD include difficulty in planning or organizing their daily life and social activities, continuing to have rigid thought patterns, and continuing to struggle with social interactions (Dubbelink, Linda, & Geurts, 2017). That being said, individuals with a diagnosis of ASD can see a decrease in their symptoms with the implementation of behavioral and psychological interventions. In a study of over 240 adults and individuals with ASD, those who were 31 years of age and older displayed fewer maladaptive behaviors and experienced more improvement in their behaviors over time (Shattuck et al., 2007). This evidence suggests that, although the ASD diagnosis is fairly stable throughout the lifespan, it is possible for symptoms to decrease with proper interventions and time.

The development of and cause for ASD is not yet fully understood as to why we see such a wide array of differences across several domains including the severity of the symptoms present in each client. These differences seen among different age groups also affect diagnosis as well, and it is important to note that there are also age-related factors to consider when diagnosing ASD.

Appropriate Age of Diagnosis

Early diagnosis is a crucial component of positive outcomes for children with ASD. Parents generally begin to recognize autistic-related problems in their child between 12 and 36 months of age (Chakrabarti, 2009; Kishore & Basu, 2011). However, the latency period between parents' first concern of ASD and the time of receiving a diagnosis is often several years (Chakrabarti, 2009). There are several factors that affect the age at diagnosis and likelihood of being referred for an evaluation. Factors that generally lead to early diagnosis include more severe autism symptomology, living in an urban area, income above poverty level, and specific behaviors such as toe walking, hand flapping, and sustained odd play (Mandell, Novak, & Zubritsky, 2005).

Many tools have been developed to assess ASD symptoms in young children under 3 years of age, which is a crucial period in which many children could capitalize on early intervention programs. Although it is hypothesized by some that ASD symptoms are present from birth (e.g., Planche 2010), many of these symptoms are not observable until the child is older. Tools specialized for early detection have been developed to assess ASD symptoms in children as young as 12 months of age with increased validity and reliability in tools for children between 2 and 3 years of age. Clinicians and physicians are able to appropriately use screening tools and assessments to find similarities or clusters of symptoms associated with ASD. These screening tools save time by flagging the individuals that are considered to be at risk for ASD.

Screening Methods

Screening methods are typically the first line in a series of assessment or tools used by clinicians or physicians and are usually given to clients at a specific developmental wellness checkpoints (generally 18 and 24 months of age). Evidence is generated through the use of parent-report and other-report measures to differentiate at-risk children. Follow-up measures and screeners with more specific criteria are then given to at-risk children to further clarify the presenting concerns. This screening approach requires regular developmental surveillance to differentiate individuals with ASD from other developmental or mental health disorders. Clinicians and other behavioral professionals are encouraged to use the screening tools, measures, and procedures in this section to aid in their ability to differentiate clients considered to be at risk for ASD from typically developing children.

It is recommended that clinicians use screening tools that are empirically supported and that have been standardized across large populations. The sensitivity and specificity of each developmental screening tool allows the clinician to identify the known ASD-like symptoms present in the client as ASD is believed to encompass a continuum of symptomology and associated neurobehavioral and cognitive irregularities. In general, ASD screening methods were developed to gather information regarding the symptom presentation endorsed by independent observers (e.g., parent, teacher, other caregiver) that help the clinician identify specific ASD markers in an individual. Below is a list of recommended screening measures frequently used by clinicians or medical professionals in the assessment of ASD. While there are several additional tools that look at developmental delays more broadly, and other ASD specific tools that still require further validation, these are the most commonly used and empirically validated tools for ASD screening (Table 1).

Modified Checklist for Autism in Toddlers, Revised (M-CHAT-R)

One of the most common ASD screening tools used is the M-CHAT. The M-CHAT is a 20-item parent-report tool designed for screening children from ages 16 to 30 months for ASD. The M-CHAT relies on information gathered from the perspective of the parent regarding a number of

Assessment of Autism Spectrum Disorders

Table 1 Recommended screening measures for autism spectrum disorder

Screening tools	Informant	Format	Age range	Time to administer
Modified Checklist for Autism in Toddlers, Revised (M-CHAT-R), (Robins, Fein, & Barton, 2009)	Parent	Rating scale	16–30 months	10 min
Early Screening of Autistic Traits (ESAT), (Swinkels et al., 2006)	Parent	Rating scale	0–36 months	10 min
First Year Inventory (FYI), (Baranek, Watson, Crais, & Reznick, 2003)	Parent	Rating scale	12 months	20–30 min

developmental domains including sensory, motor, and social development. The parent is asked to answer each question with either a "yes" or "no" answer. These responses are then scored to determine if the client is at risk for ASD. Depending on the score, an additional follow-up has been developed to further differentiate potential ASD symptoms from other typical or non-typical development. The M-CHAT was designed to be administered at 18 and 24 month wellness visits to pediatricians or other primary care practitioners. Advantages to using the M-CHAT include being available for free online, wide use among practitioners, and good psychometric properties.

Early Screening of Autistic Traits (ESAT)

The ESAT is a 14-item screening tool administered by a behavioral professional, which gathers information from the parent's perspective. This screening instrument and procedure may be administered to children between 0 and 36 months of age but is typically used with children at 14–15 months of age. The items on the ESAT are used to highlight important areas of play behavior and social development such as pretend play, joint attention, and eye contact. The ESAT is also available for free online but is not as widely used as the M-CHAT in the United States; however, the tool still has sufficient psychometric properties.

First Year Inventory (FYI)

The FYI is a parent-report questionnaire given to children at 12 months of age. The report consists of 63 questions and is used to determine irregularities in social communication and sensory domains. The questions are based on a retrospective video analysis of children diagnosed with ASD and the behavioral markers that were exhibited at 12 months of age (Baranek et al., 2003). The FYI is one of the few tools that has been developed for children as young as 12 months of age; however, the FYI is a lengthy screening tool, and further research is needed to improve its sensitivity and specificity.

One of the primary goals of clinicians in the screening phase of assessment is to accurately identify children who have ASD symptoms and differentiate them from those who do not meet the criteria of ASD based on the symptoms described. An additional goal from a health perspective is to use screening methods in order to identify individuals that should be referred for a comprehensive ASD assessment. Therefore it is important to use measures that have a very low false-positive. After the individual has positively screened for symptomology associated with ASD, a comprehensive ASD evaluation should be recommended by the clinician which includes a full battery of measures used to identify ASD symptomology. There are several different types of assessment that should be included in a comprehensive evaluation as detailed in the next section.

Types of Assessment

This section outlines the components that are needed for an ASD assessment. By having a wide range of different measures, the assessor is better able to conceptualize the case and form a diagnostic impression of the child using a multi-method and multi-informant approach. Therefore, it is strongly recommended that when conducting a comprehensive diagnostic assessment for ASD, you include self-report measures of behaviors and emotional functioning, observational measures, cognitive measures, language measures, and measures of adaptive skills.

Assessment Components

Self-report measures and interviews The first component that is most often administered across all assessors is obtaining self-report questionnaires and conducting an interview. This information provides assessors with a developmental history of the child as well as current issues observed by the parent, teacher, or other caregiver. These typically include things such as social skills, anxious or depressive symptoms, repetitive behaviors, and any special interests as well as abnormalities in attaining developmental milestones.

Observational measures Assessors typically include a self-report measure of behavioral observations from their time spent with the child or include an assessment that is specifically designed to elicit specific behavioral responses. Additionally, many assessors use behavioral measures such as the Autism Diagnostic Observation Schedule (ADOS; Lord et al., 2000). The ADOS assesses multiple components of ASD including social skills, eye contact, restrictive or repetitive behaviors, and verbal skills in a play-/interaction-based evaluation of skills and deficits. Observational measures are a crucial part of a comprehensive diagnostic evaluation and should be used to elicit those skills, specifically social communication skills, which we would expect based on developmental level.

Cognitive ability/intelligence The next component that is often included within an ASD battery is a measure of cognitive ability or intelligence such as a Wechsler Intelligence Scale for Children Fifth Edition (WISC-V) or Stanford Binet Fifth Edition (SB-5). This allows the assessor to determine whether or not the ASD diagnosis includes intellectual disabilities or if there are any components of intelligence that are at a higher than average or below average level of functioning such as working memory or visual-spatial skills. Additionally, in many US states, a dual diagnosis of ASD and intellectual disability provides the family with a wider array of support and options for improving their child's functioning. However, many children with low functioning ASD are considered to be un-testable due to an inability to obtain a baseline on traditional cognitive measures. While other tools may be used to estimate cognitive age equivalents (e.g., Bayley-3) such tools were not designed or validated for such uses.

Language A measure of language abilities is included in the battery as a way to determine long-term outcome as the two are often correlated (Ozonoff, Goodlin-Jones, & Solomon, 2005). As one of the most common deficits in children with ASD, many children on the ASD spectrum also receive speech/language therapy. By including an assessment of language, clinicians can better conceptualize their language abilities and develop recommendations that are more individualized and appropriate.

Adaptive behavior The final core component included in an ASD comprehensive diagnostic assessment is a measure or series of measures assessing adaptive behavior. This is typically a parent-/caregiver-report measure completed by the parent(s), teachers, and/or other caregivers such as daycare providers, after-school providers, etc. Measures of adaptive behavior are not only important because they are components consistent with the DSM-5 diagnostic criteria for assessing intellectual disabilities but they also help to determine the level of support that is required in order to perform daily tasks (Ozonoff et al., 2005).

Although the different components described above are strongly recommended when conducting a comprehensive diagnostic assessment for ASD, many assessors often only include self-report measures, behavioral observations, and a measure of intelligence. Reasons for this will be further discussed within this chapter, but this becomes problematic because it does not provide the parent with a full picture of their child's functioning and affects the ability of clinicians to develop appropriate interventions. A more comprehensive assessment allows the clinician to better understand the symptom presentation and more accurately provide a diagnosis of ASD and treatment recommendations that are individualized.

Assessment Tools

The assessment tools used in a comprehensive diagnostic evaluation of ASD are focused approaches that require empirical support and have the ability to accurately measure targeted behaviors within a specific population. Each assessment tool needs to be "fit for purpose," and the information generated needs to have the potential to produce findings that could help each clinician in understanding the symptomology of each client and offer incremental validity in the diagnostic process. When selecting the correct assessment tool to use for a given situation, a clinician must identify a valid test that correctly differentiates the individuals that meet the criteria for a diagnosis from those who do not meet the criteria. Materials, forms, and the proper training and competence are also crucial components of a comprehensive ASD assessment, and each can help the clinician to identify clinically relevant information. Ideally, each measure that a clinician uses should be standardized with a large group, and the measure should also be representative of the population that is being tested.

Clinicians should rely heavily on empirically supported tools that have been used in previous assessments of ASD. A number of assessment tools have been updated or modified throughout the years, while other assessment tools are deemed to be outdated or obsolete. Therefore, it is the responsibility of the clinician to know whether or not an assessment tool is up-to-date and applicable to the ASD population. Some assessment tools have been standardized for use within specific age ranges, and clinicians should always follow the appropriate age guidelines to ensure test reliability and validity. In some assessments, it may be necessary to use more broad assessment tools that are not specific to ASD. In these cases, the measure should add reasonable additional support and fill in the gaps left by other assessment tools already in use.

The primary objective of each clinician is to accurately measure and correctly diagnose ASD. Consequently, it is of utmost importance to measure each client's presenting symptoms that are associated with ASD. This goal can be accomplished through the use of a comprehensive ASD assessment battery. Each ASD assessment battery should assess the client's cognitive abilities, communication abilities, and adaptive skills in addition to potential ASD symptomology. These abilities are assessed using several diagnostic assessments of ASD symptoms including interviews, rating scales, observation scales, and additional assessment tools.

Diagnostic Assessments of Autism Symptoms: Interviews

Diagnostic interviews for the assessment of ASD symptoms are an area of assessment that have some of the most variability from one clinician to the next; however, this is one of the most crucial pieces to making an accurate diagnostic decision. The reason for such variability is the time and resources that most of the well-validated interviews take to administer. As an example, one of the most common semistructured interviews is the Autism Diagnostic Interview-Revised (ADI-R) which can take anywhere from about 90 min to over 150 min to administer depending on the age of the client and other family factors. Because of this, many clinicians in practice will develop their own style of a more unstructured interview. While this may save time, it is often at the expense of diagnostic reliability and validity. Below are some of the well-validated interviews for ASD which include algorithms for scoring and assist

Table 2 Recommended diagnostic interviews for autism spectrum disorder

Diagnostic interviews	Informant	Format	Age range	Time to administer
Autism Diagnostic Interview – Revised (ADI-R), (Rutter, Le Couteur, & Lord, 2003)	Parent	Semi-structured interview	Mental age > 2.0	90–150 min
Diagnostic interview for Social and Communication Disorders (DISCO), (Wing, 2003)	Parent	Semi-structured interview	All ages	120–180 min
Developmental, Dimensional and Diagnostic Interview (3di), (Skuse et al., 2004)	Parent	Computer-assisted interview	Early childhood to adult	45–120 min

in differential diagnostic decisions. While the ADI-R and Diagnostic Interview for Social and Communication Disorders (DISCO) are the most common diagnostic interviews, each with good psychometric properties and validation, the unique style and psychometric properties of the Developmental, Dimensional and Diagnostic Interview (3di) make it an interesting alternative. It is strongly recommended that all clinicians include some type of structured or semi-structured interview to their core diagnostic assessment. While several brief tools are being developed for the same purpose, they currently do not hold the same reliability and validity as these measures (Table 2).

Diagnostic Assessments of Autism Symptoms: Rating Scales

Rating scales are often used in the process of diagnostic decision-making for ASD; however, the over-reliance on such tools is one of the main causes and arguments for the misdiagnosis of ASD. First, one must determine if the checklist or rating scale is meant to be used as a screener or a diagnostic tool. There are significant differences between the sensitivity and specificity of such tools and other psychometric properties. The tools listed below are meant to be used as tools to assist in diagnostic decision-making; however, clinicians need to balance the weight that is placed on such tools in comparison to other tools and the informant of those tools. Overall, such rating scales are often a measure of parental or teacher beliefs about the behaviors of a child and are not sufficient alone to make any diagnostic decisions. The rating scales listed below include measures beginning in early development through adulthood and include forms for parents, teachers, and other caregivers. It is often useful to gain multiple perspectives throughout the diagnostic process to see convergence of evidence across differing environments with different people. These are all well-validated measures that are recommended as a piece of information to be included in the overall core diagnostic assessment (Table 3).

Diagnostic Assessments of Autism Symptoms: Observation Scales

Observational measures are a unique and useful tool in the assessment of ASD. These measures help to compare clinical observations (in analog and more naturalistic environments) to the norms for that population. The Autism Diagnostic Observation Schedule (ADOS-2) is often a core component of a competent and comprehensive assessment for ASD and includes a direct assessment by the clinician in a variety of play and interaction analogs to help guide a more objective assessment of ASD symptomology. The Childhood Autism Rating Scale (CARS-2) and Checklist for Autism Spectrum Disorder (CASD) are useful tools to help summarize all clinical observations, information gathered from various informants, and testing data into a central and more objective rating of symptomology. These two types of observation tools (direct assessment and clinician ratings) can be used independently but offer greater diagnostic reliability and validity when used in tandem (Table 4).

Table 3 Recommended diagnostic rating scales for autism spectrum disorder

Diagnostic rating scales	Informant	Format	Age range	Time to administer
Autism Spectrum Rating Scales (ASRS), (Goldstein & Naglieri, 2010)	Parent/teacher	Rating scale	2–18 years	20 min
Baby and Infant Screen for Children with Autism Traits (BISCUIT), (Matson, Boisjoli, & Wilkins, 2007)	Parent/caregiver	Interview-based rating scale	17–37 months	30 min
Social Communication Questionnaire (SCQ), (Rutter, Bailey, & Lord, 2003)	Parent	Rating scale	4 to adult; mental age > 2.0	10 min
Autism Spectrum Disorders battery-Child Version (ASD-C), (Matson & González, 2007)	Parent/caregiver	Interview-based rating scale	2–18	30 min
Autism Spectrum Disorders battery-Adult Version (ASD-A), (Matson, Terlonge, & González, 2006)	Direct care staff/caregiver	Interview-based rating scale	18+	30 min
PDD Behavior Inventory (PDDBI), (Cohen & Sudhalter, 2005)	Parent/teacher	Rating scale	1.5–12.5 years	20–45 min

Table 4 Recommended diagnostic observation scales for autism spectrum disorder

Diagnostic observation scales	Informant	Format	Age range	Time to administer
Autism Diagnostic Observation Schedule (ADOS-2), (Lord, Rutter, DiLavore, & Risi, 2012)	Clinician-direct assessment	Clinical semi-structured observation	12 months to adult	40–60 min
Childhood Autism Rating Scale (CARS-2), (Schopler, Reichler, & Renner, 2010)	Clinician observational assessment	Clinician observation rating scale	2 to adult	5–10 min (after sufficient data has been collected)
Checklist for Autism Spectrum Disorder (CASD), (Mayes, 2012)	Clinician observational assessment	Clinician rating scale	1–17	15 min (after sufficient data has been collected)

Assessments of Cognitive Abilities

Due to the high rate of intellectual impairments and cognitive idiosyncrasies found in ASD, cognitive assessment is a crucial component to any ASD assessment. Developmental assessments are often useful for children within the first several years of life and often include not only assessment of cognitive abilities but language and motor abilities as well. There are many intellectual assessments available for older children and adults; however, the tools listed in Table 5 are the most used and well-validated tools for this specific population. The Stanford Binet-5 is often a highly recommended tool for ASD assessments due to better precision for intellectual impairments and the distinct cognitive profiles that are exhibited (e.g., Butter & Arendt, 2012). Additionally, as many individuals with ASD are nonverbal or have significant verbal deficits, a nonverbal assessment of intellectual functioning is often warranted, such as by using the Leiter-3, the most well-validated measure for this population. Although traditional cognitive assessments include measures of nonverbal abilities, these often require verbal instructions and/or verbal responses, whereas the Leiter-3 is a truly nonverbal assessment without the need for verbal instructions or verbal responses. It is important to note, however, that it is only an assessment of their nonverbal abilities and not an indicator of their overall intellectual functioning. However, it can sometimes be used in conjunction with other cognitive assessments.

Assessments of Communication Abilities

Assessments of an individual's communication abilities attempt to identify their language expression and language comprehension in comparison to typically developing peers. Due to the high

Table 5 Recommended cognitive assessments for autism spectrum disorder

Cognitive assessments	Informant	Format	Age range	Time to administer
Bayley Scales of Infant and Toddler Development (Bayley-3), (Bayley, 2005)	Clinician-direct assessment	Developmental assessment	1–42 months	30–90 min
Mullen Scales of Early Learning, (Mullen, 1995)	Clinician-direct assessment	Developmental assessment	Birth to 68 months	15–60 min
Stanford Binet-5, (Roid, 2003)	Clinician-direct assessment	Intelligence assessment	2–85+ years	60 min
Wechsler Scales of Intelligence (WPPSI-IV, WISC-V, WAIS-IV), (Wechsler, 2014)	Clinician-direct assessment	Intelligence assessment	2.5–90+ years	30–90 min
Differential Ability Scales (DAS-II), (Elliott, 2007)	Clinician-direct assessment	Intelligence assessment	2.5–17 years	45–60 min
Leiter International Performance Scale (Leiter-3), (Roid & Miller, 2013)	Clinician-direct assessment	Nonverbal intelligence assessment	3–75+ years	20–45 min

rate of language impairment in ASD, this is also a crucial piece to a comprehensive diagnostic assessment. Depending on the age and verbal ability of the individual, there are several assessments that have been well-validated for this population ranging from birth to adulthood. The traditional language assessments (PLS-5 and CELF-5) are comprehensive language assessments that assess several areas of expressive and receptive language use and understanding. With individuals with more limited language skills (either due to age or language impairment), receptive/expressive vocabulary assessments can often be useful tools in approximating an individual's language capacity in comparison to same-aged peers. Finally, the *Bracken Basic Concept Scale* is a unique assessment that straddles academic and vocabulary assessment and can be a useful tool for assessing readiness for school settings. This tool also has a special use in differentiating between basic core concepts such as colors, shapes, and numbers that are more concrete and primed for rote memorization from more abstract concepts such as social and self-awareness concepts, time, and quantity (Table 6).

Assessments of Adaptive Behavior Skills

Individuals with ASD often have significant deficits in skills of independence and general adaptive behavior. This is due not only to the high comorbidity rate with intellectual disabilities but is generally exhibited as a deficit for individuals with average cognitive functioning as well. These assessments generally include self or other reports regarding activities of daily living, daily self-care, as well as communication, social, and motor skills. The two recommended tools (ABAS-3 and Vineland-3) have both been recently updated to include socially relevant items. Another commonly used tool, the Scales of Independent Behavior-Revised (SIB-R; Bruininks, Woodcock, Weatherman, & Hill, 1996), is not recommended as the items included in this measure are severely dated and do not represent adaptive behavior skills that are socially relevant to our time (e.g., the use of white/yellow pages). The SIB-R was published in 1996 and has not been updated since and therefore would be an insufficient tool to use in the assessment of adaptive behavior (Table 7).

Additional Areas of Assessment

The core of an ASD assessment should focus on an individual's cognitive abilities, communication abilities, and adaptive behavior skills. In addition, executive functioning, working memory, central coherence, theory of mind, issues with eating and drinking, and sleep difficulties may also be assessed as part of a comprehensive

Table 6 Recommended language assessments for autism spectrum disorder

Language assessments	Informant	Format	Age range	Time to administer
PLS-5 (Preschool Language Scales), (Zimmerman, Steiner, & Pond, 2011)	Clinician-direct assessment	Language assessment	Birth to 7 years	45–60 min
CELF-5 (Clinical Evaluation of Language Fundamentals), (Wiig, Semel, & Secord, 2013)	Clinician-direct assessment	Language assessment	5–21 years	30–45 min
PPVT-4/EVT-2 (Peabody Picture Vocabulary Test/ Expressive Vocabulary Test), (Dunn & Dunn, 2007)	Clinician-direct assessment	Vocabulary assessment	2.5–90+ years	10–20 min each
ROWPVT-4/EOWPVT-4 (Receptive/Expressive One-Word Picture Vocabulary Test) (Gardner, 2010)	Clinician-direct assessment	Vocabulary assessment	2–70+ years	15–25 min
CCC-2 (Children's Communication Checklist) (Bishop, 2006)	Parent/caregiver	Rating scale	4–16 years	5–10 min
Bracken Basic Concept Scales (Receptive-3/ Expressive), (Bracken, 2006)	Clinician-direct assessment	Pre-academic vocabulary assessment	3–6 years	20–40 min each

Table 7 Recommended adaptive behavior measures for autism spectrum disorder

Adaptive behavior measures	Informant	Format	Age range	Time to administer
Adaptive Behavior Assessment System (ABAS-3), (Harrison & Oakland, 2015)	Parent/caregiver/ teacher/self	Rating scale	Birth to 89 years	15–20 min
Vineland Adaptive Behavior Scales (Vineland-3), (Sparrow, Cicchetti, & Balla, 2005)	Parent/caregiver/ teacher	Rating scale	Birth to 90 years	20–60 min

ASD assessment battery. For adult clients it may also be beneficial to measure the client's ability to live independently through assessments that focus on the independent functioning and vocational skills of the client. By assessing these additional areas, a clinician can offer more targeted recommendations that can inform future treatment or intervention options.

Assessments of Motor Skills

Motor skill assessments are used to assess challenges associated with the developmental and use of both fine and gross motor skills. A number of age-appropriate muscle developmental sequences may be assessed including those related to eating, locomotion, and engagement in other daily living skills depending on developmental level. Deficits in fine motor dexterity, handwriting, and the manipulation of objects are assessed by a number of measures currently in use. Such assessments can provide information regarding an individual's development of fine and gross motor skills. The overarching goal of each assessment of motor skills is to measure the client's gross and fine motor skills in relation to typically developing peers. While many of the tools discussed include measures of motor skills (e.g., Bayley-3, Mullen, ABAS-3, and Vineland-3), additional assessment may be required by occupational and physical therapists.

Assessments of Executive Functioning

Assessments of executive functioning measure a person's abilities on tasks related to planning, working memory, attention, inhibition, monitoring, and initiation. Furthermore, executive functions are used in the planning and sequencing of complex behaviors. The client's ability to pay attention to several components at once is often part of the executive functioning assessment tasks. Measurement of susceptibility to distraction or interference and inhibition of inappropriate response tendencies are also components of an executive functioning assessment. Finally, the client's ability to sustain behavioral output for a prolonged period of time can also be measured during lengthier assessments and may offer additional information of interest to clinicians developing treatment and intervention plans.

Assessments of Central Coherence

Central coherence theory suggests that there may be deficits in ASD populations in terms of a specific perceptual cognitive style and capacity to grasp the larger concept. Assessments of central coherence use tasks like block design, embedded figure test (EFT), hierarchical figures, motion coherence, partial occlusion, planning drawing, radial frequency search task (RFST), sentence completion, and visual illusions to test the client's ability to grasp larger more complex concepts. Deficits in central coherence may be addressed through appropriate intervention planning and therefore may be of interest to clinicians.

Assessments of Theory of Mind

Theory of mind measures a client's ability to attribute various mental states to oneself and others and the understanding that others have their own unique desires, beliefs, intentions, and perspectives. Theory of mind is captured by assessment tasks related to character intention and novel comic-strip tasks. In such tasks, the client is asked to interpret the mental states of the characters involved in the task and is then asked to describe events from the perspective of the characters during each phase of the task. Assessment of deficits in theory of mind may aid the differential diagnosis of more complex cases.

Assessments of Issues with Eating and Drinking

Assessments of an individual's eating and drinking patterns help identify clients with atypical eating and drinking routines. Food selectivity is one common issue found in individuals with ASD, which has a direct and often adverse impact on the individual, in terms of the nutritional value of food that is consumed. Inadequate levels of nourishment can have adverse effects and negatively impact an individual's health and behavior in a broad range of areas. Other common comorbid conditions related to eating and drinking that may need to be addressed are symptoms of pica, rumination disorder, and repetitive behaviors such as polydipsia.

Assessments of Sleep Difficulties

Assessments of sleep difficulties attempt to highlight sleep disturbances related to sleep latency, duration, and quality in individuals with ASD. It is estimated that individuals with developmental disabilities (including ASD) are four times more likely to suffer from sleep disturbances than typically developing peers (Cotton & Richdale, 2006). The proper assessment and treatment of sleep difficulties can greatly improve the effectiveness of other behavioral and developmental interventions that are implemented. Ultimately, it is the combination of multiple areas of assessment that makes up an appropriate assessment for the diagnosis of ASD.

Diagnosing ASD

The level of evidence needed to support a diagnosis of ASD varies greatly across different assessment settings. For example, it is not uncommon for a diagnosis from a school or primary care physician to be based solely on parent report, brief screening measures, and brief observations. The diagnostic evidence needed to make a diagnosis also varies widely among those that work specifically in the fields of psychology, psychiatry, and related mental health fields. An evaluation for ASD should be comprehensive and interdisciplinary; however, access to such services is limited by family resources, geographic location, and a paucity of clinicians that specialize in ASD assessment. There are many barriers that lie in the way of receiving appropriate evaluations, and clinicians that specialize in ASD assessment have a duty to decrease these barriers and provide appropriate assessment with the aim of providing better access to interventions, resources, and knowledge for parents/families.

Children that have screened positive for ASD, or other developmental disorders in which ASD is a concern for the family or primary care clinician, should be referred for a comprehensive diagnostic evaluation which includes assessment of all of the following domains: developmental history, ASD diagnostic assessment, cognitive assessment, language assessment, and adaptive behavior assessment (Ozonoff, et al., 2005) as well as assessment or screening for common comorbid conditions such as anxiety, attention issues, and various behavioral and medical conditions. These screenings may suggest further assessment or referral but are not necessary for making a diagnosis of ASD; however, they are crucial in the development of treatment and intervention plans for the individual and their family. Additional assessment may be warranted in other areas including executive functioning, academic functioning, and comorbid psychopathology if deficits or concerns arise during the evaluation process. These assessments will vary depending on the age and level of functioning of the individual.

Core Considerations

There are three primary considerations when conducting a comprehensive ASD assessment. These considerations can help ensure that all components of the diagnosis have been attended to.

Developmental trajectory First, it is important to note that one of the criteria for a diagnosis of ASD is that the disorder is lifelong, typically first presenting in childhood and then continuing throughout development. Oftentimes what happens in children with ASD is that they fail to meet a particular developmental milestone or they do not develop a certain skill such as language, which then negatively affects further development of additional skills (Ozonoff, et al., 2005). Therefore, obtaining information from parents or other caregivers present during the child's developmental stages is incredibly important. This allows the assessor to determine if the disorder had been lifelong or if symptoms become apparent later in life, which could be due to a different reason for the development of these ASD-type symptoms.

Using multiple sources When conducting an ASD assessment, it is important to assess from a wide range of areas and informants. As stated earlier, obtaining behavioral data from parents, teachers, and other caregivers gives you an idea of what behaviors are seen based on the context (i.e., at home or at school), and it is also important to include clinician ratings as well (Ozonoff, et al., 2005). For example, a parent with an older child diagnosed with ASD may be more aware of symptoms exhibited by a younger child. However, the teacher reports typical behaviors at school in terms of social interactions, cognitive abilities, and academic achievement, and you as the assessor do not observe any ASD-specific behaviors that the mother is reporting. By gathering a comprehensive multi-informant assessment, you are better able to determine whether or not the individual meets the criteria for a diagnosis of ASD.

Multidisciplinary teams Although obtaining developmental information and multi-informant behavioral data is incredibly useful in determining an ASD diagnosis, including other professionals from psychology, psychiatry, pediatrics, occupational therapy, or speech therapy can give you a wider, more detailed picture of the symptoms (Ozonoff, et al., 2005). By creating a multidisciplinary or interdisciplinary team, the assessment and treatment outcomes become more comprehensive and more streamlined.

The aforementioned considerations allow the clinician performing the assessment to have a better sense of what symptoms the child has been experiencing and provide them with a more comprehensive idea of what recommendations to make and ways to improve the child's functioning through the use of a best practice model.

Best Practices

As previously mentioned, multiple organizations and disciplines have developed guidelines and practice parameters for assessing ASD. Commonalities found between these best practices include the importance of early screenings for autism, the use of empirically validated assessments, the need to assess multiple areas of functioning through multidisciplinary or interdisciplinary teams, and a focus on family-centered care and valuing parental input in the assessment process. While the tools recommended by each discipline may vary, the overall goals remain the same: to provide a valuable and accurate assessment to best serve the client and their family taking into account the individual differences of the client.

Best practices across disciplines highlight the importance of interdisciplinary or multidisciplinary work in the assessment of ASD, and several locations in the United States and Canada provide such teams (e.g., large children's hospitals, the Autism Treatment Network). However, not all families have access to these services, and the provision of interdisciplinary teams with a specialty in ASD is difficult to find in many geographic regions. Unfortunately, this means that many families will not have access to services that fully incorporate these best practices. This does not mean, however, that families should settle for "subpar" services or rely solely on their primary care physician who likely has little experience in diagnosing and treating ASD. Instead, clinical psychologists with expertise in ASD should attempt to collaborate with other disciplines in smaller interdisciplinary or multidisciplinary teams to include primary care physicians, psychology, speech-language pathologists, occupational and physical therapists, and other developmental specialists that are involved in the care of the child. This requires additional effort by all disciplines to increase communication and learn the roles of each within the team. The inclusion of these, and other relevant disciplines, is important considering the myriad of comorbid conditions and deficits that children and families with ASD face.

Challenges in Establishing an ASD Diagnosis

There are a number of challenges that many clinicians face when assessing for ASD. Arguably the most difficult job a clinician is tasked with is the final decision and diagnosis, which is of the utmost importance. Clinical experience helps clinicians make informed decisions about diagnoses by gathering accurate information through the use of reliable testing procedures, testing materials, and training methods. However, if the assessment is not able to deliver a valid profile of the relevant issues associated with each client, clinicians are not able to accurately diagnosis the client. Therefore, it is crucial that each measure used in an ASD assessment is empirically supported.

Literacy may also play a role in ASD assessment. To be considered valid, the raw data collected from each assessment should accurately reflect the client's true abilities on the day of testing. Barriers associated with the client's reading ability sometimes make it harder for the clinician to accurately assess the client (e.g., the use of rating scales). To combat this problem, clinicians should always state any conflicting opinions or observations gathered during the testing procedures. The clinician can then describe and communicate these observations in their final report. This process ensures that a client's abilities are not underestimated and the client does not receive a diagnosis of ASD when ASD is not present.

Another potential problem is the overuse of an assessment tool in a specific period of time. Typically, a concern for older clients after the client has received a number of independent assessments in short period of time. The data gathered from subsequent assessments can be misleadingly and suggest improvement. Instead, the client may be experiencing positive practice effects. That is why it is important to request all examination reports associated with each client at the beginning of your assessment process. A number of measures used in a typical ASD assessment process may generate practice effects and are not designed for repeated use within a short period of time. It is important that clinicians realize that most intelligence measures are unreliable if they are repeated too frequently. If used repeatedly, these measures tend to overestimate the client's ability due to their familiarity with the materials.

Standardization and norms are also potential problems often associated with ASD assessment batteries. For example, if the assessment tool being used during the assessment process was not normed on an ASD population, the clinician may not be able to accurately measure the client's presenting symptomology. Inconsistency regarding test reliability is a major concern because each assessment tool should, ideally, be normed within the population it attempts to measure.

Typical challenges faced by a clinician when administering an ASD assessment include selecting the appropriate assessment measures with appropriate standardization and determining the client's ability to understand the assessment material. Additionally, comorbid diagnoses such as anxiety, depression, ADHD, and intellectual disability can further affect severity of symptoms and influence the clinician's ability to determine an appropriate diagnosis.

Comorbidity

Obtaining a diagnosis of ASD based on the wide range of assessments suggested is very difficult. However, when attempting to obtain diagnostic clarification between a neurodevelopmental diagnosis such as ASD versus a mental health diagnosis becomes even more difficult. Consequently, ASD assessment tools are typically standardized on populations with specific exclusion criteria regarding significant comorbidity issues meaning that each assessment was standardized on clients without major comorbidity concerns (e.g., no symptoms of anxiety or depression). Unfortunately, these previous restrictions somewhat limit the standardization data related to a number of individuals who have currently received an ASD diagnosis. Unfortunately, numerous studies indicate surprisingly high rates of comorbidities diagnosed within ASD populations, making the assessment process more complex. That being said, the assessments for ASD used under best clinical practice should still be administered with the caveat that the measures may be affected by other comorbid disorders and may therefore not be an accurate representation of the individual's functioning.

Adults with ASD are at an increased risk for a host of comorbid conditions including (but not limited to) seizures, feeding problems, insomnia, and gastrointestinal abnormalities. In fact, population-based studies suggest adults with ASD suffer from approximately 11 comorbid medical conditions and symptomatology, regardless of the level of intellectual functioning (Jones et al., 2016). Included in these comorbid conditions, adults with high-functioning ASD typically experience significantly higher rates of sleep disturbances than neuro-typical peers (e.g., difficulty with sleep-onset latency, poor sleep efficiency, and self-reported feelings of restlessness) (Baker & Richdale, 2015). This also emphasizes the continuation of sleep disturbances from childhood into adulthood while controlling for additional influences such as anxiety/depression and intellectual functioning.

Recently the field has increasingly recognized the role that comorbidities play in ASD, with a rapid expansion in research addressing these issues and their relevance to both the assessment and intervention processes (Mannion, Leader, & Healy 2013; Matson & Williams 2014). Careful consideration should focus on the limiting factors associated with the known comorbidity issues and potential overlap of symptomology. This increased understanding could have beneficial implications, especially if the clinician is planning to use a measure to evaluate specific aspects of a given population.

Implications

A worthwhile and achievable goal for each clinician is greater consistency through the use of improving measurement tools in ASD clinical trials. To assist in this process, it would be beneficial for each clinician to recognize the benefits and drawbacks of the existing measures used as part of an ASD assessment battery. Only after thoroughly assessing the existing measures of an ASD assessment battery can a clinician be better prepared to assess the symptomatology present in each client.

Clinicians must be able to make the necessary decisions regarding the proper diagnosis of each client. By generating a communal road map or set of guidelines that is shared among clinicians, future clinicians are better able to accurately diagnose ASD in individuals who have the disorder. These guidelines should also be beneficial as an established standard for the review process of academic journals and granting agencies. New instruments and assessment approaches that add to the field are frequently being developed and marketed. Some of these are new assessment tools based off of new developments in the field, while others are merely updated versions of older assessment tools and scales. These new measures could potentially be able to fill gaps from what is missing on the market today. By improving current approaches and providing novel approaches to ASD assessments, we are better able to uncover previously neglected areas of functioning. This increase in the ability to accurately measure and diagnose ASD is of great benefit to both the client and clinician.

Clinicians dedicate their time to maximizing benefits and ensuring the appropriateness of each assessment tool of the assessment battery. Data gathered from the various components of the assessment process can be directed to generate swift answers to clinically relevant questions. The impact of this research could create a robust foundation that further establishes the criteria needed to diagnose ASD accurately and reliably.

References

American Psychiatric Association. (1980). *Diagnostic and statistical manual of mental disorders* (3rd ed.). Washington, DC: Author.

Baker, E. K., & Richdale, A. L. (2015). Sleep patterns in adults with a diagnosis of high-functioning autism spectrum disorder. *Sleep, 38*(11), 1765–1774.

Baranek, G. T., Watson, L. R., Crais, E., & Reznick, S. (2003). *First Year Inventory (FYI) 2.0*. Chapel Hill, NC: University of North Carolina.

Bayley, N. (2005). *Bayley scales of infant development* (3rd ed.). San Antonio, TX: Psychological Corporation.

Bishop, D. (2006). *Children's communication checklist* (2nd ed.). San Antonio, TX: Harcourt Assessment.

Bracken, B. A. (2006). *Bracken basic concept scale, Receptive* (3rd ed.). San Antonio, TX: Psychological Corporation.

Bruininks, R. H., Woodcock, R. W., Weatherman, R. F., & Hill, B. K. (1996). *Scales of independent behavior-revised*. Itasca, IL: Riverside Publishing Company.

Butter, E., & Arendt, R. (2012, May). Cognitive profile in higher functioning children with an autism Spectrum disorder. Presented at the annual international meeting for autism research in Toronto, Ontario, Canada.

Centers for Disease Control and Prevention. (2014). Prevalence of autism spectrum disorder among children aged 8 years: Autism and developmental disabilities monitoring network, 11 sites, United States, 2010. *Morb Mortal Wkly Rep Surveill Summ, 63*(2), 1–21.

Chakrabarti, S. (2009). Early identification of autism. *Indian Pediatrics, 46*, 412–414.

Cohen, I. L., & Sudhalter, V. (2005). *PDD behavior inventory (PDDBI)*. Lutz, FL: Psychological Assessment Resources.

Cotton, S., & Richdale, A. (2006). Brief report: Parental descriptions of sleep problems in children with autism, down syndrome, and Prader–Willi syndrome. *Research in Developmental Disabilities, 27*(2), 151–161.

Dubbelink, O., Linda, M. E., & Geurts, H. M. (2017). Planning skills in autism spectrum disorder across the lifespan: A meta-analysis and meta-regression. *Journal of Autism and Developmental Disorders, 47*(4), 1148–1165. https://doi.org/10.1007/s10803-016-3013-0

Dunn, L. M., & Dunn, D. M. (2007). *PPVT-4: Peabody picture vocabulary test*. Minneapolis, MN: Pearson Assessments. American Guidance Service.

Elliott, C. D. (2007). *Differential Ability Scales, 2nd edition: Introductory and technical handbook*. San Antonio, TX: The Psychological Corporation

Filipek, P. A., Accardo, P. J., Ashwal, S., Baranek, G. T., Cook, E. H., Dawson, G., & Volkmar, F. R. (2000). Practice parameter: Screening and diagnosis in autism. *Neurology, 55*, 468–479.

Filipek, P. A., Accardo, P. J., Baranek, G. T., Cook, E. H., Jr., Dawson, G., Gordon, B., et al. (1999). The screening and diagnosis of autistic spectrum disorders.

Journal of Autism and Developmental Disorders, 29, 439–484.

Gardner, M. F. (2010). *Receptive One-Word Picture Vocabulary Test (ROWPVT)*. East Aurora, NY: Slosson Educational Publications.

Ghanizadeh, A. (2012). Co-morbidity and factor analysis on attention deficit hyperactivity disorder and autism spectrum disorder DSM-IV-derived items. *Journal of research in medical sciences: the official journal of Isfahan University of Medical Sciences, 17*(4), 368.

Goldin, R. L., Matson, J. L., Tureck, K., Cervantes, P. E., & Jang, J. (2013). A comparison of tantrum behavior profiles in children with ASD, ADHD and comorbid ASD and ADHD. *Research in Developmental Disabilities, 34*(9), 2669–2675.

Goldstein, S., & Naglieri, J. A. (2010). *Autism Spectrum Rating Scales (ASRS)*. North Tonawanda, NY: Multi-Health Systems.

Gotham, K. O. (2010). Defining and quantifying severity of impairment in autism spectrum disorders across the lifespan.

Harrison, P. L., & Oakland, T. (2015). *Adaptive behavior assessment system* (3rd ed.). San Antonio, TX: Psychological Corporation.

Johnson, C. P. (2008). Recognition of autism before age 2 years. *Pediatrics in Review, 29*(3), 86.

Jones, K. B., Cottle, K., Bakian, A., Farley, M., Bilder, D., Coon, H., & McMahon, W. M. (2016). A description of medical conditions in adults with autism spectrum disorder: A follow-up of the 1980s Utah/UCLA Autism Epidemiologic Study. *Autism, 20*(5), 551–561.

Kishore, M. T., & Basu, A. (2011). Early concerns of mothers of children later diagnosed with autism: Implications for early identification. *Research in Autism Spectrum Disorders, 5*, 157–163.

Klaiman, C., Fernandez-Carriba, S., Hall, C., & Saulnier, C. (2015). Assessment of autism across the lifespan: A way forward. *Current Developmental Disorders Reports, 2*(1), 84–92. https://doi.org/10.1007/s40474-014-0031-5

Lord, C., Risi, S., Lambrecht, L., Cook, E. H., Leventhal, B. L., DiLavore, P. C., & Rutter, M. (2000). The autism diagnostic observation schedule—Generic: A standard measure of social and communication deficits associated with the spectrum of autism. *Journal of Autism and Developmental Disorders, 30*(3), 205–223.

Lord, C., Rutter, M., DiLavore, P. C., & Risi, S. (2012). *Autism Diagnostic Observation Schedule (ADOS)*. Los Angeles: Western Psychological Services.

Mandell, D. S., Novak, M. M., & Zubritsky, C. D. (2005). Factors associated with age of diagnosis among children with autism spectrum disorders. *Pediatrics, 116*, 1480–1486.

Mannion, A., Leader, G., & Healy, O. (2013). An investigation of comorbid psychological disorders, sleep problems, gastrointestinal symptoms and epilepsy in children and adolescents with autism spectrum disorder. *Research in Autism Spectrum Disorders, 7*(1), 35–42.

Matson, J. L., Boisjoli, J., & Wilkins, J. (2007). *The baby and infant screen for children with autIsm traits (BISCUIT)*. Baton Rouge, LA: Disability Consultants, LLC.

Matson, J. L., & González, M. L. (2007). *Autism Spectrum Disorders diagnosis child version (ASD-C)*. Baton Rouge, La: Disability Consultants, LLC.

Matson, J. L., Terlonge, C., & González, M. L. (2006). *Autism Spectrum Disorders diagnosis adult version (ASD-A)*. Baton Rouge, LA: Disability Consultants, LLC..

Matson, J. L., & Williams, L. W. (2014). The making of a field: The development of comorbid psychopathology research for persons with intellectual disabilities and autism. *Research in Developmental Disabilities, 35*(1), 234–238.

Mayes, S. D. (2012). *Checklist for Autism Spectrum Disorder (CASD)*. Los Angeles, CA: Western Psychological Services, LLC.

Mullen, E. M. (1995). *Mullen scales of early learning*. Circle Pines, MN: AGS.

Ozonoff, S., Goodlin-Jones, B. L., & Solomon, M. (2005). Evidence-based assessment of autism spectrum disorders in children and adolescents. *Journal of Clinical Child & Adolescent Psychology, 34*(3), 523–540. https://doi.org/10.1207/s15374424jccp3403_8

Planche, P. (2010). La réaction à la nouveauté : Un indice de dépistage précoce de l'autisme ? *Annales Médico-psychologiques, revue psychiatrique, 168*, 578–583.

Robins, D. L., Fein, D., & Barton, M. (2009). *Modified checklist for autism in toddlers, revised, with follow-up (M-CHAT-R/F) TM*.

Roid, G. H. (2003). *Stanford-Binet intelligence scales* (5th ed.). Itasca, IL: Riverside.

Roid, G. H., & Miller, L. J. (2013). *Leiter 3 international performance scale, revised*. Wood Dale, IL: Stoelting Co.

Rutter, M., Bailey, A., & Lord, C. (2003). *Social Communication Questionnaire (SCQ)*. Los Angeles, CA: Western Psychological Services.

Rutter, M., Le Couteur, A., & Lord, C. (2003). *Autism Diagnostic Interview-Revised (ADI-R)*. Los Angeles, CA: Western Psychological Services.

Schopler, E., Reichler, R. J., & Renner, B. R. (2010). *The childhood autism rating scale (CARS)*. Los Angeles, CA: Western Psychological Services.

Shattuck, P. T., Seltzer, M. M., Greenberg, J. S., Orsmond, G. I., Bolt, D., Kring, S., & Lord, C. (2007). Change in autism symptoms and maladaptive behaviors in adolescents and adults with an autism spectrum disorder. *Journal of Autism and Developmental Disorders, 37*(9), 1735–1747. https://doi.org/10.1007/s10803-006-0307-7

Skuse, D., Warrington, R., Bishop, D., Chowdhury, U., Lau, J., Mandy, W., & Place, M. (2004). The developmental, dimensional and diagnostic interview (3di): A novel computerized assessment for autism spectrum disorders. *Journal of the American Academy of Child and Adolescent Psychiatry, 43*(5), 548–558.

Sparrow, S. S., Cicchetti, D. V., & Balla, D. A. (2005). *Vineland adaptive behavior scales* (2nd ed.). Circle Pines, MN: American Guidance Service.

Swinkels, S. H., Dietz, C., van Daalen, E., Kerkhof, I. H., van Engeland, H., & Buitelaar, J. K. (2006). Screening for autistic spectrum in children aged 14 to 15 months. I: The development of the Early Screening of Autistic Traits Questionnaire (ESAT). *Journal of Autism and Developmental Disorders, 36*(6), 723–732.

Volkmar, F. R., Cook, E. H., Jr., Pomeroy, J., Realmuto, G., & Tanguay, P. (1999). Practice parameters for the assessment and treatment of children, adolescents, and adults with autism and other pervasive developmental disorders. *Journal of the American Academy of Child & Adolescent Psychiatry, 38*, 32S–54S.

Wechsler, D. (2014). *Wechsler scales of intelligence*. San Antonio, TX: Psychological Corporation.

Wiig, E. H., Semel, E. M., & Secord, W. (2013). *CELF 5: Clinical evaluation of language fundamentals*. Pearson/PsychCorp. Bloomington, MN: Pearson.

Wing, L. (2003). *Diagnostic interview for social and communication disorders* (11th ed.). Bromley, United Kingdom: Centre for Social and Communication Disorders.

Wing, L., & Potter, D. (2002). The epidemiology of autistic spectrum disorders: Is the prevalence rising? *Developmental Disabilities Research Reviews, 8*(3), 151–161.

Zimmerman, I. L., Steiner, V. G., & Pond, R. E. (2011). *PLS-5: Preschool language scales*. San Antonio, TX: NCS Pearson. Pearson/PsychCorp.

Assessing Bipolar Disorder and Major Depression

Johnny L. Matson and Claire O. Burns

Pediatric bipolar disorder and major depression are topics which have received a marked increase in attention by the mental health community in recent years. This group of disorders, when present, is very serious and debilitating. Also, symptoms can wax and wane for many years. Thus, identification and treatment are very important. One of the greatest concerns regarding this mental health condition is misidentification, often through the application of symptoms that do not truly represent pediatric mood disorders. A variety of symptoms have been reported in the literature. A brief review of the behaviors which have been described in the literature to characterize pediatric mood disorders follows. This section is followed by relevant topics in diagnosis and methods used to identify major depression and bipolar disorder.

Symptoms

Tillman et al. (2008) studied 257 children and adolescents who were 6–16 years of age. These participants had all been diagnosed with bipolar I disorder. The purpose of the study was to establish what percentage of the children and adolescents had experienced psychotic symptoms. These authors reported that 76% of the clients evinced psychosis, 39% had delusions, and 32% had both types of symptoms. Visual hallucinations were the most common hallucinations, while the most common delusion was grandiosity. The presence of psychotic symptoms did not differ by age. Hafeman et al. (2013) studied 707 children 6–12 years of age for symptoms of bipolar disorder. Bipolar I and bipolar II diagnosed children did not differ on manic symptoms, but they were different from children with no bipolar diagnosis.

Van Meter, Burke, Kowatch, Findling, and Youngstrom (2016) studied bipolar symptoms in a very large group: 2226 children and adolescents. The most common symptoms were increased energy (79%), irritability (77%), mood lability (26%), distractibility (74%), goal-directed activity (72%), euphoric mood (64%), and pressured speech (63%). Other common symptoms included hyperactivity, racing thoughts, grandiosity, poor judgment, less sleep, bizarre laughter, and flight of ideas. Among the youth with bipolar disorder, over half displayed each of these symptoms. Irritability was a commonly noted symptom of pediatric bipolar disorder and was also noted in a sample of 6–16-year-olds in India (Tiwari, Agarwal, Aryce, Gupta, & Mahour, 2016).

J. L. Matson · C. O. Burns (✉)
Department of Psychology, Louisiana State University, Baton Rouge, LA, USA
e-mail: Cburn26@lsu.edu

Researchers have also reported that social skills excesses and deficits are common among children and youth with bipolar disorder. Benarous, Mikita, Goodman, and Stringaris (2015) note that this behavior symptom profile exists even when manic symptoms do not meet the full criteria for a manic episode. These authors studied 5325 individuals through the British Child and Adolescent Mental Health Survey. The more pronounced the manic symptoms, the greater the observed social deficits.

Suicide attempts are also an issue that warrants consideration for obvious reasons. The identification of risk factors is particularly important. Goldstein et al. (2012) note that 18% of a sample of 413 youth with bipolar disorder had attempted suicide. Greater numbers of weeks with depression, substance use disorder, mixed symptoms of mood disorder, and the use of more psychosocial services predicted suicide attempts.

All in all, more studies are needed that look specifically at key symptoms of pediatric bipolar disorder. Many assessment and treatment studies list the symptoms being addressed. However, symptom expression is not the primary research question. This issue is further underscored by the fact that many of the "bipolar symptoms" treated do not conform to the DSM criteria nor do they conform to many of the scale that are used to diagnose the disorder.

Those engaged in clinical practice have also followed this approach, confusing a range of symptoms, many which do not correspond in many cases to published criteria in recognized diagnostic manuals and tests. Additionally, researchers have concluded that symptoms used to diagnose pediatric bipolar disorder vary widely across studies (Van Meter, Burke, Kowatch, Findling, & Youngstrom, 2016). While not as pronounced, this is also a problem with childhood major depression. This fact should be a concern to anyone reading this volume. To enhance the systematic study of symptom expression, the development of standardized methods is critical. Also important to address are various factors that impact diagnosis. These issues are discussed below.

Diagnosis

A variety of factors should be considered in the diagnostic process for major depression and bipolar disorder. Relevant variables to consider include history (generally defined here as risk factors), diagnostic issues such as symptom selection, comorbid conditions, and specific tests to aid in diagnosis. The importance of a comprehensive evaluation cannot be overemphasized. Hafeman et al. (2013), for example, found considerable overlap in symptoms for bipolar I, bipolar II, and bipolar disorder – not otherwise specified in 707 children 6–12 years of age. For example, parental psychiatric history and a parental diagnosis of mania were more common in children who received a bipolar diagnosis versus typically developing children. Symptom overlap for bipolar disorder with major depression is also pronounced, particularly when manic symptoms are excluded from the picture. These points confirm the need for a multimethod, careful and systematic approach to problem identification and differential diagnosis.

Diagnosing depressive disorders is particularly difficult with children. As Carlson (2000) points out, children with internalizing disorders rarely seek help. Rather, they must depend on caregivers to reach out to mental health professionals. Additionally, while 2 weeks of depressive symptoms qualify as a mood disorder, parents rarely refer that quickly.

Bipolar Disorder

A variety of factors have been associated with the development of bipolar disorder in children. The biological factors and environmental events can be useful for identifying children who should be monitored and/or evaluated. These data can also, in the congregate, help establish whether a diagnosis of bipolar disorder is or is not warranted. Among the environmental variables that should be considered are stressful life events. McCraw and Parker (2017) found that the bipolar group in their study, while younger than controls, exhibited higher rates of psychological and physical trauma. These problems included physical and psychological abuse and neglect. Additional problems were associated with bipolar disorder into adulthood, including substance abuse, difficulty developing and maintaining social relationships, and legal and financial difficulties. These traumatic childhood events can also lead to anxiety and related social dysfunction. Other social difficulties that could be implicated include the person's ability to cooperate, be appropriately assertive and responsible, and demonstrate self-control (Feldman, Tung, & Lee, 2017). The effects of early life adversity in the development of depressive symptoms are further underscored by Kendler and Aggen (2017). Finally, emotional labeling errors with respect to angry or sad faces have also been associated with pediatric bipolar disorder (Hanford, Sassi, & Hall, 2016).

For periods where mania is not present, a number of symptoms across major depression and pediatric bipolar disorder overlap. Behaviors such as a drop in school performance, lack of motivation, an inability to concentrate, low self-esteem, pessimism, and somatic disturbances such as headaches and stomach pain may be present. Also, Carlson (2000) notes that switch rates of mania symptoms are much more frequent in children than in adults. In instances where mania is present, researchers have suggested that symptoms such as deficits in learning may occur (Dickstein, Axelson, Weissman, Yen, & Goldstein, 2016). Additionally, Frazier et al. (2011) point out that multiple measures over a brief period may be necessary to identify mania in children.

Childhood and adolescence is not a monolith with respect to symptom presentation. Safer, Zito, and Safer (2012) reviewed the existing literature on mania symptom presentation on standardized bipolar measures such as the Young Mania Rating Scale. They reported that 63% of inpatient children diagnosed with bipolar disorder were aggressive, while only 24% of an adolescent group similarly diagnosed exhibited aggression. Compared to adults, children had less grandiosity, less sleep disturbance, more motor activity, and less disruptive behavior. Luckenbaugh, Findling, Leverich, Pizzcerello, and Post (2009) have also explored age as a factor in symptom presentation. They note that brief and extended periods of mood lability issues and decreased sleep problems were the earliest precursors of adolescent bipolar disorders. Symptoms of depression appeared late, demonstrating a gradual progression in symptoms. Assuming this point can be confirmed, it provides an excellent diagnostic marker for differentiating major depression from pediatric bipolar disorder. The importance of such findings is unscored by Stringaris, Santosh, Leibenluft, and Goodman (2010) who stress that classic bipolar disorder is rare in children and adolescents. They also call into question the widespread use of bipolar disorder – not otherwise specific – which they emphasize is associated with a number of other externalizing disorders.

Fristad and colleagues (2016) have also addressed differentiating subtypes of childhood mood disorder: mood dysregulation disorder versus bipolar disorder – not otherwise specified. They found that most characteristics of bipolar disorder were present relatively equally in these two groups. However, mania was much more likely to be present in the latter versus the former group.

Hutchinson, Beresford, Robinson, and Ross (2010) have also investigated symptoms that may differentiate symptoms of bipolar disorder in young children. They looked at mood dysregulation in story completion tasks. The children were 3.5–6 years of age and divided into a bipolar group and a typically developing group. Those children in the clinical group had content including violence or bizarreness descriptors. This finding was not the case for the typically developing group. The authors suggest that this symptom presentation is similar to what might be observed in adolescents and adults.

Uchida et al. (2015) have analyzed how bipolar disorder can be differentiated from major depression in children. Their general conclusions were that severity of symptoms was greater for the bipolar group. These behaviors included a range of depression symptoms and a high rate of comorbidity with respect to other mental health conditions. Of course, mania symptoms for bipolar disorder would differentiate the conditions also. In another study looking at characteristics of bipolar disorder, inflammatory markers such as stomach and bowl symptoms were evident in young adults and adolescents (Goldstein et al., 2015). At this point however, we would consider these results to be preliminary. Having said that, the bipolar diagnosis is generally considered to be valid for children and adolescents. Whether the disorder, as noted earlier, is rare or not is still open to question. Part of this is due to differences among researchers in how childhood bipolar disorder is defined (Mitchell et al., 2016). Considerable variability exists across studies.

Donfrancesco et al. (2014) also question current diagnostic practices as applied to pediatric bipolar disorder. They note that Italian children displayed greater symptoms in the category of elevated mood compared to children from the USA. Conversely, the US sample had greater elevations on flight of ideas. These differences underscore the inconsistencies that exist when diagnosing pediatric bipolar disorder. While differences exist with major depression in children, they are not as pronounced. A variety of factors may lead to this development. Confusion over criteria for bipolar disorder may be greater than what is observed with major depression. Similarly, the lack of consistency in diagnosis may be greater for the bipolar group, and the methods of diagnosing bipolar disorder may be less well developed than for major depression in children and adolescents. Also, bipolar disorder symptoms may extend into symptoms that typically characterize other mental health conditions such as personality disorders (Paris, 2014). Similarly, Bayes et al. (2016) further highlight this issue in their efforts to differentiate bipolar disorder from borderline personality disorder. These authors report considerable success in this regard. However, the data also suggest that progress in differential diagnosis is still a work in progress.

Birmaher and associates (2014) also discuss the diagnostic trajectories of children diagnosed with bipolar disorder. They discuss how euthymic mood states among groups of youth (mean age of 12 years) vary over time from severe to mild. They note that these symptoms may be present for extended periods of time, which therefore needs to be monitored.

Findling et al. (2013) have also looked at the trajectory of manic symptoms in children 6–12 years of age. While the majority of children saw decreases in manic symptoms over a 24-month span, there were also children who experienced an increase or stabilization of manic symptoms. Efforts to identify predictor variables for these trends are underway but required considerably more research.

Major Depression

Researchers have also identified diagnostic issues for children and adolescents with major depression. An area where difficulty in differential diagnosis may result is where the cutoff between depression and subthreshold symptoms exists. Wesselhoeft, Heierbang, Kragh-Sorensen, Sorensen, and Bilenberg (2016) studied 3421 children 8–10 years of age. They found no difference in life stressors, anxiety problems, or conduct disorders. However, children with a diagnosis of major depression were more impaired in functional skills than the subclinical groups. Suicidal behavior constitutes a significant problem even in very young children (Martin et al., 2016).

As previously noted, the onset of symptoms of mood disorders may be gradual and cumulative. Additionally, symptoms may wax and wane with time. Thus, the clinician may expect different symptom profiles to indicate not primarily the severity of a disorder but the stage of the disorder in its overall course. Nadkarni and Fristad (2010), for example, note that when manic symptoms are transient in children, they may present a particularly salient set of symptoms for the eventual development of bipolar disorder. Findling et al. (2010) refer to this phenomenon as diagnostic evolution.

Comorbidity

What is becoming more evident as the field of childhood mental health matures is that co-occurring forms of psychopathology are common in children and adults. In this subsection of our chapter, a few examples of these comorbidities are described as they occur among children and adolescents with major depression and bipolar disorder. Yen et al. (2016) note that as comorbid conditions worsen, the severity of depression and mania symptoms increases. The interplay between core symptoms for children and adolescents who display comorbid symptoms has been infrequently studied; therefore, a great deal more research is needed on this topic.

For both major depression and bipolar disorder, anxiety disorders are common (McCraw & Parker, 2017). This phenomenon has been a common knowledge among clinicians and researchers for some time and includes generalized anxiety disorder, PTSD, social phobia, agoraphobia, and obsessive-compulsive disorder. Thus, mood disorders may be considered a risk factor for a range of anxiety-related conditions. Pavlova et al. (2016) also noted that childhood mistreatment was related to the development of these anxiety symptoms in children with bipolar disorder.

Quek, Tam, Zhang, and Ho (2017) studied a sample of 51,272 children and adolescents to assess the comorbidity of depression and obesity. They found that being depressed was a risk factor for obesity. They also noted that when depression was more severe, the risk for obesity was greater. Finally, they note that being female and being from a non-Western culture were also risk factors for obesity and depression co-occurring.

A variety of other comorbid conditions have been reported in combination with bipolar disorder. Amerio and colleagues (2016) present a review of studies that address the co-occurrence of bipolar disorder and obsessive-compulsive disorder in children. ADHD has also been reported in pediatric bipolar disorder cases (Marangoni, DeChiara, & Faedda, 2015). Collins (2014) further reported an overlap between these two disorders and stresses that such co-occurrences are very common. She also noted that a considerable overlap in symptom for these disorders exist, including risky behavior, psychomotor agitation, impulsivity, emotional volatility, higher rates of motor activity, and sleep issues. Finally, Faedden et al. (2016) also stress the comorbid presentation of ADHD and major depression and discuss methods for discriminating between the two disorders.

Bipolar disorder has also been linked to conditions such as Tourette syndrome (Shim & Kwon, 2014). In their case study, these authors report that the child also experienced a bout of major depression. Further underscoring potential medical comorbidities that children with mood disorders display is a study by Salpekar, Gaurav, and Hauptman (2015). They note that epilepsy commonly occurs along with major depression in children.

The important takeaway is that when diagnosing major depression and/or bipolar disorder in children and adolescents, a broad range of co-occurring disorders should be screened. This approach not only has value in assessment but has major implications for the development of treatment protocols.

Onset

A number of articles have been published on the onset of childhood mood disorders and a variety of factors have been addressed. For example, Udal and colleagues (2012) found that children with bipolar disorder who developed the condition very early in life (i.e., early onset) displayed marked deficits in executive functioning and processing speed. These deficits were also evidence in an ADHD sample. Additionally, where ADHD was comorbid with bipolar disorder, the deficits in executive functioning and processing speed were the most pronounced.

Age also been shown to have a major effect on core symptoms of bipolar disorder and comorbidities. Comorbid ADHD dissipated as children age. Excessive motor activity, aggression, and irritability also decreased among children and adolescents diagnosed with bipolar disorders. Symptoms of depression, however, increased as the children got older (Demeter et al., 2013). Preisig et al. (2016) looked at the early onset of bipolar disorder and major depressive disorder. Children whose parents had early onset bipolar disorder were at greater risks for the condition as well as for substance abuse. However, status of any type of mood disorders of parents did not affect rates of major depression in their children. These types of data have led researchers to further refine the earliest symptoms that are present.

Researchers are attempting to identify a prodromal bipolar condition similar to early onset psychosis. Another reason for early and more precise diagnosis is emphasized by Hong et al. (2016). They conclude that people who go for long durations without being diagnosed with bipolar disorder are likely to have a higher frequency of relapse. These authors underscore the need for improved clinician recognition of symptoms of mood disorders at younger ages. Serra et al. (2015) further emphasize the importance of being able to distinguish between bipolar disorder and major depression early on. Addressing social skills may also prove to be very important to consider because deficits in this area have been shown to be precursors to major depression in children (Feldman, Tung, & Lee, 2017). What is also evident is that the line of research on early onset needs a great deal of additional development.

Tests of Major Depression

We do not suggest that the measures described below are a complete list of all available assessment methods, but the scales covered are certainly representative. For this section and for the scales for bipolar disorder which follow, instruments have been broken down into three sections. These sections include tests that address core symptoms of the disorder, studies that use criteria to assess for the core symptoms, and secondary measures which cover symptoms that are not core for a diagnosis but which often occur alongside the core symptoms. For major depression, 18 tests are reviewed in category one, one set of criteria is reviewed, and three secondary scales are discussed (see Tables 1 and 2).

Table 1 Major depression measures for children and adolescents

Scales
1. Beck Depression Inventory
2. Bellevue Index of Depression
3. Center for Epidemiologic Studies Depression Scale (CES-D)
4. Children's Depression Inventory (CDI)
5. Children's Depression Inventory-short form
6. Children's Depression Scale
7. Children's Depression Screener (ChIlD-S)
8. Children's Depression Self-Rating Scale-Revised
9. Depression Indicator Assessment Battery
10. Depression Observation Schedule
11. Depression Self-Rating Scale
12. Depression Symptom Checklist
13. Dysthymic Checklist
14. Hopelessness Scale for Children
15. Personality Inventory for Children
16. Revised Child Anxiety and Depression Scale (RCADS)
17. Kiddie - Schedule for Affective Disorders and Schizophrenia (Kiddie-SADS)
18. Short Mood and Feelings Questionnaire
Criteria
19. DSM-III and IV
Secondary scales
20. Matching Familiar Figures Test
21. My Standards Questionnaire

Table 2 Bipolar disorder measures for children and adolescents

Scales
1. Child Behavior Checklist- Mania Scale
2. Child Bipolar Questionnaire (CBQ)
3. Children's Depression Rating Scale- Revised (CDRS-R)
4. *Children's Interview for Psychiatric Syndromes (ChIPs)*- Mania Subscale
5. Child Mania Rating Scale- Parent
6. General Behavior Inventory- Revised (GBI-R)
7. Kiddie - Schedule for Affective Disorders and Schizophrenia (Kiddie-SADS)
8. Young Mania Rating Scale (YMRS)
Neuroimaging
9. Functional magnetic resonance imaging (fMRI)
Criteria
10. Bipolar At-Risk (BAR) criteria
Secondary measures
11. Barratt Impulsiveness Scale

Beck Depression Inventory

The Beck Depression Inventory (Beck, Steer, & Brown, 1996) is a well-studied measure that was largely developed for adults. However, McLean, Su, Carpenter, and Foa (2017) utilized it as an outcome measure with 61 female adolescents who had been sexually assaulted. In addition to assessing for depression, symptoms of post-traumatic stress disorder (PTSD) were also addressed. A similar approach was used by Chang, Kaczkurkin, McLean, and Foa (2017). Again in addressing sexual abuse experiences of children and adolescent, they used the Beck Depression Inventory to address emotional regulation, PTSD, and depression. Roberts, Andreus, Lewinsohn, and Hops (1990) also used the Beck Depression Inventory. Their sample also consisted of adolescents: about 10,000 9–12th graders. They used the measure as part of a battery designed to identify individuals with depression. These authors concluded that the Beck Depression Inventory should not be used alone as a method of detecting adolescents with depression or as a treatment outcome measure. However, it was endorsed as a screener. Having said that, the child version of the scale, which is discussed below (Children's Depression Inventory), is far more popular for children and adolescents.

Bellevue Index of Depression

The Bellevue Index of Depression is a semistructured interview for children or their parents (Kazdin, French, Unis, & Esveldt-Dawson, 1983). It includes 26 items, all measuring core symptoms of major depression such as crying and losing interest in activities. Children assessed using this scale were 5–13 years old. This measure is one of the several that has not caught on with researchers and clinicians.

Center for Epidemiologic Studies Depression Scale

A scale which received considerable research attention in the 1990s was the Center for Epidemiologic Studies Depression Scale (CES-D; Radloff, 1977). As the name implies, this measure was used largely as a measure of depressive symptoms in children and adolescents. Fendrich, Weissman, and Warner (1990) used the measure with 220 children and adolescents 12–18 years of age. They report good reliability and validity with the measure, but they note that the measure lacks specificity. Roberts et al. (1990) also studied this measure, in their case with 9–12th graders. They report good internal consistency and test-retest reliability. Radloff (1991) tested high school and college students and also reported good reliability. Roberts, Lewinsohn, and Seeley (1991) noted that the Center for Epidemiologic Studies Depression Scale should not be used as a stand-alone scale for diagnosis. Finally, Costello and Angold (1988), in a review of several childhood depression measures, state that the scale was easy to administer and placed few cognitive demands such as comparing and remembering several statements at a time. Thus, the measure has been well studied and appears to be a good option for assessing major depression among children and adolescents.

Children's Depression Inventory

Perhaps the most extensively researched and used measure of depression in youth is the Children's Depression Inventory (CDI; Muris, Mannens, Peters, & Meesters, 2017). Developed by Marica Kovacs in 1985, the scale consists of 27 items that address core features of depression such as self-blame, insomnia, loss of appetite, and school adjustment issues (Kovacs, 1992). These authors tested 187 children 8–12 years of age and demonstrated that the scale was promising. Lobovits and Handel (1985) used the CDI to establish rates of major depression in latency-aged kids. They report that the instrument is a useful screener and that in comparing the scale scores to DSM-III, they further established the measure's validity. Similarly, internal consistency and test-retest reliability for over 1000 children 8–16 years of age were good (Smucker, Craighead, Craighead & Green, 1986). The newest version of the CDI, the Children's Depression Inventory 2 (CDI-2) was published in 2003 (Kovacs & Staff, 2003).

Derivois, Cenat, Joseph, Karray, and Chahraoui (2017) also studied this measure. They used the CDI with 128 children and adolescents between 7 and 18 years of age. They found that the measure was useful in identifying major depression in children. The CDI was used by Gasso et al. (2017) to assess 83 children and adolescents. In their study they investigated potential genetic factors related to depression. Freira et al. (2017) also studied the CDI for a population of overweight adolescents. The measure was used successfully at pretest and posttest to assess the efficacy of treatment.

Saylor, Finch, Spirito, and colleagues (1984) described a validity study using the CDI. They compared a DSM-III symptoms checklist to CDI scores for 185 children and adolescents between 7 and 16 years of age. Additionally, they calculated test-retest, split-half, and Kuder-Richardson reliability coefficients. The authors report that similar diagnostic profiles for depressed and nondepressed children based on the DSM-III checklist and the CDI scores. Also, good reliability and internal consistency for the CDI were reported. In a similar study, the CDI's validity was compared to DSM-III, self-concept, and learned helplessness (Saylor, Finch, Jr., Baskin, & Kelley, 1984). The authors note considerable overlap in the constructs that were measured.

The CDI has also been compared to the Children's Depression Scale. Moretti, Fine, Haley, and Marriage (1985) studied 60 inpatient children and adolescents between 8 and 17 years of age. All of these patients were referred for possible depression. They used the CDI in this study to validate the notion that children and adolescents can accurately report depression symptoms. Reynolds, Anderson, and Bartelli (1985) also underscore the reliability and validity of the CDI for self-reporting of depression. In this study, 166 children from 3rd to 6th grade in elementary schools in Wisconsin were included.

Other measures such as the Bellevue Index of Depression and the Depression Symptom Checklist have also been used in combination with the CDI. Kazdin et al. (1983) tested 104 inpatient children on the CDI. Based on test-retest data, the authors concluded that children as well as parents report stability in symptoms over time. They also reported that parent ratings were more accurate than ratings by the children. Fundudis et al. (1991) report far less positive findings with the CDI. They report that the scale had only moderate discrimination ability for identifying depression.

As time has gone on, the CDI has become an accepted measure for diagnosing depression in children and adolescents. These early studies focused on establishing the psychometric properties of the scale with respect to stability of scores, the reliability of parent and child informants, the ability to discriminate children and adolescents who do or do not have major depression, and as a means of accurately testing depression symptoms. Thus, recent studies have focused on different issues. As an example, Gomez-Baya, Mendoza, Paino, Sanchez, and Romero (2017) report on the development of a short form for the CDI in Spanish with 63 adolescents.

Child Depression Scale

The Reynolds Child Depression Scale (RCDS), developed by Bill Reynolds, is another widely used method of assessing depression symptoms of children and adolescents (Reynolds, 1989). It is a self-report scale originally developed to evaluate symptoms of depression in 8–13-year-old children. The scale has 30 items which were based on DSM-III criteria and symptoms described in the literature. Reynolds, Anderson, and Bartell (1985) report good reliability and validity with the Childhood Depression Scale. Similarly, Moretti et al. (1985) also report good reliability for this test.

Children's Depression Screener (ChlID-S)

Another childhood depression scale is the Children's Depression Screener (ChlID-S), developed by Frühe and colleagues (2012). Allgaier et al. (2014) describe using the measure for 79 psychiatric patients who were 9–12 years of age. The measure includes eight items. These authors concluded that the test was a valid screener for depression. They further underscore the brevity and shows how rapidly a child can be evaluated.

Children's Depression Rating Scale-Revised (CDRS-R)

The Children's Depression Rating Scale-Revised Version (CDRS-R) has also been put forward as a potential measure of major depression (Poznanski, et al., 1984). These authors state that their scale is designed to measure the severity of depression symptoms in 6–12-year-olds. The original scale items were based on clinical experience and included weeping, evaluating self-esteem, suicidal thoughts, depressed mood, issues with homework, fatigue, physical complaints, and similar symptoms of major depression. A few minor changes were made to the test including scoring based on nonverbal behavior. The paper is largely descriptive, but the authors suggest that the CDRS-R may be useful for assessing primary and secondary depression. In an independent study, Asarnow and Carlson (1985) using the original version of the scale also endorsed its usefulness and suggest that it may be a valuable tool for identifying children and adolescents with depression.

Children's Depression Scale (CDS)

Kazdin (1987) evaluated the Children's Depression Scale (to be distinguished from the Children's Depression Scale created by Reynolds et al., 1985) for 185 psychiatric 7–12-year-old inpatients along with the children's parents. They report the development of good reliability and agreement with accepted diagnostic criteria. The scale has 66 items with each item printed on a separate card. The 60 children who participated in the study were asked to place each card into one of five boxes that range from agree to disagree. Parent report, in particular, proved to be accurate in identifying depressive symptoms compared to their children.

Depression Indicator Assessment Battery

This scale was designed to assess depression and related issues such as self-concept and self-esteem. Borges, Baptista, and de Oliviera Serpa (2017) tested 8–18-year-olds (n = 976). The population was a general sample obtained from local schools and also from mental health facilities in Brazil. The study demonstrated good internal consistency. However, this is one of the scales that has not been consistently studied and developed.

Depression Observation Schedule (DOS)

Sanders, Dodds, Johnston, and Cash (1992) studied clinic and non-clinic sample which ranged in age from 7 to 14. Thirty of these children were described as depressed, 27 had conduct disorders, and 16 were typically developing children. The DOS included behaviors on depressed and angry affect and positive and aversive content. Ratings were based on 10-min observations that were divided in 30, 20-s blocks. The data collected was used to support theories focused on family problem solving.

Depression Self-Rating Scale for Children (DSRSC)

The Depression Self-Rating Scale for Children (DSRSC) (Birleson, 1981) is another measure developed to tap into symptoms of depression. Birleson, Hudson, Buchanan, and Wolff (1987) endorse the value of this scale. These researchers also point to the ease of administration. Fundudis et al. (1991) report only moderate ability to discriminate between children with and without major depression. A more robust endorsement of the scale is the recognition that it was as useful as the well-recognized CDI.

Depression Symptom Checklist

The Depression Symptom Checklist was studied with 104 children who were 5–13 years of age (Kazdin et al., 1983). The scale had ten items based on DSM-III. Scores range from 1 to 10 depending on the number of items endorsed.

Dysthymic Checklist

Yet another childhood depression scale is the Dysthymic Checklist. The measure was based on DSM-III with 14 items rated on a three-point scale (Moretti et al., 1985). This measure is outdated at this point and has not been studied further. The use of the Dysthymic Checklist was primarily employed as an additional criterion measure. However, while the checklist is no longer in use, it does provide a template for checklists that might be devised from diagnostic criteria to help diagnose child and adolescent major depression in the future.

Hopelessness Scale for Children

Another scale which has failed to gain traction is the Hopelessness Scale for Children (Beck, Weissman, Lester, & Trexler, 1974). This is unfortunate since research has shown that in the course of studying 262, 6–13-year-old psychiatric patients, good psychometrics were established (Kazdin, Rodgers, & Colbus, 1986). The researchers report that the scale was internally consistent and test-retest reliability over 6 weeks was good.

Personality Inventory for Children (PIC)

This test was first described by Wirt, Lachar, Klinedinst, and Seat (1984) and later studied by Reynolds, Anderson, and Bartell (1985). In this latter paper, 166, 3rd to 6th graders were assessed by their parents. This measure is a large scale (600 true/false items) that measures a range of psychopathology including depression. They reported good test-retest reliability with a small group of typically developing individuals. Little further development of the scale has occurred.

Revised Child Anxiety and Depression Scale (RCADS)

A scale which has fared better in the empirical literature is the Revised Child Anxiety and Depression Scale (RCADS) (Chorpita, Moffitt, & Gray, 2005). Piqueras, Martin-Vivar, Sandin, San Luis, and Pineda (2017) recently published an excellent and exhaustive review of this scale. For the reader who is interested in the RCADS, it is highly recommended that they read this review. The authors note that 146 studies were identified and included in their review. Piqueras et al. (2017) state that the criteria for the empirical studies included were papers published in Spanish or English. Studies were included if they were focused on psychometrics of the scale or were used to assess treatment outcomes. These authors looked at the reliability of the total score and of the six subscales: major depression, generalized anxiety, separation anxiety, social anxiety, panic disorder, and obsessive-compulsive disorder. Piqueras et al. (2017) conclude that studies demonstrate robust reliability across countries, language, and setting where children and adolescents were evaluated.

Chorpita, Yim, Moffitt, Umemoto, and Francis (2000) publish one of the first studies reported on the RCADS. The scale was an adaptation of the Spence Anxiety Scale (Spence, 1997) and included 56 items from the original scale. Seven items on excessive worry were added. Also, 11 depression items from DSM-IV were added. Children and adolescents from grades 3 to 12 in Hawaii were assessed. Thirteen schools and 1641 participants were included. A factor analysis was performed and yielded the six categories which were described above. For study two of the paper, 246 children from the same area as the first study were recruited. They found good results on reliability for the total score and all subscales. To study the validity, total and subscale scores on the RCADS were correlated with the CDI. The highest correlation with the CDI was the major depression subscale of the RCADS. This outcome was the best possible solution with regard to validating the measure for identifying pediatric depression.

Ebesutani et al. (2011) have also addressed the psychometrics of the RCADS. In this case, parents versus children and adolescents (see above) completed the form. Their sample had 976 individuals. Parents also completed the Child Behavior Checklist. The authors reported high internal consistency, test-retest reliability, and strong divergent and convergent on the Child Behavior Checklist. Stevanovic, Bagheri, Atilola, and Vostanis (2017) have also endorsed the soundness of the RCADS. In their paper, children and adolescents from 11 countries were tested. Most items proved to be relevant and the use of the RCADS cross-culturally was endorsed.

Kiddie Schedule for Affective Disorder and Schizophrenia (Kiddie-SADS)

The Kiddie-SADS (Puig-Antich & Chambers, 1978) is a somewhat different standardized assessment of depression. It is a substantial structural assessment for 6–17-year-olds that is administered in an interview format. The test is based on an adult measure called the Schedule for Affective Disorder and Schizophrenia. The Kiddie-SADS items cover DSM-III symptoms for a broad range of disorder including major depression and bipolar disorder. One form of the scale measures past episodes of psychopathology, while a second form addresses parent status. Orvaschel, Puig-Antich, Chambers, Tabrizi, and Johnson (1982) assessed 17 youngsters who were 6–11 years old at the initial interview and 8–13 years old at the time of the second interview. They reported consistent findings from test to retest. However, the authors note that this was an initial pilot study. The sample size was far too small, and the application of appropriate statistics and research design features was not used.

Later studies have addressed these psychometric concerns. In one such study, 55 outpatients and 11 typically developing children and adolescents between 7 and 17 years of age were studied (Kaufman et al., 1997). They report excellent inter-item and test-retest reliability. Danielson, Youngstrom, Findling, and Calabrese (2003) used the Kiddie-SADS and the General Behavior Inventory. The overall takeaway from this study was that the authors accept the psychometrics of the Kiddie-SADS as a viable measure of childhood depression. This point is further underscored by Jarbin, Andersson, Rastom, and Ivarsson (2017) who noted that the Kiddie-SADS is "one of the most commonly used standardized diagnostic interviews used in child and adolescent psychiatry." Having said that, we would emphasize that structured interviews are not frequently used in clinical practice. They are cumbersome, require a great deal of time to administer, and require a highly trained interviewer. On the positive side, this approach provides perhaps the most consistent means of interviewing for depression and bipolar disorder that is available for youth.

Short Mood and Feelings Questionnaire (SMFQ)

The final measure of core symptoms of major depression which will be covered is the SMFQ. This test consists of 13 items which is rated as true, sometimes true, or not true (Angold et al., 1995; Angold, Erkanli, Silberg, Eaves, & Costello, 2002). Angold et al. (2002) report cutoff scores for the measure, while Angold et al. (1995) report good reliability and convergence with the CDI.

A number of scales to measure major depression in children and adolescents emerged in the 1980s and 1990s. The CDI appears to have the most widespread use, followed by the RCADS. A substantial number of measures were described in a few studies but did not appear to develop momentum among clinicians and researchers.

The psychometrics fidelity of scales appears to be the only one factor that has fostered these developments. How early on the scale was described, ease of administration, whether the scale was a priority for funding agencies, persistence of the investigators, and other factors also appear to have shaped these developments.

Criteria

The DSM-III and IV have been used as the reference for a substantial number of studies and are presumed to be used very frequently in clinical practice to establish a diagnosis of major depression in children and adolescents. Lobovits and Handal (1985), for example, used these criteria to establish reliable and valid diagnosis of depression in conjunction with the CDI and the Personality Inventory for Children. Similarly, 24 emotionally disturbed youth from 7 to 15 years of age were tested on DSM-III criteria compared to the CDI (Kendall, Stark, & Adam, 1990; Saylor, Finch, Jr., Furey, Baskin, & Kelly, 1984). And Kazdin et al. (1986) look at overt symptoms of depression while comparing DSM-III diagnoses obtained using clinical information and direct interviews compared to direct observations. Finally, we mention that DSM-III was used as an anchor to measure depression while evaluating the Center for Epidemiologic Studies Depression Scale.

Secondary Scales

Matching Familiar Figures Test

Kendall, Stark, and Adam (1990) evaluated 47 6th graders, 17 of whom had a diagnosis of depression. The Matching Familiar Figures Test (Kagan, 1964) was ancillary and was used to assess self-evaluation styles. They also used the *My Standards Questionnaire* to address this same concept.

Another example of using secondary measures to address major depression in children and adolescents is described by Chang et al. (2017) to evaluate how self-perception and emotion regulation were related to depression symptoms.

Overall, a large number of major depression measures have been developed for children and adolescents. The RCADS and especially the CDI have emerged as popular, well-studied measures. These measures should typically be used with DSM-V diagnostic criteria when making a diagnosis. DSM-V waits validation, but DSM-III and DSM-IV criteria have been proven to be useful in the diagnostic process and to have good reliability and validity. The secondary measures appear to be more a means to establish theoretical hypotheses and ways children and adolescents thinks and view the world. These factors are not to be minimized but have less to do with prognostic diagnostic issues than many of the other studies reviewed.

Tests of Bipolar Disorders

A number of measures designed to address pediatric bipolar disorder are substantial but have fewer scales and have been studied less frequently than measures for major depression. This current state of affairs is likely due to several factors. First, the study of bipolar disorders in children and adolescents is a more current development than for major depression. Second, the disorder is far less common than major depression. Third, the adult literature is better developed for major depression. In general, the child mood disorder literature has been largely modeled after the adult literature. Fourth, it has taken time to develop people with expertise in the child and adolescent mood disorders literature, particularly for bipolar disorder. A brief review of specific tests and some research designed to support these scales follows.

Child Behavior Checklist-Mania Scale (CBCL-MS)

This subscale of the Child Behavior Checklist (Achenbach, 1991) has 19 items. Papachristou and colleagues (2013) studied 2230 Dutch adolescents and report good reliability and validity. In a follow-up study, Zappitelli, Pereira, and Isabel (2015) studied 424, 6–17-year-olds who the author described as at risk for bipolar disorders who lived in Brazil. These authors report good sensitivity for this subscale as a means of identifying bipolar disorder. Ratheesh and colleagues (2015), in a review of the study on bipolar disorder in children and adolescents, also underscored the utility of the CBLC-MS. Finally, Southammakosane et al. (2013) studied 32 adolescents who ranged from 12 to 18 years old and who reported a much more outcome. They concluded that new scales be developed that do a better job of identifying pediatric bipolar disorder.

Child Bipolar Questionnaire (CBQ)

A rapid screener for assessing bipolar disorder in children and youth has been reported by Papolos, Hennen, Cockerham, Thode, and Youngstrom (2006). The primary goal of their study was to report reliability and validity. Both inter-rater and test-retest reliability were good. Also, the measure had good specificity and sensitivity when compared to the bipolar disorders scale for the Kiddie-SADS. These authors were enthusiastic about these initial results but suggest that further development is needed. Miguez et al. (2013) did just that. They also compared the scale to the Kiddie-SADS and found good agreement on bipolar disorder items.

Children's Depression Rating Scale-Revised (CDRS-R)

Frazier and colleagues (2007) compared the Children's Depression Rating Scale-Revised (Poznanski & Mokros, 1996) across four groups divided by age: 4–7, 8–10, 11–13, and 14–17 years of age. These youth had been seen at an outpatient clinic and included 1014 patients. They stress the value of this scale for measuring bipolar disorders across age groups.

Children's Interview for Psychiatric Syndromes (ChIPs)

The ChIPS (Weller, Weller, Fristad, Rooney, & Schecter, 2000) is another measure often utilized. For example, Hunt et al. (2005) assessed 391 psychiatric inpatients. They compared this instrument to the Kiddie-SADS and the Mania Rating Scale. The authors were generally positive about this scale, but it is not one of the primary bipolar measures at this point.

Child Mania Rating Scale-Parent

The Child Mania Rating Scale-Parent was tested with 150 parents of children who had been previously diagnosed with bipolar disorder, ADHD, or typically developing youth. These researchers report that it correlated highly with the full Child Mania Rating Scale in identifying young people into the three categories noted above (Henry, Pavuluri, Youngstrom, & Birmaher, 2008).

General Behavior Inventory-Revised (GBI-R)

One study that examined the General Behavior Inventory (Depue, 1987) included 813 parents who completed the parent version of the test (Freeman, et al., 2012). Settings for the examinations occurred included a medical school and a mental health center. The authors suggest that the scale was useful for identifying bipolar symptoms. Ratheesh et al. (2015) in a review of the pediatric diagnostic disorder also endorse the utility of the scale for identifying bipolar disorders. In addition, Youngstrom, Frazier, Demeter, Calabrese, and Findling (2008) tested 637 youth and found that parents in particular were good at identifying elevated mood, high energy, irritability, and cycling of symptoms of mania. Ong et al. (2017) studied the General Behavior Inventory with 681 caregivers of children being seen at a mental health outpatient clinic. They report that the test demonstrated good utility in distinguishing pediatric bipolar disorder from other childhood mental health conditions.

Kiddie Schedule for Affective Disorders and Schizophrenia (Kiddie-SADS)

A number of studies noted above describe the Kiddie-SADS as an anchor measure to diagnose bipolar disorder (e.g., Reichart et al., 2004; Tillman et al., 2008). The same pattern has emerged in research on major depression for children and adolescents. Thus, this structured interview is based on these studies and in our view is a well-accepted method of differential diagnosis for mood disorder of youth. A few specific studies that exemplify the psychometric of the Kiddie-SADS follow.

Youngstrom et al. (2004) investigated 642 children and adolescents between 5 and 17 years of age (over 40% had a bipolar disorder diagnosis). Their main conclusion was the parents were more accurate reporters of bipolar symptoms than the children themselves or their teachers. As such, these results are similar to results of other studies using different measure of mood disorders in children and youth. Another psychometric study of the Kiddie-SADS, this time in Persian, was reported by Shahrivar, Kousha, Moallemi, Tehrani-Doost, and Alaghband-Rad (2010). They studied 102 young people (mean age of 15.3 years) who were inpatients at a psychiatric hospital. They report finding good reliability and validity with the scale.

Axelson et al. (2004) have taken a somewhat different approach. In a nod to the brevity, they extracted 14 items from the Kiddie-SADS that measured bipolar disorder and then added an item on mood lability. They then assessed 22 individuals residing in a bipolar outpatient clinic and 23 controls. The authors concluded that this new "subscale" of the Kiddie-SADS had good sensitivity and specificity.

Mood Disorder Questionnaire- Adolescent Version (MDQ-A)

The MDQ-A (Wagner, Emslie, Findling, Gracious, & Reed, 2004) is another pediatric bipolar measure that has received some attention. In one study, 76 adolescents 13–18 years old were evaluated (Miguez et al., 2013). They report moderate test-retest reliability and poor agreement between parents and child report. Conversely, Lee et al. (2014) found that the Korean version of the MDQ-A had "fair to good" agreement for making bipolar diagnosis in 92 youngsters diagnosed with bipolar disorder using the General Behavior Inventory and the Adolescent General Behavior Inventory.

Young Mania Rating Scale (YMRS)

The final test of bipolar disorder core symptoms is the YMRS (Young, Biggs, Ziegler, & Meyer, 1978). In one study with 1014 young people who were 4–17 years of age, good psychometrics were reported. The author suggest that the test provided a distinct measure of mania, with good internal consistency (Frazier et al., 2007). In another study of this sort, Serrano, Ezpeleta, Alda, Matali, and San (2011) describe psychometrics in a Spanish version of the YMRS. They assessed 100 children and adolescents in an effort to discriminate mania from ADHD. The authors note that this distinction is important because of the high rate of comorbidity of the two disorders.

Neuroimaging

Functional magnetic resonance imaging (fMRI) studies have also been published as a means of better understanding the nature of pediatric bipolar disorder. Pavuluri, Passarotti, Parnes, Fitzgerald, and Sweeney (2010) published one such study. They tested 14 people who were typically developing and 17 individuals with mania or hypomania (mean age of 14 years). The fMRI was administered twice: 14 weeks apart. A matching test was used as a standard stimulus. Participants linked neutral, positive, or negative words to colors. Fifty words were used. The bipolar group was slower and less accurate than controls. fMRI data has also been collected by Stoddard et al. (2016). They assessed adults from 105 years old: 39 with bipolar disorder and 78 typically developing individuals. The bipolar groups had more difficulties than the typically developing groups in visual processing, responding, and attention. No differences across ages were noted. This area of study is in its infancy. However, it is likely to receive much more attention in the future.

Criteria

Bipolar At-Risk Criteria

The Bipolar At-Risk Criteria were administered to 35, 15–24-year-olds who were receiving neutral health services in a study by Bechdolf and colleagues (2014). They were compared to 35 controls. Symptoms taped included mania, depression, genetic risk factors, and cyclothymic features. They found that these criteria were useful in identifying bipolar disorders prior to the onset of mania/hypomanic. Criteria have not been frequently studied in the literature with children and adolescents. Given the widespread use of DSM-V criteria, research on its reliability and validity are needed.

Secondary Scales

Barrat Impulsiveness Scale

There is also some research on the Barratt Impulsiveness Scale (Patton, Stanford, Barratt, 1995). Nandagopal et al. (2011) tested 31 children with bipolar disorder, 30 individuals with ADHD, and 25 typically developing individuals. The function of this assessment was to establish the level of impulsivity in adolescents with bipolar disorder relative to the other two groups that were studied. They found that impulsivity was elevated for both the bipolar groups and for individuals who had ADHD. Non-planning impulsivity was especially pronounced in the bipolar groups.

Conclusions

There are an impressive number of tests and diagnostic criteria that have been developed to assess mood disorder in children and adolescents. Most of these assessment methods dated to the 1980s. A great deal of research activity occurred during this decade, particularly with respect to instruments and other methods designed to assess major depression. More scale and studies have been developed for this problem, but bipolar disorder has also received a good deal of attention. Research on these topics continues, but many scales have fallen by the wayside over time.

Based on the available information, there is little reason not to include at least one checklist or the Kiddie-SADS in a diagnostic workup. The latter, a structured interview, may be particularly helpful when the clinician is trying to determine if major depression or bipolar disorder should be diagnosed. The Kiddie-SADS has proven to be quite useful for diagnosing both conditions. Given the widespread use of DSM criteria to aid in diagnosis, a top priority should be studied that establishes symptom checklists based on DSM-V that can help in accurately diagnosing depression, bipolar disorder, and related mood disorders. Solid diagnostic methods are currently available, but a good deal or additional research is needed.

References

Achenbach, T. M. (1991). Manual for Child Behavior Checklist/ 4–18 and 1991 Profile. Burlington: University of Vermont Department of Psychiatry.

Allgaier, A.-K., Krick, K., Opitz, A., Saravo, B., Romanos, M., & Schulte-Korne, G. (2014). Improving early detection of childhood depression in mental health care: The children's depression screener (Child-S). *Psychiatry Research, 217,* 248–252.

Amerio, A., Tonna, M., Odone, A., Stubbs, B., & Ghaemi, S. N. (2016). Comorbid bipolar disorder and obsessive-compulsive disorder in children and adolescents: Treatment implications. *Australian and New Zealand Journal of Psychiatry, 50,* 594–596.

Angold, A., Costello, E. J., Messer, S. C., Pickles, A., Winder, F., & Silver, D. (1995). Development of a short questionnaire for use in epidemiological studies of depression in children and adolescents. *International Journal of Research Methods in Psychiatric Research, 5,* 1–12.

Angold, A., Erkanli, A., Silberg, J., Eaves, L., & Costello, E. J. (2002). Depression scale scores in 8-17 year olds: Effects of age and gender. *Journal of Child Psychology and Psychiatry, 43,* 1052–1063.

Asarnow, J. R., & Carlson, G. A. (1985). Depression self-rating scale: Utility with child psychiatric inpatients.

Journal of Consulting and Clinical Psychology, 53, 491–499.

Axelson, D., Birmaher, B. J., Brent, D., Wassick, S., Hoover, C., Bridge, J., & Ryan, W. (2004). A preliminary study of the Kiddie Schedule for affective disorders and schizophrenia for school-age children mania rating scale for children and adolescents. *Journal of Child and Adolescent Psychopharmacology, 13*, 463–470.

Bayes, A. J., McClure, G., Fletcher, K., Roman Ruiz del Moral, Y. E., Hadzi-Pavlovic, D., Stevenson, J. L., … Parker, G. B. (2016). Differentiating the bipolar disorders from borderline personality disorder. *Acta Psychiatrica Scandiavica, 133*, 187–195.

Bechdolf, A., Ratheesh, A., Cotton, S. M., Nelson, B., Chanen, A. M., Betts, J., … & McGorry, P. D. (2014). The predictive validity of bipolar at-risk (prodromal) criteria in help-seeking adolescents and young adults: a prospective study. *Bipolar disorders, 16*(5), 493–504.

Beck, A. T., Weissman, A., Lester, D., & Trexler, L. (1974). The measurement of pessimism: The Hopelessness Scale. *Journal of Consulting and Clinical Psychology, 42*, 861–865.

Beck, A. T., Steer, R. A., & Brown, G. K. (1996). *Manual for the beck depression inventory-II*. San Antonio, TX: Psychological Corporation.

Benarous, X., Mikita, N., Goodman, R., & Stringaris, A. (2015). Distinct relationships between social aptitude and dimensions of manic-like symptoms in youth. *European Child and Adolescent Psychiatry*. https://doi.org/10:10071500787-015-0800-7.

Birleson P. (1981) The Validity of Depressive Disorder in Childhood and the Development of a Self-Rating Scale: A Research Report. *Journal of Child Psychology and Psychiatry, 22*, 73/88.

Birleson, P., Hudson, I., Buchanan, D. G., & Wolff, S. (1987). Clinical evaluation of a self-rating scale for depressive disorder in childhood (Depression Self-Rating Scale). *Journal of Child Psychology and Psychiatry, 28*, 43–60.

Birmaher, B., Gill, M. K., Axelson, D. A., Goldstein, B. I., Goldstein, T. R., Yu, H., … Keller, M. B. (2014). Longitudinal trajectories and associated baseline predictors in youths with bipolar spectrum disorders. *American Journal of Psychiatry, 171*, 990–999.

Borges, L., Baptista, M. N., & de Oliviera Serpa, A. L. (2017). Structural analysis of depression indicators Scale- Children and Adolescents (BAID-IJ): A bifactor-ESEM approach. *Trends in Psychology, 25*, 545–552.

Carlson, G. A. (2000). The challenge of diagnosing depression in childhood and adolescence. *Journal of Affective Disorders, 61*, 53–58.

Chang, C., Kaczkurkin, A. N., McLean, C. P., & Foa, E. B. (2017). Emotion regulation is associated with PTSD and depression among female adolescent survivors of childhood sexual abuse. *Psychological Trauma: Theory, Research, Practice, and Policy.*. https://doi.org/10.1037/tra0000306

Chorpita, B. F., Yim, L., Moffitt, C., Umemoto, L. A., & Francis, S. E. (2000). Assessment of symptoms of DSM-IV anxiety and depression in children: A revised child anxiety and depression scale. *Behaviour Research and Therapy, 38*, 835–855.

Chorpita, B. F., Moffitt, C., & Gray, J. (2005). Psychometric properties of the Revised Child Anxiety and Depression Scale in a clinical sample. *Behaviour Research and Therapy, 43*, 309–322.

Collins, A. M. (2014). Childhood attention-deficit/hyperactivity disorder and bipolar Mania: Neurobiology of symptoms and treatments. *The Journal for Nurse Practitioners, 10*, 16–21.

Costello, E. J., & Angold, A. (1988). Scales to assess child and adolescent depression: Checklists, screens, and nets. *Journal of the American Academy of Child and Adolescent Psychiatry, 27*, 726–737.

Danielson, C. K., Youngstrom, E. A., Findling, R. L., & Calabrese, J. R. (2003). Discriminative validity of the General Behavior Inventory using youth report. *Journal of Abnormal Child Psychology, 31*, 29–39.

Depue, R. (1987). General behavior inventory. Ithaca, NY: *Department of Psychology, Cornell University*.

Demeter, C. A., Youngstrom, E. A., Carlson, G. A., Frazier, T. W., Rowles, B. M., Lingler, J., … Findling, R. L. (2013). Age differences in the phenomenology of pediatric bipolar disorder. *Journal of Affective Disorders, 147*, 295–303.

Derivois, D., Cenat, J. M., Joseph, N. E., Karray, A., & Chahraoui, K. (2017). Prevalence and determinants of post-traumatic stress disorder, anxiety, and depression symptoms in street children survivors of the 2010 earthquake in Haiti, four years after. *Child Abuse and Neglect, 67*, 174–181.

Dickstein, D. P., Axelson, D., Weissman, A. B., Yen, S., & Goldstein, B. (2016). Cognitive flexibility and performance in children and adolescents with threshold and sub-threshold bipolar disorder. *European Child and Adolescent Psychiatry, 25*, 625–638.

Donfrancesco, R., Marano, A., Innocenzi, L., Toni, A., DeLelio, A., Milone, A., … DelBello, M. P. (2014). A comparison of bipolar disorders in children in Italy and the United States. *Journal of Affective Disorders, 159*, 53–55.

Ebesutani, C., Chorpita, B. F., Higa-McMillan, C. K., Nakamura, B. J., Regan, J., & Lynch, R. E. (2011). A psychometric analysis of the Revised Child Anxiety and Depression Sclaes- Parent version in a school sample. *Journal of Abnormal Child Psychology, 39*, 173, 185.

Faedden, G. L., Ohashi, K., Hernandez, M., McGreenery, C. E., Grant, M. C., Baroni, A., … Teicher, M. H. (2016). Actigraph measures discriminate pediatric bipolar disorder from Attention-Deficit/Hyperactivity disorder and typically developing control. *Journal of Child Psychology and Psychiatry, 57*, 706–716.

Feldman, J. S., Tung, I., & Lee, S. S. (2017). Social skills mediate the association of ADHD and depression in preadolescents. *Journal of Psychopathology and Behavioral Assessment, 39*, 79–91.

Fendrich, M., Weissman, M. M., & Warner, V. (1990). Screening for depressive disorder in children and adolescents: Validating the Center for Epidemiologic Studies Depression Scale for children. *American Journal of Epidemiology, 131,* 538–551.

Findling, R. L., Jo, B., Frazier, T. W., Youngstrom, E. A., Demeter, C. A., Fristad, M. A., ... Horwitz, S. M. (2013). The 24-month course of manic symptoms in children. *Bipolar Disorders, 15,* 669–679.

Findling, R. L., Youngstrom, E. A., Fristad, M. A., Birmaher, B., Kowatch, R. A., Arnold, E., ... Horwitz, S. M. (2010). Characteristics of children with elevated symptoms of mania: The longitudinal assessment of manic symptoms (LAMS) study. *The Journal of Clinical Psychiatry, 71,* 1664–1672.

Frazier, T. W., Demeter, C. A., Youngstrom, E. A., Calabreses, J. R., Stransbrey, R. J., McNamara, N. K., & Findling, R. L. (2007). Evaluation and comparison of psychometric instruments for pediatric bipolar spectrum disorders in four age groups. *Journal of Child and Adolescent Psychopharmacology, 17,* 853–866.

Frazier, T. W., Youngstrom, E. A., McCue-Horwitz, S., Demeter, C. A., Fristad, M. A., ... Findling, R. L. (2011). Relationship of persistent manic symptoms to the diagnosis of pediatric bipolar spectrum disorders. *The Journal of Clinical Psychiatry, 72,* 846–853.

Freeman, A. J., Youngstrom, E. A., Frazier, E. A., Youngstrom, T. W., Kogos, J., ... Findling, R. (2012). Portability of a screener for pediatric bipolar disorder in a diverse setting. *Psychological Assessment, 24,* 341–351.

Freira, S., Lemos, M. S., Williams, G., Riberio, M., Pena, F., & deCeau Machado, M. (2017). Effect of motivational interviewing on depression scale scores of adolescents with obesity and overweight. *Psychiatric Research, 252,* 340–345.

Fristad, M. A., Wolfson, H., Perez, A. G., Youngstrom, E. A., Arnold, E. L., Birmaher, B., ... the LAMS Group. (2016). Disruptive mood dysregulation disorder and bipolar disorder not otherwise specified: Fraternal or identical twins. *Journal of Child and Adolescent Psychopharmacology, 26,* 138–146.

Frühe, B., Allgaier, A. K., Pietsch, K., Baethmann, M., Peters, J., Kellnar, S., ... & Schulte-Körne, G. (2012) Children's Depression Screener (ChilD-S): development and validation of a depression screening instrument for children in pediatric care. *Child Psychiatry & Human Development, 43*(1), 137–151.

Fundudis, T., Berney, T. P., Kolvin, I., Famuyiwa, O. O., Barrett, L., Bhate, S., & Tyrer, S. P. (1991). Reliability and validity of two self-rating scales in the assessment of childhood depression. *The British Journal of Psychiatry, Supplement* (11), 36–40.

Gasso, P., Rodriguez, N., Boloc, D., Blazquez, A., Torres, T., ... Fernandez-Lazaro, F. (2017). Association of regulatory TPH2 polymorphism with higher reduction in depressive symptoms in children and adolescents treated with fluoxetine. *Progress in Neuropsychopharmacology and Biological Psychiatry, 77,* 236–240.

Goldstein, B. I., Lotrich, F., Axelson, D. A., Gill, M. K., Houer, H., Goldstein, T. R., ... Birmaher, B. (2015). Inflammatory markers among adolescents and young adults with bipolar spectrum disorders. *The Journal of Clinical Psychiatry, 76,* 1556–1563.

Goldstein, T. R., Ha, W., Axelson, D. A., Goldstein, B. I., Liao, F., Gill, M. K., ... Birmaher, B. (2012). Predictors of prospectively examined suicide attempts among youth with bipolar disorder. *Archives of General Psychiatry, 69,* 1113–1122.

Gomez-Baya, D., Mendoza, R., Paino, S., Sanchez, A., & Romero, N. (2017). Latent growth curve analysis of gender differences in response styles and depressive symptoms during mid-adolescents. *Cognitive Therapy and Research, 41,* 289–303.

Hafeman, D., Axelson, D., Demeter, C., Findling, R. L., Fristad, M. A., Kowatch, R., ... Birmaher, B. (2013). Phenomenology of bipolar disorder not otherwise specified in youth: A comparison of clinical characteristics across the spectrum of manic symptoms. *Bipolar Disorders, 15,* 240–252.

Hanford, L. C., Sassi, R. B., & Hall, G. B. (2016). Accuracy of emotion labeling in children of parents diagnosed with bipolar disorders. *Journal of Affective Disorders, 194,* 226–233.

Henry, D. B., Pavulari, M. N., Youngstrom, E., & Birmaher, B. (2008). Accuracy of brief and full forms of the Child Mania Rating Scale. *Journal of Clinical Psychology, 64,* 368–381.

Hong, W., Zhang, C., Xing, M. J., Peng, D. H., Wu, Z. G., Wang, Z. W., ... Fang, Y. R. (2016). Contribution of long duration of undiagnosed bipolar disorder to high frequency of relapse: A naturalistic study in China. *Comprehensive Psychiatry, 70,* 77–81.

Hunt, J. I., Dyl, J., Armstrong, L., Litvin, E., Sheeran, T., & Sprito, A. (2005). Frequency of manic symptoms and bipolar disorder in psychiatrically hospitalized adolescents using the K-SADS Mani Rating Scale. *Journal of Child and Adolescent Psychopharmacology, 15,* 918–930.

Hutchinson, A. K., Beresford, C., Robinson, J. A., & Ross, R. G. (2010). Assessing disordered thoughts in preschoolers with dysregulated mood. *Child Psychiatry and Human Development, 41,* 479–489.

Jarbin, H., Andersson, M., Råstam, M., & Ivarsson, T. (2017). Predictive validity of the K-SADS-PL 2009 version in school-aged and adolescent outpatients. *Nordic Journal of Psychiatry, 71*(4), 270–276.

Kagan, J. (1964). Matching familiar figures test. Harvard University.

Kaufman, J., Birmaher, B., Brent, D., Flynn, C., Moreci, P., ... Ryan, N. (1997). Schedule for affective disorders and Schizophrenia for School-Age Children- Present and Lifetime Version (K-SADS-PL): Initial reliability and validity data. *Journal of the American Academy of Child and Adolescent Psychiatry, 36,* 980–988.

Kazdin, A. E. (1987). Children's Depression Scale: Validation with child psychiatric inpatients. *Journal of Child Psychology and Psychiatry, 28,* 29–41.

Kazdin, A. E., French, N. H., Unis, A. S., & Esveldt-Dawson, K. (1983). Hopelessness, depression, and suicidal intent among psychiatrically disturbed inpatient children. *Journal of the American Academy of Child Psychiatry, 22*, 157–164.

Kazdin, A. E., Rodgers, A., & Colbus, D. (1986). The hopelessness scale for children: Psychometric characteristics and concurrent validity. *Journal of Consulting and Clinical Psychology, 54*, 241–245.

Kendall, P. C., Stark, K. D., & Adam, T. (1990). Cognitive deficit or cognitive distortion in childhood depression. *Journal of Abnormal Child Psychology, 18*(3), 255–270.

Kendler, K. S., & Aggen, S. H. (2017). Symptoms of major depression: Their stability, familiality, and prediction by genetic, temperamental, and childhood environmental risk factors. *Depression and Anxiety, 34*, 171–177.

Kovacs, M. (1985). The Children's Depression Inventory (CDI). *Psychopharmacology Bulletin, 2*, 995–998.

Kovacs, M. (1992). Children's Depression Inventory. CDI. Manual. Toronto (Canada): Multi-health systems.

Kovacs, M., & Staff, M. H. S. (2003). Children's Depression Inventory 2 (CDI-2). Multi-Health Systems, Incorporated.

Lee, H.-J., Joo, Y., Youngstrom, E. A., Yum, S. Y., Findling, R. L., & Kim, H.-W. (2014). Diagnostic validity and reliability of a Korean version of the parent and adolescent general behavior inventories. *Comprehensive Psychiatry, 55*, 1730–1737.

Lobovits, D. A., & Handel, P. J. (1985). Childhood depression: Prevalence using DSM-III criteria and validity of parent and child depression scales. *Journal of Pediatric Psychology, 10*, 45–54.

Luckenbaugh, D. A., Findling, R. L., Leverich, G. S., Pizzcerello, S. M., & Post, R. M. (2009). Earliest symptoms discriminating juvenile-onset bipolar illness from ADHD. *Bipolar Disorders, 11*, 441–451.

Marangoni, C., DeChiara, L., & Faedda, G. L. (2015). Bipolar disorder and ADHD: Comorbidity and diagnostic distinctions. *Current Psychiatric Reports, 17*, 67.

Martin, S. E., Liu, R. T., Mernick, L. R., DeMarco, M., Cheek, S. M., Spirito, A., & Boekamp, J. R. (2016). Suicidal thoughts and behaviors in psychiatrically referred young children. *Psychiatric Research, 246*, 308–313.

McCraw, S., & Parker, G. (2017). The prevalence and outcomes of exposure to potentially traumatic stressful life events compared across patients with bipolar disorder and unipolar depression. *Psychiatry Research, 255*, 399–404.

McLean, C. P., Su, Y. J., Carpenter, J. K., & Foa, E. B. (2017). Changes in PTSD and depression during prolonged exposure and client-centered therapy for PTSD in adolescents. *Journal of Clinical Child and Adolescent Psychology*. Doi/abs/10.1080/15374416.2015.1012722.

Miguez, M., Weber, B., Debbane, M., Balanzin, D., Gex-Fabry, M., Raiola, F., ... Aubry, J.-M. (2013). Screening for bipolar disorder in adolescents with the Mood Disorder Questionnaire-Adolescent Version (MDQ-A) and the Child Bipolar Questionnaire (CBQ). *Early Intervention in Psychiatry, 7*, 270–277.

Mitchell, R. H. B., Timmins, V., Jordan, C., Scavone, A., Iskric, A., & Goldstein, B. I. (2016). Prevalence and correlates of disruptive mood dysregulation disorder among adolescents with bipolar disorder. *Journal of Child and Adolescent Psychopharmacology, 26*, 147–153.

Moretti, M. M., Fine, S., Haley, M. A., & Marriage, K. (1985). Childhood and adolescent depression: Child-report versus parent-report information. *Journal of the American Academy of Child Psychiatry, 24*, 298–302.

Muris, P., Mannens, J., Peters, L., & Meesters, C. (2017). The Youth Anxiety Measure for DSM-5 (YAM-5): Correlations with anxiety, fear, and depression scales in non-clinical children. *Journal of Anxiety Disorders, 51*, 72–78.

Nadkarni, R. B., & Fristad, M. A. (2010). Clinical course of children with a depressive spectrum disorder and transient manic symptoms. *Bipolar Disorders, 12*, 494–503.

Nandagopal, J. J., Fleck, D. E., Adler, C. M., Mills, N. P., Strakowski, S. M., & DelBello, M. P. (2011). Impulsivity in adolescents with bipolar disorder and/or attention-deficit/hyperactivity disorder and healthy controls as measured by the Barratt Impulsiveness Scale. *Journal of Child and Adolescent Psychopharmacology, 21*, 465–468.

Ong, M.-L., Youngstrom, E. A., Chua, J. J. X., Halverson, T. F., Horwitz, S. M., Storfer-Isser, A., ... the LAMS Group. (2017). Comparing the CASI-4R and the PGBI-18M for differentiating bipolar spectrum disorders from other outpatient diagnoses in youth. *Journal of Abnormal Child Psychology, 45*, 611–623.

Orvaschel, H., Puig-Antich, J., Chambers, W., Tabrizi, M. A., & Johnson, R. (1982). Retrospective assessment of prepubertal major depression with the Kiddie-SADS-E. *Journal of the American Academy of Child Psychiatry, 21*, 392–397.

Papachrisou, E., Ormel, J., Oldehinkel, A. J., Kyriakopoulos, M., Reinares, M., Reicheberg, A., & Frangou, S. (2013). Child Behavior Checklist- Mania Scale (CBCL-MS): Development and evaluation of a population-based screening scale for bipolar disorder. *PLoS One, 8*, 81–89.

Papolos, D., Hennen, J., Cockerham, M. S., Thode, H. C., & Youngstrom, E. A. (2006). The child bipolar questionnaire: A dimensional approach to screening for pediatric bipolar disorder. *Journal of Affective Disorders, 95*, 149–158.

Paris, J. (2014). Problems in the boundaries of bipolar disorders. *Current Psychiatric Reports, 16*, 461.

Patton, J. H., Stanford, M. S., & Barratt, E. S. (1995). Factor structure of the Barratt impulsiveness scale. *Journal of Clinical Psychology, 51*(6), 768–774.

Pavlova, B., Perroud, N., Cordera, P., Uher, R., Dayer, A., & Aubry, J.-M. (2016). Childhood maltreatment and comorbid anxiety in people with bipolar disorder. *Journal of Affective Disorders, 192*, 22–27.

Pavuluri, M. N., Passarotti, A. M., Parnes, S. A., Fitzgerald, J. M., & Sweeney, J. A. (2010). A pharmacological functional magnetic resonance imaging study probing the interface of cognitive and emotional brain systems in pediatric bipolar disorder. *Journal of Child and Adolescent Psychopharmacology, 20*, 395–406.

Piqueras, J. A., Martin-Vivar, M., Sandin, B., San Luis, C., & Pineda, D. (2017). The revised child anxiety and depression scale: A systematic review and reliability generalization meta-analysis. *Journal of Affective Disorders, 218*, 153–169.

Poznanski, E., & Mokros, H. (1996). Children's Depression Rating Scale–Revised (CDRS-R) Los Angeles: WPS.

Poznanski, E. O., Grossman, J. A., Buchsbaum, Y., Banegas, M., Freeman, L., & Gibbons, R. (1984). Preliminary studies of the reliability and validity of the Children's Depression Rating Scale. *Journal of the American Academy of Child Psychiatry, 23*, 191–197.

Poznanski, E. O., Freeman, L. N., & Mokros, H. B. (1985). Children's Depression Rating Scale-Revised. *Psychopharmacol Bull, 21*, 979–989.

Preisig, M., Strippoli, M.-P. F., Castelao, E., Merikangas, K. R., Gholam-Rezaee, M., Pierre-Marquet, P., … Vandeleun, C. L. (2016). The specificity of the familial aggregation of early-onset bipolar disorder: A controlled 10-year follow-up study of offspring of parents with mood disorder. *Journal of Affective Disorders, 190*, 26–33.

Puig-Antich, J., & Chambers, W. (1978). The schedule for affective disorders and schizophrenia for school-age children (Kiddie-SADS). New York: New York State Psychiatric Institute.

Quek, Y.-H., Tam, W. W., Zhang, M. W. B., & Ho, R. C. M. (2017). Exploring the association between childhood and adolescent obesity and depression: A meta-analysis. *Obesity Reviews, 18*, 742, 754.

Radloff, L. S. (1977). The CES-D scale: A self report depression scale for research in the general population. *Applied Psychological Measurements, 1*, 385–401.

Radloff, L. S. (1991). The use of the Center for Epidemiological Studies Depression Scale in adolescents and young adults. *Journal of Youth and Adolescents, 20*, 149–166.

Ratheesh, A., Berk, M., Davey, C. G., McGorry, P. D., & Cotton, S. M. (2015). Instruments that prospectively predict bipolar disorder- A systematic review. *Journal of Affective Disorders, 179*, 65–73.

Reichart, C. G., van der Ende, J., Wals, M., Hillegers, M. H. J., Ormel, J., Nolen, W. A., & Verhulst, F. C. (2004). The use of GBI in a population of adolescent offspring of parents with a bipolar disorder. *Journal of Affective Disorders, 80*, 263–267.

Reynolds, W. M. (1989). Reynolds child depression scale. Odessa, FL: Psychological Assessment Resources.

Reynolds, W. M., Andersen, G., & Bartell, N. (1985). Measuring depression in children: A multimethod assessment investigation. *Journal of Abnormal Child Psychology, 13*, 513–526.

Roberts, R. E., Andreus, J. A., Lewinsohn, P. M., & Hops, H. (1990). Assessment of depression in adolescents using the Center for Epidemiologic Studies Depression Scale. *Psychological Assessment: A Journal of Consulting and Clinical Psychology, 2*, 122–128.

Roberts, R. E., Lewinsohn, P. M., & Seeley, J. R. (1991). Screening for adolescent depression: A comparison of depression scales. *Journal of the American Academy of Child and Adolescent Psychiatry, 30*, 58–66.

Safer, D. J., Zito, J. M., & Safer, A. M. (2012). Age-group differences in bipolar mania. *Comprehensive Psychiatry, 53*, 1110–1117.

Salpekar, J. A., Gaurav, M., & Hauptman, A. J. (2015). Key issues in addressing the comorbidity of depression and pediatric epilepsy. *Epilepsy and Behavior, 46*, 12–18.

Sanders, M. R., Dadds, M. R., Johnston, B. M., & Cash, R. (1992). Childhood depression and conduct disorder: I. Behavioral, affective, and cognitive aspects of family problem-solving interactions. *Journal of Abnormal Psychology, 101*, 495–504.

Saylor, C. F., Finch, A. J., Jr., Furey, W., Baskin, C. H., & Kelly, M. M. (1984). Construct validity for measures of childhood depression: Application of multitrait-multimethod methodology. *Journal of Consulting and Clinical Psychology, 52*, 977–985.

Saylor, C. F., Finch, A. J., Jr., Spirito, A., & Bennett, B. (1984). The children's depression inventory: A systematic evaluation of psychometric properties. *Journal of Consulting and Clinical Psychology, 52*, 955–967.

Serra, G., Koukopoulous, A., DeChiara, L., Napoletano, F., Koukopoulos, A. E., Curto, M., … Baldessanin, R. J. (2015). Features preceding diagnosis of bipolar versus major depressive disorder. *Journal of Affective Disorders, 173*, 134–142.

Serrano, E., Ezpeleta, L., Alda, J. A., Matali, J. L., & San, L. (2011). Psychometric properties of the Young Mania Rating Scale for the identification of mania symptoms in Spanish children and adolescents with Attention Deficit/Hyperactivity Disorder. *Psychopathology, 44*, 125–132.

Shahrivar, Z., Kousha, M., Moallemi, S., Tehrani-Doost, M., & Alaghband-Rad, J. (2010). The reliability and validity of Kiddie-Schedule for affective disorders and Schizophrenia- Present and lifetime version- Persian version. *Child and Adolescent Mental Health, 15*, 97–102.

Shim, S.-H., & Kwon, Y. J. (2014). Adolescent with Tourette syndrome and bipolar disorder: A case report. *Clinical Psychopharmacology and Neuroscience, 12*, 235–239.

Smucker, M. R., Craighead, W. E., Craighead, L. W., & Green, B. J. (1986). Normative and reliability data for the Children's depression inventory. *Journal of Abnormal Child Psychology, 14*, 25–39.

Southammakosane, C., Danielyan, A., Welge, J. A., Blom, T. J., Adler, C. M., Chang, K. D., … DelBello,

M. P. (2013). Characteristics of the Child Behavior Checklist in adolescents with depression associated with bipolar disorder. *Journal of Affective Disorders, 145*, 405–408.

Spence, S. H. (1997). Structure of anxiety symptoms among children: A confirmatory factor-analytic study. *Journal of Abnormal Psychology, 106*, 280–297.

Stevanovic, D., Bagheri, Z., Atiola, O., & Vostanis, P. (2017). Cross-cultural measurement in variance of the Revised Child Anxiety and Depression Scale across world-wide societies. *Epidemiology and Psychiatric Sciences, 26* http://doi.org/10.1017/5204579601/600038x

Stoddard, J., Gotts, S. J., Brotman, M. A., Lever, S., Hsu, D., Zarate, C., ... Leibenluft, E. (2016). Aberrant intrinsic functional connectivity within and between corticostriatal and temporal-parietal networks in adults and youth with bipolar disorder. *Psychological Medicine, 46*, 1509–1522.

Stringaris, A., Santosh, P., Leibenluft, E., & Goodman, R. (2010). Youth meeting symptom and impairment criteria for mania-like episodes lasting less than four days: An epidemiological inquiry. *Journal of Child Psychology and Psychiatry, 51*, 31–38.

Tillman, R., Geller, B., Klages, T., Corrigan, M., Bolhofner, K., & Zimerman, B. (2008). Psychotic phenomena in 257 young children and adolescents with bipolar I disorder: Delusions and hallucinations (benign and pathological). *Bipolar Disorders, 10*, 45–55.

Tiwari, R., Agarwai, V., Arya, A., Gupta, P. K., & Mahour, P. (2016). An exploratory clinical study of disruptive mood dysregulation disorder in children and adolescents from India. *Asian Journal of Psychiatry, 21*, 37–40.

Uchida, M., Serra, G., Zayas, L., Kenworthy, T., Faraone, S. V., & Biederman, J. (2015). Can unipolar and bipolar pediatric major depression be differentiated from each other? A systematic review of cross-sectional studies examining differences in unipolar and bipolar depression. *Journal of Affective Disorders, 176*, 1–7.

Udal, A. H., Oygarden, B., Egeland, J., Malt, V. F., Lovdahl, H., Pripp, A. H., & Groholt, B. (2012). Executive deficits in early onset bipolar disorder versus ADHD: Impact of processing speed and lifetime psychosis. *Clinical Child Psychology and Psychiatry, 49*, 255–265.

Van Meter, A. R., Burke, C., Kowatch, R. A., Findling, R. L., & Youngstrom, E. A. (2016). Ten year updated meta-analysis of the clinical characteristics of pediatric mania and hypomania. *Bipolar Disorders, 18*, 19–32.

Wagner, K. D., Emslie, G. J., Findling, R. L., Gracious, B., & Reed, M. L. (2004). Clinic Validation of the Adolescent Mood Disorder Questionnaire (A-MDQ). In Annual Meeting of the American Psychiatric Association. New York: APA.

Weller, E. B., Weller, R. A., Fristad, M. A., Rooney, M. T., & Schecter, J. (2000). Children's interview for psychiatric syndromes (ChIPS). *Journal of the American Academy of Child & Adolescent Psychiatry, 39*(1), 76–84.

Wesselhoeft, R., Heierbang, E. R., Kragh-Sorensen, P., Sorensen, M. J., & Bilenberg, N. (2016). Major depressive disorder and subthreshold depression in prepubertal children from the Danish National Birth Cohort. *Comprehensive Psychiatry, 70*, 65–76.

Wirt, R., Lachar, D., Klinedinst, J., & Seat, P. (1984). *Multidimensional description of child personality: A manual for the personality inventory for children*. Los Angeles: Western Psychological Services.

Yen, S., Stout, R., Hower, H., Killam, M. A., Weinstock, L. M., Topor, D. R., ... Keller, M. B. (2016). The influence of comorbid disorders on the episodicity of bipolar disorder in youth. *Acta Psychiatrica Scandinavica, 133*, 324–334.

Young, R. C., Biggs, J. T., Ziegler, M. G., Meyer, D. A. (1978). A rating scale for mania: Reliability, validity, and sensitivity. *The British Journal of Psychiatry, 133*, 429–435.

Youngstrom, E. A., Findling, R. L., Danielson, C. K., & Calabrese, J. R. (2001). Discriminative validity of parent report of hypomanic and depressive symptoms on the General Behavior Inventory. *Psychological Assessment, 13*(2), 267–276.

Youngstrom, E. A., Findling, R. L., Calabrese, J. R., Gracious, B. L., Demeter, C., DelPorto Bedoya, D., & Price, M. (2004). Comparing the diagnostic accuracy of six potential screening instruments for bipolar disorder in youths aged 5 to 17 years. *Journal of the American Academy of Child and Adolescent Psychiatry, 43*, 847–858.

Youngstrom, E. A., Frazier, T. W., Demeter, C., Calabrese, J. R., & Findling, R. L. (2008). Developing a 10-items Mania Scale from the parental general behavior inventory for children and adolescents. *Journal of Clinical Psychiatry, 69*, 831–839.

Zappitelli, M. C., Pereira, M. L., & Bordin, I. A. (2015). Child Behavior Checklist-Mania Scale as a screening tool to identify children at risk for bipolar disorder. *Journal of Child and Adolescent Psychopharmacology, 25*, 448–449.

Assessment of Anxiety Disorders

Paige M. Ryan, Maysa M. Kaskas, and Thompson E. Davis III

Anxiety is an emotional and behavioral response to stressors that occurs across development and cultures. The tripartite model suggests that physiological responses (e.g., quick, shallow breathing; increased heart rate), behaviors (e.g., avoidance of anxiety-provoking situations or stimuli), and negative thoughts (e.g., belief that the outcome of a feared situation will be difficult to cope with) act in conjunction to create what we recognize as the anxiety and fear response (Lang, 1979). This response is typically thought to serve an adaptive purpose, alerting people to danger and motivating action; however, some individuals experience anxiety and fear which is severe, consistent, and impairing enough to interfere with daily functioning (e.g., academic, social, occupational); these individuals are considered to have anxiety disorders (American Psychiatric Association, 2013). Anxiety disorders are fairly common across development, with a 12-month prevalence rate as high as 25% in children and adolescents and a lifetime prevalence of approximately 30% (Demertzis & Craske, 2006; Kessler, Petukhova, Sampson, Zaslavsky, & Wittchen, 2012).

Youth with anxiety disorders experience significant impairments across important areas of functioning. Overall, both children and adults diagnosed with anxiety disorders report less satisfaction with their quality of life than their non-anxious counterparts (Barrera & Norton, 2009; Ramsawh & Chavira, 2016). Academically, anxious children experience increased impairments, an effect which is related to anxiety severity and is demonstrated across race, gender, and age (Nail et al., 2015). Toddlers and children with anxiety and anxiety disorders have significantly more impairment in their intellectual and developmental functioning (Davis, May, & Whiting, 2011; Davis, Ollendick, & Nebel-Schwalm, 2008), and anxiety and sadness have even been suggested to impact the well-being of college students (Davis, Nida, Zlomke, & Nebel-Schwalm, 2009). Mental health can significantly affect physical health, and children with anxiety disorders tend to experience poorer sleep quality in addition to overall increased medical problems in adulthood (Alfano, Beidel, Turner, & Lewin, 2006; Bardone et al., 1998). Additionally, children with anxiety disorders are prone to experiencing more social problems (e.g., being disliked by peers, being teased, being left out of events or social groups) and displaying less social competence (i.e., less and poorer quality social relationships), a trend which strengthens with the severity of their anxiety (Settipani & Kendall, 2013).

Without treatment, anxiety disorders are often pervasive and may lead to additional psychopathology (Woodward & Fergusson, 2001).

P. M. Ryan · M. M. Kaskas · T. E. Davis III (✉)
Louisiana State University, Baton Rouge, LA, USA
e-mail: ted@lsu.edu

Fortunately, treatment for anxiety disorders is often effective (Davis, May, & Whiting, 2011). For example, one common, evidence-based treatment, cognitive-behavioral therapy (CBT), reduces symptoms in roughly 65% of anxious youth (Kendall, Settipani, & Cummings, 2012). Studies have also demonstrated that the aforementioned impairments in academic and social functioning decrease along with anxiety severity, after a course of cognitive-behavioral therapy (Nail et al., 2015; Reuther, Davis, Moree, & Matson, 2011; Settipani & Kendall, 2013). Therefore, it is important to properly assess for anxiety disorders in order to provide accurate diagnoses to facilitate effective and timely intervention. This chapter will summarize research and theories on assessment as well as current assessment tools for select anxiety disorders (i.e., separation anxiety disorder, social anxiety disorder, generalized anxiety disorder, panic disorder, selective mutism, and obsessive-compulsive disorder; see Table 1) in children.

Etiology and Maintenance of Anxiety and Anxiety Disorders

Anxiety disorders develop and are maintained through a complex integration of temperamental, biological, environmental, cognitive, and behavioral factors, which may change in prominence across child development and throughout the lifespan. Understanding these factors may help facilitate more accurate diagnoses as well as inform the course of treatment. One difference in temperament, behavioral inhibition, or the tendency to withdraw from or be fearful in unfamiliar situations, is considered to be an early risk factor for development of anxiety disorders in children (Biederman et al., 2001; Rosenbaum et al., 1992). Biologically, approximately 30% of the variance in anxiety can be explained by genetic factors (Schrock & Woodruff-Borden, 2010). Additionally, it is important to take the family environment into account, as children spend a great deal of time with family members and in the home. For example, children with anxious

Table 1 Characteristic symptoms of select anxiety disorders

Disorder	Description
Separation anxiety disorder	Persistent worry, disproportionate concern, and distress about separating from an attachment figure or from the home; worries may include harm befalling the parents, the child him/herself, or the home when separated or fears that the parent will never return
Social anxiety disorder	Intense distress/fear in or anxiety about social situations or performances in which the primary concern is negative evaluation from others, typically leading to the avoidance of those situations
Generalized anxiety disorder	Persistent, uncontrollable worry across multiple domains (e.g., doing things perfectly, making good impressions on others, performance, world events) occurring more days than not that is associated with the presence of at least one physical symptom (e.g., aches and pains, feelings of restlessness, trouble concentrating)
Panic disorder	Usually unexpected anxiety reaction (i.e., panic attack) leading to intense physiological symptoms (e.g., heart palpitations, sweating, shortness of breath); the person may experience significant worry and concern about these reactions and avoid situations where these reactions could occur
Selective mutism	Consistent failure to speak in certain situations where the person is required to do so due to debilitating fear; the behavior causes significant impairment in academic, occupational, and/or social settings
Obsessive-compulsive disorder	Persistent and distressing obsessions (thoughts or impulses) and/or compulsions (repetitive compensatory behaviors) that significantly impair functioning for at least an hour per day

Adapted from Kaskas, Ryan, and Davis (in press).

parent(s) may repeatedly observe anxious behaviors (e.g., a parent worrying aloud, avoiding feared, unfamiliar, or uncertain situations) and hear negative information (e.g., suggesting or stating that a situation is unsafe or likely to end poorly). In addition to these acts of modeling anxiety, anxious parents may inadvertently reinforce their children's avoidant behavior by allowing escape from or avoidance of feared, unfamiliar, or uncertain situations (e.g., a socially anxious parent may allow a behaviorally inhibited child to avoid attending a birthday party in order to minimize distress for both parent and child; Fisak & Grills-Taquechel, 2007). Cognitively, there is significant evidence demonstrating that youth with anxiety disorders experience more negative thoughts than their nonanxious peers before entering a feared, unfamiliar, or uncertain situation (Rudy, Davis, & Matthews, 2012; Rudy, Davis, & Matthews, 2014; e.g., thinking more about possible negative outcomes, underestimating their own abilities to cope with a negative outcome if one does occur; Alfano, Beidel, & Turner, 2006; Bögels & Zigterman, 2000), while engaged in a situation (e.g., more negative thoughts about the quality of their performance; Blöte, Miers, Heyne, Clark, & Westenberg, 2014), and after leaving a situation (e.g., excessive negative rumination; Hodson, McManus, Clark, & Doll, 2008). Finally, behavioral avoidance generally promotes development and maintenance of anxiety by decreasing the possibility of a positive or neutral experience, reducing the opportunities to challenge negative cognitions, and restricting the opportunities children have to practice appropriate coping skills or strategies when faced with the cause of their fear or anxiety (Rapee, 2001).

Purposes of Assessment

Many psychologists aim to ameliorate suffering and enhance quality of life through the direct treatment of psychopathology. However, before implementation of treatments is possible, one must first accrue thorough, reliable, and valid information about clients' history of impairment and details of their symptoms in order to make informed decisions about appropriate treatment options. Assessment is useful beyond diagnostic labeling; it also works in (1) screening large groups of people to find those few individuals at risk of a disorder, (2) classifying and describing symptoms and behaviors associated with disorders, (3) identifying maintaining and environmental variables which may affect the course or severity of disorders, and (4) serving to monitor treatment outcome and mechanisms of change as they occur (Silverman & Ollendick, 2005). Overall, evidence-based assessments allow treatments to target the clients' most impairing concerns (e.g., using cognitive-behavioral therapy to address underlying anxiety rather than implementing study skills strategies to improve poor grades, which may have been the client's initial reason for seeking services) and to track symptoms and interference across domains reliably over time (i.e., to monitor treatment success; Rey, Marin, & Silverman, 2013).

Obstacles to Accurate Assessment

Comorbidity

A host of challenges face psychologists in the pursuit of accurate assessment. First, anxiety disorders are highly comorbid with other disorders and with each other. In fact, comorbidity is thought to be the rule rather than the exception, particularly in clinically referred youth, where estimated comorbidity rates are as high as 91% (Angold, Costello, & Erkanli, 1999). Among anxious youth who do present with comorbidity, other anxiety disorders are the most common secondary diagnoses, followed by depressive disorders and finally by externalizing disorders like attention-deficit/hyperactivity disorder and oppositional defiant disorder (Silverman & Ollendick, 2005). Therefore, it is particularly important to be aware of the differences between clusters of internalizing symptoms and to select assessment measures that are able to discriminate among the disorders.

Confirmation Bias

Second, psychologists must be able to consider multiple sources of information and suspend their preconceived notions in order to combat costly decision errors, such as confirmation bias. Confirmation bias occurs due to the human tendency to support one's own preliminary hunches by seeking out supporting information and neglecting or discounting contradictory information. This confirmation bias effect has been found in seasoned professionals and in students and is magnified by time pressure (Mendel et al., 2011). In order to reduce the likelihood of inaccurate diagnoses, Suhr (2015) recommends the following steps before arriving at a diagnosis: (1) restate all hypotheses (e.g., for an anxiety evaluation, hypotheses may include a specific anxiety disorder, a specific depressive disorder, social skill deficits, an expressive language deficit, below-average intellectual functioning, sleep problems, or medical conditions such as hyperthyroidism), (2) consider the baseline likelihood of each hypothesis (e.g., rate of specific anxiety disorder in youth vs. rate of hyperthyroidism), (3) consider the constructs underlying each hypothesis (e.g., developmental course and impairment across settings underlying an anxiety disorder), and (4) consider the evidence for and against each hypothesis (e.g., evaluating behavioral observations, prior diagnoses, self-report questionnaires, informant-report measures, interviews). This systematic and balanced approach ensures that clinicians slow down at the end of the assessment process and consider all possibilities (as opposed to merely supporting one's own preliminary theories, giving the most familiar or common diagnosis, or ignoring possible comorbidities).

Multiple Informants

Clinicians who assess children and adolescents face particular challenges in balancing multiple informants. As children are typically unable to report their own symptoms in a detailed and accurate manner, clinicians often rely heavily on parents and teachers to fill in the gaps. This becomes particularly important for instances in which youth display concerns in certain contexts but not others (De Los Reyes & Kazdin, 2005). For example, a child may be extremely anxious about negative evaluation from peers and struggle to answer questions in class, play group games on the playground, and eat meals in the cafeteria; this child's teacher would likely report high levels of anxiety. However, that same child may not display impairment in the home environment; if the child's parents do not regularly observe their child interact with peers, they may report minimal-to-no symptoms of social anxiety. Unsurprisingly, a recent meta-analysis of 341 studies of cross-informant correspondence of mental health symptoms in youth yielded low agreement (i.e., mean internalizing symptoms, such as anxiety and depression: $r = .25$; De Los Reyes et al., 2015), indicating that clinicians rarely receive unanimous reports of a youth's symptoms and level of impairment.

Similarly, low parent-child agreement was found using a popular semi-structured interview of anxiety disorders. Grills and Ollendick (2003) examined 165 child-parent dyads (children aged 7–16 years) that were separately the Anxiety Disorder Interview Schedule: Child and Parent versions (ADIS: C/P; semi-structured interviews which will be reviewed in detail later in the chapter). Child-parent agreement was below approximately 50% for all disorders assessed in the ADIS, but it was particularly low for internalizing disorders (between 24% and 32% for anxiety disorders and about 8% for depressive disorders). Interestingly, neither child demographic variables (e.g., age, gender) nor family factors (i.e., family conflict, parental psychopathology) were systematically related to these reporting discrepancies (Grills & Ollendick, 2003).

In spite of—or perhaps due to—low cross-informant agreement, most clinicians and researchers recommend a multi-informant approach to assessment, as careful consideration of each source increases the likelihood that no child or adolescent is missed and thus denied care (Comer & Kendall, 2004; Rey et al., 2013). However, the importance of this approach may vary with the child's developmental level, cognitive functioning, insight, motivation for change, and expressive language abilities. Edelbrock, Costello, Dulcan, Kalas, & Conover (1985) suggest that parental reports of internalizing symptoms are more reliable than self-reports from young children (i.e., aged

6–9 years), with the opposite effect shown for older children (i.e., aged 10–18 years). Regardless of the child's age, psychologists are encouraged to obtain information from a variety of sources, including the child's teacher(s), if possible. Teachers are often able to observe the child's physiological and behavioral symptoms of anxiety as well as report on impairment in the school environment (e.g., academic functioning, quality and quantity of peer relationships, presence of peer victimization or rejection). Due to the importance of this report, several structured teacher interviews and questionnaires exist to facilitate assessment of symptoms and interference in the school setting; for example, the Teacher Telephone Interview: Selective Mutism and Anxiety in the School Setting (TTI-SM; Martinez et al., 2015) serves to guide psychologists in assessing anxiety disorders, including selective mutism, in children aged 6–11 years. Of course, clinicians may have difficulty coordinating schedules in order to get a teacher on the phone for an interview. An alternative to a structured telephone interview is a questionnaire, which may be sent through the mail and completed at the teacher's earliest convenience. One popular teacher questionnaire, the Achenbach System of Empirically Based Assessment (ASEBA) Teacher Report Form, has both preschool (C-TRF, intended for children aged 1.5–5 years; Achenbach & Rescorla, 2000) and school-age (TRF, intended for youth aged 6–18 years; Achenbach, 1991) forms, and both forms contain an Anxious/Depressed Syndrome scale and an Anxiety Problems DSM-Oriented scale, which may be instrumental in the assessment process.

Multiple Methods

As with the challenge of balancing information from multiple informants, clinicians are often tasked with comparing information received from multiple methods of assessment (e.g., screeners, questionnaires, rating scales, behavioral observations, diagnostic interviews, physiological measures). Multimethod assessment is particularly recommended for anxiety disorders due to Lang's (1979) tripartite model of anxiety, which states that physiological responses (e.g., fast beating heart, quick and shallow breaths), behaviors (e.g., escape, avoidance), and cognitions (e.g., negative outcome expectancies, skewed likelihood estimates) together produce the anxiety and fear response (Davis & Ollendick, 2005). Table 2 discusses interview schedules that aid in the assessment of anxiety in children.

Assessment of physiological responses In order to directly assess for physiological responses, a clinician could measure the child's heart rate while displaying a picture or video of a purportedly feared stimulus or situation (e.g., showing a child who might have social anxiety a video of children laughing and pointing off-camera). Alternatively, an ambitious clinician might ask a child to engage in an anxiety-provoking task (e.g., reading aloud, completing a difficult test) while the child's sympathetic adrenal medullary (SAM) system functions (consisting of heart rate, blood pressure, and galvanic skin response) or hypothalamic pituitary adrenal (HPA) axis activity (e.g., measuring cortisol levels in blood, urine, or saliva) are measured (Rey et al., 2013). Of course, both of these direct methods are often impractical or even inappropriate outside of a laboratory setting, as they may appear unnecessarily intrusive in addition to being costly and lengthy procedures requiring extensive staff training and investment. Alternatively, most clinicians use substitute measures of physiological anxiety, which may include subscales on questionnaires (e.g., items asking children to report if and how often they experience bodily sensations associated with anxiety) or behavioral observations (e.g., looking for flushed cheeks, listening for shallow breaths).

Assessment of behavioral responses In order to directly assess for behavioral responses to anxiety, a clinician faces several practical and logistical obstacles, such as acquisition of feared stimuli or ability to access either technology or actors to realistically portray feared situations. Clinicians may find behavioral observations helpful in lieu

Table 2 Structured and semi-structured interviews for assessment of anxiety in youth

Interview	Age range	Select anxiety disorders	Inter-rater reliability child	Inter-rater reliability parent	Relevant studies
Anxiety Disorders Interview Schedule for DSM-IV: Child and Parent (*Semi-Structured*)	6–18 years	Separation anxiety disorder Social anxiety disorder Panic disorder Generalized anxiety disorder Obsessive-compulsive disorder	.70–.81 .80–.87 .59–1.00 .72–.82	.66–.86 .63–.87 .33–.87 .78–.82 .91	Silverman and Eisen (1992) Silverman and Nelles (1988) Silverman et al. (2001) Lyneham, Abbott, and Rapee (2007) Rapee, Barrett, Dadds, and Evans (1994)
Diagnostic Interview for Children and Adolescents (*Semi-Structured*)	6–18 years	Separation anxiety disorder Specific phobia	Combined child and parent, .94 Combined child and parent, .98		Boyle et al. (1997) Kebede, Kebede, Desta, and Alem (2000)
Schedule for Affective Disorders and Schizophrenia for School-Age Children (*Semi-Structured*)	6–18 years	Generalized anxiety disorder Separation anxiety disorder Social anxiety disorder	Combined child and parent, 1.00 Combined child and parent, .64–.75 Combined child and parent, .80		Ambrosini (2000) Shahrivar, Kousha, Moallemi, Tehrani-Doost, and Alaghband-Rad (2010) Ambrosini (2000)
NIMH Diagnostic Interview Schedule for Children Version IV (*Structured*)	9–17 years	Generalized anxiety disorder Separation anxiety disorder	Combined child and parent, 1.00 Combined child and parent, 1.00		Breton, Bergeron, Valla, Berthiaume, and St. Georges (1998) Schwab-Stone et al. (1993)

Adapted from Silverman and Ollendick (2005)

of simulating feared or anxiety-provoking situations; for example, a clinician may obtain consent from the child's parents to observe the client in the classroom or on the playground in order to track target behaviors (e.g., avoiding heights, like the monkey bars, for fear of injury or embarrassment from a fall). Rey et al. (2013) note that the presence of external observers may influence the behavior of children, even in naturalistic settings like classrooms or playgrounds. Therefore, it is important to factor in the extra time it will take to allow all children (not just the client) in the setting to habituate to the presence of adult observers before taking detailed notes or drawing premature conclusions about behavior. In-clinic tasks include social evaluative tasks (e.g., asking anxious youth to perform or tell a story in front of a group), behavioral avoidance tasks (BATs, reviewed in detail later in the chapter), and parent-child interaction tasks (e.g., measuring anxiety level and assertiveness while asking children to solve problems or puzzles with a parent; Silverman & Ollendick, 2005). Questionnaires, rating scales, and semi-structured diagnostic interviews with both children and relevant adults (e.g., parents, babysitters, teachers) are often useful in obtaining different facets of detailed information about the child's typical avoidance and escape behaviors. For example, parents may indicate on a questionnaire that the child often has temper tantrums when asked to greet a stranger; a rating scale may provide data on the frequency, intensity, and duration of the temper tantrums; and a semi-structured interview may yield more information on typical antecedents and consequences to the behavior.

Assessment of cognitive responses Clinicians must rely on self- and informant-reports of youth's anxious cognitions; however, this approach is dependent on the client's level of insight into their own thoughts and honest reporting of those cognitions. Younger children (or youth of lower intellectual, verbal, and/or developmental levels) tend to have more difficulties generally expressing their thoughts in detail (e.g., may simply state, "I thought that I was scared because I felt scared" rather than "I worried that everyone would laugh at me") and specifically connecting their thoughts to feelings and experiences (e.g., may be unable to connect the thought of "I worried that everyone would laugh at me" to the feeling of embarrassment to the experience of reading aloud at school). Older children may not have the same difficulties linking their thoughts, feelings, and experiences; however, they may censor or edit their cognitions in order to downplay impairment or avoid uncomfortable or potentially embarrassing conversations (e.g., an adolescent with obsessive-compulsive disorder may avoid mentioning a sexual obsession to an adult clinician, particularly if a parent is present). Due to the inherently private nature of cognitions, parents and teachers may be unaware of thoughts that children experience and therefore may be inaccurate, biased, or otherwise unreliable reporters. Again, multimethod assessments may help improve accuracy and detail of symptom and impairment reporting. For example, what an anxious adolescent is willing to say aloud in a semi-structured interview may be very limited compared to what the same person will report on a written measure, such as a rating scale or questionnaire.

General practical obstacles Overall, certain assessment methods may be more or less appropriate and practical in specific settings (Davis, 2012). In community health clinics or in busy hospitals, clinicians may not have time to administer or access to measures that adhere to recommended protocols for empirically supported assessment (i.e., using several report methods and reporters such as both paternal and maternal report, teacher interviews/measures, semi-structured interviews, self-reports, and direct behavioral observations; Whiteside, Sattler, Hathaway, & Douglas, 2016). Furthermore, differences in the base rate of disorders across settings (e.g., general outpatient setting versus a specialty clinic) should be considered while choosing appropriate assessment methods (Johnston & Murray, 2003). Less common disorders may merit an assessment process with multiple stages, which is a more cost- and time-efficient approach. For example, clinicians may initially administer short screener questions, particularly for disorders with lower base rates (e.g., selective mutism), followed by more comprehensive diagnostic interviews of those specific disorders where symptoms were endorsed (Kendall, Cantwell, & Kazdin, 1989).

Common Tools for Broad Assessment of Anxiety and Anxiety Disorders

Semi-structured/Structured Interviews

Anxiety Disorders Interview Schedule: Child/Parent Versions (ADIS:C/P) The ADIS:C/P is a semi-structured interview that allows clinicians to assess for anxiety disorders (including separation anxiety disorder, social anxiety disorder, generalized anxiety disorder, panic disorder, and obsessive-compulsive disorder) in addition to other internalizing disorders (e.g., persistent depressive disorder) and externalizing disorders (e.g., attention-deficit/hyperactivity disorder, oppositional defiant disorder). The ADIS:C/P also contains screening questions for less common psychological conditions, including selective mutism. The ADIS:C/P is useful not only in determining presence of anxiety disorders but also in assessing symptom and disorder severity, using a scale of 0–8, with ratings of 4 ("definitely disturbing/impairing") and higher considered to meet clinical threshold. In the case of comorbidity, disorders are ranked in descending order based on severity ratings to determine the primary (and presumably, most impairing) disorder and then secondary, tertiary, and/or other comorbid disorders (Silverman & Albano, 1996). As the child and parent versions are separately administered, both informants have opportunities to report symptom presence (i.e., answering yes or no to broad screener questions), rate severity of symptoms across domains (i.e., using the 0–8 rating scale), and freely detail examples of interference or impairment (Silverman & Ollendick, 2005). Clinicians are then able to compare interviews to form diagnostic impressions or track progress in anxiety treatments. Due to the detailed, comprehensive, and user-friendly nature of the ADIS:C/P, it is the most widely used and most commonly studied assessment measure in the youth anxiety disorders research literature; however, an updated release for *DSM-5* has yet to materialize as of the time of this chapter. Even so, the ADIS:C/P is considered to have the strongest evidence supporting its ability to provide reliable and valid diagnoses and its sensitivity to change over time with the course of treatment (Silverman, Saavedra, & Pina, 2001; Silverman & Ollendick, 2005).

Diagnostic Interview for Children and Adolescents (DICA) The DICA is a semi-structured interview with a parent version, a child version (intended for youth aged 6–12 years), and an adolescent version (intended for youth aged 13–18 years). This interview assesses for 20 psychological disorders, including all of the anxiety disorders using DSM-IV criteria in addition to disorders which were described in DSM-III-R (e.g., overanxious disorder). It covers current and lifetime (i.e., disorders for which full criteria were met in the past but are currently in remission or absent) disorders (Reich, 2000; Rey et al., 2013). Reliability of anxiety disorder diagnoses using the DICA range from $\kappa = .55$ (for disorders which are no longer described in the DSM, such as overanxious disorder) to .75 (for past history of social anxiety disorder in adolescents; Silverman & Ollendick, 2005).

Schedule for Affective Disorders and Schizophrenia for School-Aged Children (K-SADS) The K-SADS is a semi-structured interview which can be used with children aged 6–18 years and their parents; it assesses for over 30 psychological disorders, including all of the anxiety disorders and both common and rare psychiatric disorders (e.g., bipolar disorder). Three versions of the K-SADS are available: a present episode (K-SADS-PE) version to assess for frequency and severity of current psychopathology, an epidemiologic version (K-SADS-E) to assess for course of psychopathology over the child's lifetime, and finally, a present and lifetime version (K-SADS-PL) to assess for both current and lifetime symptomatology. The K-SADS uses a modular interviewing technique using screening questions to reduce administration time to an average of 90 min per assessment (Leffler, Riebel, & Hughes, 2015; Rey et al., 2013). Although the K-SADS is free to download and use, it may lack sensitivity in monitoring response to treatment and symptom change over time due to the absence of a broad assessment of symptom severity (Leffler et al., 2015). The DSM-5 version of the K-SADS is currently being unveiled at the time of this chapter and awaits further study.

Diagnostic Interview Schedule for Children Version IV (DISC-IV) The DISC-IV is a structured interview with both parent and child versions; it is designed to assess for symptoms of over 30 psychological disorders, including all of the anxiety disorders, occurring in the past year (i.e., recent diagnoses) and in the past 4 weeks (i.e., current diagnoses). Optional lifetime modules may be added, if desired (Rey et al., 2013). A computerized version of this structured interview, the C-DISC, is also available, and versions exist in both English and Spanish. Developed by the National Institute of Mental Health, the DISC is considered to be highly comprehensive and reliable. However, the highly structured nature of the DISC does not allow room for follow-up assessment of possible invalid responding or atypical symptom presentations (Leffler et al., 2015).

Questionnaires: Self-Report, Informant-Report, and Clinician Report

Achenbach System The Achenbach system is a set of broadband questionnaires measuring emotional and behavioral problems in children and adolescents that includes the Child Behavior Checklist (CBCL-1.5–5, 6–18 versions), Youth Self-Report (YSR for ages 11–18), and Teacher Report Form (TRF-1.5–5, 6–18 years). The Achenbach system is widely used by both researchers and clinicians because it offers comparable multi-informant questionnaires for a wide age range of youth. van Meter et al. (2014) recently completed a study on the psychometric properties of the Achenbach system, including the sensitivity and specificity of identification of anxious symptomatology in children. Results indicated that the CBCL and YSR "internalizing problems scales" reliably discriminated between participants with an anxiety disorder and other nonanxiety diagnoses. The study also found that "internalizing problems" T-scores greater than 69 on the CBCL or greater than 63 on the YSR had a higher likelihood of the presence of an anxiety disorder (i.e., diagnostic likelihood ratio of 1.5). Lower scores resulted in a four-fold decrease of the likelihood that an anxiety disorder is present.

Revised Children's Manifest Anxiety Scale-Second Edition (RCMAS-2) The RCMAS is one of the most widely used and researched self-report measures of anxiety disorders in youth aged 6–19 years. The RCMAS is 49 items, including 40 items about anxiety and 9 items on the defensiveness scale, which measures socially desirable responding. Unlike most other youth anxiety measures, the RCMAS utilizes a dichotomous "Yes" or "No" response, rather than a Likert scale; this may facilitate responding for younger children or those with reading or cognitive deficits (Seligman, Ollendick, Langley, & Baldacci, 2004). The psychometric properties of the RCMAS include strong reliability (ranging from .75 to .86) for the subscales and .92 for the total scale (Reynolds & Richmond, 2008).

Screen for Child Anxiety Related Emotional Disorders (SCARED) The SCARED system consists of child and parent versions; this includes 41 items and assesses symptoms of anxiety in children aged 9–18 years. It includes specific subscales for generalized anxiety disorder, panic disorder, social anxiety disorder, separation anxiety disorder, somatic symptoms, and school avoidance. Respondents rate each item on a Likert scale from "Not True" to "Very True" depending on the severity of symptoms over the past 3 months. Psychometric properties of the SCARED (both parent- and child-report) suggest generally good internal consistency (ranging from .74 to .93), test-retest reliability (ranging from .70 to .90), and moderate agreement between the parent- and child-report forms ($r = .20–.40$) (Birmaher et al., 1997).

Multidimensional Anxiety Scale for Children-Second Edition (MASC-2) The MASC-2 is a 50-item self-report questionnaire for youth aged 8–19 years. The MASC-2 includes the following scales: separation anxiety/phobias, social anxiety, obsessions and compulsions, physical symptoms, harm avoidance, and generalized anxiety disorder index. The MASC-2 also includes an inconsistency index to screen for random or contradictory patterns of responses which may invalidate the report. Internal consistency for the MASC-2 ranges from .90 to .95 for each of the subscales and demonstrates good discriminant and convergent validity (March, 2013).

State-Trait Anxiety Inventory (STAI) The STAI is a 40-item questionnaire which includes a child self-report and a parent-report version. Both versions assess general proneness to anxious behavior (i.e., 20 items measuring trait anxiety or how the child generally feels) and temporary anxiety as an affective state (i.e., 20 items measuring state anxiety or how the child feels at specific moments). The STAI asks respondents to rate each item on a four-point Likert scale ranging from "almost never" to "almost always" (Balsamo et al., 2013). Internal consistency for the measure ranges from .80 to .91. The STAI has moderate correlations with other anxiety measures but interestingly has higher correlations with depression measures. The STAI's internal consistency for both mother- and father-report ranges from .84 to .91 (Silverman & Ollendick, 2005).

Pediatric Anxiety Rating Scale (PARS) The PARS is a 50-item checklist of symptoms of anxiety in children. To complete the checklist, clinicians collect information from interviews with both the child and parent, and then the clinician scores each symptom as present or absent (yes/no) during the past week. All items endorsed by the clinician are then integrated and rated by the clinician on a seven-point scale of global severity across several dimensions of anxiety (e.g., number of symptoms, frequency, severity of distress, physical symptoms, avoidance, and interference). Psychometric properties include inter-reliability of .85 (Ginsburg, Keeton, Drazdowski, & Riddle, 2011).

Child Anxiety Sensitivity Index (CASI) The CASI is an 18-item self-report questionnaire for children aged 6–17 years. The measure assesses anxiety sensitivity, or the aversion or fear of experiencing somatic symptoms of anxiety (e.g., elevated heart rate, sweating). Anxiety sensitivity is often viewed as a transdiagnostic, predisposing factor for anxiety disorders; therefore, assessment of this variable is important to determine it as a factor in the development or maintenance of a client's anxiety (Silverman, Fleisig, Rabian, & Peterson, 1991). The CASI includes four subscales: disease concerns, unsteady concerns, mental incapacitation concerns, and social concerns. Respondents rate on a Likert scale the experience of various anxiety symptoms. Psychometric properties include an internal consistency of .87 and a test-retest reliability of .76.

Children's Automatic Thoughts Scale (CATS) The CATS is a 40-item self-report measure for children aged 7–16 years that assesses cognitions about physical threat, social threat, personal failure, and hostility. The questionnaire uses a five-point Likert scale to rate the frequency that children experience the thoughts over the past week from "not at all" to "all the time" (Schniering & Rapee, 2002). The internal consistency for the total scale is a .94 and the test-retest reliability for the total scale is a .79. The measure has also been found to be sensitive to treatment change for the physical threat and failure subscales, which are often high in youth suffering from anxiety disorders or mood disorders. The measure has also demonstrated convergent validity with both anxiety and depression measures (Schniering & Lyneham, 2007).

Selected Disorder-Specific Assessments

Obsessive-Compulsive Disorder

The Children's Yale-Brown Obsessive Compulsive Scale (CY-BOCS; Goodman et al., 1989) is a ten-item, semi-structured clinician-rated scale which may be administered to either the parent or the child. The measure separately assesses presence of obsessions and/or compulsions, yielding two subtotals for severity of each symptom cluster. Severity is rated on a scale ranging from 0 (no symptoms) to 4 (extreme symptoms), with a total range of 0–40, based on (1) the frequency and duration of symptoms, (2) interference associated with the overall disorder, (3) subjective distress experienced by the child, (4) child's degree of resistance to symptoms, and (5) overall subjective feeling of control over the intrusive, unwanted thoughts and/or compulsive compensatory behaviors (Goodman et al., 1989). According to Silverman and Ollendick (2005), scores over 15 indicate a clinically significant obsessive-compulsive disorder. The CY-BOCS is considered to be a reliable disorder-specific instrument (i.e., internal consistency of .87, inter-rater reliability ranging from .66 to .91; Silverman & Ollendick, 2005).

Social Anxiety Disorder

The Liebowitz Social Anxiety Scale for Children and Adolescents (LSAS-CA; Storch et al., 2006) is a semi-structured interview which prompts children and adolescents aged 6 to 18 years to rate their feelings in 24 specific social (e.g., making eye contact with a stranger) and performance (e.g., giving a presentation in class) situations. Youth provide their own ratings of both anxiety and avoidance for each situation; however, clinicians may adjust these ratings through the assessment process based on clinical judgment (e.g., downward adjustments of ratings for a child who tends to rate all situations very highly or appears to misunderstand the scope of the scale) and/or behavioral observation (e.g., upward adjustments of ratings for a child who blushes while verbally endorsing minimal anxiety of a specific situation). The LSAS-CA is considered to have excellent test-retest reliability (i.e., ranging from .89 to .94) and has been found to distinguish between children with social anxiety disorder and children with other anxiety disorders and between children with social anxiety disorder and those without diagnoses (Storch et al., 2006).

The Social Phobia and Anxiety Inventory (SPAI; Beidel, Turner, & Morris, 1999) is one widely used questionnaire of social anxiety disorder in individuals aged 8–17 years. It involves 32 items to assess anxiety and avoidance in social situations, including thoughts and physiological responses that occur before and during various social situations. The SPAI has demonstrated efficacy in distinguishing social anxiety disorder from other anxiety disorders, including panic disorder (Turner, Stanley, Beidel, & Bond, 1989). It is considered to have good internal consistency, high test-retest reliability, and good concurrent validity with other measures of social anxiety and behavioral observations (Capozzoli, Hayes-Skelton, Aderka, & Hofmann, 2013).

Generalized Anxiety Disorder

The Intolerance of Uncertainty Scale for Children (IUSC; Comer et al., 2009) is a 27-item self-report questionnaire designed to assess the degree of a child's intolerance of uncertainty (i.e., negative emotional, cognitive, or behavioral reactions when confronted with uncertain or ambiguous events or situations). Intolerance of uncertainty is considered a central construct and cognitive vulnerability to the development and maintenance of generalized anxiety disorder. The IUSC is appropriate for children aged 7 through 17 years and uses a five-point Likert scale ranging from "not at all" to "very much" to assess agreement with statements of intolerance of uncertainty (e.g., "I can't relax if I don't know what will happen tomorrow," "It's not fair that other kids are more sure of things"). There is also a corresponding parent-report version, which contains the same constructs, reworded to provide an informant-report (e.g., parent item "Unforeseen events upset my child greatly" to correspond with child item "Surprise events upset me greatly"; Comer et al., 2009). The measure has demonstrated sensitivity and specificity in distinguishing between youth with anxiety disorders and nonanxious control groups and between children with a primary diagnosis of generalized anxiety disorder and with other principal anxiety disorder diagnoses (such as social anxiety disorder or separation anxiety disorder; Comer et al., 2009; Read, Comer, & Kendall, 2013). The IUSC is also considered to have excellent internal consistency (i.e., Cronbach's alpha ranging from .91 to .96; Read et al., 2013).

Assessment of Anxiety Through Behavioral Observation

Behavioral avoidance is one of the most impairing aspects of anxiety and anxiety disorders. Thus, the systematic measurement and assessment of behavior is essential. Historically, the behavioral avoidance task (BAT) has been used to measure avoidance of a specific situation or stimulus (Davis et al., 2013). BATs typically involve asking the child to enter a room that contains the feared stimuli (e.g., a snake) or in which the feared situation is simulated (e.g., a video of a snake playing) or to visit a particular place/environment that elicits the fear (e.g., entering an elevator). The child is asked to engage in various, graduated approach behaviors to address the anxious or fear response and to move toward a self-identified goal (e.g., take an elevator to the 30th floor of a building). The BAT can be scored in several different ways: proximity to stimulus, latency of interaction time with feared stimulus, time spent near feared stimulus, and touching/holding the feared stimulus. In addition, most assessments include a self-reported level of distress (i.e., Subjective Units of Distress Scale, or SUDS), while some measure objective physiology (e.g., heart rate, galvanic skin response). Much like the self-report measures mentioned previously, researchers and clinicians have used the BAT to monitor treatment progress and measure treatment outcome and to explore theories related to avoidance. Additionally, evidence from studies using the BAT can be used to compare the BAT's psychometric properties to that of phobia self-report questionnaires. Castagna, Davis, and Lilly (2016) recently completed a review of the BAT literature that compares the results of 31 studies spanning from 1986 to 2016. Results suggest that the BAT might be particularly sensitive to the effects of treatment, as youth with specific phobias completed an average of 30% of the BAT at pretreatment and 60% at posttreatment (indicating observable changes in level of impairment). These effects have generally been maintained at 6-month follow-ups. However, measures of physiological anxious arousal (e.g., SUDS) are more stable, even after treatment, indicating a gap between change in behavioral avoidance (which may be more emphasized during treatment) and change in physiological responses.

Challenges of the BAT include standardization and sufficient psychometric studies to provide evidence of the task's reliability and validity. Castagna, Davis, and Lilly (2016) found high test-retest reliability of the BAT for both number of steps completed and SUDS for repeated assessments which range from 1 h to 2 weeks apart. Hamilton and King (1991) report that the BAT has a large correlation with parent ratings of phobic behavior in natural settings ($r = .52, p < 0.05$), and parents questioned indicated the BAT serves as a useful and ethical form of assessment. Practical challenges include arranging a task for more abstract fears or situations (e.g., for storm phobias, it may be difficult to arrange an appointment time when a storm is imminent). Some researchers have circumvented this issue by having children watch a video of storms for 5 min (Ollendick et al., 2009). However, difficulties remain in creating both a standardized and immersive situation (e.g., selecting appropriate content/video, day/night, outside/inside, darkness/lighting). Of note, BAT experimenter instructions often vary in the degree of demand required to complete the task (e.g., "Make this talk as interesting as possible; we will be listening" places more demand on participants than "Tell us about yourself"; Silverman & Ollendick, 2005). Variations of BATs also exist: including a paper-and-pencil version (Davis et al., 2013) and a parent-child version (Ollendick, Lewis, Cowart, & Davis, 2012).

Alternative tasks to allow for behavioral observation of anxiety include social evaluative tasks and parent-youth interaction tasks. Social evaluative tasks are often performed with individuals with social anxiety, as children are informed that the task is evaluative in nature (e.g., reading aloud) and are given basic assertiveness instructions (Beidel, Turner, & Morris, 2000; Kendall, 1994). Parent-youth interaction tasks involve parents and youth dyads engage in problem-solving situations (e.g., observations of parental involvement during moderately challenging puzzle tasks; Hudson & Rapee, 2002). Table 3 shows examples of behavioral observation tasks that have been conducted with anxious youth.

Table 3 Behavioral observation tasks with youth

Study	Age range	Task
Social evaluative task		
Beidel, Turner, and Morris (2000)	8–12 years	Role-playing with a peer; read aloud for 10 min
Kendall (1994)	9–13 years	Giving a 5-min talk, "Tell us about yourself"
Behavioral avoidance task		
Öst, Svensson, Hellstrom, and Lindwall (2001)		Approaching a leashed dog and touch for 30 s; watching videos of storms
Parent-child interaction task		
Hudson and Rapee (2002)	7–16 years	Working on a challenging puzzle with parent for 5 min
Woodruff-Borden, Morrow, Bourland, and Cambron (2002)	6–12 years	Working on unsolvable anagrams for 10 min with parent; talking with parent about themselves for 10 min
Barrett, Dadds, and Rapee (1996)	7–16 years	Working on generating solutions to problems with a parent

Adapted from Silverman & Ollendick (2005).

Future Directions

The assessment of anxiety continues to be an important yet challenging endeavor. One of these challenges involves the inherently internal nature of anxiety, making it difficult to objectively measure its occurrence, extent, and severity. Due to this, researchers and clinicians alike rely primarily on self-report measures (as reviewed here); however, children often have difficulties accurately reporting their own thoughts and linking their cognitions, behaviors, and physiological sensations to specific events, situations, and/or stimuli. Thus, adult informants such as parents and teachers are often involved in the assessment process. Although inter-rater reliability has been mixed, showcasing the difficult and inexact nature of anxiety assessment in youth, each reporter often has valuable insights into the child's behavior across settings, so this information should continue to be collected.

As the field of child psychopathology continues to progress, it is important to adjust assessment practices, both in clinical and research settings, in order to keep up with advances. For example, the DSM-5 has shifted emphasis from a categorical (i.e., the disorder is either present or absent) to a dimensional (i.e., symptoms exist along a spectrum) approach. With this shift comes an increased focus on transdiagnostic assessments and treatments, particularly for internalizing disorders, which share core characteristics (e.g., negative affect, rumination). Given this and the high rate of comorbidities in anxious youth, clinicians and researchers should carefully assess the transdiagnostic domains (e.g., anxiety sensitivity, intolerance of uncertainty) which are occurring across settings, causing the most impairment, or maintaining the underlying processes.

References

Achenbach, T. M. (1991). *Manual for the Teachers Report Form and 1991 profile*. Burlington, VT: University of Vermont, Department of Psychiatry.

Achenbach, T. M., & Rescorla, L. A. (2000). *ASEBA preschool forms & profiles*. Burlington, VT: University of Vermont, Research Center for Children, Youth and Families.

Alfano, C. A., Beidel, D. C., & Turner, S. M. (2006). Cognitive correlates of social phobia among children and adolescents. *Journal of Abnormal Child Psychology, 34*(2), 182–194. https://doi.org/10.1007/s10802-005-9012-9

Alfano, C. A., Beidel, D. C., Turner, S. M., & Lewin, D. S. (2006). Preliminary evidence for sleep complaints among children referred for anxiety. *Sleep Medicine, 7*(6), 467–473.

Ambrosini, P. J. (2000). Historical development and present status of the Schedule for Affective Disorders and Schizophrenia for School-Age Children (K-SADS). *Journal of the American Academy of Child and Adolescent Psychiatry, 39*(1), 49–58. https://doi.org/10.1097/00004583-200001000-00016

American Psychiatric Association. (2013). *Diagnostic and statistical manual of mental disorders* (5th ed.). Arlington, VA: American Psychiatric Publishing.

Angold, A., Costello, E. J., & Erkanli, A. (1999). Comorbidity. *Journal of Child Psychology and Psychiatry, 40*(1), 57–87.

Balsamo, M., Romanelli, R., Innamorati, M., Ciccarese, G., Carlucci, L., & Saggino, A. (2013). The state-trait anxiety inventory: Shadows and lights on its construct validity. *Journal of Psychopathology and Behavioral Assessment, 35*(4), 475–486. https://doi.org/10.1007/s10862-013-9354-5

Bardone, A. M., Moffitt, T. E., Caspi, A., Dickson, N., Stanton, W. R., & Silva, P. A. (1998). Adult physical health outcomes of adolescent girls with conduct disorder, depression, and anxiety. *Journal of the American Academy of Child & Adolescent Psychiatry, 37*(6), 594–601.

Barrera, T. L., & Norton, P. J. (2009). Quality of life impairment in generalized anxiety disorder, social phobia, and panic disorder. *Journal of Anxiety Disorders, 23*(8), 1086–1090.

Barrett, P. M., Dadds, M. R., & Rapee, R. M. (1996). Family treatment of childhood anxiety: A controlled trial. *Journal of Consulting and Clinical Psychology, 64*(2), 333–342.

Beidel, D. C., Turner, S. M., & Morris, T. L. (2000). Behavioral treatment of childhood social phobia. *Journal of Consulting and Clinical Psychology, 68*(6), 1072–1080.

Beidel, D. C., Turner, S. M., & Morris, T. L. (1999). Psychopathology of childhood social phobia. *Journal of the American Academy of Child & Adolescent Psychiatry, 38*(6), 643–650.

Biederman, J., Hirshfeld-Becker, D. R., Rosenbaum, J. F., Hérot, C., Friedman, D., Snidman, N., ... Faraone, S. V. (2001). Further evidence of association between behavioral inhibition and social anxiety in children. *American Journal of Psychiatry, 158*(10), 1673–1679.

Birmaher, B., Khetarpal, S., Brent, D., Cully, M., Balach, L., Kaufman, J., & Neer, S. M. (1997). The Screen for Child Anxiety Related Emotional Disorders (SCARED): Scale construction and psychometric characteristics. *Journal of the American Academy of Child & Adolescent Psychiatry, 36*(4), 545–553.

Blöte, A. W., Miers, A. C., Heyne, D. A., Clark, D. M., & Westenberg, P. M. (2014). The relation between social anxiety and audience perception: Examining Clark and Wells' (1995) model among adolescents. *Behavioral and Cognitive Psychotherapy, 42*(05), 555–567.

Bögels, S. M., & Zigterman, D. (2000). Dysfunctional cognitions in children with social phobia, separation anxiety disorder, and generalized anxiety disorder. *Journal of Abnormal Child Psychology, 28*(2), 205–211.

Boyle, M. H., Offord, D. R., Racine, Y. A., Szatmari, P., Sanford, M., & Fleming, J. E. (1997). Adequacy of interviews vs checklists for classifying childhood psychiatric disorder based on parent reports. *Archives of General Psychiatry, 54*(9), 793–799.

Breton, J., Bergeron, L., Valla, J., Berthiaume, C., & St-Georges, M. (1998). Diagnostic Interview Schedule for Children (DISC-2.25) in Quebec: Reliability findings in light of the MECA study. *Journal of the American Academy of Child and Adolescent Psychiatry, 37*(11), 1167–1174.

Capozzoli, M. C., Hayes-Skelton, S. A., Aderka, I. M., & Hofmann, S. G. (2013). Assessment of social and generalized anxiety disorder. In Handbook of assessing variants and complications in anxiety disorders (pp. 3–14). New York, NY: Springer.

Castagna, P. J., Davis, T. E., & Lilly, M. (2016). Behavioral avoidance tasks with anxious youth: A review of procedures, properties, and criticisms. *Clinical Child and Family Psychology Review*. https://doi.org/10.1007/s10567-016-0220-3

Comer, J. S., & Kendall, P. C. (2004). A symptom-level examination of parent–child agreement in the diagnosis of anxious youths. *Journal of the American Academy of Child & Adolescent Psychiatry, 43*(7), 878–886.

Comer, J. S., Roy, A. K., Furr, J. M., Gotimer, K., Beidas, R. S., Dugas, M. J., & Kendall, P. C. (2009). The intolerance of uncertainty scale for children: A psychometric evaluation. *Psychological Assessment, 21*, 402–411. https://doi.org/10.1037/a0016719

Davis, T. E., III. (2012). Where to from here for ASD and anxiety? Lessons learned from child anxiety and the issue of DSM-5. *Clinical Psychology: Science and Practice, 19*, 358–363.

Davis, T. E., III, Reuther, E., May, A., Rudy, B., Munson, M., Jenkins, W., & Whiting, S. (2013). The Behavioral Avoidance Task using Imaginal Exposure (BATIE): A paper-and-pencil version of traditional in vivo behavioral avoidance tasks. *Psychological Assessment, 25*, 1111–1119.

Davis, T. E., May, A., & Whiting, S. E. (2011). Evidence-based treatment of anxiety and phobia in children and adolescents: Current status and effects on the emotional response. *Clinical Psychology Review, 31*(4), 592–602.

Davis, T. E., Moree, B. N., Dempsey, T., Reuther, E. T., Fodstad, J. C., Hess, J. A., ... Matson, J. L. (2011). The relationship between autism spectrum disorders and anxiety: The moderating effect of communication. *Research in Autism Spectrum Disorders, 5*(1), 324–329.

Davis, T. E., Nida, R. E., Zlomke, K. R., & Nebel-Schwalm, M. S. (2009). Health-related quality of life in college undergraduates with learning disabilities: The mediational roles of anxiety and sadness. *Journal of Psychopathology and Behavioral Assessment, 31*(3), 228.

Davis, T. E., Ollendick, T. H., & Nebel-Schwalm, M. (2008). Intellectual ability and achievement in anxiety-disordered children: A clarification and extension of the literature. *Journal of Psychopathology and Behavioral Assessment, 30*(1), 43–51.

Davis, T. E., & Ollendick, T. H. (2005). Empirically supported treatments for specific phobia in children: Do efficacious treatments address the components of a phobic response?. *Clinical Psychology: Science and Practice, 12*(2), 144–160.

De Los Reyes, A., Augenstein, T. M., Wang, M., Thomas, S. A., Drabick, D. G., Burgers, D. E., & Rabinowitz, J. (2015). The validity of the multi-informant approach to assessing child and adolescent mental health. *Psychological Bulletin, 141*(4), 858–900. https://doi.org/10.1037/a0038498

De Los Reyes, A., & Kazdin, A. E. (2005). Informant discrepancies in the assessment of childhood psychopathology: A critical review, theoretical framework, and recommendations for further study. *Psychological Bulletin, 131*(4), 483–509.

Demertzis, K. H., & Craske, M. G. (2006). Anxiety in primary care. *Current Psychiatry Reports, 8*(4), 291–297.

Edelbrock, C., Costello, A. J., Dulcan, M. K., Kalas, R., & Conover, N. C. (1985). Age differences in the reliability of the psychiatric interview of the child. *Child Development*, 265–275.

Fisak, B., Jr., & Grills-Taquechel, A. E. (2007). Parental modeling, reinforcement, and information transfer: Risk factors in the development of child anxiety? *Clinical Child and Family Psychology Review, 10*(3), 213–231.

Ginsburg, G. S., Keeton, C. P., Drazdowski, T. K., & Riddle, M. A. (2011). The utility of clinicians ratings of anxiety using the Pediatric Anxiety Rating Scale (PARS). *Child & Youth Care Forum, 40*(2), 93–105. https://doi.org/10.1007/s10566-010-9125-3

Goodman, W. K., Price, L. H., Rasmussen, S. A., Mazure, C., Fleischmann, R. L., Hill, C. L., ... Charney, D. S. (1989). The Yale–Brown Obsessive–Compulsive Scale: Development, use, and reliability. *Archives of General Psychiatry, 46*, 1006–1011.

Grills, A. E., & Ollendick, T. H. (2003). Multiple informant agreement and the anxiety disorders interview schedule for parents and children. *Journal of the American Academy of Child & Adolescent Psychiatry, 42*(1), 30–40.

Hamilton, D. I., & King, N. J. (1991). Reliability of a behavioral avoidance test for the assessment of dog phobic children. *Psychological Reports, 69*(1), 18. https://doi.org/10.2466/pr0.1991.69.1.18

Hodson, K. J., McManus, F. V., Clark, D. M., & Doll, H. (2008). Can Clark and Wells' (1995) cognitive model of social phobia be applied to young people? *Behavioral and Cognitive Psychotherapy, 36*(4), 449–461.

Hudson, J. L., & Rapee, R. M. (2002). Parent-child interactions in clinically anxious children and their siblings. *Journal of Clinical Child and Adolescent Psychology, 31*(4), 548–555.

Johnston, C., & Murray, C. (2003). Incremental validity in the psychological assessment of children and adolescents. *Psychological Assessment, 15*(4), 496–507.

Kaskas, M., Ryan, P., & Davis, T. E., III. (in press). Treatment of anxiety disorders. In J. L. Matson (Ed.), *Handbook of childhood psychopathology and developmental disabilities: Treatment*. Switzerland: Springer International Publishing Group.

Kebede, M., Kebede, D., Desta, M., & Alem, A. (2000). Evaluation of the Amharic version of the Diagnostic Interview of Children and Adolescents (DICA-R) in Addis Ababa. *Ethiopian Journal of Health Development, 14*(1), 13–22.

Kendall, P. C. (1994). Treating anxiety disorders in youth: Results of a randomized clinical trial. *Journal of Consulting and Clinical Psychology, 62*, 100–110.

Kendall, P. C., Cantwell, D. P., & Kazdin, A. E. (1989). Depression in children and adolescents: Assessment issues and recommendations. *Cognitive Therapy and Research, 13*(2), 109–146.

Kendall, P. C., Settipani, C. A., & Cummings, C. M. (2012). No need to worry: The promising future of child anxiety research. *Journal of Clinical Child & Adolescent Psychology, 41*(1), 103–115.

Kessler, R. C., Petukhova, M., Sampson, N. A., Zaslavsky, A. M., & Wittchen, H. U. (2012). Twelve-month and lifetime prevalence and lifetime morbid risk of anxiety and mood disorders in the United States. *International Journal of Methods in Psychiatric Research, 21*(3), 169–184.

Lang, P. J. (1979). A bio-informational theory of emotional imagery. *Psychophysiology, 16*, 495–512.

Leffler, J. M., Riebel, J., & Hughes, H. M. (2015). A review of child and adolescent diagnostic interviews for clinical practitioners. *Assessment, 22*(6), 690–703. https://doi.org/10.1177/1073191114561253

Lyneham, H. J., Abbott, M. J., & Rapee, R. M. (2007). Interrater reliability of the anxiety disorders interview schedule for DSM-IV: Child and parent version. *Journal of the American Academy of Child and Adolescent Psychiatry, 46*(6), 731–736.

March, J. S. (2013). *Multidimensional anxiety scale for children* (2nd ed.). Toronto, Ontario, Canada: Multi-Health Systems.

Martinez, Y. J., Tannock, R., Manassis, K., Garland, E. J., Clark, S., & McInnes, A. (2015). The teachers' role in the assessment of selective mutism and anxiety disorders. *Canadian Journal of School Psychology, 30*(2), 83–101.

Mendel, R., Traut-Mattausch, E., Jonas, E., Leucht, S., Kane, J. M., Maino, K., ... Hamann, J. (2011). Confirmation bias: Why psychiatrists stick to wrong preliminary diagnoses. *Psychological Medicine, 41*, 2651–2659. https://doi.org/10.1017/S0033291711000808

Nail, J. E., Christofferson, J., Ginsburg, G. S., Drake, K., Kendall, P. C., McCracken, J. T., ... Sakolsky, D. (2015). Academic impairment and impact of treatments among youth with anxiety disorders. *Child & Youth Care Forum, 44*(3), 327–342. https://doi.org/10.1007/s10566-014-9290-x

Ollendick, T. H., Lewis, K., Cowart, M., & Davis, T. E., III. (2012). Prediction of child performance on a parent-child behavioral approach test with animal phobic children. *Behavior Modification, 36*, 509–524.

Ollendick, T. H., Öst, L. G., Reuterskiöld, L., Costa, N., Cederlund, R., Sirbu, C., ... & Jarrett, M. A. (2009). One-session treatment of specific phobias in youth:

a randomized clinical trial in the United States and Sweden. *Journal of consulting and clinical psychology, 77*(3), 504.

Öst, L. G., Svensson, L., Hellstrom, K., & Lindwall, R. (2001). One-session treatment of specific phobias in youths: A randomized clinical trial. *Journal of Consulting and Clinical Psychology, 69*, 814–824.

Ramsawh, H. J., & Chavira, D. A. (2016). Association of childhood anxiety disorders and quality of life in a primary care sample. *Journal of Developmental and Behavioral Pediatrics, 37*(4), 269–276. https://doi.org/10.1097/DBP.0000000000000296

Rapee, R. M. (2001). The development of generalized anxiety. In M. W. Vasey & M. R. Dadds (Eds.), *The developmental psychopathology of anxiety* (pp. 481–503). New York: Oxford University Press.

Rapee, R. M., Barrett, P. M., Dadds, M. R., & Evans, L. (1994). Reliability of the DSM–III–R childhood anxiety disorders using structured interview: Interrater and parent–child agreement. *Journal of the American Academy of Child and Adolescent Psychiatry, 33*(7), 984–992.

Read, K. L., Comer, J. S., & Kendall, P. C. (2013). The Intolerance of Uncertainty Scale for Children (IUSC): Discriminating principal anxiety diagnoses and severity. *Psychological Assessment, 25*(3), 722–729. https://doi.org/10.1037/a0032392

Reich, W. (2000). Diagnostic Interview for Children and Adolescents (DICA). *Journal of the American Academy of Child & Adolescent Psychiatry, 39*(1), 59–66. https://doi.org/10.1097/00004583-200001000-00017

Reuther, E. T., Davis III, T. E., Moree, B. N., & Matson, J. L. (2011). Treating selective mutism using modular CBT for child anxiety: A case study. *Journal of Clinical Child & Adolescent Psychology, 40*(1), 156–163.

Rey, Y., Marin, C. E., & Silverman, W. K. (2013). Assessment of anxiety disorders: Categorical and dimensional perspectives. In R. A. Vasa & A. K. Roy (Eds.), *Pediatric anxiety disorders* (pp. 231–267). New York: Springer.

Reynolds, C. R., & Richmond, B. O. (2008). *Revised Children's Manifest Anxiety Scale, Second Edition (RCMAS-2)*. Los Angeles: Western Psychological Services.

Rosenbaum, J. F., Biederman, J., Bolduc, E. A., Hirshfeld, D. R., Faraone, S. V., & Kagan, J. (1992). Comorbidity of parental anxiety disorders as risk for childhood-onset anxiety in inhibited children. *American Journal of Psychiatry, 149*(4), 475–481.

Rudy, B. M., Davis, T. E., & Matthews, R. A. (2012). The relationship among self-efficacy, negative self-referent cognitions, and social anxiety in children: A multiple mediator model. *Behavior Therapy, 43*(3), 619–628.

Rudy, B. M., Davis, T. E., & Matthews, R. A. (2014). Cognitive indicators of social anxiety in youth: A structural equation analysis. *Behavior Therapy, 45*(1), 116–125.

Schniering, C. A., & Lyneham, H. J. (2007). The Children's Automatic Thoughts Scale in a clinical sample: Psychometric properties and clinical utility. *Behaviour Research and Therapy, 45*(8), 1931–1940.

Schniering, C. A., & Rapee, R. M. (2002). Development and validation of a measure of children's automatic thoughts: The children's automatic thoughts scale. *Behaviour Research and Therapy, 40*(9), 1091–1109.

Schrock, M., & Woodruff-Borden, J. (2010). Parent-child interactions in anxious families. *Child and Family Behavior Therapy, 32*(4), 291–310 doi.org/10.1080/07317107.2010.515523

Schwab-Stone, M., Fisher, P., Piacentini, J., Shaffer, D., Davies, M., & Briggs, M. (1993). The Diagnostic Interview Schedule for Children-Revised Version (DISC-R): II. Test-retest reliability. *Journal of the American Academy of Child and Adolescent Psychiatry, 32*(3), 651–657.

Seligman, L. D., Ollendick, T. H., Langley, A. K., & Baldacci, H. B. (2004). The utility of measures of child and adolescent anxiety: a meta-analytic review of the Revised Children's Manifest Anxiety Scale, the State–Trait Anxiety Inventory for Children, and the Child Behavior Checklist. *Journal of Clinical Child and Adolescent Psychology, 33*(3), 557–565.

Settipani, C., & Kendall, P. (2013). Social functioning in youth with anxiety disorders: Association with anxiety severity and outcomes from cognitive-behavioral therapy. *Child Psychiatry and Human Development, 44*(1), 1–18. https://doi.org/10.1007/s10578-012-0307-0

Shahrivar, Z., Kousha, M., Moallemi, S., Tehrani-Doost, M., & Alaghband-Rad, J. (2010). The reliability and validity of Kiddie-Schedule for Affective Disorders and Schizophrenia-Present and Lifetime version-Persian version. *Child and Adolescent Mental Health, 15*(2), 97–102. https://doi.org/10.1111/j.1475-3588.2008.00518.x

Silverman, W. K., & Albano, A. M. (1996). *Anxiety Disorders Interview Schedule for Children for DSM–IV:(Child and parent versions)*. San Antonio, TX: Psychological Corporation.

Silverman, W. K., & Eisen, A. R. (1992). Age differences in the reliability of parent and child reports of child anxious symptomatology using a structured interview. *Journal of the American Academy of Child and Adolescent Psychiatry, 31*(1), 117–124.

Silverman, W. K., Fleisig, W., Rabian, B., & Peterson, R. A. (1991). Childhood anxiety sensitivity index. *Journal of Clinical Child & Adolescent Psychology, 20*(2), 162–168.

Silverman, W. K., & Nelles, W. B. (1988). The anxiety disorders interview schedule for children. *Journal of the American Academy of Child & Adolescent Psychiatry, 27*, 772–778.

Silverman, W. K., & Ollendick, T. H. (2005). Evidence-based assessment of anxiety and its disorders in children and adolescents. *Journal of Clinical Child and Adolescent Psychology, 34*(3), 380–411. https://doi.org/10.1207/s15374424jccp3403_2

Silverman, W. K., Saavedra, L. M., & Pina, A. A. (2001). Test-retest reliability of the anxiety symptoms and diagnoses with the Anxiety Disorders Interview Schedule for DSM-IV: Child and parent versions. *Journal of the American Academy of Child and Adolescent Psychiatry, 40*(8), 937–944.

Storch, E. A., Masia-Warner, C., Heidgerken, A. D., Fisher, P. H., Pincus, D. B., & Liebowitz, M. R. (2006). Factor structure of the Liebowitz Social Anxiety Scale for children and adolescents. *Child Psychiatry and Human Development, 37*(1), 25–37.

Suhr, J. (2015). Putting the data together: Empirically guided integration of assessment information. In *Psychological assessment: A problem solving approach* (pp. 221–238). New York: The Guilford Press.

Turner, S. M., Stanley, M. A., Beidel, D. C., & Bond, L. (1989). The social phobia and anxiety inventory: construct validity. *Journal of Psychopathology and Behavioral Assessment, 11*(3), 221–234.

van Meter, A., Youngstrom, E., Youngstrom, J. K., Ollendick, T., Demeter, C., & Findling, R. L. (2014). Clinical decision making about child and adolescent anxiety disorders using the Achenbach system of empirically based assessment. *Journal of Clinical Child and Adolescent Psychology, 43*(4), 552–565. https://doi.org/10.1080/15374416.2014.883930

Whiteside, S. H., Sattler, A. F., Hathaway, J., & Douglas, K. V. (2016). Use of evidence-based assessment for childhood anxiety disorders in community practice. *Journal of Anxiety Disorders, 39*, 65–70. https://doi.org/10.1016/j.janxdis.2016.02.008

Woodruff-Borden, J., Morrow, C., Bourland, S., & Cambron, S. (2002). The behavior of anxious parents: Examining mechanisms of transmission of anxiety from parent to child. *Journal of Clinical Child and Adolescent Psychology, 31*(3), 364–374.

Woodward, L. J., & Fergusson, D. M. (2001). Life course outcomes of young people with anxiety disorders in adolescence. *Journal of the American Academy of Child & Adolescent Psychiatry, 40*(9), 1086–1093.

Posttraumatic Stress Disorder

Jennifer Piscitello, Adrienne Anderson,
Sabrina Gretkierewicz, and Mary Lou Kelley

Introduction

Epidemiological studies estimate that 60% of adolescents have experienced at least one traumatic event during their childhood, with a majority reporting multiple events (McLaughlin et al., 2012). This figure is even higher in impoverished, minority children who are at greater risk for the development of negative outcomes due to inadequate financial, social, and community support (Atwoli, Stein, Koenen, & McLaughlin, 2015; Goldstein et al., 2016; Le, Holton, Romero, & Fisher, 2016). As exposure to natural disasters, war, and terrorism are increasingly prevalent, the need for accurate assessment and identification of posttraumatic reactions in youth is imperative. Although the majority of youth demonstrate resilience following exposure to a traumatic event, a significant minority develops persistent mental health problems, including posttraumatic stress disorder (PTSD).

Relative to adults, children and adolescents are particularly vulnerable because of the negative impact trauma has on their biological, psychological, and social development (Davis & Siegel, 2000; National Commission on Children and Disasters, 2010). Given children and adolescents' cognitive developmental level and nascent coping skills, they are at increased risk of developing severe psychopathology following adverse events. A recent meta-analysis conducted by Alisic et al. (2014) indicated that one in six youth exposed to a traumatic event met criteria for PTSD. This demonstrates an incontestable need for the establishment of developmentally appropriate assessment tools.

Traumatic events experienced by children and adolescents include exposure to natural and man-made disasters (including displacement); child maltreatment; family, school, and community violence; loss of a loved one; medical trauma; and war and terrorism (Fairbank, Putnam, & Harris, 2014). Children and adolescents display a range of psychological problems in response to traumatic events including anxiety, depression, and externalizing behavior problems, with posttraumatic stress (PTS) symptoms being the most common (Kelley et al., 2010; Self-Brown, Lai, Thompson, McGill, & Kelley, 2013). Youth with PTSD experience impairment across psychosocial, biological, behavioral, and cognitive functioning that can endure well into adulthood (Briggs, Nooner, & Amaya-Jackson, 2014). For example, youth exposed to trauma may experience learning and development delays, which may in turn impair academic performance and

J. Piscitello (✉) · A. Anderson · S. Gretkierewicz
M. L. Kelley
Louisiana State University, Baton Rouge, LA, USA
e-mail: jpisci2@lsu.edu

ultimately reduce lifelong productivity (Cook et al., 2017). Other negative consequences include risky health behavior (e.g., substance use), physical health conditions (e.g., heart disease), structural and functional impairments in brain functioning, and difficulty regulating emotions and behavior (Briere, Kaltman, & Green, 2008; Cook et al., 2017; Felitti et al., 1998).

There has been a proliferation of research on children's responses to traumatic events during the past two decades. This has stimulated the development of psychometrically sound assessment and diagnostic measures designed to assess PTS symptoms in youth (Leigh, Yule, & Smith, 2016). The development of reliable and valid assessment tools for accurately assessing youth at risk for experiencing PTS symptoms is essential to offering services to identified individuals. This is especially important after a large-scale event, such as a natural or man-made disaster (c.f., Lai, Alisic, Lewis, & Ronan, 2016) or exposure to ongoing war and terrorism. Thus, it is important to have empirically sound assessment methods for identifying youth who may meet clinical threshold, as well as instruments for treatment planning and measuring treatment outcomes in clinical samples (Leigh et al., 2016). Other factors to consider are the context and goals of assessment. For example, it is important to consider whether the assessment is for clinical or research purposes or whether continuous or categorical outcomes are desired. Further, it is important to select measures with strong psychometric support normed on diverse samples.

The purpose of this chapter is to provide a contextual history of the assessment and diagnosis of PTSD in youth as well as to provide a review of current diagnostic criteria. Additionally, the chapter discusses important individual, family, and community considerations for the case conceptualization, assessment, and treatment of PTSD. Finally, we review psychometrically supported tools for screening, diagnosis, and treatment of PTS symptoms in youth.

DSM-5 Criteria

Unlike previous iterations, the Fifth Edition of the *Diagnostic and Statistical Manual of Mental Disorders* (DSM-5; American Psychiatric Association, 2013) incorporates research findings that indicate children under the age of 6 often have a different presentation of PTS symptoms than older children. As such there are separate criteria for children under and above the age of 6. Each is reviewed below.

Criteria for Adolescents and Children over 6 Years Old The hallmark feature of the nosology of PTSD is that symptoms are present following exposure to a traumatic event (American Psychiatric Association, 2013). According to the DSM-5 (2013), a potentially traumatic event consists of exposure to actual or threatened death and can be experienced in a number of ways (i.e., direct exposure, witnessing or learning about a traumatic event as it is happened to a close family member or loved one). The DSM-5 includes four symptom clusters: (1) intrusive symptoms/reexperiencing, (2) avoidance, (3) changes in mood and cognition, and (4) changes in arousal and reactivity. Symptoms must be experienced for at least 1 month following the event, and disturbance must cause clinically significant distress or impairment in important areas of functioning (e.g., academic performance).

Traumatic events can be reexperienced in a number of ways (i.e., emotionally, sensory, physiologically, or behaviorally). Symptoms related to reexperiencing trauma may manifest as recurrent, intrusive memories, dreams, dissociative reactions (e.g., flashbacks), prolonged psychological distress, and physiological reactions (American Psychiatric Association, 2013). Dissociative reactions may exist on a continuum where some children may experience a complete loss of awareness of their present surroundings, while others may be able to maintain a reality orientation (Cintron, Salloum, Blair-Andrews, & Storch, 2017). In children, it may not be possible to ascertain that the frightening content in children's dreams is directly related to the traumatic event (American Psychiatric Association, 2013). Depending on the child's developmental level, he or she may not be able to describe the intrusive symptoms with the same detail and insight as an adolescent or adult.

Avoidance of distressing reminders of the traumatic event must also be present. For example, a child exposed to a traumatic hurricane may become distressed on windy or rainy days. Children tend to have difficulty reporting avoidant symptoms compared to adults but often are observed by their caretakers (Dyregrov & Yule, 2006). This may be due to children lacking the ability to describe complex cognitive symptoms (Dyregrov & Yule, 2006), making it more difficult for children to meet the avoidant criteria compared to adults. Similarly, due to cognitive immaturity, young children may be unable to accurately report changes in cognitions or mood.

Changes in arousal and reactivity may manifest as increased irritability, recklessness, hypervigilance, startle responses, difficulty concentrating, or sleep disturbance (American Psychiatric Association, 2013). Although there is substantial research associating psychophysiological reactions of PTS symptoms in adults, much less research has focused on youth (for a review see Kirsch, Wilhelm, & Goldbeck, 2011). However, increased cortisol excretion and heart rate, as well as decreased immune functioning, emerge as significant short- and long-term symptoms associated with PTS symptoms in children and adolescents (Kirsch et al., 2011).

Criteria for Children 6 Years Old and Younger Research consistently has found that the same four-factor model of PTSD outlined above is inappropriate for preschool-aged children (American Psychiatric Association, 2013; Dyregrov & Yule, 2006; La Greca, Danzi, & Chan, 2017; Scheeringa, 2008; Scheeringa, Zeanah, & Cohen, 2011). Traumatic events experienced by young children are similar to those experienced by adolescents and school-aged children and commonly include child maltreatment, car accidents, war, dog bites, invasive medical procedures, as well as home, school, and community violence (Hagan, Sulik, & Lieberman, 2016). Symptom clusters for the preschool subtype include (1) intrusive symptoms/reexperiencing, (2) avoidance *or* changes in mood and cognition, and (3) changes in arousal and reactivity. Additionally, fewer symptoms are required to make the diagnosis. Because young children are underdeveloped cognitively, reliance on report of symptoms falls primarily on parent report. This can lead to underreporting of symptoms depending on whether the parent was involved in the traumatic event as well or if they are the perpetrator.

Specifiers DSM-5 requires specifiers be indicated for two different subtypes of PTSD: with dissociative symptoms or with delayed expression. These specifiers are used regardless of age of the child. If an individual experiences symptoms of depersonalization (i.e., feelings of detachment or unreality) and derealization (i.e., feelings of unreality of surroundings), they would meet for the "with dissociative symptoms" specifier (American Psychiatric Association, 2013). Delayed onset is defined as an individual experiencing symptoms 6 months or more following the traumatic event (American Psychiatric Association, 2013). Due to the heterogeneity of youth's responses to traumatic events, clinicians must be aware of the possibility of delayed onset. For certain types of trauma, onset of PTSD symptoms may begin months or years following exposure to the traumatic event (Yule, Udwin, & Bolton, 2002). Research on delayed onset in adults suggests a more chronic trajectory, but more research is required in this area in regard to children (Boscarino & Adams, 2009; Fikretoglu & Liu, 2011).

Important Changes in Diagnostic Criteria

PTSD was first introduced into the American Psychiatric Association's *Diagnostic and Statistical Manual of Mental Disorders*, Third Edition (DSM-III), in 1980. In the DSM-III, PTSD was operationalized as a catastrophic event "beyond the range of normal human experience" (American Psychiatric Association, 1980; pp. 236). This definition was controversial due to its lack of specificity, resulting in the revision of this definition in the DSM-IV/TR (American Psychiatric Association, 2000) and further refinement in the DSM-5, limiting traumatic events to include only those that are actually life threatening (Scheeringa, 2015).

Initially, it was believed that children could not experience PTSD and therefore the criteria in the DSM-III were not applied to children and adolescents. From the DSM-III to the current iteration, the DSM-5, there have been substantial changes based on decades of empirical research and intense debate among experts to include criteria and considerations specific to children (for a review see Pai, Surris, & North, 2017). Although the DSM-IV/TR provided specific developmental considerations for children and adolescents, distinct diagnostic criteria for older and younger children were not presented. There has been two decades of substantial research on supporting the distinction (Scheeringa, 2008; Scheeringa et al., 2011). The modifications in the DSM-5 for children under the age of 6 included reducing the number of symptom clusters and number of symptoms necessary to meet diagnostic criteria. This change is based on research indicating that preschool-aged children experience similar rates of PTEs as school-aged children but were meeting DSM-IV criteria for PTSD at substantially lower rates (Scheeringa et al., 2011). Most likely this is due the inability of young children to articulate their experiences and symptoms (Scheeringa et al., 2011).

Other changes seen in the DSM-5 diagnostic criteria of PTSD included removing PTSD from the anxiety disorders to the "trauma and stressor-related disorders" domain, which covers all disorders that require "exposure to a traumatic or stressful event" (American Psychiatric Association, 2013; pp. 265). This modification in the DSM-5 was a result of research indicating that individuals who are diagnosed with PTSD not only experience anxiety symptoms (e.g., insomnia, irritability, poor concentration, behavioral and cognitive avoidance) but also experience significant depressive, dissociative, hypervigilant symptoms (Friedman et al., 2014).

Furthermore, the criterion that traumatic event must be experienced with "intense fear, horror, or helplessness" was removed in the DSM-5 as the definition led to the exclusion of individuals who experienced a traumatic event, but not with intense fear, horror, or hopelessness (Breslau & Kessler, 2001; Karam et al., 2010). Additionally, this subjective criterion added no predictive value in diagnosis (Bedard-Gilligan & Zoellner, 2008; Breslau & Kessler, 2001).

Additional changes from the DSM-IV/TR to the DSM-5 include an increase in symptom clusters from three (i.e., intrusion, avoidance, and alterations in arousal/reactivity) to four, with the addition of "negative alterations in cognition and mood." Specifiers of "chronic" and "acute" are no longer represented in the DSM-5 and have been replaced with "delayed expression" and "dissociative symptoms."

Although several assessment tools have been revised to reflect these major changes, many have not yet incorporated them. This is one important caveat to consider when selecting assessment tools for diagnostic purposes.

Etiology and Prognosis

Due to the heterogeneity of PTS reactions in children and adolescents, copious factors have been implicated in the onset and maintenance of symptoms. Therefore, when conducting an assessment, it is useful to evaluate demographic variables, psychological precursors, and environmental factors associated with increased risk following exposure to a traumatic event. In addition, assessing for the presence of risk and protective factors can also aid in identifying potential barriers to successful treatment implementation.

Pretrauma Demographic risk factors associated with the development of PTS symptoms include low socioeconomic and minority status, female gender, and younger age (Alisic et al., 2014; Trickey, Siddaway, Meiser-Stedman, Serpell, & Field, 2012; Lai, Lewis, Livings, Greca, & Esnard, 2017). Other pretrauma risk factors include temperament (e.g., irritability), prior emotional or behavioral problems, family adversity (e.g., family dysfunction, parental separation, or death), cultural characteristics (e.g., fatalistic or self-blaming coping strategies), family psychiatric history, and biological and genetic vulnerabilities (American Psychiatric Association, 2013; Nader & Fletcher, 2014). Exposure to prior trauma or multiple traumas, as is often the case with child maltreatment and violence, is associated with greater distress and a more severe and chronic trajectory (Green et al., 2000; Lam, Lyons, Griffin, & Kisiel, 2015). The presence of social support from family, peers, and teachers prior to a traumatic event has been found to buffer the deleterious effects of trauma exposure (Banks & Weems, 2014; Lai, Kelley, Harrison, Thompson, & Self-Brown, 2015).

Additional individual-level risk factors pertinent to the assessment of PTSD in children and adolescents are developmental and cognitive deficits. Individuals with intellectual, developmental, and language impairments are particularly vulnerable in the face of trauma, as they typically exhibit underdeveloped coping skills and difficulty reporting their experiences (Tomasulo & Razza, 2007). Despite this, research on the clinical assessment of PTSD in this population is scarce. Furthermore, many existing diagnostic assessment tools are not validated in children with disabilities, resulting in underreporting of symptoms and misdiagnoses (Mevissen & De Jongh, 2010). These limitations highlight the need for careful measurement selection and comprehensive assessment to ensure adequate information is collected for a diagnosis. In the following section, we provide details on assessment tools that may be most appropriate for children and adolescents with impaired intellectual functioning.

Peritrauma Children's PTS symptoms may also vary based on the event experienced (i.e., nature, cause, severity, and duration; Nader & Fletcher, 2014). For example, research assessing youth reactions following acts of terrorism and natural disasters demonstrate that the nature of the traumatic event can elicit very different symptom patterns. Following 9/11 many children experienced separation anxiety and agoraphobia symptoms in addition to PTSD (Hoven et al., 2005), while children exposed to natural disasters tend to experience comorbid depression symptoms (Lai, Auslander, Fitzpatrick, & Podkowirow, 2014; Lai, La Greca, Auslander, & Short, 2013). Further, in the case of certain traumatic events (e.g., natural disaster, war, terrorism, and other large-scale events impacting communities), broader systems (e.g., schools) are negatively affected. This severely disrupts children's sense of normalcy and routine, which is negatively correlated with symptom severity following a traumatic event (American Red Cross, 2016; Botey & Kulig, 2014; Pfefferbaum & Shaw, 2013; Prinstein, La Greca, Vernberg, & Silverman, 1996; Vernberg, 2002). Assessing the level of support children have on multiple ecological levels (e.g., individual coping abilities, parental and school-based support) is important during the assessment process and to provide helpful treatment recommendations.

Some research suggests that interpersonal trauma (e.g., assault, war) has more severe impact than non-interpersonal trauma (e.g., disasters, accidents; Alisic et al., 2014). This may be the case as interpersonal trauma tends to be more chronic, diminishes available social support (especially in cases when a perpetrator is a family member), and leads to more self-blame or other maladaptive cognitions (Alisic et al., 2014). Further, girls are more likely than boys to experience clinical levels of posttraumatic stress symptoms, but this relationship is further complicated by the type of trauma experienced. For example, in a meta-analysis, Alisic et al. (2014) found that girls with interpersonal trauma had the highest rates of PTSD and boys with non-interpersonal trauma had the lowest rates. Trickey and colleagues (2012) found that type of assessment (i.e., questionnaire v. interview), intentionality of the trauma (e.g., war, terrorism), and group v. individual trauma are significant moderators of the impact of female gender as a risk factor for PTSD. Thus, girls and boys may require different levels of support following an event and may display a different constellation of symptoms.

Posttrauma Several posttraumatic risk factors influence the onset and trajectory of significant clinical symptoms. These variables include individual (e.g., negative attributions, symptom severity, comorbid symptoms, and ineffective coping), familial (e.g., parent psychopathology, lack of social negative coping), and community (e.g., disrupted neighborhood, repeated reminders, subsequent adverse life events). Alternately, social support from family members, peers, and other adults and positive coping skills following a traumatic event have been found to be protective (Kelley et al., 2010; La Greca, Silverman, Lai, & Jaccard, 2010).

The PTS symptoms experienced by parents and caregivers significantly impact children's PTS symptom severity and recovery following a traumatic event. Research indicates that the way parents respond both to the traumatic event itself and afterward is associated with children's recovery (Dyregrov & Yule, 2006; Lai, Tiwari, Beaulieu, Self-Brown, & Kelley, 2015). Children often avoid discussing a traumatic event and its consequences, as they soon realize that doing so may upset their parents (Dyregrov & Yule, 2006). It is recommended that parent's PTS and other symptoms be assessed given the positive correlation of children and parent PTS symptoms. (Kelley et al., 2010; Lai et al., 2013; Self-Brown, Lai, Harbin, & Kelley, 2014; Vigna, Hernandez, Paasch, Gordon, & Kelley, 2009). As such, a comprehensive evaluation when assessing for PTSD should include multiple informant and self-report measures, as well as interviews and observational methods (Dyregrov & Yule, 2006; Scheeringa, 2008).

Clinical Assessment

According to the National Child Traumatic Stress Network (2004), many children and parents are reluctant to reveal trauma histories, and the clinician should take a direct approach to assessing trauma either through the use of rating scales or clinical interviews. Clinicians should provide or query about a comprehensive list of traumatic events. When directly assessing trauma in children and adolescents, an important consideration is the purpose of the assessment. For example, if the assessment is strictly for diagnostic purposes, the clinician must be careful of the potentially negative consequences associated with having a child describe a traumatic event without providing accurate trauma-informed follow-up or treatment.

When selecting appropriate assessment tools, the clinician should consider whether the measure is developmentally appropriate, assesses for multiple traumas, is supported by research findings, and is suitable for the purpose of assessment (e.g., to screen a large number of individuals at once, strictly diagnostic, research, or informing treatment). Moreover, symptoms should be assessed in a variety of domains of functioning such as physiological and cognitive (Kerig, Fedorowicz, Brown, & Warren, 2000). Diagnostic assessments should include careful consideration of factors related to all aspects of the child's ecology (Kerig et al., 2000). Assessment measures for PTSD in children take a variety of forms. These include screening measures that may be completed by children, caregivers, and other informants (e.g., teachers, medical professionals), clinical interviews, clinical observations, as well as broadband instruments for assessing comorbid symptoms.

Given that many youth with PTSD experience comorbid symptoms, it is imperative that other internalizing and externalizing symptoms are adequately assessed to accurately inform case conceptualization and treatment planning. For example, many children and adolescents, especially those experiencing multiple traumatic events, demonstrate difficulty regulating their behavior (Cook et al., 2017). Although prevelance rates vary, research suggests that approximatley 70-90% of youth with PTSD (Fan, Zhang, Yang, Mo, & Liu, 2011; Cheeringa, Zeanah, Myers, & Putnam, 2003), have at leastone other disorder, with oppositional behavior, anxiety, and depression as the most common (Kilpatrick et al., 2003).

Individuals with PTSD are at heightened risk for suicidal ideation and completion; thus a comprehensive assessment should also include suicidality. A recent meta-analysis revealed that PTSD and adolescent suicidality were strongly associated ($d = 0.70$, 95% CI 0.555–0.848; Panagioti, Gooding, Triantafyllou, & Tarrier, 2015). Because several symptoms of PTSD overlap with symptoms of depression, anxiety, and psychotic disorders, it is important to assess for disorders that may present similarly to PTSD.

Acceptable measures for assessing comorbid disorders and suicidality in youth include broadband measures such as the Child Behavior Checklist (Achenbach & Rescorla, 2001) and the Behavioral Assessment System for Children (Kamphaus & Reynolds, 2015). Semi-structured interviews include the Anxiety Disorders Interview Schedule (DiNardo, O'Brien, Barlow, Waddell, & Blanchard, 1983) and the Kiddie Schedule for Affective Disorders and Schizophrenia (Kaufman et al., 1997). Frequently used measures of specific non-PTSD symptoms include measures of depression (Children's Depression Inventory; Kovacs, 1985), anxiety (Multidimensional Anxiety Scale for Children; March, 2012), and suicidality (Columbia-Suicide Severity Rating Scale; Posner et al., 2011, Suicidal Ideation Questionnaire (Reynolds, 1987).

The following section provides a comprehensive list of PTSD assessment measures appropriate for use in young children, school-aged children, and adolescents. This is by no means an exhaustive list of all available measures. Instead, we have provided a list of the most informative for diagnostic assessment and treatment monitoring. Further reviews on PTSD measures are available (c.f., Leigh et al., 2016).

Broadband Assessment Tools

Given the prevalence of comorbid disorders in youth who exhibit PTS symptoms, best practice includes assessing broadly for psychopathology and problematic behavior. Several broadband rating scales and structured interviews are described below.

Child Behavior Checklist This is a 118-item measure that assesses parents' perceptions of children's internalizing and externalizing symptoms (Achenbach, 1966; Achenbach & Rescorla, 2001). This scale includes eight symptom domains: attention problems, delinquent problems, aggressive behavior, thought problems, withdrawn, somatic complaints, anxious/depressed, and social problems. Items are rated on a 3-point scale ("not true," "somewhat true," and "very true"). This measure can be used to aid in the diagnosis of youth who have PTS symptoms as well as other internalizing or externalizing problems. The measure includes a 14-item scale that assesses the presence of PTS symptoms. The measure has excellent psychometric properties and is often used in clinical assessment and research. Additionally, this measure contains a parallel form for youth (11–18) to report on their own symptoms. Limitations of this measure include the length and the need for scoring software to produce results.

Child Behavior Checklist (CBCL 1.5–5) This broadband measure is a parallel form of the CBCL for use by parents of preschool-aged children (Achenbach & Rescorla, 2001). The 100-item scale is used to assess a wide range of psychological symptoms and problematic behaviors (Achenbach & Rescorla, 2001). Moreover, researchers have created a modified CBCL-PTSD 15-item scale based on pre-existing items that can be used as a screening tool with children who have experienced traumatic events (Dehon & Scheeringa, 2006).

Diagnostic Interviews for Children and Adolescents

The assessment of PTS symptoms and comorbid problems includes an interview with the child, as well as the caregiver. Semi-structured interviews offer a relatively uniform, comprehensive assessment of psychological symptoms. Potential diagnostic interviews include:

Anxiety Disorders Interview Schedule for Children and Adolescents (ADIS-C/P) The ADIS is a semi-structured interview instrument primarily used to assess anxiety disorders (DiNardo et al., 1983). The ADIS includes a parent and child version so that multi-informant information is obtained. The instrument contains a PTSD module that is used to identify children's exposure to a variety of potentially traumatic events. Additionally, adolescents are asked to provide their perceived level of impairment due to PTS symptoms based on a 7-point scale. Strengths of ADIS include the addition of developmental considerations such as the use of feeling thermometers, parent and child versions, and an additional PTSD module. However, administration of the measure is time intensiveness taking between 1 and 2 h. Overall the ADIS has been found to have good reliability and validity; however, specific psychometric information on the PTSD module is lacking (Meiser-Stedman, Smith, Glucksman, Yule, & Dalgleish, 2007).

Diagnostic Interview for Children and Adolescents-Revised (DICA-R) This is a semi-structured interview utilized to assess present and lifetime diagnoses (Reich, Leacock, & Shanfield, 1994). The interview can be administered to an adolescent or parent. This interview includes a 17-item PTSD module which assesses the child's identified traumatic event and the subsequent reactions to the event. There are multiple versions of the interview: one for children 6–12 years old, a second for adolescents 13–18 years old, and a third for the parent.

Kiddie Schedule for Affective Disorders and Schizophrenia for School-Aged Children This is a 32-scale semi-structured interview that assesses a range of childhood psychopathology (Kaufman et al., 1997). In addition, the instrument assesses lifetime and present diagnoses. Questions in the PTSD module assess past or recent traumatic events; however, the clinician will only utilize one event to assess PTSD symptoms. Specifically, the length of the PTSD scale is dependent upon the amount of symptomatology endorsed by the youth. It should be noted that this instrument requires extensive training to accurately administer.

Childhood PTSD Interview (CPI) This is a structured clinical interview based on the DSM criteria in order to assist in the determination of whether a child meets criteria for a PTSD diagnosis (Fletcher, 1996). The interview begins with the clinician inquiring about the child's trauma history and then is followed by 78 questions that are answered with "yes" or "no" responses. There are two formats for this interview, a child and parent form. One strength of this interview is it can be completed in less than an hour (approximately 40 min).

Children's PTSD Inventory (CPTSD-I) The CPTSD-I is a semi-structured interview for assessing PTS symptoms in youth aged 7–18 (Saigh, 2004; Saigh et al., 2000). The interview can be used for diagnosis based on DSM-IV criteria. The measure evaluates the child's trauma history, PTSD symptoms, and associated PTSD features. This interview only takes 20 min to administer to the youth. The CPTSD-I has excellent inter-rater reliability and diagnostic agreement.

Clinician-Administered PTSD Scale for Children and Adolescents (CAPS-CA) The CAPS-CA is one of the most widely used measures for assessing PTS symptoms in youth (Nader et al., 1996; Newman et al., 2004). The CAPS assesses trauma exposure and PTS symptoms in youth between 8 and 15. In addition, CAPS measures current and lifetime PTS symptoms. The interview includes 36 questions, which identifies the child's most distressing traumatic event. The measure has good internal consistency, particularly for adolescents (Leigh et al., 2016; Saltzman, Weems, & Carrion, 2006). A revised version of this instrument is available (CAPS-CA-5; Pynoos et al., 2015), which is based on the revised DSM-5 criteria; however, limited psychometric support is available at this time. There are several strengths of the CAPS-CA including comprehensiveness and the assessment of impairment level. Limitations of the measure include time requirements (35–70 min to administer) and there is no parent version.

PTSD Rating Scales for Children and Adolescents

A number of empirically supported rating scales are available for assessing PTSD and related symptoms. These instruments are used for diagnosis and treatment planning. These assessment tools include:

PTSD Checklist The PTSD Checklist is a 21-item self-report measure utilized to assess PTSD symptoms based on DSM-5 criteria (Weathers et al., 2013). Each item is rated on a 4-point scale with 0 being "not at all true" and 4 being "extremely true." Depending on the sample, the cutoff score varies between 33 and greater, indicating likelihood of PTSD symptoms. The measure is used with a wide range of individuals including adults and adolescents. The PTSD Checklist can be used as a diagnostic tool, in treatment planning, and for monitoring symptoms. The measure has high convergent validity with other PTSD measures (Eddinger & McDevitt-Murphy, 2017) and excellent internal consistency (Boal, Vaughan, Sims, & Miles, 2017; Eddinger & McDevitt-Murphy, 2017).

Screening Tool for Early Predictors of Posttraumatic Stress Disorder (STEPP) This is a 12-item rating scale screening tool used to assess children's risk for developing PTS symptoms (Meijel et al., 2015; Winston, Kassam-Adams, Garcia-Espana, Ittenbach, & Cnaan, 2003). The STEPP contains four items answered by the child, four items answered by the caregiver, and four items completed based on the child's medical records. Items are rated dichotomously. The STEPP has a sensitivity of 0.88 for children and 0.96 for parents (Meijel et al., 2015). In addition, test-retest reliability is excellent for children and very good for parents (Meijel et al., 2015).

UCLA Posttraumatic Stress Disorder-Reaction Index This is a 20-item clinician-administered measurement used to assess the presentation of DSM-IV symptom criteria for youth between the ages of 7 and 18 (Steinberg, Brymer, Decker, & Pynoos, 2004). Each question is rated on a 5-point scale (0, the symptom is not present, to 4, the symptom is present most of the time). The measure contains three parts: the first assesses the adolescent's lifetime trauma history, the second part measures the subjective and objective features of trauma exposure, and the final part of the measure evaluates the frequency occurrence of the symptoms (Steinberg et al., 2004). The measure is only intended to assess the youth's symptoms based on one identified event and is not intended to be a diagnostic tool. This measure has been widely used in a variety of countries and populations. This measure is found to have good psychometric properties; several studies have found the measure to have good to excellent internal consistency (Nilsson et al., 2015).

Child's Reaction to Traumatic Events Scale (CRTES) The CRTES is a 23-item self-report measure used to evaluate a child's response to a traumatic event (Jones, Fletcher, & Ribbe, 2002). Each item is measured on a 4-point scale based on the frequency the child experiences the symptoms with higher scores indicating more frequent experiences. The scale contains three subscales: hyperarousal, intrusion, and avoidance. This measure has been translated to other languages as well.

Children's Revised Impact of Events Scale (CRIES) This scale was modified from the Impact of Events Scale for adults used to assess PTSD symptoms of avoidance and reexperiencing (Smith, Perrin, Dyregrov, & Yule, 2003). This is a self-report measure for youth over the age of 8. There are two versions of this measure: one version contains 8 items and the other version contains 13 items. The 8-item version contains only two subscales avoidance behaviors and reexperiencing, and the 13-item version contains a third subscale of hyperarousal. For each scale items are rated on a 4-point scale with higher scores indicating greater severity. Both scales have demonstrated adequate internal consistency with coefficients ranging from 0.75 to 0.80 (Smith et al., 2003). In addition, both scales have been found to be useful in diagnosing youth; the cutoff score for the 8-item scale is 17 and the 13-item scale is 30 (Smith et al., 2003). There are several strengths of this scale that include the translation of the scale in several languages, the ease of administration, the ability to use throughout treatment, and the free accessibility to clinicians.

Child Trauma Screening Questionnaire This is a 10-item self-report measure used to assist in the identification of children at risk for the development of PTSD (Kenardy, Spence, & Macleod, 2006). Each item is answered dichotomously, yes or no. The instrument contains two domains: hyperarousal and reexperiencing. This measure was validated with youth aged 7–16 years. Strengths of the measure include minimal time constraints to complete, the measure is available at no cost, and the measure is not impacted by practice effects allowing it to be used for re-screening purposes.

Trauma Symptom Checklist for Children (TSCC) This is a self-report measure that contains 54 items used to assess a variety of symptoms in youth (Briere, 1996). This measure assesses exposure to a variety of traumas including sexual traumas and abuse. In addition, the PTSD scale is one of six clinical scales assessed. While the administration of the measure does not require training, in order to accurately interpret the results, training is needed. There is also a parallel form for younger children.

Child PTSD Symptoms Scale (CPSS) The CPSS is a 17-item self-report measure used to assess PTSD symptoms based on DSM-IV symptom clusters in youth aged 8–18 (Foa, Johnson, Feeny, & Treadwell, 2001). Each question is rated on a 4-point scale, yielding scores that range from 0 to 51, with higher scores indicating more symptoms. Clinical cutoff scores range from 11 to 16 (Foa et al., 2001; Leigh et al., 2016). In addition, there are seven questions that address individual functioning, providing an impairment index. Overall, this scale is found to have good psychometric properties with reliability coefficients ranging from 0.70 to 0.89 for a youth experiencing a variety of traumas, such as natural disasters and sexual abuse (Nixon et al., 2013), and the CPSS has good specificity and sensitivity (Foa et al., 2001; Nixon et al., 2013). Strengths of this measure include feasibility and ease of scoring. It is available in multiple languages and is freely available to clinicians. Additionally, the CPSS can be used regularly in treatment for symptom monitoring.

NYU Child and Adolescent Stressors Checklist This is a 66-item self-report measure for assessing whether the respondent has experienced a traumatic event (Cloitre, Morin, & Silva, 2002; Mullett-Hume, Anshel, Guevara, & Cloitre, 2008). Items are rated as either "yes" or "no" as to whether the individual has experienced the potentially traumatic event. This measure is found to have good internal consistency with reported alpha coefficients at 0.75 (Havens et al., 2012).

Child Posttraumatic Cognitions Inventory This 33-item measure assesses the respondent's negative beliefs about oneself or the world and self-blame (Foa, Ehlers, Clark, Tolin, & Orsillo, 1999). The instrument has good internal consistency, test-retest reliability, and convergent validity (Foa et al., 1999). The measure is lengthy but yields useful information for symptom monitoring.

Assessing PTSD in Young Children

Given that the criteria for PTSD differ in children 6 and under from older children, the need for developmentally appropriate measures that include the DSM-5 criteria is necessary (American Psychiatric Association, 2013). Therefore, assessment methods used for assessing PTSD in young children include diagnostic interviews, observational methods, and caregiver-report measures.

Diagnostic Interviews for Young Children

Diagnostic Infant and Preschool Assessment The Diagnostic Infant and Preschool Assessment (DIPA; Scheeringa, 2004) is a semi-structured clinical interview that has been validated for use with young children aged 1–6 years. The interview is administered to caregivers and takes approximately 90 min; however, each module is administered individually potentially reducing administration time (Scheeringa & Haslett, 2010). The DIPA covers a broad range of disorders (e.g., attention-deficit/hyperactivity disorder, oppositional defiant disorder, major depressive disorder, generalized anxiety disorder, obsessive-compulsive disorder, reactive attachment disorder) and includes a thorough assessment of PTSD in young children (Scheeringa & Haslett, 2010). Questions about PTSD reflect DSM-5 criteria and query about symptom frequency and impairment. The assessment is unique in that it assesses functional impairment in five domains (with caregivers, siblings, peers, child care or school, and broadly within public settings; Scheeringa & Haslett, 2010). The measure not only assesses DSM-5 symptoms but also a PTSD Alternative Algorithm (PTSD-AA) that has been empirically supported (Scheeringa & Haslett, 2010). While psychometric properties for the overall DIPA varied, the PTSD portion resulted in test-retest reliability at 0.87 (Scheeringa & Haslett, 2010). The DIPA is available at no cost with the most but updated psychometric properties coinciding with the DSM-5 are unavailable.

Preschool Age Psychiatric Assessment The Preschool Age Psychiatric Assessment (PAPA; Egger & Angold, 2004) is a structured interview that broadly measures psychopathology in children aged 2–5 years. The PAPA assesses a wide range of externalizing and internalizing symptoms in 30 domains. The disabilities definition created by the World Health Organization's International Classification of Functioning, Disability, and Health (Egger et al., 2006; World Health Organization, 2001) is used to measure functional impairment. The interview is administered to caregivers in approximately 90 min. The PAPA demonstrated test-retest reliability ranging from kappa 0.36 to 0.79 and intraclass correlation from alpha 0.56 to 0.89 with the DSM-IV (Egger et al., 2006). Specifically, the PTSD test-retest reliability had kappa of 0.73 and intraclass correlation alpha of 0.56 with the DSM-IV (Egger et al., 2006). The PAPA is widely used clinically and within research and formal training is required to administer the PAPA.

Trauma Assessment Tools for Young Children

Traumatic Events Screening Inventory Parent Report Revised Traumatic Events Screening Inventory Parent Report Revised (TESI-PR-R; Ghosh-Ippen et al., 2002) is a caregiver screening tool validated for assessment of traumatic experiences for children 0–6 years old. The TESI-PR-R contains 24 questions that elicit "yes," "no," or "not sure" responses. Limited psychometric data is available regarding the TESI-PR-R although the measure has good internal consistency (alpha = 0.82; Chemtob, Gudiño, & Laraque, 2013). The measure is available at no cost but must be administered by qualified professionals.

Pediatric Emotional Distress Scale The Pediatric Emotional Distress Scale (PEDS; Saylor, Swenson, Stokes Reynolds, & Taylor, 1999) is a 21-item caregiver-report measure of internalizing and externalizing symptoms. It has been validated for use with children aged 2–10 (Saylor et al., 1999). Administration time is estimated at 10 min. Items are rated on a 4-point scale from "almost never" to "very often." The PEDS yields three subscales, anxious or withdrawn, fearful, and acting out, as well as a composite score. The measure has good internal consistency, inter-rater reliability, and convergent validity (Saylor et al., 1999). Some benefits include the brevity of the measure and it is available at no cost. However, it is not intended for examining PTSD symptoms per se.

Trauma Symptom Checklist for Young Children The Trauma Symptom Checklist for Young Children (TSCYC; Briere, 2005) is a 90-item screening tool for use with children aged 3–12. The instrument is completed by a caregiver and allows for assessment of multiple traumatic experiences (Briere, 2005). The TSCYC has eight clinical scales: anxiety, depression, anger/aggression, posttraumatic stress-intrusion, posttraumatic stress-avoidance, posttraumatic stress-arousal, dissociation, and sexual concerns. It also has two validity scales: response level and atypical response (Briere, 2005). The TSCYC uses a 4-point frequency scale ranging from "not at all" to "very often." The norms take into account gender and age (Briere, 2005). The TSCYC had demonstrated good psychometric properties (Gilbert, 2004). The TSCYC is based on the DSM-IV and is a relatively costly.

Young Child PTSD Screen The Young Child PTSD Screen (YCPS; Scheeringa et al., 2010) is a brief 6-item measure completed by caregivers based on DSM-5 PTSD criteria. The YCPS probes for the severity of symptoms in preschool-aged children (ages 3–6; Scheeringa et al., 2010). Although this measure is currently unpublished, reports suggest adequate psychometric properties (Scheeringa, 2012; Scheeringa et al., 2010).

Early Childhood Traumatic Stress Screen The Early Childhood Traumatic Stress Screen (ECTSS; Harris, 2016) is a 34-item caregiver-report measure assessing PTS symptoms in young children aged 1–6. The ECTSS contains four factors, arousal and hyper-reactivity, fearful attachment, intrusion and reexperiencing, and avoidance and negative cognition and mood, as well as a composite score (Harris, 2016). Although, the ECTSS has limited empirical support, it is one of the few assessment tools based on DSM-5 criteria (American Psychiatric Association, 2013; Harris, 2016). Psychometric properties include concurrent validity ranging from 0.45 to 0.81 and internal consistency reliability ranging from alpha of 0.68 to 0.85 (Harris, 2016).

Assessing PTSD in Children and Adolescents with Cognitive Delays

Due to the increased risk of experiencing potentially traumatic events by children with cognitive deficits, some research has explored assessment of PTSD for this specific population (Mevissen, Barnhoorn, Didden, Korzilius, & De Jongh, 2014; Mevissen, Didden, Korzilius, & de Jongh, 2016). Researchers utilized an adapted form of the Anxiety Disorders Interview Schedule of DSM-IV – Child version (ADIS-C PTSD) scale with children who exhibit mild to borderline intellectual disabilities (Mevissen et al., 2014, 2016). As a result, the adapted ADIS-C demonstrated good to excellent psychometric properties with this population (Mevissen et al., 2014, 2016). Additionally, research has been conducted on children with special needs broadly (Saylor, Macias, Wohlfeiler, Morgan, & Awkerman, 2009). The Pediatric Emotional Distress Scale (PEDS) was utilized within this population and demonstrated excellent interrater reliability (Saylor et al., 2009). Therefore, the ADIS-C PTSD and PEDS have both demonstrated application for children with special needs. However, due to the disparate impact experienced by children with special needs, future research is needed within this population utilizing assessment tools corresponding to DSM-5 criteria.

Future Considerations

Although numerous assessment tools are available for assessing PTSD, existing measures are limited in several ways. First, many assessment tools are based on DSM-IV criteria for PTSD and have not been updated to reflect DSM-5 criteria. Further, updated instruments frequently lack psychometric support. Thus, it is important for researchers to update measures of PTSD to reflect the revised DSM-5 criteria. As the DSM-5 provides specific criteria for young children based on research findings, updated tools capturing younger children's experiences would lead to more accurate diagnosis in this age group.

For measures that do have readily available psychometric properties, the standardization samples often lack diversity. For example, many measures were validated on samples with primarily low SES minorities, while others were validated with primarily Caucasian samples. In either case, the normative samples may bring about some limitations such as the generalizability of using measures in a differing population. Similarly, a major shortcoming is the lack of measures that capture the posttrauma experiences of individuals with developmental disabilities. It is important that measures be developed to reflect the posttrauma experiences of this population.

The predominant focus of researchers and clinicians has been on identifying and treating maladjustment experienced by youth following a traumatic event. More recent research, however, has examined factors related to children's resiliency and posttraumatic growth in response to trauma (Bonanno & Diminich, 2013; Masten, 2014; Spell et al., 2008; Tedeschi & Calhoun, 1996; Weems & Graham, 2014; Zolkoski & Bullock, 2012). We recommend that measures of resiliency and posttraumatic growth as well as protective variables be included in the assessment process, and this may help to identify psychological resources that can be strengthened.

Assessment tools for children and adolescents				
Assessment tool	Age range	Informant	Administration time	Purpose
PTSD Checklist (Weathers et al., 2013)	7–18	Child; caregiver	N/A (21 items)	Screening
Screening Tool for Early Predictors of Posttraumatic Stress Disorder (STEPP; Winston et al., 2003)	youth	Child; caregiver	5 min	Screening
UCLA Posttraumatic Stress Disorder-Reaction Index (Steinberg et al., 2004)	6–18	Child; caregiver	15 min	Diagnostic
Clinician-Administered PTSD Scale for Children and Adolescents (CAPS-CA; Nader et al., 1996)	8–15	Clinician administered to child	45 min	Diagnostic
Child's Reaction to Traumatic Events Scale (CRTES; Jones et al., 2002)	6–18	Child	10 min	Assessment of symptoms
Children's Revised Impact of Events Scale (CRIES; Smith et al., 2003)	8–18	Child	10–15 min	Assessment of PTSD symptoms and symptom monitoring
Child Trauma Screening Questionnaire (Kenardy et al., 2006)	7–16	Child	5 min	Assessment of symptoms
Trauma Symptom Checklist for Children (TSCC; Briere, 1996)	8–16	Child	20 min	Assessment of symptoms
Child PTSD Symptoms Scale (CPSS; Foa et al., 2001)	8–15	Child	10 min	Assessment; symptom monitoring
NYU Child and Adolescent Stressors Checklist (Cloitre et al., 2002; Mullett-Hume et al., 2008)	youth	Child	N/A (66 items)	Assessment of traumatic event
Anxiety Disorders Interview Schedule for Children and Adolescents (ADIS--C/P; DiNardo et al., 1983)	6–18	Child; caregiver	90 min	Diagnostic interview
Diagnostic Interview of Children and Adolescents- Revised (DICA-R; Reich et al., 1994)	7–18	Child; caregiver	90 min	Diagnostic interview
Kiddie Schedule for Affective Disorders and Schizophrenia for School-Aged Children (Kaufman et al., 1997)	7–17	Child; caregiver	90 min	Diagnostic interview

Assessment tools for children and adolescents				
Assessment tool	Age range	Informant	Administration time	Purpose
Childhood PTSD Interview (CPI; Fletcher, 1996)	7–18	Child; caregiver	40 min	Diagnostic interview
Children's PTSD Inventory (CPTSD-I; Saigh et al., 2000; Saigh, 2004)	6–18	Child	20 min	Assessment of symptoms
Child Post Traumatic Cognitions Inventory (Foa et al., 1999)	6–18	Child	N/A (33 items)	Assessment of symptoms; treatment planning
Child Behavior Checklist (CBCL; Achenbach & Rescorla, 2001)	6–18	Caregiver	20 min	Screening of symptoms

Assessment tools for young children				
Assessment tool	Age range	Format and informant	Administration time	Purpose
Diagnostic Infant and Preschool Assessment (DIPA; Scheeringa, 2004)	1–6	Caregiver; diagnostic interview	100 min	Diagnosis
Preschool Age Psychiatric Assessment (PAPA; Egger & Angold, 2004)	2–5	Caregiver; diagnostic interview	90 min	Diagnosis
Traumatic Events Screening Inventory Parent Report Revised. (TESI-PR-R; Ghosh-Ippen et al., 2002	0–6	Caregiver; screening tool	NA (24 items)	Assessment of traumatic experiences
Pediatric Emotional Distress Scale (PEDS; Saylor et al., 1999).	2–10	Caregiver; screening tool	10 min	Assessment of symptoms
Trauma Symptom Checklist for Young Children (TSCYC; Briere, 2005)	3–12	Caregiver; screening tool	20 min	Assessment of symptoms
Child Behavior Checklist (CBCL 1.5–5; Achenbach & Rescorla, 2001; Dehon & Scheeringa, 2006)	1.5–5	Caregiver; screening tool	10–20 min	Screening for symptoms
Young Child PTSD Screen (YCPS; Scheeringa, 2010)	3–6	Caregiver; screening tool	NA (6 items)	Screening for treatment referral
Early Childhood Traumatic Stress Screen (ECTSS; Harris, 2016)	1–6	Caregiver; screening tool	NA (34 items)	Assessment of symptoms

References

Achenbach, T. M. (1966). The classification of children's psychiatric symptoms: A factor-analytic study. *Psychological Monographs: General And Applied, 80*(7), 1–37.

Achenbach, T. M., & Rescorla, L. A. (2001). *Manual for ASEBA school-age forms and profiles*. Burlington, NJ: University of Vermont, Research Center for Children, Youth, & Families.

Alisic, E., Zalta, A. K., van Wesel, F., Larsen, S. E., Hafstad, G. S., Hassanpour, K., & Smid, G. (2014). Rates of post-traumatic stress disorder in trauma-exposed children and adolescents: Meta-analysis. *The British Journal of Psychiatry, 204*, 335–340.

American Psychiatric Association. (1980). *Diagnostic and statistical manual of disorders* (3rd ed.). Washington, DC: American Psychiatric Association.

American Psychiatric Association. (2000). *Diagnostic and statistical manual of mental disorders: DSM-IV-TR*. Washington, DC: American Psychiatric Association.

American Psychiatric Association (APA). (2013). Diagnostic and statistical manual of mental disorders: Fifth edition. American Psychiatric Association, Washington.

American Red Cross (2016). Helping kids cope with disaster. Retrieved from https://redcrosschat.org/2016/11/10/helping-kids-cope-with-disaster/.

Atwoli, L., Stein, D. J., Koenen, K. C., & McLaughlin, K. A. (2015). Epidemiology of posttraumatic stress disorder: Prevalence, correlates and consequences. *Current Opinion in Psychiatry, 28*(4), 307.

Banks, D. M., & Weems, C. F. (2014). Family and peer social support and their links to psychological distress among hurricane-exposed minority youth. *American Journal of Orthopsychiatry, 84*(4), 341.

Bedard-Gilligan, M., & Zoellner, L. A. (2008). The utility of the A1 and A2 criteria in the diagnosis of PTSD. *Behavior Research and Therapy, 46*, 1062–1069.

Boal, A. L., Vaughan, C. A., Sims, C. S., & Miles, J. N. (2017). Measurement invariance across administration mode: Examining the posttraumatic stress disorder (PTSD) checklist. *Psychological Assessment, 29*(1), 76.

Bonanno, G. A., & Diminich, E. D. (2013). Annual research review: Positive adjustment to adversity— Trajectories of minimal-impact resilience and emergent resilience. *Journal of Child Psychology and Psychiatry, 54*(4), 278–401.

Boscarino, J. A., & Adams, R. E. (2009). PTSD onset and course following the world trade center disaster: Findings and implications for future research. *Social Psychiatry and Psychiatric Epidemiology, 44*(10), 887–898.

Botey, A. P., & Kulig, J. C. (2014). Family functioning following wildfires: Recovering from the 2011 slave lake fires. *Journal of Child and Family Studies, 23*(8), 1471–1483.

Breslau, N., & Kessler, R. C. (2001). The stressor criterion in DMS-IV posttraumatic stress disorder: An empirical investigation. *Biological Psychiatry, 50*, 699–704.

Briere, J. (1996). *Trauma symptom checklist for children(TSCC): Professional manual*. Odessa, FL: Psychological Assessment Resources.

Briere, J. (2005). *Trauma symptom checklist for young children (TSCYC): Professional manual*. Odessa, FL: Psychological Assessment Resources, Inc.

Briere, J., Kaltman, S., & Green, B. L. (2008). Accumulated childhood trauma and symptom complexity. *Journal of Traumatic Stress, 21*(2), 223–226.

Briggs, E. C., Nooner, K., & Amaya-Jackson, L. M. (2014). In M. Friedman, T. M. Keane, & P. A. Resick (Eds.), *Handbook of PTSD: Science and practice* (pp. 391–406). New York, NY: Guilford Press.

Chemtob, C. M., Gudiño, O. G., & Laraque, D. (2013). Maternal posttraumatic stress disorder and depression in pediatric primary care: Association with child maltreatment and frequency of child exposure to traumatic events. *JAMA Pediatrics, 167*(11), 1011–1018.

Cintron, G., Salloum, A., Blair-Andrews, Z., & Storch, E. A. (2017). Parents' descriptions of young children's dissociative reactions after trauma. *Journal of Trauma & Dissociation*, 1–14.

Cloitre, M., Morin, N., & Silva, R. (2002). *The NYU child and adolescent stressors checklist—Revised (CASC)*. Unpublished manuscript.

Cook, A., Spinazzola, J., Ford, J., Lanktree, C., Blaustein, M., Cloitre, M., ... Mallah, K. (2017). Complex trauma in children and adolescents. *Psychiatric Annals, 35*(5), 390–398.

Davis, L., & Siegel, L. J. (2000). Posttraumatic stress disorder in children and adolescents: A review and analysis. *Clinical Child and Family Psychology Review, 3*(3), 135–154.

Dehon, C., & Scheeringa, M. S. (2006). Screening for preschool posttraumatic stress disorder with the child behavior checklist. *Journal of Pediatric Psychology, 31*(4), 431–435.

DiNardo, P. A., O'Brien, G. T., Barlow, D. H., Waddell, M. T., & Blanchard, E. B. (1983). Reliability of DSM-III anxiety disorder categories using a new structured interview. *Archives of General Psychiatry, 40*, 1070–1074.

Dyregrov, A., & Yule, W. (2006). A review of PTSD in children. *Child and Adolescent Mental Health, 11*(4), 176–184.

Eddinger, J. R., & McDevitt-Murphy, M. E. (2017). A confirmatory factor analysis of the PTSD checklist 5 in veteran and college student samples. *Psychiatry Research, 255*, 219–224.

Egger, H. L., & Angold, A. (2004). The preschool age psychiatric assessment (PAPA): A structured parent interview for diagnosing psychiatric disorders in preschool children. In *Handbook of infant, toddler, and preschool mental health assessment* (pp. 223–243). Oxford/New York, NY: Oxford University Press.

Egger, H. L., Erkanli, A., Keeler, G., Potts, E., Walter, B. K., & Angold, A. (2006). Test-retest reliability of the preschool age psychiatric assessment (PAPA). *Journal of the American Academy of Child & Adolescent Psychiatry, 45*(5), 538–549.

Fairbank, J. A., Putnam, F. W., & Harris, W. W. (2014). Child traumatic stress: Prevalence, trends, risk and impact. In M. Friedman, T. M. Keane, & P. A. Resick (Eds.), *Handbook of PTSD: Science and practice* (pp. 121–145). New York, NY: Guilford Press.

Fan, F., Zhang, Y., Yang, Y., Mo, L., & Liu, X. (2011). Symptoms of posttraumatic stress disorder, depression, and anxiety among adolescents following the 2008 Wenchuan earthquake in China. *Journal of Traumatic Stress, 24*(1), 44–53.

Felitti, V. J., Anda, R. F., Nordenberg, D., Williamson, D. F., Spitz, A. M., Edwards, V., ... Marks, J. S. (1998). Relationship of childhood abuse and household dysfunction to many of the leading causes of death in adults: The adverse childhood experiences (ACE) study. *American Journal of Preventive Medicine, 14*(4), 245–258.

Fikretoglu, D., & Liu, A. (2011). Prevalence, correlates, and clinical features of delayed-onset posttraumatic stress disorder in a nationally representative military sample. *Social Psychiatry and Psychiatric Epidemiology, 47*, 1359–1366.

Fletcher, K. (1996). Psychometric review of the childhood PTSD interview. In B. H. Stamm (Ed.), *Measurement of stress, trauma, and adaptation* (pp. 87–89). Lutherville, MD: Sidran Press.

Foa, E. B., Ehlers, A., Clark, D. M., Tolin, D. F., & Orsillo, S. M. (1999). The posttraumatic cognitions inventory (PTCI): Development and validation. *Psychological Assessment, 11*(3), 303.

Foa, E. B., Johnson, K. M., Feeny, N. C., & Treadwell, K. R. H. (2001). The child PTSD symptom scale: A preliminary examination of its psychometric properties. *Journal of Clinical Child Psychology, 30*, 376–384.

Friedman, M. J., Resick, P. A., & Keane, T. M. (2014). PTSD from DSM-III to DSM-5: Progress and challenges. In M. Friedman, T. M. Keane, & P. A. Resick (Eds.), Handbook of PTSD: Science and practice (pp. 3–20). New York, NY: Guilford Press.

Ghosh-Ippen, C., Ford, J., Racusin, R., Acker, M., Bosquet, K., Rogers, C., & Edwards, J. (2002). Trauma events screening inventory-parent report revised. San Francisco: The Child Trauma Research Project of the Early Trauma Network and The National Center for PTSD Dartmouth Child Trauma Research Group.

Gilbert, A.M. (2004). *Psychometric properties of the Trauma Symptom Checklist for Young Children* (Unpublished doctoral dissertation). Alliant University, San Diego, CA.

Goldstein, R. B., Smith, S. M., Chou, S. P., Saha, T. D., Jung, J., Zhang, H., ... Grant, B. F. (2016). The epidemiology of DSM-5 posttraumatic stress disorder in the United States: Results from the National Epidemiologic Survey on alcohol and related conditions-III. *Social Psychiatry and Psychiatric Epidemiology, 51*(8), 1137–1148.

Green, B. L., Goodman, L. A., Krupnick, J. L., Corcoran, C. B., Petty, R. M., Stockton, P., & Stern, N. M. (2000). Outcomes of single versus multiple trauma exposure in a screening sample. *Journal of Traumatic Stress, 13*(2), 271–286.

Hagan, M. J., Sulik, M. J., & Lieberman, A. F. (2016). Traumatic life events and psychopathology in a high risk, ethnically diverse sample of young children: A person-centered approach. *Journal of Abnormal Child Psychology, 44*(5), 833–844.

Harris, S. E. (2016). *Development of the Early Childhood Traumatic Stress Screen* (Unpublished Doctoral Dissertation). Marquette University, Milwaukee, Wisconsin.

Havens, J. F., Gudino, O. G., Biggs, E. A., Diamond, U. N., Weis, J. R., & Cloitre, M. (2012). Identification of trauma exposure and PTSD in adolescent psychiatric inpatients: An exploratory study. *Journal of Traumatic Stress, 25*(2), 171–178.

Hoven, C. W., Duarte, C. S., Lucas, C. P., Wu, P., Mandell, D. J., Goodwin, R. D., ... Musa, G. J. (2005). Psychopathology among new York City public school children 6 months after September 11. *Archives of General Psychiatry, 62*(5), 545–551.

Jones, R. T., Fletcher, K., & Ribbe, D. R. (2002). Child's Reaction to Traumatic Events Scale-Revised (CRTES-R): A self-report traumatic stress measure. Available from Russell T. Jones, PhD, Professor, Department of Psychology, Stress and Coping Lab, 4102 Derring Hall, Virginia Tech University, Blacksburg, VA 24060.

Kamphaus, R. W., & Reynolds, C. R. (2015). Behavior Assessment System for Children – Third Edition (BASC-3): Behavioral and Emotional Screening System (BESS). Bloomington, MN: Pearson.

Karam, E. G., Andrews, G., Bromet, E., Petukhova, M., Rusico, A. M., Salamoun, M., Sampson, N., Stein, D. J., Alsono, J., Andrade, L.H, et al. (2010). The role of criterion A2 in the DSM-IV Diagnosis of posttraumatic stress disorder. Biological Pyschiatry, 68, 465–473.

Kaufman, J., Birmaher, B., Brent, D., Rao, U. M. A., Flynn, C., Moreci, P., ... Ryan, N. (1997). Schedule for affective disorders and schizophrenia for school-age children-present and lifetime version (K-SADS-PL): Initial reliability and validity data. *Journal of the American Academy of Child & Adolescent Psychiatry, 36*, 980–988.

Kelley, M. L., Self-Brown, S., Le, B., Bosson, J. V., Hernandez, B. C., & Gordon, A. T. (2010). Predicting posttraumatic stress symptoms in children following hurricane Katrina: A prospective analysis of the effect of parental distress and parenting practices. *Journal of Traumatic Stress, 23*(5), 582–590.

Kenardy, J., Spence, S., & Macleod, A. (2006). Screening for posttraumatic stress disorder in children after accidental injury. *Pediatrics, 118*, 1002–1009.

Kerig, P. K., Fedorowicz, A. E., Brown, C. A., & Warren, M. (2000). Assessment and intervention for PTSD in children exposed to violence. *Journal of Aggression, Maltreatment & Trauma, 3*(1), 161–184.

Kilpatrick, D. G., Ruggiero, K. J., Acierno, R., Saunders, B. E., Resnick, H. S., & Best, C. L. (2003). Violence and risk of PTSD, major depression, substance abuse/dependence, and comorbidity: Results from the National Survey of adolescents. *Journal of Consulting and Clinical Psychology, 71*(4), 692.

Kirsch, V., Wilhelm, F. H., & Goldbeck, L. (2011). Psychophysiological characteristics of PTSD in children and adolescents: A review of the literature. *Journal of Traumatic Stress, 24*(2), 146–154.

Kovacs, M. (1985). The children's depression inventory (CDI). *Psychopharmacology Bulletin, 21*, 995–998.

La Greca, A. M., Danzi, B. A., & Chan, S. F. (2017). DSM-5 and ICD-11 as competing models of PTSD in preadolescent children exposed to a natural disaster: Assessing validity and co-occurring symptomatology. *European Journal of Psychotraumatology, 8*(1), 1310591.

La Greca, A. M., Silverman, W. K., Lai, B., & Jaccard, J. (2010). Hurricane-related exposure experiences and stressors, other life events, and social support: Concurrent and prospective impact on children's persistent posttraumatic stress symptoms. *Journal of Consulting and Clinical Psychology, 78*(6), 794.

Lai, B. S., Alisic, E., Lewis, R., & Ronan, K. R. (2016). Approaches to the assessment of children in the context of disasters. *Current Psychiatry Reports, 18*(5), 45.

Lai, B. S., Auslander, B. A., Fitzpatrick, S. L., & Podkowirow, V. (2014). Disasters and depressive symptoms in children: A review. *Child & Youth Care Forum, 43*(4), 489–504.

Lai, B. S., Kelley, M. L., Harrison, K. M., Thompson, J. E., & Self-Brown, S. (2015). Posttraumatic stress, anxiety, and depression symptoms among children after hurricane Katrina: A latent profile analysis. *Journal of Child and Family Studies, 24*(5), 1262–1270.

Lai, B. S., La Greca, A. M., Auslander, B. A., & Short, M. B. (2013). Children's symptoms of posttraumatic stress and depression after a natural disaster: Comorbidity and risk factors. *Journal of Affective Disorders, 146*(1), 71–78.

Lai, B. S., Lewis, R., Livings, M. S., Greca, A. M., & Esnard, A. M. (2017). Posttraumatic stress symptom trajectories among children after disaster exposure: A review. *Journal of Traumatic Stress, 30*(6), 571–582.

Lai, B. S., Tiwari, A., Beaulieu, B. A., Self-Brown, S., & Kelley, M. L. (2015). Hurricane Katrina: Maternal depression trajectories and child outcomes. *Current Psychology, 34*(3), 515–523.

Lam, A., Lyons, J. S., Griffin, G., & Kisiel, C. (2015). Multiple traumatic experiences and the expression of traumatic stress symptoms for children and adolescents. *Residential Treatment for Children & Youth, 32*(2), 167–181.

Le, M. T., Holton, S., Romero, L., & Fisher, J. (2016). Polyvictimization among children and adolescents in low-and lower-middle-income countries: A systematic review and meta-analysis. *Trauma, Violence, & Abuse,* 1524838016659489.

Leigh, E., Yule, W., & Smith, P. (2016). Measurement issues: Measurement of posttraumatic stress disorder in children and young people–lessons from research and practice. *Child and Adolescent Mental Health, 21*(2), 124–135.

March, J. S. (2012). *Manual for the multidimensional anxiety scale for children-(MASC 2)*. North Tonawanda, NY: MHS.

Masten, A. S. (2014). Global perspectives on resilience in children and youth. *Child Development, 85*, 6–20.

McLaughlin, K. A., Greif Green, J., Gruber, M. J., Sampson, N. A., Zaslavasky, A. M., & Kessler, R. C. (2012). Childhood adversities and the first onset of psychiatric disorders in a national ample of US adolescents. *Archives of General Psychiatry, 69*(11), 1151–1160.

Meiser-Stedman, R., Smith, P., Glucksman, E., Yule, W., & Dalgleish, T. (2007). Parent and child agreement for acute stress disorder, post-traumatic stress disorder and other psychopathology in a prospective study of children and adolescents exposed to single-event trauma. *Journal of Abnormal Child Psychology, 35*, 191–201.

Mevissen, L., Barnhoorn, E., Didden, R., Korzilius, H., & De Jongh, A. (2014). Clinical assessment of PTSD in children with mild to borderline intellectual disabilities: A pilot study. *Developmental Neurorehabilitation, 17*(1), 16–23.

Mevissen, L., & De Jongh, A. (2010). PTSD and its treatment in people with intellectual disabilities: A review of the literature. *Clinical Psychology Review, 30*(3), 308–316.

Mevissen, L., Didden, R., Korzilius, H., & de Jongh, A. (2016). Assessing posttraumatic stress disorder in children with mild to borderline intellectual disabilities. *European Journal of Psychotraumatology, 7*, 1–9.

Mullett-Hume, E., Anshel, D., Guevara, V., & Cloitre, M. (2008). Cumulative trauma and posttraumatic stress disorder among children exposed to the 9/11 world trade center attack. *American Journal of Orthopsychiatry, 78*(1), 103–108.

Nader, K., & Fletcher, K. E. (2014). Childhood posttraumatic stress disorder. In *Child psychopathology*. New York, NY: Guilford.

Nader, K. K. O., Newman, E., Weathers, F. W., Kaloupek, D. G., Kriegler, J. A., & Blake, D. D. (1996). *National center for PTSD clinician-administered PTSD scale for children and adolescents (CAPS-CA) interview booklet and interview guide*. Los Angeles, CA: Western Psychological Services.

National Child Traumatic Stress Network, & Child Sexual Abuse Task Force and Research & Practice Core. (2004). *How to implement trauma-focused cognitive behavioral therapy*. Durham, NC/Los Angeles, CA: National Center for Child Traumatic Stress.

National Commission on Children and Disasters (2010). Report to the President and Congress Phillips, J. (2015). PTSD in DSM-5: Understanding the changes. *Psychiatric Times, 32*(9), 1–5.

Newman, E., Weathers, F. W., Nader, K., Kaloupek, D. G., Pynoos, R. S., & Blake, D. D. (2004). *Clinician-administered PTSD scale for children and adolescents (CAPS-CA)*. Los Angeles, CA: Western Psychological Services.

Nilsson, D., Nordenstam, C., Green, S., Wetterhall, A., Lundin, T., & Svedin, C. G. (2015). Acute stress among adolescents and female rape victims measured by ASC-kids: A pilot study. *Nordic Journal of Psychiatry, 69*(7), 539–545.

Nixon, R., Meiser-Stedman, R., Dalgleish, T., Yule, W., Clark, D. M., Perrin, S., & Smith, P. (2013). The child PTSD symptom scale: An update and replication of its psycho-metric properties. *Psychological Assessment, 25*, 1025–1031.

Pai, A., Surris, A. M., & North, C. S. (2017). Posttraumatic stress disorder in the DSM-5: Controversy, change, and conceptual considerations. *Behavioral Sciences, 7*(1), 7.

Panagioti, M., Gooding, P. A., Triantafyllou, K., & Tarrier, N. (2015). Suicidality and posttraumatic stress disorder (PTSD) in adolescents: A systematic review and meta-analysis. *Social Psychiatry and Psychiatric Epidemiology, 50*(4), 525–537.

Pfefferbaum, B., & Shaw, J. A. (2013). Practice parameter on disaster preparedness. *Journal of the American Academy of Child & Adolescent Psychiatry, 52*(11), 1224–1238.

Posner, K., Brown, G. K., Stanley, B., Brent, D. A., Yershova, K. V., ... Mann, J. J. (2011). The Columbia-suicide severity rating scale: Initial validity and internal consistency findings from three multisite studies with adolescents and adults. *American Journal of Psychiatry, 168*, 1266–1277.

Prinstein, M. J., La Greca, A. M., Vernberg, E. M., & Silverman, W. K. (1996). Children's coping assistance: How parents, teachers, and friends help children cope after a natural disaster. *Journal of Clinical Child Psychology, 25*(4), 463–475.

Pynoos, R. S., Weathers, F. W., Steinberg, A. M., Marx, B. P., Layne, C. M., Kaloupek, D. G., ... Kriegler, J. A. (2015). Clinician-Administered PTSD scale for DSM-5 – Child/Adolescent version. Scale available from the National Center for PTSD at www.ptsd.va.gov

Reich, W., Leacock, N., & Shanfield, C. (1994). *Diagnostic inter-view for children and adolescents-revised (DICA-R)*. St. Louis, MO: Washington University.

Reynolds, W. M. (1987). *Suicidal ideation questionnaire (SIQ)*. Odessa, FL: Psychological Assessment Resources.

Saigh, P. A. (2004). *The children's posttraumatic stress disorder inventory*. San Antonio, TX: Psychological Corp.

Saigh, P. A., Yasik, A. E., Oberfield, R. A., Green, B. L., Halamandaris, P. V., Rubenstein, H., ... McHugh, M. (2000). The children's PTSD inventory: Development and reliability. *Journal of Traumatic Stress, 13*, 369–380.

Saltzman, K. M., Weems, C. F., & Carrion, V. G. (2006). IQ and posttraumatic stress disorder in children that experience interpersonal violence. *Child Psychiatry and Human Development, 36*, 261–272.

Saylor, C. F., Macias, M., Wohlfeiler, M., Morgan, L., & Awkerman, N. G. (2009). Exposure to potentially traumatic life events in children with special needs. *Child Psychiatry and Human Development, 40*(3), 451–465.

Saylor, C. F., Swenson, C. C., Stokes Reynolds, S., & Taylor, M. (1999). The pediatric emotional distress scale: A brief screening measure for young children exposed to traumatic events. *Journal of Clinical Child Psychology, 28*(1), 70–81.

Scheeringa, M. S. (2004). Posttraumatic stress disorder. In *Handbook of infant, toddler, and preschool mental health assessment* (pp. 377–397). New York, NY: Oxford University Press.

Scheeringa, M. S. (2008). Developmental considerations for diagnosing PTSD and acute stress disorder in preschool and school-age children. *American Journal of Psychiatry, 165*, 1237–1239.

Scheeringa, M. S. (2010). Young child PTSD checklist. New Orleans, LA: Tulane University.

Scheeringa, M. (2012). Young child PTSD screen. Measurement instrument database for the social science. Retrieved from www.midss.ie

Scheeringa, M. S. (2015). Untangling psychiatric comorbidity in young children who experienced single, repeated, or hurricane Katrina traumatic events. *Child & Youth Care Forum, 44*(4), 475–492.

Scheeringa, M. S., & Haslett, N. (2010). The reliability and criterion validity of the diagnostic infant and preschool assessment: A new diagnostic instrument for young children. *Child Psychiatry & Human Development, 41*(3), 299–312.

Scheeringa, M. S., Zeanah, C. H., Myers, L., & Putnam, F. W. (2003). New findings on alternative criteria for PTSD in preschool children. *Journal of the American Academy of Child & Adolescent Psychiatry, 42*, 561–570.

Scheeringa, M., Scheeringa, M. S., Cohen, J. A., Deblinger, E., Mannarino, A. P., Steer, R. A., ... Guthrie, D. (2010). *Young child PTSD screen*. Orleans, LA: Tulane Univ (http://www.infantinstitute.org/MikeSPDF/YCPS_versFeb2011.pdf)

Scheeringa, M. S., Zeanah, C. H., & Cohen, J. A. (2011). PTSD in children and adolescents: Toward an empirically based algorithm. *Depression and Anxiety, 28*(9), 770–782.

Self-Brown, S., Lai, B. S., Thompson, J. E., McGill, T., & Kelley, M. L. (2013). Posttraumatic stress disorder symptom trajectories in hurricane Katrina affected youth. *Journal of Affective Disorders, 147*(1), 198–204.

Self-Brown, S., Lai, B., Harbin, S., & Kelley, M. L. (2014). The impact of parental posttraumatic stress disorder symptom trajectories on the long-term outcomes of youth following hurricane Katrina. *International Journal of Public Health, 59*(6), 957.

Smith, P., Perrin, S., Dyregrov, A., & Yule, W. (2003). Principal components analysis of the impact of event scale with children in war. *Personality and Individual Differences, 34*, 315–322.

Spell, A. W., Kelley, M. L., Wang, J., Self-Brown, S., Davidson, K. L., Pellegrin, A., ... Baumeister, A. (2008). The moderating effects of maternal psychopathology on children's adjustment post–hurricane Katrina. *Journal of Clinical Child & Adolescent Psychology, 37*(3), 553–563.

Steinberg, A. M., Brymer, M. J., Decker, K. B., & Pynoos, R. S. (2004). The University of California at Los Angeles post-traumatic stress disorder reaction index. *Current Psychiatry Reports, 6*, 96–100.

Tedeschi, R. G., & Calhoun, L. G. (1996). The posttraumatic growth inventory: Measuring the positive legacy of trauma. *Journal of Traumatic Stress, 9*(3), 455–471.

Tomasulo, D. J., & Razza, N. J. (2007). Posttraumatic stress disorders. In R. Fletcher, E. Loschen, C. Stavrakaki, & M. First (Eds.), *Diagnostic manual-intellectual disability: A textbook of diagnosis of mental disorders in persons with intellectual disability* (pp. 365–378). Kingston, NY: National Association for the Dually Diagnosed.

Trickey, D., Siddaway, A. P., Meiser-Stedman, R., Serpell, L., & Field, A. P. (2012). A meta-analysis of risk factors for post-traumatic stress disorder in children and adolescents. *Clinical Psychology Review, 32*(2), 122–138.

van Meijel, E. P., Gigengack, M. R., Verlinden, E., Opmeer, B. C., Heij, H. A., Goslings, J. C., ... Lindauer, R. J. (2015). Predicting posttraumatic stress disorder in children and parents following accidental child injury: Evaluation of the screening tool for early predictors of posttraumatic stress disorder (STEPP). *BMC Psychiatry, 15*(1), 113.

Vernberg, E. M. (2002). Intervention approaches following disasters. In A. M. La Greca, W. K. Silverman, E. M.

Vernberg, & M. C. Roberts (Eds.), *Helping children cope with disasters and terrorism* (pp. 55–72). Washington, DC: American Psychological Association.

Vigna, J. F., Hernandez, B. C., Paasch, V., Gordon, A. T., & Kelley, M. L. (2009). Positive adjustment in youth post-katrina: The impact of child and maternal social support and coping. In K. Cherry (Ed.), *Lifespan perspectives on natural disasters*. New York, NY: Springer.

Weathers, F. W., Litz, B. T., Keane, T. M., Palmieri, P. A., Marx, B. P., & Schnurr, P. P. (2013). *The PTSD checklist for DSM-5 (PCL-5). Scale available from the National Center for PTSD*. Boston, MA: National Center for PTSD.

Weems, C. F., & Graham, R. A. (2014). Resilience and trajectories of posttraumatic stress among youth exposed to disaster. *Journal of Child and Adolescent Psychopharmacology, 24*(1), 2–8.

Winston, F. K., Kassam-Adams, N., Garcia-Espana, F., Ittenbach, R., & Cnaan, A. (2003). Screening for risk of persistent posttraumatic stress in injured children and their parents. *Journal of the American Medical Association, 290*, 643–649.

World Health Organization. (2001) *The World Health Report 2001: Mental health—new understanding, new hope*. Geneva: World Health Organization.

Yule, W., Udwin, O., & Bolton, D. (2002). Mass transportation disasters. In: A. M. La Greca, W. K. Silverman, E. M. Vernberg, & M. C. Roberts (Eds.), Helping children cope with disasters and terrorism (pp. 223–240). Washington, DC: American Psychological Association.

Zolkoski, S. M., & Bullock, L. M. (2012). Resilience in children and youth: A review. *Children and Youth Services Review, 34*(12), 2295–2303.

Tics and Tourette's Syndrome

W. Jason Peters and Johnny L. Matson

Introduction

Tics are typically defined or described as sudden, rapid, repetitive, and purposeless vocalizations or motor movements (Cath et al., 2011; Cohen, Leckman, & Bloch, 2013). Additionally, tics generally occur in bouts and tend to vary in regard to frequency, intensity, and type. Different types of tics include motor, phonic (vocal), sensory, and cognitive tics. Motor tics are often seen as fragments of typical motor movements, generally involve discrete muscle groups, and appear to occur out of context (Leckman, Yeh, & Cohen, 2001). Phonic tics involve the movement of air through the mouth, nose, or pharynx and consist of any noise produced by such air movement (Cath et al., 2011). These types of tics are sometimes referred to as vocal tics; however, because not all tics of this type are produced via movement of the vocal cords, the term phonic is preferred. Sensory tics refer to sensations that may often precede other tics (Leckman, 2003). These types of tics typically involve the experience of unpleasant, or uncomfortable, somatosensory sensations somewhere within the body (e.g., abdominal discomfort, stabbing pain, tiredness,

W. J. Peters (✉) · J. L. Matson
Department of Psychology, Louisiana State University, Baton Rouge, LA, USA
e-mail: wpeter7@lsu.edu

itch, etc.). Lastly, cognitive tics, which primarily occur in adolescents and adults, refer to repetitive thoughts (Cath et al., 1992). These thoughts are generally not motivated by anxiety or feelings of anxiety but instead occur in response to an urge to act upon salient or provocative stimuli in the environment.

Other defining characteristics of tics include complexity (i.e., simple or complex), duration, whether they occur in isolation or multiply occur, and location (Cath et al., 2011; Cohen et al., 2013). Simple tics generally involve a single muscle contraction, such as in simple motor tics involving the eyes (e.g., eye blinking) or in simple phonic tics involving brief vocalizations comprised of single sounds (e.g., grunting; Cohen et al., 2013). Complex tics, as opposed to simple tics, may involve several muscles or groups of muscles (e.g., hand or arm gestures) or the utterance of whole words or phrases. According to Cath et al. (2011), tics can be isolated (i.e., originating from one anatomical location) or occur at multiple locations.

Tics and tic disorders generally onset during childhood with a mean age of onset at 5 years and follow a pattern of waxing and waning over time (Cath et al., 2011; Cohen et al., 2013; Leckman et al., 1998). According to Leckman et al. (1998), tic severity is at its worst at approximately 10 years of age. However, most individuals experience a reduction in regard to tic frequency and

© Springer International Publishing AG, part of Springer Nature 2018
J. L. Matson (ed.), *Handbook of Childhood Psychopathology and Developmental Disabilities Assessment*, Autism and Child Psychopathology Series,
https://doi.org/10.1007/978-3-319-93542-3_13

severity as they age, with approximately 80% of individuals no longer experiencing any impairment as a result of tics by the age of 18 (Cath et al., 2011; Leckman et al., 1998; Pappert, Goetz, Louis, Blasucci, & Leurgans, 2003). Alternatively, an estimated 20% of individuals either do not improve or worsen in regard to their tic severity (Cath et al., 2011). According to Cohen et al. (2013), simple motor tics are usually the first to appear in the individual, followed by simple phonic tics. Additionally, motor tics typically progress from simple tics to more complex tics over time (Leckman et al., 1998). According to Cath et al. (2011), while it is fairly common for motor tics to present without concomitant phonic tics, it is rare (i.e., less than 5% of individuals) for phonic tics to present without motor tics.

According to the *Diagnostic and Statistical Manual of Mental Disorders, Fifth Edition* (DSM-5), at present, there are three main tic disorders including Tourette's disorder, persistent (chronic) motor and vocal tic disorder (PMVTD), and provisional tic disorder (American Psychiatric Association (APA), 2013). Diagnoses are based on the presence and duration of tics, the age of onset, and the absence of any known cause (e.g., medical); however, all three disorders differ somewhat in regard to their diagnostic criteria. While all three disorders require age of onset prior to age 18 years, they differ in regard to the type of tics as well as the duration in which tics have been present. For example, a diagnosis of provisional tic disorder requires that tics have been present for less than 1 year since onset, while both Tourette's disorder, otherwise known as Tourette's syndrome (TS), and PMVTD require that tics have been present for at least 1 year. Additionally, a diagnosis of TS requires the presence of both multiple motor tics and at least one phonic (vocal) tic, whereas a diagnosis of PMVTD requires that either motor or phonic tics, but not both, are present. Similar to TS, a diagnosis of provisional tic disorder does not require the presence of either type of tic alone. According to the DSM-5, the tic disorders are arranged in a hierarchy, with TS at the top followed by PMVTD and provisional tic disorder, such that if individuals meet criteria for one tic disorder, they can no longer meet criteria for another tic disorder further below on the hierarchy (APA, 2013). For example, an individual who meets criteria and is diagnosed with PMVTD can no longer be diagnosed with provisional tic disorder.

Tics are somewhat common in childhood, with up to approximately 18% of children developing a motor tic at some point during childhood (Peterson, Pine, Cohen, & Brook, 2001). However, the prevalence of tics declines over the life span as an estimated 1% of adults engage in tics. Prevalence estimates for tic disorders and TS typically range from 0.3% to 3% (APA, 2013; Freeman et al., 2000; Khalifa & Knorring, 2005), with some researchers suggesting higher estimates at approximately 18% (Robertson, 2003). More recent research suggests that the estimated prevalence of TS ranges from 0.08% to 0.52%, with population-based epidemiological studies demonstrating higher prevalence estimates than those based on clinical samples (Scharf et al., 2015). However, some researchers agree that a number of individuals with TS may not have been identified and diagnosed, therefore lowering prevalence estimates (Bruun & Budman, 1997; Freeman et al., 2000; Peterson & Cohen, 1998). In regard to gender differences, males are typically more likely to experience tics and be diagnosed with a tic disorder, with approximate male-to-female ratios ranging from 2:1 to 4.3:1 (APA, 2013; Freeman et al., 2000; Robertson, 2003).

Comorbidities

Tics frequently present and are commonly associated with other psychopathology including attention-deficit/hyperactivity disorder (ADHD) and obsessive-compulsive disorder (OCD), among others. According to Hirschtritt et al. (2015), a majority of individuals with tics and TS experience comorbid psychopathology with an estimated lifetime prevalence of 85.7%. Additionally, a majority of those individuals (57.7%) with comorbid disorders experienced two or more. One of the most common comorbid disorders among individuals with tics and tic disorders is ADHD (Cath et al., 2011; Freeman, 2007; Lebowitz et al., 2012). According to Simpson, Jung, and Murphy (2011), individuals diagnosed with ADHD may have an elevated risk for developing an associated tic disorder. Further, tic disorders may occur at slightly greater rates among adults with ADHD (Spencer et al., 2001). Alternatively, individuals diagnosed with a tic disorder may also be at higher risk for developing ADHD (Freeman, 2007; Simpson et al., 2011). Previous researchers have found that ADHD onset often precedes onset of TS and, interestingly, may lead to earlier onset of TS (Comings, 2000; Freeman, 2007). Additionally, the presence of comorbid ADHD is associated with higher levels of disruptive behavior as well as psychosocial impairments (Cath et al., 2011; Gorman et al., 2010; Sukhodolsky et al., 2003). Further, individuals with comorbid ADHD and tic disorders experience higher levels of psychosocial stress (Lebowitz et al., 2012).

Another one of the most common comorbid disorders among individuals with tics and tic disorders is that of OCD (Cath et al., 2011; Hirschtritt et al., 2015; Lebowitz et al., 2012). Much like individuals with comorbid ADHD, individuals with comorbid tics and OCD are at risk for poorer psychosocial outcomes and poor quality of life (Cath et al., 2011; Gorman et al., 2010). The presence of comorbid OCD is also associated with greater tic severity and higher levels of internalizing problems (e.g., anxiety or depression; Lebowitz et al., 2012). Further, symptoms of OCD in individuals with TS tend to worsen with age and are more likely to persist than the individual's tics (Bloch et al., 2006). Tics and tic disorders are also commonly associated with anxiety, depression, autism, and externalizing problems such as disruptive behavior or anger (Cavanna et al., 2015; Eapen, Fox-Hiley, Banerjee, & Robertson, 2004; Hirschtritt et al., 2015; Huisman-van Dijk, van de Schoot, Rijkeboer, Mathews, & Cath, 2016). Given the high rates of comorbid disorders in individuals with tics and tic disorders and their associated difficulties (e.g., poor outcomes, psychosocial impairment, etc.), it is particularly important to assess and account for these comorbid conditions.

Associated Characteristics and Difficulties

Tics and tic disorders are often associated with functional impairments across a number of domains, poorer quality of life, and reduced psychosocial functioning (Cavanna et al., 2013; Conelea, Woods, Zinner, et al., 2011; McGuire et al., 2015; O'Hare, Helmes, et al., 2016). For example, Storch et al. (2007) found a majority of parents reporting tic-related impairment in at least one domain for their children with TS, with many reporting impairment in two or more. Additionally, these concerns can be exacerbated when comorbid disorders, such as ADHD or OCD, are present (Cavanna et al., 2013). However, findings regarding the relationship between tics and quality of life have been mixed. For example, while some researchers have demonstrated significant associations between tic severity and poorer quality of life or impairment (Conelea, Woods, Zinner, et al., 2011; Cutler, Murphy, Gilmour, & Heyman, 2009; Eddy et al., 2011), others have failed to find such an association (Bernard et al., 2009; Eddy et al., 2011). McGuire et al. (2015), in an attempt to evaluate how different dimensions of tics, such as severity, type, frequency, intensity, complexity, and others, demonstrated that these characteristics of tics significantly predicted impairment. However, those characteristics of tics that predicted impairment differed according to rater (i.e., clinician, parent, child), suggesting that the many aspects of tic phenomenology are emphasized differently in regard to conceptualizing impairment across raters. Other researchers have demonstrated similar differences between parent- and child-rated impairment (Cavanna et al., 2013).

In addition to experiencing significant impairment or poorer quality of life as a result of tics, individuals exhibiting tics are also subject to significant bullying, teasing, harassment, and stigmatization (Malli, Forrester-Jones, & Murphy, 2016). Many aspects of tic disorders and TS may make it more likely that an individual will experience these difficulties as a result. For example, according to Malli et al. (2016), many tics are highly visible and difficult to conceal unlike other problems or difficulties. Additionally, the individual engaging in tics may be perceived by an observer as being responsible for and able to control their tics. As a result, the individual exhibiting tics may be held accountable for their actions, and others may react negatively (i.e., become angry). Further, tics are considered disruptive to interpersonal communication and social interactions, as well as visually displeasing. Taken together, this suggests a need for anti-stigma interventions for this population as it is apparent that a number of misconceptions exist about tics and individuals with tic disorders.

Many individuals with TS and other tic disorders experience premonitory urges, which are sometimes referred to as sensory tics. Premonitory urges are uncomfortable sensations such as aches, itching, tension, pressure, etc. that occur immediately prior to engaging in tics (Cath et al., 2011; Reese et al., 2014; Steinberg et al., 2010). According to Steinberg et al. (2010), these sensations are often described as unpleasant or aversive. Additionally, many individuals with TS and tic disorders indicate that premonitory urges may, in fact, be more distressing than tics themselves (Reese et al., 2014). Some researchers have suggested that premonitory urges may play an important role in tics and their maintenance as tics may be negatively reinforced by the removal of the uncomfortable sensations associated with the urges upon completion of tics (Woods et al., 2008). Similarly, other researchers have suggested that the execution of the tic is a conscious and intentional decision by the individual so as to relieve the uncomfortable sensations associated with the premonitory urge (Lang, 1991). According to Leckman (2003), children typically do not experience this intentionality associated with their tics. Additionally, they either rarely experience premonitory urges or are unaware of their presence prior to approximately age 10 years, while a majority of adults report awareness of premonitory urges and sensations preceding their tics.

Treatment of Tourette's Syndrome and Tic Disorders

In regard to treatment for individuals with TS and tic disorders, the primary method of intervention is pharmacological in nature (O'Hare, Helmes, et al., 2016; Robertson, 2012). Pharmacological interventions are primarily intended to reduce the severity of tics; however, they vary in regard to their efficacy and are often associated with adverse side effects (O'Hare, Eapen, et al., 2016; Robertson, 2012; Woods, Conelea, & Himle, 2010). Alternative treatments for individuals with TS and tic disorders do exist such as behavioral interventions and deep brain stimulation (Maciunas et al., 2007; Scahill et al., 2006; Woods et al., 2010). However, these interventions also vary in regard to their efficacy in treating individuals with TS and tic disorders and are primarily used in conjunction with pharmacological interventions. While treatment is undoubtedly an important aspect of working with individuals with TS and tic disorders, a discussion of treatment is outside of the scope of this chapter.

Assessment Methods

Within the last 30–40 years, a number of rating scales, interviews, and screening instruments have been developed to assess the presence and characteristics (e.g., type, frequency, complexity, severity) of tics. A significant body of research has been developed surrounding tics and tic disorders, such as TS, and these methods of assessment have been an integral part of that literature. The following sections describe and review these assessment methods.

Rating Scales

Rating scales are a widely used and popular method for assessing a number of concerns including anxiety, depression, challenging behaviors, social skills, and many more. Generally, rating scales consist of items designed to represent and measure a particular construct, and those items are typically based on how often an individual engages in a particular behavior. On average, rating scales are comprised of between 25 and 75 items and take between 10 and 30 min to administer (Matson & Wilkins, 2009). Normative data, which are used to evaluate the individual's scores, are generally based on age and gender. Additionally, rating scales generally take a multi-informant approach, where parents, teachers, or other persons familiar with the individual being assessed provide ratings on the individual's behavior.

Rating scales and their use have several advantages. For example, rating scales have the ability to rate and assess less frequent behaviors. Additionally, they can be used in settings where resources (e.g., time) may be limited, due to their efficiency. While there are advantages to using rating scales, it is important to note that there are also some limitations. For example, the assessment of behavior using rating scales may not reliably or accurately capture the changing nature of behavior as rating scales typically focus on the individual's current or recent levels of behavior. This suggests the need for follow-up evaluations. An additional concern is that ratings may vary across multiple informants. The use of multiple informants may therefore provide an inaccurate representation of the individual's behavior. Further, rating scales may be subject to a rater's opinions or biases in regard to the individual being assessed. Therefore, it is strongly suggested that other assessment methods (e.g., direct observation) be used in combination with rating scales.

Yale Global Tic Severity Scale

The Yale Global Tic Severity Scale (YGTSS; Leckman et al., 1989) is a semi-structured interview designed to assess for the presence and severity of motor and phonic tics. It is one of the most widely used rating scales for tics and tic disorders and is recommended for use by international guidelines (Cath et al., 2011). The YGTSS assesses the presence of motor and phonic tics across five separate dimensions including frequency, intensity, number, complexity, and level of interference (Leckman et al., 1989). Items on the YGTSS are rated on a six-point ordinal scale, ranging from 0 to 5, with each point being accompanied by a descriptive anchor statement and relevant examples. Additionally, the YGTSS provides an additional scale designed to measure the cumulative toll the individual experiences as a result of tics. This scale provides an overall rating of impairment based on the impact of tics experienced by the individual over the past week, including impact on peer and/or social relationships, self-esteem and self-perception, or ability to perform in a vocational or academic setting. The YGTSS can be administered to multiple informants (e.g., parents, teachers, etc.); however, it requires a trained assessor, usually a clinician, to administer the interview (Leckman et al., 1989). Originally appearing in English, the YGTSS has been translated and validated into several languages including Korean (Chung et al., 1998), Polish (Stefanoff & Wolańczyk, 2004), Spanish (García-López et al., 2008), and Chinese (Wang, Qi, Li, Zhao, & Li, 2012).

Research on the YGTSS has demonstrated good psychometric properties including good internal consistency across the motor, phonic, and total tic severity scores, as well as good interrater and test-retest reliability (Leckman et al., 1989; Storch et al., 2005; Walkup, Rosenberg, Brown, & Singer, 1992). Previous research has also established convergent validity, with the YGTSS demonstrating moderate-to-strong relationships with other measures of tics and tic severity (Leckman et al., 1989; Walkup et al., 1992). Further, strong divergent validity has been demonstrated for the YGTSS as evinced by small-to-moderate associations with measures of ADHD, OCD, depression, and aggression (Leckman et al., 1989; Storch et al., 2005). Factor analyses on the YGTSS have demonstrated a two-factor solution consistent with the original design of the scale (Leckman et al., 1989; Storch, Murphy, et al., 2007). However, while these analyses demonstrated that the motor and phonic tics subscales represent separate but related dimensions, results also suggested that the item measuring overall impairment may capture impairments primarily related to phonic tics (Storch, Murphy, et al., 2007).

The YGTSS is one of the most widely used measures of tics and tic severity and has been used across a number of different types of research. For example, the YGTSS has been used in clinical pharmacotherapy trials as an outcome measure of tic severity (Gadow, Sverd, Nolan, Sprafkin, & Schneider, 2007; Howson et al., 2004; Packer-Hopke & Motta, 2014). Additionally, the YGTSS has been used to correlate current levels of tic severity with behavioral and social competence (Capriotti, Brandt, Turkel, Lee, & Woods, 2014; Conelea, Woods, & Brandt, 2011; Himle et al., 2014; Lewin et al., 2012) as well as biomarkers (Fahim et al., 2010; Lemay, Lê, Richer, & Montreal Tourette Study Group, 2010).

Shapiro Tourette Syndrome Severity Scale

The Shapiro Tourette Syndrome Severity Scale (STSS; Shapiro, Shapiro, Young, & Feinberg, 1988), previously known as the Tourette Syndrome Severity Scale, is a rating scale designed to evaluate the initial severity and change in severity of tics and TS as well as the level of interference. The STSS consists of five questions, each rated by the individual being assessed or an informant, as well as a clinician, on an ordinal scale ranging from 0 (i.e., "none") to 9 (i.e., "very severe"). The questions on the STSS ask the individual to rate to what degree tics are noticeable to others, interfere with functioning, elicit comments or curiosity from others, and cause the individual to appear odd or bizarre (Shapiro et al., 1988). The final question on the STSS asks whether the individual is hospitalized, homebound, or incapacitated. Responses to these questions provide a global severity score. Unlike other measures (e.g., the YGTSS), the STSS does not assess the frequency or the complexity of tics. According to Shapiro et al. (1988), administration of the STSS typically requires less than 5 min.

Previous research on the STSS has demonstrated adequate psychometric properties for the measure. According to Walkup et al. (1992), the STSS demonstrates good interrater reliability. Additionally, internal consistency analyses have indicated that the STSS is excellent in this regard (Shapiro et al., 1988). Further, moderate-to-strong convergent validity with other measures examining tic severity, as well as adequate divergent validity with severity measures of ADHD and OCD, has also been indicated (Walkup et al., 1992). The STSS has been used as an outcome measure for tics and TS in clinical pharmacotherapy trials examining and comparing the effects of pimozide, haloperidol, and placebo (Shapiro et al., 1989; Shapiro & Shapiro, 1984).

Rush Video-Based Tic Rating Scale

The Rush Video-Based Tic Rating Scale (RVBTRS; Goetz, Tanner, Wilson, & Shannon, 1987) is a rating scale that uses a video-based filming protocol to rate the presence of tics, their severity, as well as the number of body areas involved. The RVBTRS assesses both motor and phonic tics. The filming protocol of the RVBTRS involves a 10-min film which makes use of two separate views under two different conditions. According to the scale developers (Goetz et al., 1987), the individual being assessed is filmed while relaxed, both with and without an examiner in the room. Originally, the RVBTRS was scored using a method combining scores in regard to tic frequency, tic distribution (e.g., body areas involved), and tic severity, each with a different scaling method (Goetz et al., 1987). For example, tic severity was rated on a scale ranging from 0 to 5, while the tic distribution scale ranged from 0 to 11. However, this scoring method has since been revised. Currently, the RVBTRS maintains the original scoring domains including frequency of motor and phonic tics, severity of motor and phonic tics, and number of body areas involved, but, instead of different scaling methods across domains, all domains are rated on a scale ranging from 0 to 4 with descriptive, fixed anchor points (Goetz, Pappert, Louis, Raman, & Leurgans, 1999).

Analyses of the psychometric properties for the RVBTRS have demonstrated excellent interrater reliability across all domains (Goetz et al., 1987). Additionally, moderate convergent validity has been demonstrated with other tic rating scales such as the STSS, the Tourette Syndrome

Global Scale, and the YGTSS (Goetz et al., 1987, 1999,). Further, psychometric analyses have demonstrated adequate structural validity for the RVBTRS (Goetz et al., 1987). According to Martino et al. (2017), analyses regarding divergent validity have not been conducted for the RVBTRS, demonstrating a potential weakness of this measure. Additionally, the use of audiovisual equipment for this measure has not yet been clearly standardized. Previous research using the RVBTRS has used the scale as an outcome measure in a clinical pharmacotherapy trial (Onofrj, Paci, D'andreamatteo, & Toma, 2000) as well as a longitudinal study examining the long-term outcome of TS (Pappert et al., 2003). Additionally, the RVBTRS has demonstrated use as a measure to assess tic inhibitory potential, which refers to an individual's ability to actively suppress tics (Ganos et al., 2012).

Tourette Syndrome-Clinical Global Impression Scale

The Tourette Syndrome-Clinical Global Impression (TS-CGI; Leckman, Towbin, Ort, & Cohen, 1988) is a rating scale that assesses the severity and overall impact of tics. The TS-CGI is one of a number of scales together known as the Clinical Global Impression of Severity scales. These are commonly used to assess symptom severity in individuals with psychiatric disorders. The items on the TS-CGI are each rated on a seven-point, Likert-type scale that ranks current symptom severity, ranging from "extremely severe" to "normal." Additionally, information for the TS-CGI ratings are based on interviews with the individual being assessed and/or their caregiver, in addition to direct examination and observation (Leckman et al., 1988). Similar to the STSS, the TS-CGI does not assess the individual dimensions of tics such as frequency or complexity. Psychometric analyses have indicated that the TS-CGI demonstrates good interrater reliability (Walkup et al., 1992). The TS-CGI also demonstrates moderate convergent validity with measures such as the YGTSS and STSS in addition to good divergent validity with measures of ADHD and OCD. Previous research has used the TS-CGI as an initial measure of tic severity (Gadow et al., 2007; Gadow, Sverd, Sprafkin, Nolan, & Ezor, 1995), as well as a measure for responsiveness to treatment in clinical pharmacotherapy trials (Budman et al., 2008; McConville et al., 1992).

Tourette's Disorder Scale

The Tourette's Disorder Scale (TODS; Shytle et al., 2003) is a rating scale that evaluates a number of symptoms including tics, aggression, hyperactivity, obsessions, compulsions, inattention, and mood/emotional disturbances, in addition to their severity. The TODS is comprised of 15 items, with each item rated between 0 and 10 along an ordinal scale. For each item on the TODS, raters are asked to what extent has the individual being assessed been bothered by that symptom with a score of 0 corresponding to "not at all," a score of 2 corresponding to "a little," a score of 5 corresponding to "moderately," a score of 8 corresponding to "markedly," and a score of 10 corresponding to "extremely" (Shytle et al., 2003). An overall total score for the TODS, ranging from 0 to 150, is generated by summing all item scores. Additionally, the TODS provides four separate subscale scores including aggression (five items), ADHD (four items), OCD (four items), and tics (two items). Currently, the TODS appears as two separate versions with one based on parent ratings (TODS-PR) and the other based on clinician ratings (TODS-CR). According to Shytle et al. (2003), parents are asked to base their ratings on observations of the individual's symptoms during the past week, and clinicians are asked to base their ratings on information gathered from the parent as well as the individual regarding their symptoms in reference to the same time frame.

Analyses regarding the psychometric properties of the TODS have indicated that the internal consistency is high for both versions of the measure (Shytle et al., 2003). However, follow-up analyses have demonstrated a lower internal consistency value for the tics subscale (0.64; Storch et al., 2004). According to Shytle et al. (2003), interrater reliability for items on the TODS ranged from moderate to good, with the item assessing motor tics demonstrating the highest value (0.79). Additionally, analyses have indicated that agreement between both versions of the TODS is high. Good convergent validity has been established as evidenced by positive associations between the TODS total score and the YGTSS severity score (Storch et al., 2004). Divergent validity with subscales of the Conners Parent Rating Scale has also been established. Lastly, both exploratory and confirmatory factor analyses have supported a four-factor structure consistent with the subscales on the TODS (Shytle et al., 2003; Storch et al., 2004). Research using the TODS has been limited; however, it has been used to examine changes in tic and related symptoms over time in response to aerobic exercise intervention (Packer-Hopke & Motta, 2014).

Tourette Syndrome Global Scale

The Tourette Syndrome Global Scale (TSGS; Harcherik, Leckman, Detlor, & Cohen, 1984) is a multidimensional scale designed to assess symptoms of TS and social functioning. It is primarily intended for use by clinicians who have prior experience with individuals with TS, as well as knowledge of TS symptomatology. According to the developers of the scale, information for ratings are based on clinician observation, in addition to parent and school reports on the individual's symptoms over the past week (Harcherik et al., 1984). The TSGS consists of eight dimensions, each of which is rated individually and is summed to create an overall global score. The eight dimensions of the TSGS are separated into two major domains measuring tics and aspects of social functioning, respectively. The first domain primarily assesses the frequency and degree of disruption of tics (Harcherik et al., 1984). The tics domain is comprised of four dimensions including simple motor tics, complex motor tics, simple phonic tics, and complex phonic tics. The social functioning domain primarily assesses areas related to social functioning and is also comprised of four dimensions including motor restlessness, behavioral problems, level of school functioning, and level of occupational functioning. Each domain contributes equally to their respective domain score, which then contributes equally to the total global score (Harcherik et al., 1984). The overall global score ranges from 0 (no symptoms) to 100 (worst possible symptoms).

Psychometric analyses indicate that the TSGS demonstrates good interrater reliability across all dimensions with the exception of the motor restlessness domain (Harcherik et al., 1984). Convergent validity with the Children's Global Assessment Scale (Shaffer et al., 1983), a measure of psychiatric symptoms and their severity, has also been established. Unfortunately, analyses regarding internal consistency and divergent validity have not been conducted (Martino et al., 2017); therefore, caution in using the TSGS is recommended. The TSGS has been primarily used as an outcome measure of tic severity in intervention trials (Müller-Vahl et al., 2002; O'Connor et al., 2009; Sallee, Nesbitt, Jackson, Sine, & Sethuraman, 1997), as well as observational studies examining the prevalence and characteristics of tics (Chee & Sachdev, 1997) and the relationship between metacognitions and tic onset (O'Connor, St-Pierre-Delorme, Leclerc, Lavoie, & Blais, 2014).

Global Tic Rating Scale

The Global Tic Rating Scale (GTRS; Gadow & Paolicell, 1986) is a rating scale that assesses the current frequency and severity of tics. The GTRS consists of nine total items, with five measuring tic frequency and the remaining four measuring the severity of tics. Additionally, the items measuring tic frequency are further subdivided into three items measuring motor tics and two measuring phonic tics, both verbal and nonverbal. Clinicians, parents or caregivers, and teachers can all provide separate ratings on the current presence, frequency, and severity of tics for the GTRS (Gadow & Paolicell, 1986). Items on the GTRS are rated on a four-point, Likert-type scale based on the frequency with which the individual exhibits their tic behavior, ranging from zero (not at all) to three (very much). Item ratings are subsequently summed to create three separate indices measuring both the frequency of motor and phonic tics and overall tic severity.

Analyses regarding the psychometric properties of the GTRS have been limited. While interrater reliability values for the motor tic frequency and the tic severity indices were good, the phonic tic index demonstrated only moderate interrater reliability (Nolan, Gadow, & Sverd, 1994). However, these data were based only on teacher ratings using the GTRS. According to Gadow et al. (2007), convergent validity with the YGTSS was low, demonstrating a potential weakness of the measure. At present, analyses regarding internal consistency and divergent validity have not been conducted (Martino et al., 2017). Research using the GTRS has been limited to one intervention trial examining the effects of immediate-release methylphenidate in a sample of children with comorbid ADHD and TS (Gadow et al., 2007).

Motor Tic, Obsessions and Compulsions, Vocal Tic Evaluation Survey

The Motor tic, Obsessions and compulsions, Vocal tic Evaluation Survey (MOVES; Gaffney, Sieg, & Hellings, 1994) is a rating scale measuring the severity of five sets of symptoms including both motor and phonic tics, obsessions, compulsions, and others (e.g., echolalia, coprolalia, etc.), each of which is a separate subscale. The MOVES is based on self-report and consists of 20 items, each rated on a four-point ordinal scale with anchor points ranging from zero (never) to three (always). According to Gaffney et al. (1994), the MOVES can be completed by individuals ranging in age from childhood to adulthood. Available psychometric data indicates that the MOVES demonstrates acceptable convergent validity with the total tic severity scores from the YGTSS and STSS (Gaffney et al., 1994). Similar to the GTRS, internal consistency and divergent validity analyses have not been conducted (Martino et al., 2017). Additional analyses examining the MOVES' utility as a screening instrument have indicated good sensitivity and specificity, as well as high positive and negative predictive values (Gaffney et al., 1994). The MOVES has been used to compare tic severity between individuals with TS and comorbid TS and ADHD (Haddad, Umoh, Bhatia, & Robertson, 2009). Additionally, researchers have used the MOVES as a measure of change in response to repetitive transcranial magnetic stimulation as an intervention for individuals with TS (Münchau et al., 2002; Orth et al., 2005).

Parent Tic Questionnaire

The Parent Tic Questionnaire (PTQ; Chang, Himle, Tucker, Woods, & Piacentini, 2009) is an inventory designed to evaluate the presence, frequency, and intensity of both motor and phonic tics. The PTQ is comprised of 2 separate lists composed of 14 common motor and 14 common phonic tics. Upon indicating the presence for each tic over the past week, parents provide ratings regarding their frequency and intensity. Frequency ratings for each endorsed tic are made using a four-point, Likert-type scale ranging from one (weekly) to four (constantly). Additionally, intensity ratings are made using the same scale ranging from one to four, where higher ratings are associated with higher intensity (Himle et al., 2012). Scores for each endorsed tic are calculated by summing frequency and intensity ratings, which range from zero (tic absent) to eight (maximum frequency and intensity; Conelea, Woods, Zinner, et al., 2011). Three separate severity scores (e.g., motor, phonic, and total) are created by summing the individual tic scores.

Psychometric analyses have indicated that the PTQ demonstrates excellent internal consistency, as well as good test-retest reliability (Chang et al., 2009). Additionally, the PTQ correlates highly with the YGTSS, indicating strong convergent validity. Further, divergent validity between the PTQ and measures of OCD as well as inattention has also been established (Chang et al., 2009; Espil, Capriotti, Conelea, & Woods, 2014). Prior research has used the PTQ as a secondary outcome measure following behavioral intervention (Himle et al., 2012; Piacentini et al., 2010), a predictor of tic-related impairment (Espil et al., 2014), and a measure of tic severity in a sample of peer-victimized youth (Zinner, Conelea, Glew, Woods, & Budman, 2012).

Tourette Syndrome Symptom List

The Tourette Syndrome Symptom List (TSSL; Cohen, Leckman, & Shaywitz, 1985) is a scale designed to assess the frequency and disruption of tics as well as related behaviors. The TSSL is comprised of a list of 41 symptoms, which are rated on a six-point, Likert-type scale with anchor points defined by the frequency with which that particular symptom is occurring ranging from 0 (i.e., "not at all or symptom-free") to 5 (i.e., "almost always"; Müller-Vahl et al., 2010). The 41 symptoms on the TSSL measure 36 types of tics, with the remaining 5 measuring related, non-tic behaviors. According to Cohen et al. (1985), the TSSL was designed and intended to assist raters, primarily parents, in daily or weekly ratings of tics. Scores from the 41 items are summed to create a total score, which can be used to compare the frequencies and disruptions of tics on a week-to-week basis. Additionally, the number of symptoms within each subdomain on the TSSL is counted over the course of a week (Cohen et al., 1985).

Although originally designed to be used with parents or caregivers as raters, the TSSL has been used as a self-report measure of tic frequency (Sallee et al., 1997). Additionally, previous research has used the TSSL as a secondary outcome measure in intervention trials examining the efficacy of medication (Sallee et al., 1997) or deep brain stimulation (Maciunas et al., 2007) in treating TS and when evaluating health-related quality of life (Müller-Vahl et al., 2010). According to Martino et al. (2017), the psychometric properties for the TSSL have not been formally evaluated demonstrating a significant weakness in using the TSSL.

Hopkins Motor and Vocal Tic Scale

The Hopkins Motor and Vocal Tic Scale (HMVTS; Walkup et al., 1992) is a rating scale that is comprised of a series of linear, visual analog scales on which raters rank each tic symptom, both motor and phonic. Each tic symptom is ranked while taking into consideration several characteristics of tics including its frequency, intensity, impairment, and interference. One of the strengths of the HMVTS is that it utilizes an individualized approach and can be changed to reflect the individual's current tic symptoms (Walkup et al., 1992). Both parents or caregivers and clinicians are required to provide separate ratings on the individual's current tic symptoms. Raters are told that each linear scale ranges from 0 (i.e., "no tics") to ten (i.e., "most severe") and that each scale can be divided into four ranges including mild, moderate, moderately severe, and severe (Walkup et al., 1992). Additionally, raters are instructed to consider the severity of tics in reference to the past week. Three final scores for both motor and phonic tics are derived based on parent report, clinician observation, and an overall assessment. Scores use a five-point, ordinal scale ranging from 1 (i.e., "no tics") to 5 (i.e., "severe"). According to the scale developers, it is permissible to use divisions of 0.5 in the final scores (Walkup et al., 1992).

Psychometric analyses of the HMVTS have revealed that it demonstrates excellent interrater reliability for both the motor and phonic tic scores (Walkup et al., 1992). Additionally, the HMVTS demonstrates high convergent validity with other measures of tics and tic severity including the YGTSS, STSS, and TS-CGI. Lastly, the HMVTS also demonstrates high divergent validity with severity measures for ADHD and OCD (Walkup et al., 1992). Use of the HMVTS by other researchers has been limited, however, as it has only been used as a measure of responsiveness to change in an intervention trial (Singer et al., 1995).

Premonitory Urge for Tics Scale

The Premonitory Urge for Tics Scale (PUTS; Woods, Piacentini, Himle, & Chang, 2005) is a self-report rating scale designed to evaluate premonitory urges and their current presence and frequency. The PUTS originally consisted of ten items; however, the final item was ultimately removed after analyses demonstrated that it did not correlate well with other items and the total score (Woods et al., 2005). Currently, the PUTS is comprised of nine items, each rated on a four-point, ordinal scale ranging from one (not at all true) to four (very much true). A total score, created by adding each item score, reflects the presence and frequency of premonitory urges where higher scores indicate more premonitory urges. Additionally, the total score reflects relief that individuals may experience after tics occur (Woods et al., 2005). Originally appearing in English, the PUTS has been translated into and validated in Hebrew (Steinberg et al., 2010) and Italian (Gulisano, Calì, Palermo, Robertson, & Rizzo, 2015).

Analyses regarding the psychometric properties of the PUTS have indicated good internal consistency and test-retest reliability (Woods et al., 2005). Additionally, concurrent validity with the total severity score and individual subscale scores on the YGTSS was established as evidenced by significant, positive correlations (Reese et al., 2014; Woods et al., 2005). Further, analyses have not supported associations between the PUTS and measures of ADHD or intellectual abilities, demonstrating divergent validity. The majority of the research using the PUTS has examined its development and validation (Gulisano et al., 2015; Reese et al., 2014; Steinberg et al., 2010; Woods et al., 2005); however, it has also been used to examine the relationship between premonitory urges and sensory gating (Sutherland Owens, Miguel, & Swerdlow, 2011), as well as interoceptive awareness (Ganos et al., 2015).

Child Tourette's Syndrome Impairment Scale

The Child Tourette's Syndrome Impairment Scale (CTIM; Storch, Lack, et al., 2007) is a rating scale designed to measure the impact a child's tics or other comorbid difficulties (e.g., anxiety, depression, etc.) have on their daily activities at school, home, or during social activities. The CTIM is primarily a parent-rated measure; however, a child self-report version has recently been developed (Cloes et al., 2016). For the parent version (CTIM-P), parents are asked to rate to what extent their child's tics have impacted or caused difficulties across a number of areas (e.g., "doing household chores") over the past month (Storch, Lack, et al., 2007). The child version (CTIM-C) asks children to rate how tics have impacted their own functioning across the same areas and tasks (Cloes et al., 2016). Both versions of the CTIM consist of 37 items, each rated on a four-point, Likert-type scale ranging from 0 (not at all) to 3 (very much). Additionally, the CTIM is composed of two separate subscales, or dimensions, measuring tic impairment and non-tic impairment, respectively (Storch, Lack, et al., 2007).

Psychometric analyses have indicated that the CTIM demonstrates excellent internal consistency for both tic and non-tic items (Storch, Lack, et al., 2007). Additionally, the CTIM demonstrates convergent validity with the YGTSS and Child Behavior Checklist (CBCL; Achenbach & Rescorla, 2001), as indicated by significant associations between scores. Further, analyses have demonstrated agreement across both versions of this scale, as well as across both dimensions within each version (Cloes et al., 2016). The CTIM has been used in research examining quality of life (Cavanna et al., 2013) as well as suicidal thoughts and behaviors in children with TS (Storch et al., 2015), both as a primary and secondary measure, respectively, of impairment associated with tics.

Screening Instruments

Autism-Tics, Attention-Deficit/ Hyperactivity Disorder, and Other Comorbidities Inventory

The autism-tics, attention-deficit/hyperactivity disorder, and other comorbidities inventory (A-TAC; Hansson et al., 2005) is a comprehensive screening instrument designed to assess for different symptoms across several disorders including tic disorders, developmental coordination disorders, ASD, and ADHD, among others. It is primarily used in epidemiological research (Larson et al., 2014) and can be administered by either professionals or trained lay assessors (Larson et al., 2013). Additionally, the A-TAC inventory can be administered either in person or over the telephone. The original version of the A-TAC inventory was composed of 178 items; however, it currently consists of 264 items divided into 20 separate modules each intended to measure a separate set of symptoms (e.g., motor control, concentration and attention, language, etc.; Larson et al., 2014). These modules are designed to provide dimensional ratings on a number of different systems as well as the problem load associated with each set of symptoms (Larson et al., 2010). Originally, each item on the A-TAC inventory had four possible responses: "yes" or "yes, previously," each of which was scored as a 1; "yes, to some extent," which was scored as a 0.5; and "no," which was scored as a 0 (Hansson et al., 2005). Currently, the A-TAC items have only three possible responses after removal of the "yes, previously" response (Larson et al., 2010).

The present version of the A-TAC inventory makes use of a gate structure, whereby "gate" items are used to determine which modules need to be administered in full (Larson et al., 2010). According to Larson et al. (2014), the gate items, of which there are 96, are intended to predict salient features of a particular module. This is one of the advantages of the A-TAC inventory in that it allows for the possibility that not all modules will require administration in full, therefore saving time. The additional items within each module beyond the gate items are only administered if one or more of the gate items are endorsed, either partially (i.e., "yes, to some extent") or fully (i.e., "yes"; Larson et al., 2010). Beyond the 96 gate items, the A-TAC consists of items which are used to identify specific symptoms within each module as well as items intended to address other associated concerns such as subjective suffering, psychosocial dysfunction, whether the problems are currently occurring, and age of onset. The tics module specifically consists of three gate items and five follow-up items.

Previous research on the A-TAC inventory has demonstrated good psychometric properties including good interrater and test-retest reliability (Hansson et al., 2005), as well as good to excellent sensitivity and specificity (Larson et al., 2013). Additionally, previous research on the gate items specifically has also demonstrated good values for sensitivity (Larson et al., 2010). The A-TAC inventory has also demonstrated convergent validity with the CBCL (Halleröd et al., 2010). Research on the tics module has demonstrated moderate interrater reliability (Larson et al., 2014), moderate sensitivity, and excellent specificity and predictive validity (Larson et al., 2013).

Proxy Report Questionnaire for Parents and Teachers

The Proxy Report Questionnaire for Parents and Teachers (PRQPT; Linazasoro, Van Blercom, & Ortiz De Zárate, 2006) is a screening instrument comprised of two yes/no questions. It can be completed by either parents or teachers and is designed to be the first step in a two-stage screening procedure. According to Cubo et al. (2011), the PRQPT includes a brief description of tics and the most common types of tics followed by two questions asking parents or teachers whether or not the individual being assessed exhibits tics or has done so previously. The second step in this two-stage procedure consists of direct behavioral observation performed by trained raters. Previous research on the PRQPT indicates that it demonstrates moderate to excellent sensitivity and specificity, depending on the rater (i.e., parent, teacher, or observer; Cubo et al., 2011). The PRQPT has primarily been used as a screening instrument in epidemiological research (Cubo et al., 2013).

Apter 4-Questions Screening

The Apter 4-questions screening (Apter 4-q; Apter et al., 1993) is a questionnaire designed to assess for the presence of tics across an individual's lifetime. It is composed of four questions where the respondent is required to answer either yes or no. Although originally designed as a self-report, the Apter 4-q has also been used in instances where teachers have served as the informant (Hornsey, Banerjee, Zeitlin, & Robertson, 2001). One of the advantages of this measure is that it is brief and quick to administer (i.e., less than 2 min). Previous research has demonstrated that the measure has poor specificity and excellent sensitivity, indicating that the Apter 4-q is better able to identify individuals exhibiting tics than those who are not (Apter et al., 1993). The Apter 4-q has been primarily used in epidemiological studies examining the prevalence of tics and tic disorders (Apter et al., 1993;

Hornsey et al., 2001). Data from those studies have been in agreement with previous estimates regarding the prevalence of tics and tic disorders supporting the potential utility of the Apter 4-q in the assessment of tics in this manner. Due to its high sensitivity and low specificity, it is recommended that the Apter 4-q be used as a screening instrument (Martino et al., 2017).

Conclusion

Typically, tics are defined as sudden, rapid, repetitive, and purposeless motor movements or vocalizations (Cath et al., 2011; Cohen et al., 2013). Defining characteristics of tics include complexity (i.e., simple or complex), frequency, intensity, duration, whether they occur in isolation or multiply occur, location, and type (i.e., motor, phonic, sensory, and cognitive). Tics and tic disorders typically onset in childhood and tend to wax and wane in regard to severity over time, often reaching peak severity at approximately the age of 10 (Leckman et al., 1998). Further, tics and tic disorders are often comorbid with other psychopathology including ADHD and OCD (Cath et al., 2011; Hirschtritt et al., 2015). This chapter described and reviewed a number of different assessment measures for tics and tic disorders and presented evidence supporting their use.

Overall, the majority of assessment methods for tics and tic disorders reviewed here consisted of rating scales, semi-structured interviews, and screening instruments primarily designed to assess for the presence of tics. Additionally, other characteristics of tics including severity, frequency, and type were also commonly assessed. Other measures also assessed premonitory urges and psychosocial impairments which are additional characteristics associated with tics. Most measures made use of ordinal or Likert-type scales with some exceptions including a filming protocol (i.e., RVBTRS; Goetz et al., 1987) or linear, visual analog scales (i.e., HMVTS; Walkup et al., 1992). For many of the measures reviewed, previous research has demonstrated adequate to excellent psychometric properties indicating their potential utility in the assessment of tics and tic disorders. However, a number of measures either did not demonstrate adequate psychometrics or research regarding their psychometric properties was lacking. Given that the majority of these measures have been used in research outside of their original development and by researchers other than the developers, this highlights the need for these analyses to be carried out. It is also important to note that many of these scales were developed prior to the last two decades, suggesting a potential need for follow-up analyses of these measures to confirm or disconfirm their continued utility in assessing tics and tic disorders.

References

Achenbach, T. M., & Rescorla, L. A. (2001). *Manual for the Achenbach system of empirically based assessment school-age forms profiles*. Burlington, VT: Aseba.

American Psychiatric Association. (2013). *Diagnostic and statistical manual of mental disorders* (5th ed.). Washington, DC: American Psychiatric Association.

Apter, A., Pauls, D. L., Bleich, A., Zohar, A. H., Kron, S., Ratzoni, G., ... Cohen, D. J. (1993). An epidemiologic study of Gilles de la Tourette's syndrome in Israel. *Archives of General Psychiatry, 50*(9), 734–738.

Bernard, B. A., Stebbins, G. T., Siegel, S., Schultz, T. M., Hays, C., Morrissey, M. J., ... Goetz, C. G. (2009). Determinants of quality of life in children with Gilles de la Tourette syndrome. *Movement Disorders, 24*(7), 1070–1073.

Bloch, M. H., Peterson, B. S., Scahill, L., Otka, J., Katsovich, L., Zhang, H., & Leckman, J. F. (2006). Adulthood outcome of tic and obsessive-compulsive symptom severity in children with Tourette syndrome. *Archives of Pediatrics & Adolescent Medicine, 160*(1), 65–69.

Bruun, R. D., & Budman, C. L. (1997). The course and prognosis of Tourette syndrome. *Neurologic Clinics, 15*(2), 291–298.

Budman, C., Coffey, B. J., Shechter, R., Schrock, M., Wieland, N., Spirgel, A., & Simon, E. (2008). Aripiprazole in children and adolescents with Tourette disorder with and without explosive outbursts. *Journal of Child and Adolescent Psychopharmacology, 18*(5), 509–515.

Capriotti, M. R., Brandt, B. C., Turkel, J. E., Lee, H.-J., & Woods, D. W. (2014). Negative reinforcement and premonitory urges in youth with Tourette syndrome: An experimental evaluation. *Behavior Modification, 38*(2), 276–296.

Cath, D. C., Hedderly, T., Ludolph, A. G., Stern, J. S., Murphy, T., Hartmann, A., ... Rizzo, R. (2011).

European clinical guidelines for Tourette syndrome and other tic disorders. Part I: Assessment. *European Child & Adolescent Psychiatry, 20*(4), 155–171.
Cath, D. C., Hoogduin, C. A. L., Van de Wetering, B. J. M., Van Woerkom, T., Roos, R. A. C., & Rooymans, H. G. M. (1992). Tourette syndrome and obsessive-compulsive disorder: An analysis of associated phenomena. *Advances in Neurology, 58*, 33–41.
Cavanna, A. E., Luoni, C., Selvini, C., Blangiardo, R., Eddy, C. M., Silvestri, P. R., … Termine, C. (2013). Parent and self-report health-related quality of life measures in young patients with Tourette syndrome. *Journal of Child Neurology, 28*(10), 1305–1308.
Cavanna, A. E., Selvini, C., Luoni, C., Eddy, C. M., Ali, F., Blangiardo, R., … Termine, C. (2015). Measuring anger expression in young patients with Tourette syndrome. *Children's Health Care, 44*(3), 264–276. https://doi.org/10.1080/02739615.2014.896216
Chang, S., Himle, M. B., Tucker, B. T., Woods, D. W., & Piacentini, J. (2009). Initial psychometric properties of a brief parent-report instrument for assessing tic severity in children with chronic tic disorders. *Child & Family Behavior Therapy, 31*(3), 181–191.
Chee, K. Y., & Sachdev, P. (1997). A controlled study of sensory tics in Gilles de la Tourette syndrome and obsessive-compulsive disorder using a structured interview. *Journal of Neurology, Neurosurgery & Psychiatry, 62*(2), 188–192. https://doi.org/10.1136/jnnp.62.2.188
Chung, S. J., Lee, J. S., Yoo, T. I., Koo, Y. J., Jeon, S. I., Kim, B. S., & Hong, K. E. (1998). Development of the Korean form of Yale Global Tic Severity Scale: A validity and reliability study. *Journal of Korean Neuropsychiatric Association, 37*(5), 942–951.
Cloes, K. I., Barfell, K. S. F., Horn, P. S., Wu, S. W., Jacobson, S. E., Hart, K. J., & Gilbert, D. L. (2016). Preliminary evaluation of child self-rating using the Child Tourette Syndrome Impairment Scale. *Developmental Medicine & Child Neurology, 59*(3), 284–290.
Cohen, D. J., Leckman, J. F., & Shaywitz, B. A. (1985). The Tourette syndrome and other tics In D. Shaffer (Eds.), *The Clinical Guide to Child Psychiatry* (pp. 3–28). New York, NY: Macmillan.
Cohen, S. C., Leckman, J. F., & Bloch, M. H. (2013). Clinical assessment of Tourette syndrome and tic disorders. *Neuroscience & Biobehavioral Reviews, 37*(6), 997–1007.
Comings, D. E. (2000). *Attention-deficit/hyperactivity disorder with Tourette syndrome*. Washington, DC: American Psychiatric Press, Inc.
Conelea, C. A., Woods, D. W., & Brandt, B. C. (2011). The impact of a stress induction task on tic frequencies in youth with Tourette Syndrome. *Behaviour Research and Therapy, 49*(8), 492–497.
Conelea, C. A., Woods, D. W., Zinner, S. H., Budman, C., Murphy, T., Scahill, L. D., … Walkup, J. (2011). Exploring the impact of chronic tic disorders on youth: Results from the Tourette Syndrome Impact Survey. *Child Psychiatry & Human Development, 42*(2), 219–242.
Cubo, E., Sáez Velasco, S., Delgado Benito, V., Ausín Villaverde, V., Maria Trejo Gabriel y Galán, J., Martín Santidrián, A., … Benito-León, J. (2011). Validation of screening instruments for neuroepidemiological surveys of tic disorders. *Movement Disorders, 26*(3), 520–526.
Cubo, E., Trejo, J., Ausín, V., Sáez, S., Delgado, V., Macarrón, J., … Benito-León, J. (2013). Association of tic disorders with poor academic performance in Central Spain: A population-based study. *The Journal of Pediatrics, 163*(1), 217–223.
Cutler, D., Murphy, T., Gilmour, J., & Heyman, I. (2009). The quality of life of young people with Tourette syndrome. *Child: Care, Health and Development, 35*(4), 496–504.
Eapen, V., Fox-Hiley, P., Banerjee, S., & Robertson, M. (2004). Clinical features and associated psychopathology in a Tourette syndrome cohort. *Acta Neurologica Scandinavica, 109*(4), 255–260.
Eddy, C. M., Cavanna, A. E., Gulisano, M., Agodi, A., Barchitta, M., Calì, P., … Rizzo, R. (2011). Clinical correlates of quality of life in Tourette syndrome. *Movement Disorders, 26*(4), 735–738.
Eddy, C. M., Rizzo, R., Gulisano, M., Agodi, A., Barchitta, M., Calì, P., … Cavanna, A. E. (2011). Quality of life in young people with Tourette syndrome: A controlled study. *Journal of Neurology, 258*(2), 291–301.
Espil, F. M., Capriotti, M. R., Conelea, C. A., & Woods, D. W. (2014). The role of parental perceptions of tic frequency and intensity in predicting tic-related functional impairment in youth with chronic tic disorders. *Child Psychiatry & Human Development, 45*(6), 657–665.
Fahim, C., Yoon, U., Das, S., Lyttelton, O., Chen, J., Arnaoutelis, R., … Evans, A. C. (2010). Somatosensory–motor bodily representation cortical thinning in Tourette: Effects of tic severity, age and gender. *Cortex, 46*(6), 750–760.
Freeman, R. D. (2007). Tic disorders and ADHD: Answers from a world-wide clinical dataset on Tourette syndrome. *European Child & Adolescent Psychiatry, 16*(9), 15–23.
Freeman, R. D., Fast, D. K., Burd, L., Kerbeshian, J., Robertson, M. M., & Sandor, P. (2000). An international perspective on Tourette syndrome: Selected findings from 3500 individuals in 22 countries. *Developmental Medicine & Child Neurology, 42*(7), 436–447.
Gadow, K. D., & Paolicell, L. (1986). Global tic rating scale. In *Stony brook*. New York, NY: State University of New York Department of Psychiatry.
Gadow, K. D., Sverd, J., Nolan, E. E., Sprafkin, J., & Schneider, J. (2007). Immediate-release methylphenidate for ADHD in children with comorbid chronic multiple tic disorder. *Journal of the American Academy of Child & Adolescent Psychiatry, 46*(7), 840–848.
Gadow, K. D., Sverd, J., Sprafkin, J., Nolan, E. E., & Ezor, S. N. (1995). Efficacy of methylphenidate for

attention-deficit hyperactivity disorder in children with tic disorder. *Archives of General Psychiatry, 52*(6), 444–455.

Gaffney, G. R., Sieg, K., & Hellings, J. (1994). The MOVES: A self-rating scale for Tourette's syndrome. *Journal of Child and Adolescent Psychopharmacology, 4*(4), 269–280.

Ganos, C., Garrido, A., Navalpotro-Gómez, I., Ricciardi, L., Martino, D., Edwards, M. J., ... Bhatia, K. P. (2015). Premonitory urge to tic in Tourette's is associated with interoceptive awareness. *Movement Disorders, 30*(9), 1198–1202.

Ganos, C., Kahl, U., Schunke, O., Kühn, S., Haggard, P., Gerloff, C., ... Münchau, A. (2012). Are premonitory urges a prerequisite of tic inhibition in Gilles de la Tourette syndrome? *Journal of Neurology, Neurosurgery & Psychiatry, 83*(10), 975–978.

García-López, R., Perea-Milla, E., Romero-González, J., Rivas-Ruiz, F., Ruiz-García, C., Oviedo-Joekes, E., & Mulas-Bejar, M. (2008). Adaptación al español y validez diagnóstica de la Yale Global Tics Severity Scale. *Revista de Neurologia, 46*, 261–266.

Goetz, C. G., Pappert, E. J., Louis, E. D., Raman, R., & Leurgans, S. (1999). Advantages of a modified scoring method for the Rush Video-Based Tic Rating Scale. *Movement Disorders, 14*(3), 502–506.

Goetz, C. G., Tanner, C. M., Wilson, R. S., & Shannon, K. M. (1987). A rating scale for Gilles de la Tourette's syndrome: Description, reliability, and validity data. *Neurology, 37*(9), 1542–1542.

Gorman, D. A., Thompson, N., Plessen, K. J., Robertson, M. M., Leckman, J. F., & Peterson, B. S. (2010). Psychosocial outcome and psychiatric comorbidity in older adolescents with Tourette syndrome: Controlled study. *The British Journal of Psychiatry, 197*(1), 36–44.

Gulisano, M., Calì, P., Palermo, F., Robertson, M., & Rizzo, R. (2015). Premonitory urges in patients with Gilles de la Tourette syndrome: An Italian translation and a 7-year follow-up. *Journal of Child and Adolescent Psychopharmacology, 25*(10), 810–816.

Haddad, A. D. M., Umoh, G., Bhatia, V., & Robertson, M. M. (2009). Adults with Tourette's syndrome with and without attention deficit hyperactivity disorder. *Acta Psychiatrica Scandinavica, 120*(4), 299–307.

Halleröd, S. L. H., Larson, T., Stahlberg, O., Carlström, E., Gillberg, C., Anckarsäter, H., ... Gillberg, C. (2010). The Autism—Tics, AD/HD and other Comorbidities (A-TAC) telephone interview: Convergence with the Child Behavior Checklist (CBCL). *Nordic Journal of Psychiatry, 64*(3), 218–224.

Hansson, S. L., Röjvall, A. S., Rastam, M., Gillberg, C., & Anckarsäter, H. (2005). Psychiatric telephone interview with parents for screening of childhood autism–tics, attention-deficit hyperactivity disorder and other comorbidities (A–TAC). *The British Journal of Psychiatry, 187*(3), 262–267.

Harcherik, D. F., Leckman, J. F., Detlor, J., & Cohen, D. J. (1984). A new instrument for clinical studies of Tourette's syndrome. *Journal of the American Academy of Child Psychiatry, 23*(2), 153–160.

Himle, M. B., Capriotti, M. R., Hayes, L. P., Ramanujam, K., Scahill, L., Sukhodolsky, D. G., ... Piacentini, J. (2014). Variables associated with tic exacerbation in children with chronic tic disorders. *Behavior Modification, 38*(2), 163–183.

Himle, M. B., Freitag, M., Walther, M., Franklin, S. A., Ely, L., & Woods, D. W. (2012). A randomized pilot trial comparing videoconference versus face-to-face delivery of behavior therapy for childhood tic disorders. *Behaviour Research and Therapy, 50*(9), 565–570.

Hirschtritt, M. E., Lee, P. C., Pauls, D. L., Dion, Y., Grados, M. A., Illmann, C., ... Tourette Syndrome Association International Consortium for Genetics. (2015). Lifetime prevalence, age of risk, and genetic relationships of comorbid psychiatric disorders in Tourette syndrome. *JAMA Psychiatry, 72*(4), 325–333.

Hornsey, H., Banerjee, S., Zeitlin, H., & Robertson, M. (2001). The prevalence of Tourette syndrome in 13-14-year-olds in mainstream schools. *Journal of Child Psychology and Psychiatry, 42*(8), 1035–1039.

Howson, A. L., Batth, S., Ilivitsky, V., Boisjoli, A., Jaworski, M., Mahoney, C., & Knott, V. J. (2004). Clinical and attentional effects of acute nicotine treatment in Tourette's syndrome. *European Psychiatry, 19*(2), 102–112.

Huisman-van Dijk, H. M., van de Schoot, R., Rijkeboer, M. M., Mathews, C. A., & Cath, D. C. (2016). The relationship between tics, OC, ADHD and autism symptoms: A cross-disorder symptom analysis in Gilles de la Tourette syndrome patients and family-members. *Psychiatry Research, 237*, 138–146.

Khalifa, N., & Knorring, A.-L. (2005). Tourette syndrome and other tic disorders in a total population of children: Clinical assessment and background. *Acta Paediatrica, 94*(11), 1608–1614.

Lang, A. (1991). Patient perception of tics and other movement disorders. *Neurology, 41*(2 Part 1), 223–223.

Larson, T., Anckarsäter, H., Gillberg, C., Stahlberg, O., Carlström, E., Kadesjö, B., ... Gillberg, C. (2010). The autism-tics, AD/HD and other comorbidities inventory (A-TAC): Further validation of a telephone interview for epidemiological research. *BMC Psychiatry, 10*(1), 1.

Larson, T., Lundström, S., Nilsson, T., Selinus, E. N., Rastam, M., Lichtenstein, P., ... Kerekes, N. (2013). Predictive properties of the A-TAC inventory when screening for childhood-onset neurodevelopmental problems in a population-based sample. *BMC Psychiatry, 13*(1), 233.

Larson, T., Selinus, E. N., Gumpert, C. H., Nilsson, T., Kerekes, N., Lichtenstein, P., ... Lundström, S. (2014). Reliability of Autism-Tics, AD/HD, and other Comorbidities (A–TAC) Inventory in a Test-Retest Design. *Psychological Reports, 114*(1), 93–103.

Lebowitz, E., Motlagh, M., Katsovich, L., King, R., Lombroso, P., Grantz, H., ... Leckman, J. (2012). Tourette syndrome in youth with and without obsessive compulsive disorder and attention deficit hyperactivity disorder. *European Child & Adolescent Psychiatry, 21*(8), 451–457. https://doi.org/10.1007/s00787-012-0278-5

Leckman, J. F. (2003). Phenomenology of tics and natural history of tic disorders. *Brain and Development, 25*, S24–S28.

Leckman, J. F., Riddle, M. A., Hardin, M. T., Ort, S. I., Swartz, K. L., Stevenson, J., & Cohen, D. J. (1989). The Yale global tic severity scale: Initial testing of a clinician-rated scale of tic severity. *Journal of the American Academy of Child & Adolescent Psychiatry, 28*(4), 566–573.

Leckman, J. F., Towbin, K. E., Ort, S. I., & Cohen, D. J. (1988). Clinical assessment of tic disorder severity. In *Tourette's syndrome and tic disorders* (pp. 55–78). New York, NY: Wiley.

Leckman, J. F., Yeh, C.-B., & Cohen, D. J. (2001). Tic disorders: When habit forming neural systems form habits of their own? *Chinese Medical Journal-Taipei, 64*(12), 669–692.

Leckman, J. F., Zhang, H., Vitale, A., Lahnin, F., Lynch, K., Bondi, C., ... Peterson, B. S. (1998). Course of tic severity in Tourette syndrome: The first two decades. *Pediatrics, 102*(1), 14–19.

Lemay, M., Lê, T.-T., Richer, F., & Montreal Tourette Study Group. (2010). Effects of a secondary task on postural control in children with Tourette syndrome. *Gait & Posture, 31*(3), 326–330.

Lewin, A. B., Murphy, T. K., Storch, E. A., Conelea, C. A., Woods, D. W., Scahill, L. D., ... Walkup, J. T. (2012). A phenomenological investigation of women with Tourette or other chronic tic disorders. *Comprehensive Psychiatry, 53*(5), 525–534.

Linazasoro, G., Van Blercom, N., & Ortiz De Zárate, C. (2006). Prevalence of tic disorder in two schools in the Basque country: Results and methodological caveats. *Movement Disorders, 21*(12), 2106–2109.

Maciunas, R. J., Maddux, B. N., Riley, D. E., Whitney, C. M., Schoenberg, M. R., Ogrocki, P. J., ... Gould, D. J. (2007). Prospective randomized double-blind trial of bilateral thalamic deep brain stimulation in adults with Tourette syndrome. *Journal of Neurosurgery, 112*, 1004–1014.

Malli, M., Forrester-Jones, R., & Murphy, G. (2016). Stigma in youth with Tourette's syndrome: A systematic review and synthesis. *European Child & Adolescent Psychiatry, 25*(2), 127–139. https://doi.org/10.1007/s00787-015-0761-x

Martino, D., Pringsheim, T. M., Cavanna, A. E., Colosimo, C., Hartmann, A., Leckman, J. F., ... Martinez-Martin, P. (2017). Systematic review of severity scales and screening instruments for tics: Critique and recommendations. *Movement Disorders, 32*(3), 467–473.

Matson, J. L., & Wilkins, J. (2009). Psychometric testing methods for children's social skills. *Research in Developmental Disabilities, 30*(2), 249–274.

McConville, B. J., Sanberg, P. R., Fogelson, M. H., King, J., Cirino, P., Parker, K. W., & Norman, A. B. (1992). The effects of nicotine plus haloperidol compared to nicotine only and placebo nicotine only in reducing tic severity and frequency in Tourette's disorder. *Biological Psychiatry, 31*(8), 832–840.

McGuire, J. F., Park, J. M., Wu, M. S., Lewin, A. B., Murphy, T. K., & Storch, E. A. (2015). The impact of tic severity dimensions on impairment and quality of life among youth with chronic tic disorders. *Children's Health Care, 44*(3), 277–292. https://doi.org/10.1080/02739615.2014.912944

Müller-Vahl, K., Dodel, I., Müller, N., Münchau, A., Reese, J. P., Balzer-Geldsetzer, M., ... Oertel, W. H. (2010). Health-related quality of life in patients with Gilles de la Tourette's syndrome. *Movement Disorders, 25*(3), 309–314.

Müller-Vahl, K. R., Schneider, U., Koblenz, A., Jöbges, M., Kolbe, H., Daldrup, T., & Emrich, H. M. (2002). Treatment of Tourette's syndrome with Δ9-tetrahydrocannabinol (THC): A randomized crossover trial. *Pharmacopsychiatry, 35*(02), 57–61.

Münchau, A., Bloem, B. R., Thilo, K. V., Trimble, M. R., Rothwell, J. C., & Robertson, M. M. (2002). Repetitive transcranial magnetic stimulation for Tourette syndrome. *Neurology, 59*(11), 1789–1791.

Nolan, E. E., Gadow, K. D., & Sverd, J. (1994). Observations and ratings of tics in school settings. *Journal of Abnormal Child Psychology, 22*(5), 579–593.

O'Connor, K. P., Laverdure, A., Taillon, A., Stip, E., Borgeat, F., & Lavoie, M. (2009). Cognitive behavioral management of Tourette's syndrome and chronic tic disorder in medicated and unmedicated samples. *Behaviour Research and Therapy, 47*(12), 1090–1095.

O'Connor, K., St-Pierre-Delorme, M.-È., Leclerc, J., Lavoie, M., & Blais, M. T. (2014). Meta-cognitions in Tourette syndrome, tic disorders, and body-focused repetitive disorder. *The Canadian Journal of Psychiatry, 59*(8), 417–425. https://doi.org/10.1177/070674371405900804

O'Hare, D., Eapen, V., Helmes, E., McBain, K., Reece, J., & Grove, R. (2016). Recognising and treating Tourette's syndrome in young Australians: A need for informed multidisciplinary support. *Australian Psychologist, 51*(3), 238–245. https://doi.org/10.1111/ap.12170

O'Hare, D., Helmes, E., Eapen, V., Grove, R., McBain, K., & Reece, J. (2016). The impact of tic severity, comorbidity and peer attachment on quality of life outcomes and functioning in Tourette's syndrome: Parental perspectives. *Child Psychiatry and Human Development, 47*(4), 563–573. https://doi.org/10.1007/s10578-015-0590-7

Onofrj, M., Paci, C., D'andreamatteo, G., & Toma, L. (2000). Olanzapine in severe Gilles de la Tourette syndrome: A 52-week double-blind cross-over study vs. low-dose pimozide. *Journal of Neurology, 247*(6), 443–446.

Orth, M., Kirby, R., Richardson, M. P., Snijders, A. H., Rothwell, J. C., Trimble, M. R., ... Münchau, A. (2005). Subthreshold rTMS over pre-motor cortex has no effect on tics in patients with Gilles de la

Tourette syndrome. *Clinical Neurophysiology, 116*(4), 764–768.

Packer-Hopke, L., & Motta, R. W. (2014). A preliminary investigation of the effects of aerobic exercise on childhood Tourette's syndrome and OCD. *The Behaviour Therapist, 37*, 188–192.

Pappert, E. J., Goetz, C. G., Louis, E. D., Blasucci, L., & Leurgans, S. (2003). Objective assessments of longitudinal outcome in Gilles de la Tourette's syndrome. *Neurology, 61*(7), 936–940.

Peterson, B. S., & Cohen, D. J. (1998). The treatment of Tourette's syndrome: Multimodal, developmental intervention. *The Journal of Clinical Psychiatry, 59*(Suppl 1), 62–72.

Peterson, B. S., Pine, D. S., Cohen, P., & Brook, J. S. (2001). Prospective, longitudinal study of tic, obsessive-compulsive, and attention-deficit/hyperactivity disorders in an epidemiological sample. *Journal of the American Academy of Child & Adolescent Psychiatry, 40*(6), 685–695.

Piacentini, J., Woods, D. W., Scahill, L., Wilhelm, S., Peterson, A. L., Chang, S., ... Walkup, J. T. (2010). Behavior therapy for children with Tourette disorder: A randomized controlled trial. *JAMA, 303*(19), 1929–1937.

Reese, H. E., Scahill, L., Peterson, A. L., Crowe, K., Woods, D. W., Piacentini, J., ... Wilhelm, S. (2014). The premonitory urge to tic: Measurement, characteristics, and correlates in older adolescents and adults. *Behavior Therapy, 45*(2), 177–186.

Robertson, M. M. (2003). Diagnosing Tourette syndrome: Is it a common disorder. *Journal of Psychosomatic Research, 55*(1), 3–6.

Robertson, M. M. (2012). The Gilles de la Tourette syndrome: The current status. *Archives of Disease in Childhood-Education and Practice, 97*(5), 166–175.

Sallee, F. R., Nesbitt, L., Jackson, C., Sine, L., & Sethuraman, G. (1997). Relative efficacy of haloperidol and pimozide in children and adolescents with Tourette's disorder. *The American Journal of Psychiatry, 154*(8), 1057–1062.

Scahill, L., Erenberg, G., Berlin, C. M., Budman, C., Coffey, B. J., Jankovic, J., ... Mink, J. (2006). Contemporary assessment and pharmacotherapy of Tourette syndrome. *NeuroRx, 3*(2), 192–206.

Scharf, J. M., Miller, L. L., Gauvin, C. A., Alabiso, J., Mathews, C. A., & Ben-Shlomo, Y. (2015). Population prevalence of Tourette syndrome: A systematic review and meta-analysis. *Movement Disorders, 30*(2), 221–228.

Shaffer, D., Gould, M. S., Brasic, J., Ambrosini, P., Fisher, P., Bird, H., & Aluwahlia, S. (1983). A children's global assessment scale (CGAS). *Archives of General Psychiatry, 40*(11), 1228–1231.

Shapiro, A. K., & Shapiro, E. (1984). Controlled study of pimozide vs. placebo in Tourette's syndrome. *Journal of the American Academy of Child Psychiatry, 23*(2), 161–173.

Shapiro, A. K., Shapiro, E. S., Young, J. G., & Feinberg, T. E. (1988). Measurement in tic disorders. In A. K. Shapiro, E. S. Shapiro, J. G. Young, & T. E. Feinberg (Eds.), *Gilles de la Tourette syndrome* (2nd ed., pp. 451–480). New York, NY: Raven Press.

Shapiro, E., Shapiro, A. K., Fulop, G., Hubbard, M., Mandeli, J., Nordlie, J., & Phillips, R. A. (1989). Controlled study of haloperidol, pimozide, and placebo for the treatment of Gilles de la Tourette's syndrome. *Archives of General Psychiatry, 46*(8), 722–730.

Shytle, R. D., Silver, A. A., Sheehan, K. H., Wilkinson, B. J., Newman, M., Sanberg, P. R., & Sheehan, D. (2003). The Tourette's Disorder Scale (TODS) development, reliability, and validity. *Assessment, 10*(3), 273–287.

Simpson, H. A., Jung, L., & Murphy, T. K. (2011). Update on attention-deficit/hyperactivity disorder and tic disorders: A review of the current literature. *Current Psychiatry Reports, 13*(5), 351.

Singer, H. S., Brown, J., Quaskey, S., Rosenberg, L. A., Mellits, E. D., & Denckla, M. B. (1995). The treatment of Attention-Deficit Hyperactivity Disorder in Tourette's syndrome: A double-blind placebo-controlled study with clonidine and desipramine. *Pediatrics, 95*(1), 74–81.

Spencer, T. J., Biederman, J., Faraone, S., Mick, E., Coffey, B., Geller, D., ... Wilens, T. (2001). Impact of tic disorders on ADHD outcome across the life cycle: Findings from a large group of adults with and without ADHD. *American Journal of Psychiatry, 158*(4), 611–617.

Stefanoff, P., & Wolańczyk, T. (2004). Validity and reliability of polish adaptation of Yale Global Tic Severity scale (YGTSS) in a study of Warsaw schoolchildren aged 12-15. *Przeglad Epidemiologiczny, 59*(3), 753–762.

Steinberg, T., Baruch, S. S., Harush, A., Dar, R., Woods, D., Piacentini, J., & Apter, A. (2010). Tic disorders and the premonitory urge. *Journal of Neural Transmission, 117*(2), 277–284.

Storch, E. A., Hanks, C. E., Mink, J. W., McGuire, J. F., Adams, H. R., Augustine, E. F., ... Murphy, T. K. (2015). Suicidal thoughts and behaviors in children and adolescents with chronic tic disorders. *Depression and Anxiety, 32*(10), 744–753.

Storch, E. A., Lack, C. W., Simons, L. E., Goodman, W. K., Murphy, T. K., & Geffken, G. R. (2007). A measure of functional impairment in youth with Tourette's syndrome. *Journal of Pediatric Psychology, 32*(8), 950–959.

Storch, E. A., Murphy, T. K., Fernandez, M., Krishnan, M., Geffken, G. R., Kellgren, A. R., & Goodman, W. K. (2007). Factor-analytic study of the Yale Global Tic Severity Scale. *Psychiatry Research, 149*(1), 231–237.

Storch, E. A., Murphy, T. K., Geffken, G. R., Sajid, M., Allen, P., Roberti, J. W., & Goodman, W. K. (2005). Reliability and validity of the Yale Global Tic Severity Scale. *Psychological Assessment, 17*(4), 486.

Storch, E. A., Murphy, T. K., Geffken, G. R., Soto, O., Sajid, M., Allen, P., ... Goodman, W. K. (2004).

Further psychometric properties of the Tourette's Disorder Scale-Parent Rated Version (TODS-PR). *Child Psychiatry & Human Development, 35*(2), 107–120.

Sukhodolsky, D. G., Scahill, L., Zhang, H., Peterson, B. S., King, R. A., Lombroso, P. J., … Leckman, J. F. (2003). Disruptive behavior in children with Tourette's syndrome: Association with ADHD comorbidity, tic severity, and functional impairment. *Journal of the American Academy of Child & Adolescent Psychiatry, 42*(1), 98–105.

Sutherland Owens, A. N., Miguel, E. C., & Swerdlow, N. R. (2011). Sensory gating scales and premonitory urges in Tourette syndrome. *The Scientific World Journal, 11*, 736–741.

Walkup, J. T., Rosenberg, L. A., Brown, J., & Singer, H. S. (1992). The validity of instruments measuring tic severity in Tourette's syndrome. *Journal of the American Academy of Child & Adolescent Psychiatry, 31*(3), 472–477.

Wang, S., Qi, F., Li, J., Zhao, L., & Li, A. (2012). Effects of Chinese herbal medicine Ningdong granule on regulating dopamine (DA)/serotonin (5-TH) and gamma-amino butyric acid (GABA) in patients with Tourette syndrome. *Bioscience Trends, 6*(4), 212–218.

Woods, D. W., Conelea, C. A., & Himle, M. B. (2010). Behavior therapy for Tourette's disorder: Utilization in a community sample and an emerging area of practice for psychologists. *Professional Psychology: Research and Practice, 41*(6), 518.

Woods, D. W., Piacentini, J., Chang, S., Deckersbach, T., Ginsburg, G., Peterson, A., … Wilhelm, S. (2008). *Managing Tourette syndrome: A behavioral intervention for children and adults therapist guide*. Oxford/New York, NY: Oxford University Press.

Woods, D. W., Piacentini, J., Himle, M. B., & Chang, S. (2005). Premonitory Urge for Tics Scale (PUTS): Initial psychometric results and examination of the premonitory urge phenomenon in youths with tic disorders. *Journal of Developmental & Behavioral Pediatrics, 26*(6), 397–403.

Zinner, S. H., Conelea, C. A., Glew, G. M., Woods, D. W., & Budman, C. L. (2012). Peer victimization in youth with Tourette syndrome and other chronic tic disorders. *Child Psychiatry & Human Development, 43*(1), 124–136.

Aggression and Conduct Disorders

Laura C. Thornton and Paul J. Frick

Nature of Serious Conduct Problems

Definitions

Conduct problems and aggression are symptoms of two diagnoses in the fifth edition of the *Diagnostic and Statistical Manual of Mental Disorders* (DSM-5; American Psychiatric Association, 2013): Oppositional Defiant Disorder (ODD) and Conduct Disorder (CD). They are grouped in the category of disruptive, impulse control, and conduct disorders, which are all defined by problems in the self-control of emotions and/or behaviors that violate the rights of others or that bring the individual in conflict with societal norms.

The diagnostic criteria for ODD include three types of symptoms: angry-irritable mood (e.g., loses temper, angry/resentful), argumentative/defiant behavior (e.g., argues with adults, defiant/noncompliant), and vindictiveness (American Psychiatric Association, 2013).

Typically developing children may of ODD to some degree, which requires several key considerations in deciding whether the behaviors are symptomatic of ODD (Frick & Nigg, 2012). That is, the individual must show at least four symptoms over the preceding 6 months, and the persistence and frequency of the symptoms should exceed what is normative for an individual's age, sex, and culture. Importantly, these behaviors must contribute to substantial impairment for the individual, such as causing problems for a child at school or leading to problems in a person's social relationships. The disorder is considered "mild" in severity if it is confined to one setting (e.g., only at home), but it is considered "moderate" if the symptoms are present in at two settings, and it is considered "severe" if it appears in three or more settings (American Psychiatric Association, 2013).

CD is defined as a persistent and repetitive pattern of behavior which violates the rights of others or that violates major age appropriate societal norms or rules (American Psychiatric Association, 2013). Four types of symptoms of CD define this disorder: aggression to people and animals (e.g., fighting, bullying), destruction of property (e.g., fire setting, vandalism), deceitfulness or theft (e.g., conning, shoplifting), and serious violations of rules (e.g., truancy, running away from home). The DSM-5 recognizes that the aggressive and antisocial behavior associated with CD can vary in the severity and in their

L. C. Thornton
Boys Town National Research Hospital, Omaha, NE, USA

P. J. Frick (✉)
Louisiana State University, Baton Rouge, LA, USA

Australian Catholic University, Brisbane, Australia
e-mail: pfrick@lsu.edu

underlying causes. Specifically, it allows for three potential specifiers to the diagnosis. First, it distinguishes between a "mild" form of the disorder in which the child shows few if any conduct problems in excess of those required to make the diagnosis and the conduct problems cause relatively minor harm to others (e.g., lying, staying out after dark without permission) and a "severe" form in which the child shows many conduct problems in excess of those needed to make the diagnosis and the conduct problems cause considerable harm to others (e.g., rape, physical cruelty). In between is considered a disorder of "moderate" severity. Second, the DSM-5 distinguishes individuals within those with CD based on the timing of the onset. That is, the childhood-onset subtype is characterized by at least one symptom of the disorder being present before 10 years, whereas the adolescent-onset subtype is characterized by no symptoms being present before the age of 10 years. Third, the DSM-5 includes a specifier for those "with limited prosocial emotions" that is defined by the presence of significant numbers of callous-unemotional (CU) traits (e.g., callous-lack of empathy, absence of guilt and remorse, failure to show concern over performance in important activities, shallow or deficient emotions).

Clinical Importance

A recent meta-analysis of epidemiological studies suggests that world prevalence of ODD in youth (ages 6–18 years) is 3.3% and the prevalence of CD is 3.2% (Canino, Polanczyk, Bauermeister, Rohde, & Frick, 2010). Further, the meta-analysis reported that prevalence estimates did not vary greatly across countries or continents, with the caveat that the majority of studies included in the analysis were conducted in Europe and North America. In community samples, the levels of conduct problems appears to decrease from preschool to school-age years (Maughan, Rowe, Messer, Goodman, & Meltzer, 2004) but then later increases during adolescence (Loeber, Burke, Lahey, Winters, & Zera, 2000). However, the differences vary somewhat across the different types of conduct problems, such that mild forms of physical aggression (e.g., fighting) decrease in across development, whereas nonaggressive and covert antisocial behavior (e.g., lying and stealing) and serious aggression (e.g., armed robbery and sexual assault) increase in prevalence from childhood to adolescence (Loeber & Hay, 1997). While boys generally show higher rates of conduct problems in girls, this male predominance appears to be emerge after preschool (Loeber et al., 2000; Maughan et al., 2004) and is greatest prior to adolescence (Silverthorn & Frick, 1999).

Conduct problems are one of the most common causes for referral to mental health services in children and adolescents (Kazdin, Whitley, & Marciano, 2006; Kimonis, Frick, & McMahon, 2014). This is likely due to the fact that conduct problems can place a child at risk for involvement with the legal system (Frick, Stickle, Dandreaux, Farrell, & Kimonis, 2005), as well as risk for being rejected by peers and being suspended or expelled from school (Dodge et al., 2003; Frick, 2012). Conduct problems can have effects beyond childhood and adolescence, with research suggesting that conduct problems in childhood predict mental health (e.g., substance use), legal (e.g., being arrested), educational (e.g., dropping out of school), occupational (e.g., poor job performance), social (e.g., poor marital adjustment), and physical health (e.g., poor respiration) problems in adulthood (Odgers et al., 2007, 2008)

Thus, it is clear that serious conduct problems are relatively prevalent in children and adolescents, and they can lead to significant impairments in the child throughout the life-span. As a result, they represent a significant mental problem and are very common referrals for assessment and treatment in various child mental health settings. However, it is also important to note that not all children with conduct problems, even those who meet criteria for the more severe diagnosis of CD, uniformly have poor outcomes. Thus, it is important for clinical assessment to consider various predictors of which youth with serious conduct problems are at most risk for future problems, so that these children and adolescents can receive effective treatments.

One consistent predictor of which children with CD are most likely to have stable problems throughout adolescence and into adulthood are those whose serious conduct problems begin early in development. That is, one subgroup of children with CD (i.e., childhood-onset type) begin exhibiting mild conduct problems associated with ODD (e.g., oppositional behavior, temper tantrums) as early as preschool or early elementary school, and these behavior problems tend to increase in rate and severity throughout childhood and into adolescence (Frick & Viding, 2009). This is in contrast to youth who do not show significant behavior problems in childhood, but they begin exhibiting significant antisocial and delinquent behavior coinciding with the onset of adolescence (Moffitt, 2006). Importantly, youth in the childhood-onset group are more likely to continue to exhibit antisocial and criminal behavior into adulthood. For example, in a birth cohort of children in New Zealand who were followed from birth to adulthood (age 32 years), boys whose conduct problems started prior to adolescence were more likely to be convicted of a violent offense as an adult (32.7%), compared to those who began exhibiting conduct problems starting in adolescence (10.2%) and those who did not exhibit serious conduct problems in childhood or adolescence (0.4%; Odgers et al., 2008).

Another important subgroup of children with CD are those who show significant levels of callous-unemotional (CU) traits. Youth who show these traits often show more severe and stable behavior problems (Frick, Ray, Thornton, & Kahn, 2014a; Ray, Thornton, Frick, Steinberg, & Cauffman, 2016). Further, they are more likely to be aggressive and, more specifically, to show aggression that is both premeditated and instrumental (for personal gain or dominance; Fanti, Frick, & Georgiou, 2009; Frick et al., 2003; Kruh, Frick, & Clements, 2005 ; Lawing, Frick, & Cruise, 2010) and to show aggression that results in greater harm to others (Kruh et al., 2005; Lawing et al., 2010). Importantly, children with serious conduct problems and elevated CU traits appear to show poorer treatment outcomes to many traditional mental health interventions (Frick, Ray, Thornton, & Kahn, 2014b; Hawes, Price, & Dadds, 2014; Wilkinson, Waller, & Viding, 2015). All of these findings led to the DSM-5 to include CU traits in its definition of CD by including the specifier "with limited prosocial emotions."

Etiology

There are two overarching findings from research on the causes of serious conduct problems that are critically important for guiding clinical assessments. First, research has clearly suggested that serious conduct problems are often a result of a host of different risk factors both within the child (e.g., biological, cognitive, and personality risk factors) and risk factors in the child's social ecology (e.g., family, peer, and neighborhood risk factors; Frick & Viding, 2009). Second, there seem to be several different common pathways through which children develop serious conduct problems, each involving somewhat different risk factors and each requiring a different approach to treatment. These different developmental pathways generally correspond to the clinical important subgroups of youth with CD included in the DSM-5 specifiers (Frick, 2016).

Specifically, the childhood-onset and adolescent-onset subtypes of CD not only show very different life course trajectories as noted above, but they also differ on a number of dispositional and contextual risk factors that seem to implicate different developmental processes leading to the disruptive behaviors of the two groups (Frick & Viding, 2009; Moffitt, 2006). To summarize these findings, childhood-onset CD seems to be more strongly related to neuropsychological (e.g., deficits in executive functioning) and cognitive (e.g., low intelligence) deficits. Also, children who show the childhood-onset pattern seem to show more temperamental and personality risk factors, such as impulsivity, attention deficits, and problems in emotional regulation. This group also shows higher rates of family instability, more family conflict, and parents who use less effective parenting strategies. When children within the adolescent-onset group differ from control children without conduct problems, it is often in showing higher levels of rebelliousness and being more rejecting of conventional values and status hierarchies (Dandreaux & Frick, 2009; Moffitt, 2006).

Based on these differences, Moffitt (2006) proposed that children in the childhood-onset group develop their serious conduct problems through a transactional process involving a difficult and vulnerable child (e.g., impulsive, with verbal deficits) who experiences an inadequate rearing environment (e.g., poor parental supervision, poor quality schools). This dysfunctional transactional process disrupts the child's socialization leading to poor social relations with persons both inside (e.g., parents and siblings) and outside (e.g., peers and teachers) the family. These disruptions lead to enduring vulnerabilities in the child's ability to regulate his or her emotions and behavior that can negatively affect the child's psychosocial adjustment across the lifespan. In contrast, children in the adolescent-onset pathway show an exaggeration of the normative process of adolescent rebellion. That is, most adolescents show some level of rebelliousness to parents and other authority figures (Brezina & Piquero, 2007). This rebelliousness is part of a process by which the adolescent begins to develop his or her autonomous sense of self and his or her unique identity. According to Moffitt (2006), the child in the adolescent-onset group engages in antisocial and delinquent behaviors as a misguided attempt to obtain a subjective sense of maturity and adult status in a way that is maladaptive (e.g., breaking societal norms) but encouraged by an antisocial peer group. Given that their behavior is viewed as an exaggeration of a process specific to adolescence, and not due to an enduring vulnerability, their antisocial behavior is less likely to persist beyond adolescence. However, they may still have impairments that persist into adulthood due to the consequences of their adolescent antisocial behavior (e.g., a criminal record, dropping out of school, substance abuse; Odgers et al., 2008).

As noted above, the DSM-5 also includes the specifier for CD "with limited prosocial emotions" for those who meet criteria for CD but who show a number of CU traits over an extended time period (i.e., at least 12 months) and in multiple relationships and settings. As with the childhood- vs. adolescent-onset distinction, there is substantial research to suggesting that youth with CD with and without elevated CU traits show very different genetic, cognitive, emotional, and social characteristics, again suggesting different causes to the antisocial behavior across the two groups. Research on these different risk factors were the subject of a comprehensive review by Frick et al., (2014b) who found several key differences between the two groups of children with conduct problems. First, behavioral genetic research suggests that the genetic influences on childhood-onset conduct problems are considerably stronger in those high on CU traits compared to those who show normative levels of these traits. Second, children and adolescents with serious conduct problems and CU traits also show an insensitivity to punishment cues, which include responding more poorly to punishment cues after a reward-dominant response set is primed, responding more poorly to gradual punishment schedules, and underestimating the likelihood that they will be punished for misbehavior relative to other youth with serious conduct problems. Third, children and adolescents with serious conduct problems and elevated CU traits endorse more deviant values and goals in social situations, such as viewing aggression as a more acceptable means for obtaining goals, blaming others for their misbehavior, and emphasizing the importance of dominance and revenge in social conflicts. Fourth, children and adolescents with elevated CU traits also show reduced emotional responsiveness in a number of situations including showing weaker responses to cues of distress in others, less reactivity to peer provocation, less fear of novel and dangerous situations, and less anxiety over the consequences of their behavior relative to other youths with serious conduct problems. Fifth, conduct problems tend to have a different association with parenting practices depending on whether or not the child or adolescent shows elevated levels of CU traits. Specifically, harsh, inconsistent, and coercive discipline is more strongly associated with conduct problems in youth with normative levels of CU traits relative to youth with elevated CU traits, whereas low warmth in parenting appears to be more highly associated with conduct problems in youth with elevated CU traits.

These findings led Frick and Viding (2009) to proposed that children with serious conduct problems and elevated CU traits, but not other children with serious conduct problems, have a temperament (i.e., fearless, insensitive to punishment, low responsiveness to cues of distress in others) that can interfere with the normal development of conscience and place the child at risk for a particularly severe and aggressive pattern of antisocial behavior. In contrast, children and adolescents with childhood-onset antisocial behavior with normative levels of CU traits do not typically show problems in empathy and guilt. In fact, Frick and Viding (2009) noted that they appear to be highly reactive to emotional cues in others and they are highly distressed by the effects of their behavior on others. Thus, the antisocial behavior in this group does not seem to be easily explained by deficits in conscience development. Further, this group that does not show elevated levels of CU traits displays higher levels of emotional reactivity to provocation from others. The conduct problems in this group are strongly associated with hostile/coercive parenting. Based on these findings, Frick and Viding (2009) proposed that children in this group show a temperament characterized by strong emotional reactivity combined with inadequate socializing experiences that do not help them to develop the skills needed to adequately regulate their emotional reactivity. The resulting problems in emotional regulation can result in the child committing impulsive and unplanned aggressive and antisocial acts, for which he or she may feel remorseful afterward but for which he or she may still have difficulty controlling in the future.

Clinical Assessment

This very brief summary of research on serious conduct problems in children and adolescence (see Frick, 2016 for a more extended review) has a number of important implications for clinical assessments. In discussing these implications, it is important to recognize that clinical assessments can serve a variety of purposes and the use of specific assessment tools should align with these goals. In the sections below, we focus on two of the most common reasons that children with serious conduct problems undergo a psychological assessment: for making diagnoses and for treatment planning. That is, when a child or adolescent with serious conduct problems is referred for psychological testing, the two most common questions that the testing is supposed to address are does this child need treatment (i.e., making a diagnosis), and, if so, what type of treatment is most likely to be effective (i.e., treatment planning)?

Assessment for Diagnosis

In the context of this chapter, "making a diagnosis" of a child with serious behavior problems in not synonymous with determining if he or she meets DSM criteria for a conduct problem diagnosis, such as ODD or CD. Instead, we use a broader definition of "diagnosis" to refer to the determination of whether the child or adolescent is showing behavior problems that warrant treatment. There are several important considerations for making this determination.

First, it is important to rule out the possibility of an inappropriate referral due to unrealistic parental or teacher expectations. That is, it is necessary to determine whether or not the youth is exhibiting levels of conduct problems that are atypical in type and frequency for his or her age. Second, it is important to assess the degree of impairment that is associated with a child's conduct problems. As noted above, children with conduct problems can range greatly in the severity of their problem behavior, ranging from children who show oppositional and defiant behaviors only at home to children who show severe aggression that results in substantial harm to others in the community. Determining the severity of the child's behavior not only can determine whether or not a child needs treatment but how intensive the treatment should be. Third, due the fact that serious conduct problems can lead to a host of problematic outcomes for the child, it is critical to at least screen for a wide variety of behavioral, emotional, social, and academic problems that can further document the need for treatment.

There are three primary assessment methods that can be used to accomplish these goals associated with diagnosis: behavior rating scales, structured diagnostic interviews, and behavioral observations. Each of these methods has specific strengths and weaknesses that they bring to the assessment process, and we summarize these in the following paragraphs.

Behavior Rating Scales Behavior rating scales are a core part of an assessment battery for assessing children and adolescents with serious conduct problems. A variety of rating scales are commercially available and have useful characteristics for meeting the goals of making a diagnosis (Frick, Barry, & Kamphaus, 2010). First, most behavior rating scales assess a range of conduct problems that differ in severity and that can be completed by adults who observe the youth in important psychosocial contexts (i.e., parents and teachers) and by the youth himself or herself. Having multiple informants who see the child in different settings can provide important information on the pervasiveness of the child's behavior problems, as well as help detect potential biases in the report of any single informant. Although most behavior rating scales have similar content across different raters, such as the Achenbach System of Empirically Based Assessment (ASEBA; Achenbach & Rescorla, 2001, 2000)) or Conners Rating Scales, Third Edition (CRS-3; Conners, 2008), a few scales assess for very different content across raters. For example, the Behavior Assessment System for Children, Third Edition (BASC-3; Reynolds & Kamphaus, 2015) has similar content for the teacher and parent versions. However, the content of the self-report version is quite different. Specifically, the child does not rate his or her own level of conduct problems, but the self-report provides more extended coverage of the child's attitudes (e.g., attitudes toward parents and teachers), his or her self-concept (e.g., self-esteem and sense of inadequacy), and his or her social relationships.

Second, rating scales provide some of the best norm-referenced data on a child's behavior. This allows for the assessment to determine how the ratings of the child's behavior compare to the ratings of other children. Such information is critical for determining whether the child's conduct problems are abnormal relative to other children of the same age and sex. For example, the standardization sample for the ASEBA (Achenbach & Rescorla, 2000, 2001) is representative of the 48 contiguous United States for SES, gender, ethnicity, region, and urban-suburban-rural residence. Thus, a child's level of conduct problems as rated on the ASEBA can be compared to the ratings of other children of the same age and gender from the very large and representative standardization sample.

Third, most behavior rating scales provide a time-efficient method for screening a large number of important psychological domains that may be influenced by a child's conduct problems, such as anxiety, depression, social problems, and family relationships. Thus, rating scales can be very useful in providing a broad screening of some of the most common co-occurring problems that are displayed by children and adolescent with serious conduct problems. It is important to note, however, that rating scales vary somewhat on how well they assess the various co-occurring conditions. For example, the ASEBA does not include separate depression and anxiety scales, nor does it include a hyperactivity scale. In a similar vein, rating scales vary how well the scales match DSM definitions of children's emotional and behavioral problems. The ASEBA (Achenbach, 2013) and the CRS-3 (Conners, 2008) standard subscales do not conform closely to DSM diagnoses, but they both include scoring algorithms for supplementary DSM-5-oriented scales. However, rating scales developed by Gadow and Sprafkin (2002), such as the Child Symptom Inventory-5 (CSI-5), Early Childhood Inventory-5 (ECI-5), and the Child and Adolescent Symptom Inventory-5 (CASI-5), were specifically developed to correspond closely to DSM criteria.

Interviews Another assessment technique that can play an important role in the diagnosis of children and adolescent with serious conduct problems are interviews. Interviews can be divided into two broad categories: unstructured clinical interviews and structured diagnostic interviews.

Conducting a clinical interview with a parent is particularly important for the assessment of conduct problems for several reasons. First, clinical interviews allow for an individualized method for assessing the type, severity, and impairment associated with the child's behavior problems, including how long the problems have been displayed by the child and whether they have changed in their frequency and severity over time. Second, a clinical interview with a parent helps to assess stressors that may be occurring in the family (e.g., parental divorce, parental substance abuse) that may be related to the child's behavior problems. Third, the unstructured interview can assess typical parent–child interactions, especially interactions involving parental behaviors that may make the conduct problems more likely to occur (e.g., yelling at the child) and parental behaviors in response to the child's behavior that either increase (i.e., give the child attention) or decrease (i.e., ignore) the likelihood that the conduct problems will reoccur. Finally, the unstructured interview allows the parent to describe previous attempts to reduce the child's conduct problems, both formal (e.g., seeking mental health counseling) and informal (e.g., change in discipline strategies).

Because the unstructured interview allows for obtaining highly individualized information about a specific child, it requires highly trained clinicians to conduct these interviews, and it is often difficult to obtain reliable information in this format. As a result, structured interview schedules were developed to improve the reliability of the information that is obtained during a clinical interview. Two structured diagnostic interviews that are frequently used in the assessment of children with conduct problems are the Diagnostic Interview Schedule for Children (DISC-IV; Shaffer, Fisher, Lucas, Dulcan, & Schwab-Stone, 2000) and the Diagnostic Interview for Children and Adolescents (DICA; Reich, 2000). These structured interviews provide a format for obtaining parent and youth reports on the symptoms that comprise the criteria for ODD and CD according to DSM-IV-TR (American Psychiatric Association, 2000). Thus, they provide the most direct method for assessing the actual criteria of these diagnoses. Both the DISC-IV and DICA are being updated to reflect the changes in criteria for the disorders included in the DSM-5 (American Psychiatric Association, 2013).

Structured interviews provide standardized question and answer formats which results in much higher reliability compared to unstructured clinical interviews. For example, a stem question is asked (e.g., "Does your child get into fights?"), and follow-up questions are only asked if the stem question is answered affirmatively (e.g., "Is this only with his or her brothers and sisters?" and "Does he or she usually start these fights?"). Further, most structured interviews assess many other types of problems in adjustment beyond conduct problems, such as attention-deficit/hyperactivity disorder, depressive disorders, and anxiety disorders. Therefore, structured interviews can be helpful in assessing possible comorbid conditions that are often present in youth with conduct problems, although not in as time efficient a manner as behavior rating scales. In fact, structured interviews can become particularly lengthy if a child has a large number of problems. In these cases, many stem questions are answered affirmatively requiring the administration of extensive follow-up questions. As a result, administration time can range widely from 45 min for children and adolescents with few problems to over 2 h for youths with many problems in adjustment (Frick et al., 2010).

Another limitation in structure interviews relative to behavior rating scales is that structured interviews often do not provide strong normative information on a child's behavior. Instead, structured interviews typically focus on assessing how much the child's behavior problems lead to impairments in his or her social and academic functioning. However, a relative advantage of the structure interview is that most include standard questions that assess the age at which a child's behavioral difficulties began to emerge (onset) and how long (persistence) they have caused problems for the child. The assessment of age of onset of the child's behavior problems, as well as the duration of any other problems in adjustment, allows for a determination of the temporal ordering of a child's problems, such as whether the child's conduct problems predated his or her emotional difficulties. Such information may aid in determining whether the emotional distress is best conceptualized as a result of the impairments caused by the child's conduct problems (e.g., distress over peer rejection or disciplinary infractions at school).

Thus, structured interviews provide several pieces of important information for determining if a child with conduct problems needs treatment and they do so in a reliable manner. However, as noted above, they also include some critical limitations (e.g., lack of normative information, time-consuming). In addition, most structured interviews do not have formats for obtaining teacher information, and it is difficult to obtain reliable information on structured interviews using the child's report for young children below the age of 9 (Frick et al., 2010). Of greatest concern, however, is that there is evidence that the number of symptoms reported declines within an interview schedule. Specifically, parents and youth tend to report more symptoms for disorders that are assessed early in the interview, regardless of which diagnoses are assessed first (Jensen, Watanabe, & Richters, 1999; Piacentini et al., 1999). This is likely due to the stem/follow-up format that makes it increasingly clear to informants that the interview becomes longer the more symptoms that are endorsed. This is a very critical limitation, given that conduct problems are often assessed last in most of the available interview schedules and, as a result, could be underreported as a result of this limitation.

Behavioral Observation The third critical assessment method that can be used for making a diagnosis of a child with serious behavior problems are behavioral observations. Observing a child's or adolescent's behavior in a natural setting (e.g., home, school, playground) can provide important information for the assessment process for several reasons. First, observations are not filtered through the perception of an informant. Second, observations provide information on the youth's environmental context. For example, behavioral observations can indicate how others in the child's environment (e.g., parents, teachers, peers) respond to the child's behavior, which is important for identifying factors that may be maintaining or exacerbate these behaviors.

Two widely used observation procedures available for assessing children with conduct problems in younger (3–8 years) children are the Behavioral Coding System (BCS; McMahon & Forehand, 2003) and the Dyadic Parent–Child Interaction Coding System (DPICS; Eyberg, Nelson, Ginn, Bhuiyan, & Boggs, 2013). The BCS and the DPICS place the parent-child dyad in standard situations that vary in the degree to which parental control is required, ranging from a free-play situation to a parent-directed activity such as completing math problems or cleaning up toys. Each task typically lasts 5–10 min. The coding system scores a variety of parent and child behaviors, particularly parental antecedents (e.g., commands) or consequences (e.g., use of verbal hostility) to the child's behavior. Scores from both the BCS and the DPICS have been shown to differentiate clinic-referred children with conduct problems from non-referred children (Eyberg et al., 2013; Griest, Forehand, Wells, & McMahon, 1980).

It is important to note that most observations systems require very extensive training to achieve reliable coding of parent and child behaviors (e.g., 20–25 h for the BCS). Such intensive trainings often limit the usefulness of these systems in many clinical settings (Frick et al., 2010). However, simplified versions of both the DPICS and the BCS have been developed to reduce training demands and are more useful for most clinical settings (Eyberg, Bessmer, Newcomb, Edwards, & Robinson, 1994; McMahon & Estes, 1994). Indeed, negative parental attention (coded from the simplified version of the BCS) during a structured child-directed play task predicted higher levels of parent-reported conduct problems concurrently and at a 6-year follow-up, which supports the predictive validity of this abbreviated coding system (Fleming, McMahon, & King, 2017).

Several behavioral observational systems have been developed for use in school settings (Nock & Kurtz, 2005). Both the BCS (McMahon & Forehand, 2003) and the DPICS (Eyberg et al., 2013) have been modified for use in the classroom to assess child behavior (Breiner & Forehand, 1981; Jacobs et al., 2000). An adaptation of the DPICS, the REDSOCS (Revised Edition of the School Observation Coding System), has been utilized in several samples of children (Bagner, Boggs, & Eyberg, 2010; Jacobs et al., 2000). REDSOCS coding is done in 10-s intervals and several disruptive behaviors (e.g., whining, crying, yelling, aggression) are coded. Of most importance, noncompliant behavior is coded when a youth does not initiate or attempt to comply with a teacher command (either direct or indirect) 5 s following the command. Off-task behavior is coded for the child who is not attending to the material or task at hand (e.g., getting out of seat, talking out of turn, day dreaming).

The BASC-3-Student Observation System (SOS; Reynolds & Kamphaus, 2015) is similar to the REDSOCS in that it provides a system for observing children's behavior in the classroom using a momentary time-sampling procedure. With the purchase of an application for a smartphone, tablet, or laptop, the observations can be entered directly into a digital database that can be integrated with the results of the parent and teacher ratings on the BASC-3. The SOS specifies 65 behaviors that are commonly displayed in the classroom and includes both adaptive (e.g., "follows directions" and "returns material used in class") and maladaptive (e.g., "fidgets in seat" and "teases others") behaviors. The observation period in the classroom is 15 min, which is divided into 30 intervals of 30 s each. The child's behavior is observed for 3 s at the end of each interval, and the observer codes all behaviors that were observed during this time window. Although the newest version of the SOS has not been extensively tested, scores from the earlier version of this observation system differentiated students with conduct problems from other children (Lett & Kamphaus, 1997).

Similar to the SOS, the Direct Observation Form from the Achenbach System (ASEBA-DOF; McConaughy & Achenbach, 2009) was designed to observe students ages 5–14 years for 10-minute periods in the classroom. Three types of information are recorded. First, at the end of each minute during the observational period, the child's behavior is coded as being on- or off-task for 5 s. Second, at the end of the observational period, the observer writes a narrative of the child's behavior throughout the 10-minute observational period, noting the occurrence, duration, and intensity of specific problems. Third, again at the end of the observational period, the observer codes 96 behaviors on a 4-point scale (0 = "behavior was not observed," through 3 = "definite occurrence of behavior with severe intensity or for greater than 3-minute duration"). These ratings can be summed into Total Problem, Internalizing, and Externalizing behavior composites.

One limitation in observational systems is the difficulty in obtaining an adequate sample of a child's behavior. That is, it is sometimes hard to know if the child's behavior during the observation period was representative of his or her typical way of behaving. Further, it is often hard to observe covert conduct problems (e.g., lying and stealing) and low base rate conduct problems (e.g., fighting) that are often the most severe and, as a result, the most critical for determining need for treatment. Further, observations are subject to reactivity, such that a child's behavior can change because the child knows that he or she is being observed (Aspland & Gardner, 2003).

Summary Taken together, it is critical to carefully assess the types and severity of a child's conduct problems, as well as common co-occurring problems in adjustment, to determine if a child or adolescent requires treatment for their behavior problems. Behavior rating scales, unstructured and structured interviews, and behavioral observations all can aid in this process, but each has their unique strengths and weaknesses. Therefore, typical assessments of children with conduct problems should include multiple methods of assessment that capitalize on the strengths of these different approaches.

Assessment for Treatment Planning

Once it is determined that a child needs treatment, then it is a critical to develop a clear case conceptualization of the most likely causes of the child's behavior problems that can then be targeted in an intervention. A key area of research for guiding these conceptualizations is the work documenting some of the common developmental pathways that lead to serious conduct problems in children and adolescents. As reviewed previously, children with conduct problems can fall into childhood-onset or adolescent-onset pathways, depending on the age at which their significant antisocial and aggressive behavior started. Further, important differences exist in the risk factors to conduct problems for children with and without elevated levels of CU traits (Frick et al., 2014a). Knowledge of the characteristics of children in these different pathways can aid case conceptualizations by providing a set of working hypotheses about the most likely causes of the child's conduct problems (Frick et al., 2010; McMahon & Frick, 2005).

For example, for youth whose serious conduct problems did not emerge until adolescence, it is reasonable to hypothesize based on the available literature that they may be less likely to be aggressive, have intellectual deficits, have temperamental vulnerabilities, and have comorbid ADHD. However, the adolescent-onset youths' association with deviant peer groups, as well as factors that may contribute to the deviant peer group affiliation (e.g., lack of parental monitoring and supervision), would be important to assess for youth in this pathway. In contrast, for youth whose serious conduct problems began prior to adolescence, one would expect more cognitive and temperamental vulnerabilities, comorbid ADHD, and more serious problems in family functioning. For youth in this childhood-onset group who do not exhibit high levels of CU traits, verbal intelligence deficits would be more likely, as well as difficulties regulating emotions, leading to higher levels of anxiety, depression, and aggression involving anger. In contrast, for a youth with childhood-onset conduct problems who exhibits high levels of CU traits, the cognitive deficits are more likely to involve a lack of sensitivity to punishment, and the temperamental vulnerabilities are more likely to involve a preference for dangerous and novel activities and a failure to express many types of emotion. Assessing the level and severity of aggressive behavior, especially the presence of instrumental aggression, would be critical for children and adolescents in this group as well.

Most clinicians recognize that people do not fall neatly into the prototypes that are suggested by research (see also Fairchild, Goozen, Calder, & Goodyer, 2013). As such, these descriptions are meant to help generate hypotheses around which to organize an evidence-based assessment and develop a clear case conceptualization as to the most likely causes of the child's behavior problems and the most effective targets to intervention. For example, for the child or adolescent with serious conduct problems in which the assessment leads to a conceptualization that is most consistent with the adolescent-onset pathway, interventions should be considered that focus on enhancing identity development in adolescents and increasing contact with prosocial peers, such as mentoring programs (Grossman & Tierney, 1998) or programs that provide structured after-school activities (Mahoney & Stattin, 2000). In contrast, for the child or adolescent with serious conduct problems whose behavior problems started early in childhood but without elevated levels of CU traits, interventions should be considered that focus on anger control (Larson & Lochman, 2005) or that focus on reducing harsh and ineffective parenting (Forgatch & Patterson, 2010) in an effort to help the child develop better emotional and behavioral regulation strategies. In contrast, young children with elevated CU traits may benefit from interventions that focus on enhancing parental warmth and help parents to coach the child to recognize other emotions (Frick, 2012; Hawes et al., 2014;

Wilkinson et al., 2015). Older children and adolescents with elevated CU traits may benefit from interventions that focus on reward-oriented approaches that target the self-interests of the adolescent in order to encourage prosocial behavior in the youth (Caldwell, Skeem, Salekin, & Van Rybroek, 2006).

Assessing Age of Onset From these descriptions, it is clear that several crucial pieces of information are important to gather from an assessment to help in developing these case conceptualizations to guide treatment recommendations. First, one crucial piece of information is determining the age at which the serious conduct problems first began to be displayed by the child, which helps to determine whether the child fits more with the childhood-onset or adolescent-onset pathway. As noted above, both unstructured and structured clinical interviews provide some of the best ways of obtaining this information on the onset of a child's behavior problems. However, one complicating factor is that research has not been consistent on the exact age at which to make this distinction or even whether this distinction should be based on chronological age or on the pubertal status of the child (Moffitt, 2006). For example, the DSM-5 criteria for conduct disorder (American Psychiatric Association, 2013) makes the distinction between children who begin showing severe conduct problems before age 10 (i.e., childhood onset) and those who do not show severe conduct problems until age 10 or older (i.e., adolescent onset). However, other research studies have used age 11 (Robins, 1966) or age 14 (Patterson & Yoerger, 1993; Tibbetts & Piquero, 1999) to define the start of adolescent onset. Thus, onset of severe conduct problems before age 10 seems to be clearly considered childhood onset and onset after age 13 clearly adolescent onset. However, classifying children whose severe conduct problems onset between the ages of 11 and 13 is less clear and likely depend on the level of physical, cognitive, and social maturity of the child.

Another important issue when assessing age of onset of a child's conduct problems relates to the accuracy of a parent or youth report. Three findings from research can help in interpreting such reports on the child's history of problem behavior. First, the longer the time frame involved in the retrospective report (e.g., a parent of a 17-year-old reporting on preschool behavior vs. a parent of a 6-year-old reporting on preschool behavior), the less accurate the report is likely to be (Green, Loeber, & Lahey, 1991). Second, although a parental report of the exact age of onset may not be very reliable over time, typical variations in years are usually small, and the relative rankings within symptoms (e.g., which symptom began first) and within a sample (e.g., which children exhibited the earliest onset of behavior) seem to be fairly stable (Green et al., 1991). Therefore, these reports should be viewed as rough estimates of the timing of onset and not as exact dating procedures. Third, there is evidence that combining informants (e.g., such as a parent or youth) or combining sources of information (e.g., self-report and school/clinical/police records), and taking the earliest reported age of onset from any source, provide an estimate that shows somewhat greater validity than any single source of information alone (Lahey et al., 1999).

Assessing Callous-Unemotional Traits In addition to age of onset of the child's conduct problems, the presence of elevated levels of CU traits is also important for treatment planning. As noted above, the DSM-5 included in the diagnosis of conduct disorder a specifier called "with limited prosocial emotions," and the criteria for this specifier provide guidance for the clinical assessment of CU. That is, according to the DSM-5, significant levels of CU traits are defined as two or more of the following characteristics that are shown by the child persistently (12 months or longer) and in multiple relationships or settings:

- Lack of remorse or guilt
- Callous-lack of empathy
- Unconcerned about performance
- Shallow or deficient affect

These symptoms were selected for inclusion in the specifier, and the diagnostic cutoff used to designate elevated levels of these traits (i.e., two or more symptoms), was chosen based on extensive secondary data analyses across several large samples of youth in different countries (Kimonis et al., 2015). These four criteria consistently were the best indicators of the overall construct of CU traits in factor analyses across samples, and the presence of two or more symptoms, if shown persistently, designated a more severely impaired group of antisocial youth across these samples.

CU traits can be assessed in unstructured clinical interviews. In addition, these traits correspond closely to the affective dimension of psychopathy (Hare & Neumann, 2008). As a result, measures for assessing psychopathic features in youth can be used to assess these traits, such as the Psychopathy Checklist: Youth Version (PCL-YV; Forth, Kosson, & Hare, 2003). The PCL-YV is a widely used clinician-rated checklist with a long history of use in largely forensic samples of adolescents (Kotler & McMahon, 2010). However, because it was designed largely for institutionalized adolescents, its utility for assessing children or for assessing children and adolescents in other mental health settings has not been firmly established. Further, its format as a clinician-rated checklist requires a highly trained clinician to administer and score the measure.

To overcome these limitations, the Antisocial Process Screening Device (APSD; Frick & Hare, 2001) was developed to assess the same content as the PCL-YV but using a behavior rating scale format that is completed by parents and teachers. A self-report version of this scale is also available for older children and adolescents (Muñoz & Frick, 2007). Unfortunately, the APSD, like the PCL-YV, was developed to assess the broader construct of psychopathy, and, as a result, it includes only six items directly assessing CU traits. Further, it only has three response options for rating the frequency of the behaviors. The few items, the limited range in response options, and the fact that ratings of CU traits are negatively skewed in most samples resulted in the APSD scores showing poor internal consistency in many samples (Poythress, Dembo, Wareham, & Greenbaum, 2006).

To overcome the APSD's limitations, the Inventory of Callous-Unemotional Traits (ICU) was developed to provide a more extended assessment of CU traits (Kimonis et al., 2008). The ICU was developed specifically to assess the four items that are included in the with limited prosocial emotions specifier. Items were developed to have six items (three positively and three negatively worded items) to assess each of the four symptoms. These 24 items were then placed on a 4-point Likert scale that could be rated from 0 (not at all true) to 3 (definitely true). Versions for parent, teacher, and self-report were developed to encourage multi-informant assessments. The ICU has a number of positive qualities for assessing CU traits. The larger number of items and its extended response format has resulted in a 24-item total score that is internally consistent in many samples, with Cronbach's alpha ranging between 0.77 and 0.89 (Frick & Ray, 2015). Further, there is a preschool version for use with children as young as age 3 (Ezpeleta et al., 2013). The ICU has been translated into over 20 languages with substantial support for its validity across these translations (Ciucci, Baroncelli, Franchi, Golmaryami, & Frick, 2014; Fanti et al., 2009; Kimonis et al., 2008). However, these positive qualities need to be weighed against the lack of a large and representative normative sample being available for the ICU and with empirically derived cutoffs only being available for only certain versions of the scale (Kimonis, Fanti, & Singh, 2014).

Conclusions

In conclusion, research has accumulated showing that children with serious conduct problems can vary greatly in the severity of their behavior and in the most likely causes of their behavior problems. This research is critical for guiding clinical assessments of children and adolescents with conduct problems that seek to determine the need for treatment (i.e., making a diagnosis) and that seek to determine the most likely treatment that would be of benefit to the child or adolescent. In this chapter, we attempted to outline the key findings from research and their implications for conducting an evidence-based approach to psychological assessment. We also summarized some of the key methods used in the assessment of children and adolescent with serious conduct problems, highlighting the strengths and weaknesses of the various methods and making practical recommendations for their use.

One overarching issue that emerged from this review is the importance of integrating the most current research findings on the causal pathways to serious conduct problems to both assessment and treatment (Frick, 2012). As noted above, research has uncovered several common developmental pathways to serious conduct problems that show very different risk factors (Frick et al., 2014a, 2014b). As knowledge of these pathways advances, it will be important for the methods of assessing children with serious conduct problems to advance as well. As a recent example, our review suggested that research has supported the importance of elevated CU traits for designating a clinically important subgroup of children and adolescents with serious conduct problems. Thus, it is important for research to continue to develop better ways of assessing these traits in a way that can inform clinical decisions in various settings (Frick & Ray, 2015).

Another broad issue that emerged from our review is that many assessments of children with serious conduct problems require a comprehensive assessment that covers multiple aspects of the youth's adjustment (e.g., conduct problems, anxiety, learning problems), that is assessed in multiple settings (e.g., home and school), and that uses multiple methods for assessing the key areas of psychological adjustment (Frick et al., 2010; McMahon & Estes, 1997; McMahon & Frick, 2005). Because of this, more research is needed into how such assessments can be conducted in the most time-efficient manner, such as using a multistage assessment procedure that starts with more time-efficient measures (e.g., broadband behavior rating scales and unstructured clinical interviews), followed by more time-intensive measures (e.g., structured interviews and behavioral observations) when indicated (McMahon & Estes, 1997; McMahon & Frick, 2005; Nock & Kurtz, 2005).

Further, methods for integrating the various measures collected as part of a comprehensive assessment into a clear case conceptualization are needed, especially given that information obtained from the different methods often don't agree with each other (De De Los Reyes & Kazdin, 2005). Several strategies for integrating and interpreting information from comprehensive assessments have been proposed (Frick et al., 2010; McMahon & Forehand, 2005; Wakschlag & Danis, 2004). For example, Frick et al. (2010) outlined a multistage strategy for integrating results from a comprehensive assessment into a clear case conceptualization to guide treatment planning. First, the clinician should document all clinically significant findings regarding the youth's adjustment (e.g., elevations on ratings scales, diagnoses from structured interviews, and problem behaviors from observations). Second, the clinician should look for convergent findings across these methods. Third, the clinician should attempt to explain, using available research as much as possible, any discrepancies in the assessment results. For instance, a finding that a child and parent are reporting high rates of anxiety but not the teacher may be explained by research suggesting that teachers may not be aware of a student's level of anxiety in the classroom (Achenbach, McConaughy, & Howell, 1987). Fourth, the clinician should then develop a profile of the areas of most concern for the child and develop a coherent explanation for the child's conduct problems, again using existing research as much as possible. Although this approach to interpreting results of a comprehensive assessment is promising, much more research is needed to guide this process of integrating data from comprehensive assessments.

Finally, a critical implication of the various causal factors that can lead to serious conduct problems is that successful intervention needs to be both comprehensive, targeting the many different risk factors that lead to the child's behavior problem, and individualized, targeting the unique factors that seem to be playing a role in the development and maintenance of the behavior problems for the individual child. As a result, there is not likely to be any single "best" treatment for serious conduct problems. Instead, interventions must be tailored to the individual needs of the child with serious conduct problems, and these needs will likely differ depending on the specific mechanisms underlying the child's behavioral disturbance. As outlined in this chapter, successful psychological assessments are critical for matching the child's specific needs to the most effective treatment. However, more research is needed on the most effective and cost-efficient approaches to treatment that successfully use this assessment information to provide comprehensive and individualized interventions for children and adolescents with serious conduct problems (Alexander, Waldron, Robbins, & Neeb, 2013; Burns et al., 2003; Zajac, Randall, & Swenson, 2015).

References

Achenbach, T. M. (2013). *DSM-oriented guide for the Achenbach System of Empirically Based Assessment (ASEBA)*. Burlington, VT: University of Vermont Research Center for Children, Youth, and Families.

Achenbach, T. M., McConaughy, S. H., & Howell, C. T. (1987). Child/adolescent behavioral and emotional problems: Implications of cross-informant correlations for situational specificity. *Psychological Bulletin, 101*(2), 213–232.

Achenbach, T. M., & Rescorla, L. (2001). *ASEBA school-age forms & profiles*. Aseba Burlington. Retrieved from http://aseba.com/ordering/ASEBA%20Reliability%20and%20Validity-School%20Age.pdf

Achenbach, T. M., & Rescorla, L. A. (2000). *ASEBA preschool forms & profiles*. Burlington, VT: University of Vermont, Research Center for Children, Youth and Families Retrieved from http://www.aseba.org/ordering/ASEBA%20Reliability%20%26%20Validity-Preschool%20.pdf

Alexander, J. F., Waldron, H. B., Robbins, M. S., & Neeb, A. A. (2013). *Functional family therapy for adolescent behavior problems*. American Psychological Association. Retrieved from http://psycnet.apa.org/psycinfo/2012-31348-000/

American Psychiatric Association. (2000). *DSM-IV-TR: Diagnostic and statistical manual of mental disorders, text revision* (p. 75). Washington, DC: American Psychiatric Association.

American Psychiatric Association. (2013). *DSM-5*. American Psychiatric Association. Washington, DC: American Psychiatric Assocation.

Aspland, H., & Gardner, F. (2003). Observational measures of parent-child interaction: An introductory review. *Child and Adolescent Mental Health, 8*(3), 136–143.

Bagner, D. M., Boggs, S. R., & Eyberg, S. M. (2010). Evidence-based school behavior assessment of externalizing behavior in young children. *Education & Treatment of Children, 33*(1), 65–83 https://doi.org/10.1353/etc.0.0084

Breiner, J., & Forehand, R. (1981). An assessment of the effects of parent training on clinic-referred childrens school behavior. *Behavioral Assessment, 3*(1), 31–42.

Brezina, T., & Piquero, A. R. (2007). Moral beliefs, isolation from peers, and abstention from delinquency. *Deviant Behavior, 28*(5), 433–465.

Burns, B. J., Howell, J. C., Wiig, J. K., Augimeri, L. K., Welsh, B. C., Loeber, R., & Petechuk, D. (2003). Treatment, Services, and Intervention Programs for Child Delinquents. Child Delinquency Bulletin Series. Retrieved from http://eric.ed.gov/?id=ED474859

Caldwell, M., Skeem, J., Salekin, R., & Van Rybroek, G. (2006). Treatment response of adolescent offenders with psychopathy features: A 2-year follow-up. *Criminal Justice and Behavior, 33*(5), 571–596 https://doi.org/10.1177/0093854806288176

Canino, G., Polanczyk, G., Bauermeister, J. J., Rohde, L. A., & Frick, P. J. (2010). Does the prevalence of CD and ODD vary across cultures? *Social Psychiatry and Psychiatric Epidemiology, 45*(7), 695–704 https://doi.org/10.1007/s00127-010-0242-y

Ciucci, E., Baroncelli, A., Franchi, M., Golmaryami, F. N., & Frick, P. J. (2014). The association between callous-unemotional traits and behavioral and academic adjustment in children: Further validation of the inventory of callous-unemotional traits. *Journal of Psychopathology and Behavioral Assessment, 36*(2), 189–200.

Conners, C. K. (2008). *Conners third edition (Conners 3)* (3rd ed.). Los Angeles, CA: Western Psychological Services Retrieved from http://v-psyche.com/doc/MENTAL%20ABILITY/Conners%203-2.doc

Dandreaux, D. M., & Frick, P. J. (2009). Developmental pathways to conduct problems: A further test of the childhood and adolescent-onset distinction. *Journal of Abnormal Child Psychology, 37*(3), 375 https://doi.org/10.1007/s10802-008-9261-5

De Los Reyes, A., & Kazdin, A. E. (2005). Informant discrepancies in the assessment of childhood psychopathology: A critical review, theoretical framework, and recommendations for further study. *Psychological Bulletin, 131*(4), 483.

Dodge, K. A., Lansford, J. E., Burks, V. S., Bates, J. E., Pettit, G. S., Fontaine, R., & Price, J. M. (2003). Peer rejection and social information-processing factors in the development of aggressive behavior problems in children. *Child Development, 74*(2), 374–393.

Eyberg, S. M., Bessmer, J. L., Newcomb, K., Edwards, D., & Robinson, E. A. (1994). *Dyadic parent-child coding system-II (DPICS-II)*. Corte Madera, CA: Select.

Eyberg, S. M., Nelson, M. M., Ginn, N. C., Bhuiyan, N., & Boggs, S. R. (2013). *Dyadic parent–child interaction coding system: Comprehensive manual for research and training*. Gainesville, FL: PCIT International.

Ezpeleta, L., de la Osa, N., Granero, R., Penelo, E., & Domènech, J. M. (2013). Inventory of callous-unemotional traits in a community sample of preschoolers. *Journal of Clinical Child & Adolescent Psychology, 42*(1), 91–105 https://doi.org/10.1080/15374416.2012.734221

Fairchild, G., Goozen, S. H., Calder, A. J., & Goodyer, I. M. (2013). Research review: Evaluating and reformulating the developmental taxonomic theory of antisocial behaviour. *Journal of Child Psychology and Psychiatry, 54*(9), 924–940.

Fanti, K. A., Frick, P. J., & Georgiou, S. (2009). Linking callous-unemotional traits to instrumental and non-instrumental forms of aggression. *Journal of Psychopathology and Behavioral Assessment, 31*(4), 285–298 https://doi.org/10.1007/s10862-008-9111-3

Fleming, A. P., McMahon, R. J., & King, K. M. (2017). Structured parent-child observations predict development of conduct problems: The importance of parental negative attention in child-directed play. *Prevention Science, 18*(3), 257–267.

Forgatch, M. S., & Patterson, G. R. (2010). Parent management training – Oregon model: An intervention for antisocial behaviors in children and adolescents. In *Evidenced-based psychotherapies for children and adolescents* (2nd ed., pp. 159–178). New York, NY: Guilford.

Forth, A. E., Kosson, D., & Hare, R. D. (2003). *The hare PCL: Youth version*. Toronto, ON: Multi-Health Systems.

Frick, P. J. (2012). Developmental pathways to conduct disorder: Implications for future directions in research, assessment, and treatment. *Journal of Clinical Child & Adolescent Psychology, 41*(3), 378–389 https://doi.org/10.1080/15374416.2012.664815

Frick, P. J. (2016). Current research on conduct disorder in children and adolescents. *South African Journal of Psychology, 46*(2), 160–174.

Frick, P. J., Barry, C. T., & Kamphaus, R. W. (2010). *Clinical assessment of child and adolescent personality and behavior* (3rd ed.). Springer US. Retrieved from http://www.springer.com/us/book/9780387896427

Frick, P. J., Cornell, A. H., Doug, S., Dane, H. E., Barry, C. T., & Loney, B. R. (2003). Callous-unemotional traits and developmental pathways to severe conduct problems. *Developmental Psychology, 39*(2), 246–260 https://doi.org/10.1037/0012-1649.39.2.246

Frick, P. J., & Hare, R. D. (2001). *APSD – Antisocial process screening device*. Toronto, ON: Multi-Health Systems Retrieved from https://downloads.mhs.com/product.aspx?gr=saf&prod=apsd&id=overview

Frick, P. J., & Nigg, J. T. (2012). Current issues in the diagnosis of attention deficit hyperactivity disorder, oppositional defiant disorder, and conduct disorder. *Annual Review of Clinical Psychology, 8*(1), 77–107 https://doi.org/10.1146/annurev-clinpsy-032511-143150

Frick, P. J., & Ray, J. V. (2015). Evaluating callous-unemotional traits as a personality construct. *Journal of Personality, 83*(6), 710–722 https://doi.org/10.1111/jopy.12114

Frick, P. J., Ray, J. V., Thornton, L. C., & Kahn, R. E. (2014a). Annual research review: A developmental psychopathology approach to understanding callous-unemotional traits in children and adolescents with serious conduct problems. *Journal of Child Psychology and Psychiatry, and Allied Disciplines, 55*(6), 532–548 https://doi.org/10.1111/jcpp.12152

Frick, P. J., Ray, J. V., Thornton, L. C., & Kahn, R. E. (2014b). Can callous-unemotional traits enhance the understanding, diagnosis, and treatment of serious conduct problems in children and adolescents? A comprehensive review. *Psychological Bulletin, 140*(1), 1–57 https://doi.org/10.1037/a0033076

Frick, P. J., Stickle, T. R., Dandreaux, D. M., Farrell, J. M., & Kimonis, E. R. (2005). Callous–unemotional traits in predicting the severity and stability of conduct problems and delinquency. *Journal of Abnormal Child Psychology, 33*(4), 471–487 https://doi.org/10.1007/s10648-005-5728-9

Frick, P. J., & Viding, E. (2009). Antisocial behavior from a developmental psychopathology perspective. *Development and Psychopathology, 21*(4), 1111–1131 https://doi.org/10.1017/S0954579409990071

Gadow, K. D., & Sprafkin, J. (2002). *Childhood Symptom Inventory-4 screening and norms manual*. Stonybrook, NY: Checkmate Plus.

Green, S. M., Loeber, R., & Lahey, B. B. (1991). Stability of mothers' recall of the age of onset of their child's attention and hyperactivity problems. *Journal of the American Academy of Child & Adolescent Psychiatry, 30*(1), 135–137.

Griest, D. L., Forehand, R., Wells, K. C., & McMahon, R. J. (1980). An examination of differences between nonclinic and behavior-problem clinic-referred children and their mothers. *Journal of Abnormal Psychology, 89*(3), 497.

Grossman, J. B., & Tierney, J. P. (1998). Does mentoring work? An impact study of the Big Brothers Big Sisters program. *Evaluation Review, 22*(3), 403–426.

Hare, R. D., & Neumann, C. S. (2008). Psychopathy as a clinical and empirical construct. *Annual Review of Clinical Psychology, 4*, 217–246.

Hawes, D. J., Price, M. J., & Dadds, M. R. (2014). Callous-unemotional traits and the treatment of conduct problems in childhood and adolescence: A comprehensive review. *Clinical Child and Family Psychology Review, 17*(3), 248–267 https://doi.org/10.1007/s10567-014-0167-1

Jacobs, J. R., Boggs, S. R., Eyberg, S. M., Edwards, D., Durning, P., Querido, J. G., ... Funderburk, B. W. (2000). Psychometric properties and reference point data for the revised edition of the school observation coding system. *Behavior Therapy, 31*(4), 695–712.

Jensen, P. S., Watanabe, H. K., & Richters, J. E. (1999). Who's up first? Testing for order effects in structured interviews using a counterbalanced experimental design. *Journal of Abnormal Child Psychology, 27*(6), 439–445.

Kazdin, A. E., Whitley, M., & Marciano, P. L. (2006). Child–therapist and parent–therapist alliance and therapeutic change in the treatment of children referred for oppositional, aggressive, and antisocial behavior. *Journal of Child Psychology and Psychiatry, 47*(5), 436–445 https://doi.org/10.1111/j.1469-7610.2005.01475.x

Kimonis, E. R., Fanti, K. A., Frick, P. J., Moffitt, T. E., Essau, C., Bijttebier, P., & Marsee, M. A. (2015). Using self-reported callous-unemotional traits to cross-nationally assess the DSM-5 "With Limited Prosocial Emotions" specifier. *Journal of Child Psychology and Psychiatry, and Allied Disciplines, 56*(11), 1249–1261 https://doi.org/10.1111/jcpp.12357

Kimonis, E. R., Fanti, K. A., & Singh, J. P. (2014). Establishing cut-off scores for the parent-reported inventory of callous-unemotional traits. *Archives of Forensic Psychology, 1*(1), 27–48.

Kimonis, E. R., Frick, P. J., & McMahon, R. J. (2014). Conduct and oppositional defiant disorders. In E. J. Mash & R. A. Barkley (Eds.), *Child psychopathology* (3rd ed., pp. 145–179). New York, NY: Guilford.

Kimonis, E. R., Frick, P. J., Skeem, J. L., Marsee, M. A., Cruise, K., Munoz, L. C., ... Morris, A. S. (2008). Assessing callous–unemotional traits in adolescent offenders: Validation of the inventory of callous–unemotional traits. *International Journal of Law and Psychiatry, 31*(3), 241–252 https://doi.org/10.1016/j.ijlp.2008.04.002

Kruh, I. P., Frick, P. J., & Clements, C. B. (2005). Historical and personality correlates to the violence patterns of juveniles tried as adults. *Criminal Justice and Behavior, 32*(1), 69–96 https://doi.org/10.1177/0093854804270629

Kotler, J. S., & McMahon, R. J. (2010). Assessment of child and adolescent psychopathy. In R. T. Salekin & D. R. Lynam (Eds.), Handbook of child and adolescent psychopahthy (pp. 79–112.). New York: Guilford.

Lahey, B. B., Goodman, S. H., Waldman, I. D., Bird, H., Canino, G., Jensen, P., ... Applegate, B. (1999). Relation of age of onset to the type and severity of child and adolescent conduct problems. *Journal of Abnormal Child Psychology, 27*(4), 247–260.

Larson, J., & Lochman, J. E. (2005). *Helping schoolchildren cope with anger: A cognitive-behavioral intervention* (1st ed.). New York, NY: Guilford.

Lawing, K., Frick, P. J., & Cruise, K. R. (2010). Differences in offending patterns between adolescent sex offenders high or low in callous—Unemotional traits. *Psychological Assessment, 22*(2), 298–305 https://doi.org/10.1037/a0018707

Lett, N. J., & Kamphaus, R. W. (1997). Differential validity of the BASC student observation system and the BASC teacher rating scale. *Canadian Journal of School Psychology, 13*(1), 1–14.

Loeber, R., Burke, J. D., Lahey, B. B., Winters, A., & Zera, M. (2000). Oppositional defiant and conduct disorder: A review of the past 10 years, part I. *Journal of the American Academy of Child and Adolescent Psychiatry, 39*(12), 1468–1484 https://doi.org/10.1097/00004583-200012000-00007

Loeber, R., & Hay, D. (1997). Key issues in the development of aggression and violence from childhood to early adulthood. *Annual Review of Psychology, 48*, 371–410 https://doi.org/10.1146/annurev.psych.48.1.371

Mahoney, J. L., & Stattin, H. (2000). Leisure activities and adolescent antisocial behavior: The role of structure and social context. *Journal of Adolescence, 23*(2), 113–127.

Maughan, B., Rowe, R., Messer, J., Goodman, R., & Meltzer, H. (2004). Conduct disorder and oppositional defiant disorder in a national sample: Developmental epidemiology. *Journal of Child Psychology and Psychiatry, and Allied Disciplines, 45*(3), 609–621.

McConaughy, S. H., & Achenbach, T. M. (2009). *Manual for the ASEBA direct observation form*. Burlington, VT: University of Vermont, Research Center for Children, Youth, & Families.

McMahon, R. J., & Estes, A. (1994). *Fast track parent-child interaction task: Observational data collection manuals*. Unpublished. Seattle, WA: University of Washington.

McMahon, R. J., & Estes, A. (1997). Conduct problems. In E. J. Mash & L. G. Terdal (Eds.), *Assessment of childhood disorders* (3rd ed., pp. 130–193). New York, NY: Guilford Press.

McMahon, R. J., & Forehand, R. L. (2003). Helping the Noncompliant Child: Family-based treatment for oppositional behavior (2nd ed.). New York, NY: Guilford Press.

McMahon, R. J., & Forehand, R. (2005). Helping the noncompliant child: Second Edition: Family-based treatment for oppositional behavior. Retrieved June 14, 2017, from https://www.guilford.com/books/Helping-the-Noncompliant-Child/McMahon-Forehand/9781593852412

McMahon, R. J., & Frick, P. J. (2005). Evidence-based assessment of conduct problems in children and adolescents. *Journal of Clinical Child and Adolescent Psychology, 34*(3), 477–505.

Moffitt, T. E. (2006). Life-course-persistent versus adolescence-limited antisocial behavior. In D. Cicchetti & D. J. Cohen (Eds.), *Developmental psychopathology* (pp. 570–598). Wiley https://doi.org/10.1002/9780470939406.ch15

Muñoz, L. C., & Frick, P. J. (2007). The reliability, stability, and predictive utility of the self-report version of the antisocial process screening device. *Scandinavian Journal of Psychology, 48*(4), 299–312 https://doi.org/10.1111/j.1467-9450.2007.00560.x

Nock, M. K., & Kurtz, S. M. (2005). Direct behavioral observation in school settings: Bringing science to practice. *Cognitive and Behavioral Practice, 12*(3), 359–370.

Odgers, C. L., Caspi, A., Broadbent, J. M., Dickson, N., Hancox, R. J., Harrington, H., ... Moffitt, T. E. (2007). Prediction of differential adult health burden by conduct problem subtypes in males. *Archives of General*

Psychiatry, *64*(4), 476–484 https://doi.org/10.1001/archpsyc.64.4.476

Odgers, C. L., Moffitt, T. E., Broadbent, J. M., Dickson, N., Hancox, R. J., Harrington, H., ... Caspi, A. (2008). Female and male antisocial trajectories: From childhood origins to adult outcomes. *Development and Psychopathology, 20*(2), 673–716.

Patterson, G. R., & Yoerger, K. (1993). Developmental models for delinquent behavior. Retrieved from http://psycnet.apa.org/psycinfo/1993-97503-008

Piacentini, J., Roper, M., Jensen, P., Lucas, C., Fisher, P., Bird, H., ... Dulcan, M. (1999). Informant-based determinants of symptom attenuation in structured child psychiatric interviews. *Journal of Abnormal Child Psychology, 27*(6), 417–428.

Poythress, N. G., Dembo, R., Wareham, J., & Greenbaum, P. E. (2006). Construct validity of the Youth Psychopathic Traits Inventory (YPI) and the Antisocial Process Screening Device (APSD) with justice-involved adolescents. *Criminal Justice and Behavior, 33*(1), 26–55.

Ray, J. V., Thornton, L. C., Frick, P. J., Steinberg, L., & Cauffman, E. (2016). Impulse control and callous-unemotional traits distinguish patterns of delinquency and substance use in justice involved adolescents: Examining the moderating role of neighborhood context. *Journal of Abnormal Child Psychology, 44*, 599–611 https://doi.org/10.1007/s10802-015-0057-0

Reich, W. (2000). Diagnostic interview for children and adolescents (DICA). *Journal of the American Academy of Child & Adolescent Psychiatry, 39*(1), 59–66.

Reynolds, C., & Kamphaus, R. (2015). *Behavioral assessment system for children—Third edition (BASC-3)* (3rd ed.). Minneapolis, MN: Pearson.

Robins, L. N. (1966). *Deviant children grown up, a sociological and psychiatric study of sociopathic personality*. Baltimore, MD: Williams & Wilkins Retrieved from http://eric.ed.gov/?id=ED018885

Shaffer, D., Fisher, P., Lucas, C. P., Dulcan, M. K., & Schwab-Stone, M. E. (2000). NIMH Diagnostic Interview Schedule for Children Version IV (NIMH DISC-IV): Description, differences from previous versions, and reliability of some common diagnoses. *Journal of the American Academy of Child & Adolescent Psychiatry, 39*(1), 28–38.

Silverthorn, P., & Frick, P. J. (1999). Developmental pathways to antisocial behavior: The delayed-onset pathway in girls. *Development and Psychopathology, 11*(1), 101–126.

Tibbetts, S. G., & Piquero, A. R. (1999). The influence of gender, low birth weight, and disadvantaged environment in predicting early onset of offending: A test of Moffitt's interactional hypothesis. *Criminology, 37*(4), 843–878.

Wakschlag, L., & Danis, B. (2004). Assessment of disruptive behavior in young children: A clinical-developmental framework. In *Handbook of Infant, Toddler and Preschool Mental Health Assessment* (pp. 421–440). New York, NY: Oxford University Press.

Wilkinson, S., Waller, R., & Viding, E. (2015). Practitioner review: involving young people with callous unemotional traits in treatment–does it work? A systematic review. *Journal of Child Psychology and Psychiatry*. Retrieved from http://onlinelibrary.wiley.com/doi/10.1111/jcpp.12494/pdf

Zajac, K., Randall, J., & Swenson, C. C. (2015). Multisystemic therapy for externalizing youth. *Child and Adolescent Psychiatric Clinics of North America, 24*(3), 601–616.

Behavioral Assessment of Self-Injury

Timothy R. Vollmer, Meghan Deshais, Kimberly N. Sloman, and Carrie S. W. Borrero

Introduction

This is an update of a chapter (Vollmer, Sloman, & Borrero, 2009) from a prior version of this volume (Matson, 2009). Self-injurious behavior (SIB) is a behavior disorder that can range in severity from self-inflicted mild bruising and abrasions to life- threatening tissue damage (Carr, 1977). The focus of this chapter is on SIB displayed by individuals with intellectual and developmental disabilities (I/DD), including autism. Although SIB occurs in psychiatric patients (e.g., self-mutilation) and in some otherwise typically developing adolescents and adults (e.g., self-cutting), these variations of SIB will not be the focus here. In addition, this chapter will focus on assessment rather than treatment. Finally, the specific focus is behavioral assessment rather than medical, biological, or psychiatric (diagnostic) assessment.

The numerous forms (topographies) of SIB described in clinical reports and scientific publications include self-hitting, head banging, self-biting, self-scratching, self-pinching, self-choking, eye gouging, hair pulling, and many others (Iwata et al., 1994). Although there are clear genetic and biological correlates with the disorder (e.g., Lesch & Nyhan, 1964), the majority of SIB appears to be learned behavior. Not including tics and related behavior, most of human behavior can be compartmentalized as either operant or reflexive (and respondent) behavior. There is no empirical evidence that SIB occurs in a fashion similar to a tic or nervous twitch.

The vast majority of evidence suggests that SIB is operant behavior controlled by either automatic (non-socially mediated) or socially mediated consequences. There is some evidence that a minority of SIB could be reflexive, but that evidence is indirect and will not be the focus of this chapter. The only evidence to date supporting SIB as reflexive behavior is found in the research on biting by various species that occurs in response to severe aversive stimulation (e.g., Hutchinson, 1977). Specifically, laboratory research has shown that many species of animals, including humans, will bite down on virtually whatever is available when certain kinds of aversive stimulation such as shock or loud noise are

T. R. Vollmer (✉)
Psychology Department, University of Florida, Gainesville, FL, USA
e-mail: vollmera@ufl.edu

M. Deshais
Caldwell University, Caldwell, NJ, USA

K. N. Sloman
Florida Institute of Technology, Melbourne, FL, USA

C. S. W. Borrero
Kennedy Krieger Institute, Baltimore, MD, USA

presented. Conceivably then, some self-biting might occur in response to either unconditioned or conditioned aversive stimuli.

The clearest evidence supports the notion that SIB is operant behavior strengthened (reinforced) by consequences to the behavior. The behavior is often so severe and so disturbing that care providers tend to act immediately and decisively to end an episode or bout of self-injury. Although well meaning, actions to end an episode of SIB might inadvertently reinforce the behavior. For example, one common care provider response is to give attention in the form of reprimands or comfort statements when severe behavior occurs (e.g., Sloman et al., 2005; Thompson & Iwata, 2001).

Social attention might serve as a source of *socially mediated positive reinforcement* for the SIB. Research has shown that even reprimands can serve as positive reinforcement, despite a clear intent of the care provider to scold or punish the behavior (e.g., Fisher, Ninness, Piazza, & Owen-DeSchryver, 1996). Other care providers may be inclined to comfort or nurse the individual following episodes of SIB (e.g., Fischer, Iwata, & Worsdell, 1997). Similarly, care providers may attempt to figure out what the individual "is upset about" and begin handing over tangible items including food, drinks, favorite toys, or activities (e.g., Marcus & Vollmer, 1996).

Conversely, escape from or avoidance of social interaction might serve as a source of *socially mediated negative reinforcement* for SIB. A common response of care providers is to move away from and terminate ongoing activity when SIB occurs, thus allowing escape or avoidance of an interaction that normally would have ensued. For example, dozens of behavioral assessment studies have shown that escape and avoidance of instructional activities, self-care activity, and daily living activity can reinforce SIB (e.g., Iwata, Pace, Kalsher, Cowdery, & Cataldo, 1990; Steege et al., 1990; Vollmer, Marcus, & Ringdahl, 1995). Similarly, some studies have shown that escape from close proximity during medical examinations (Iwata et al., 1990) or even during regular social interaction can reinforce SIB.

Not all SIB is reinforced by the actions of other people. In some cases, SIB produces its own source of reinforcement, independent of the social environment. In fact, some individuals with SIB will sit in a room alone for extended time periods engaging in repetitive SIB, even though the behavior produces no social reaction. In these cases, SIB is maintained by automatic reinforcement, meaning that no social mediation is required for the reinforcement. The specific sources of automatic reinforcement are not as well understood as the specific sources of socially mediated reinforcement, but there is some evidence that SIB can be automatically reinforced by pain attenuation (e.g., Fisher et al., 1998), attenuation of itching skin (e.g., Cowdery, Iwata, & Pace, 1990), pleasing self-stimulation (e.g., Lovaas, Newsom, & Hickman, 1987), and production of endogenous opiates (e.g., Sandman et al., 1983), among other possible sources.

Some individuals with SIB also engage in self-restraint, a form of behavior that can sometimes be puzzling to care providers. An individual is said to be self-restraining when they are engaging in a behavior that appears to be incompatible with SIB. For example, individuals may wrap their hands in clothing, sit on their hands, cross their legs, or lean against surfaces in the environment. Fisher and Iwata (1996) proposed four potential hypotheses about the relationship between SIB and self-restraint: (1) self-restraint and SIB are maintained by the same reinforcer, (2) self-restraint and SIB are maintained by different reinforcers, (3) SIB is reinforced by access to self-restraint, and (4) self-restraint is reinforced by escape from the aversive ramifications of SIB. Self-restraint can present unique challenges during behavioral assessments of SIB. Researchers have suggested that self-restraint and SIB frequently have an inverse relationship (Smith, Iwata, Vollmer, & Pace, 1992). Therefore, if self-restraint is permitted to occur during an assessment, it may be difficult to observe SIB for the purposes of determining why the individual engages in SIB. When conducting behavioral assessments with individuals who self-restrain, it might be necessary to evaluate levels of SIB when the individual is permitted to self-restrain as well as when the individual is blocked from self-restraining (Rooker & Roscoe, 2005; Scheithauer, O'Connor, & Toby, 2015).

One general purpose of a behavioral assessment of SIB is to identify which types of reinforcement are maintaining SIB in a given case. It cannot be assumed that SIB that looks similar in two different individuals serves the same function for both individuals. Conversely, similar forms of reinforcement can maintain SIB that looks very different in topography (e.g., head hitting by one individual and self-biting by another individual). Even one form of SIB displayed by a single person can serve multiple functions (Smith, Iwata, Vollmer, & Zarcone, 1993). Complications such as these underscore the need for individualized behavioral assessments. Typically, assessment components aimed at identifying the operant function of SIB involve some combination of interviews and checklists given to care providers, direct observation by a trained observer, or a functional analysis in which hypothesized reinforcers are tested. Identifying the specific source of reinforcement has powerful implications for treatment. For example, if SIB is reinforced by social attention, care providers can be taught to minimize attention following SIB and to reinforce some alternative attention-getting behavior.

A second general (but related) purpose of a behavioral assessment of SIB is to identify situations correlated with the occurrence of SIB. If SIB is most likely to occur during particular activities or kinds of activities, an intervention or further assessment may be focused on that particular activity or set of activities. Interviews and checklists, direct observation, and functional analyses are also used for this purpose.

A third general purpose of a behavioral assessment of SIB is to provide a baseline of the severity of the behavior in terms of response rate or tissue damage incurred. In so doing, the effects of behavioral or medical treatments can be compared to the period prior to intervention. Again, interviews and checklists, direct observation, and functional analyses are used for this purpose. In addition, severity charts and scales can be used to document changes in wound appearance (Self-Injury Trauma (SIT) scale; Iwata, Pace, Kissel, Nau, & Farber, 1990) and wound size (Wilson, Iwata, & Bloom, 2012).

This chapter is divided into sections describing behavioral assessment formats for SIB. The first section will describe variations of interview and checklist approaches to assessment. The second section will describe variations of descriptive analysis methods conducted via direct observation of SIB. The third section will describe variations of functional analysis methods. The fourth section will describe variations of severity scales and charts. The fifth section will describe the use of protective equipment for SIB. All sections will include a discussion of advantages and disadvantages of assessment formats.

Indirect Assessments

Indirect assessments are used to identify relevant characteristics of SIB, without directly observing the behavior. The assessment typically occurs at a different time and place from the actual occurrence of the self-injury. Indirect assessments rely on reports in the form of records (e.g., school discipline referrals, medical records), interviews (e.g., O'Neill et al., 1997), questionnaires (e.g., Iwata, DeLeon, & Roscoe, 2013), checklists (e.g., Van Houten & Rolider, 1991), or rating scales (e.g., Durand & Crimmins, 1988). Table 1 lists several commonly used forms of indirect assessment questionnaires, checklists, and rating scales. The information gathered from indirect assessments may be used to develop treatments for self-injury or to provide a foundation for a more direct assessment. In weighing benefits and limitations of indirect assessments, most practitioners recommend that they should not be used as a sole source of information but rather in conjunction with direct assessment methods (e.g., Zarcone, Rodgers, Iwata, Rourke, & Dorsey, 1991).

The primary advantage of indirect assessments is that they offer a time-efficient alternative to direct assessment methods (e.g., descriptive and experimental analyses). In most cases, the assessment can be administered within 15 minutes. This is in contrast to most direct

Table 1 Commonly used indirect assessments

Commonly used indirect assessment methods	
Child behavior checklist (CBCL)	Achenbach (1991)
Aberrant behavior checklist (ABC)	Aman, Singh, Stewart, and Field (1985)
Motivational assessment scale (MAS)	Durand and Crimmins (1988)
Functional analysis screening tool (FAST)	Iwata and DeLeon (1996)
Problem behavior questionnaire (PBQ)	Lewis, Scott, and Sugai (1994)
Functional assessment for multiple causality	Matson et al. (2003)
Questions about behavioral function (QABF)	Matson and Vollmer (1995)
Functional assessment interview (FAI)	O'Neill et al., 1997
Behavior problems inventory (BPI)	Rojahn, Matson, Lott, Esbensen, & Smalls, 2001

assessment methods, which may take several days or even weeks to complete. Second, the assessments may be administered by individuals who require relatively little training on the methods. This is in contrast to direct assessment procedures that may require sophisticated professionals to implement. Third, indirect assessments may be useful when SIB is too dangerous to allow in a direct assessment (e.g., severe forms of pica, forceful head banging). This is in contrast to procedures that require direct observation or possibly even temporary exacerbation of the SIB. Fourth, the behavior could occur too infrequently to reliably observe. Thus, direct assessment via behavioral observation is not an option for some cases of SIB. Fifth, indirect assessments may provide some preliminary information, such as operational definitions or correlated environmental events, that will be needed to conduct subsequent direct assessments. Collectively, these advantages of indirect assessments suggest there is some utility to the general method. Nonetheless some limitations of the approach should also be considered.

The primary limitation of indirect assessments is that all information is correlational, even if accurately reported by the respondent. For example, a respondent might report that SIB frequently produces attention. However, recent research has shown that dangerous behavior commonly produces attention from care providers (Thompson & Iwata, 2001) even if the attention is not serving as reinforcement for the behavior (St. Peter et al., 2005). In short, dangerous behavior such as SIB is likely to induce various social reactions by care providers. By merely identifying those common consequences to behavior, a behavioral assessment falls short of necessarily identifying cause-and-effect variables.

A secondary limitation of indirect assessments involves the reliance on human report, especially when the human report is given long after the SIB event or events have occurred. In short, the information obtained may not be accurate. There are several factors that may contribute to the inaccuracy of indirect assessments. First, the individual providing the information (respondent) may not be able to recall all of the relevant information about the behavioral episode or episodes. Second, the respondent may not have enough experience with the behavior. For example, a staff member may only work with a client for a limited time and therefore has only observed a few instances of the behavior. Third, the respondent may provide biased responses. For example, a teacher may report that a student is consistently reprimanded following SIB (with the teacher believing that is the correct response) but fails to report that the student also consistently receives a break from academic tasks (believing that to be an incorrect response). Such erroneous information might lead to a false hypothesis regarding attention as reinforcement while ignoring the possible hypothesis of escape from academic tasks as reinforcement.

Indirect assessments should be conducted with informants who are commonly present when the behavior occurs and who are familiar with the person who engages in the SIB. In most cases, the indirect assessments are conducted with the individual's parents, teachers, or other caregivers. During indirect assessments, informants are generally asked questions related to the form and patterns of the SIB, possible antecedent (events that tend to occur prior to SIB), and consequent events (events that tend to occur as a result of

SIB). Numerous indirect assessment methods exist and range from unstructured interviews to standardized psychometric instruments. A majority of these indirect assessments attempt to identify possible sources of reinforcement for problem behavior including social positive reinforcement (e.g., access to attention, access to preferred items or activities), social negative reinforcement (e.g., avoidance of academic tasks, escape from other people), and automatic/sensory reinforcement or reinforcement that is not socially mediated (e.g., sensory stimulation, attenuation of painful stimuli). For example, in the Motivation Analysis Rating Scale (MARS) designed by Weiseler, Hanson, Chamberlain, and Thompson (1985), informants are asked to rate statements such as "When the self-injurious behavior occurs, the resident is trying to get something he wants." The Motivational Assessment Scale (MAS) developed by Durand and Crimmins (1988) includes several questions aimed at identifying relevant events that precede the problem behavior. For example, the informant is asked to rate questions such as "Does the behavior occur when any request is made of this person?" or "Does the behavior occur when you take away a favorite toy, food, or activity?" Affirmative answers to these questions may indicate that the behavior is influenced by escape from tasks and access to tangible reinforcers, respectively. Other indirect assessments, such as the Questions About Behavioral Function (QABF), include components to identify both antecedent and consequent events (e.g., Matson & Vollmer, 1995).

By comparing assessment results from two independent informants (inter-rater reliability), or with the same informant over time (test-retest reliability), the reliability of indirect measures may be assessed. For instance, the assessment could be administered to both a parent and a teacher, and then the outcomes would be compared. Or, for example, the assessment could be administered to the teacher at one point in time and then again at another point in time. The reliability studies on indirect assessments have yielded mixed results (e.g., Durand and Crimmins (1988); Arndorfer, Miltenberger, Woster, Rortvedt, & Gaffaney, 1994; Zarcone, Rodgers, Iwata, Rourke, & Dorsey, 1991). Durand and Crimmins (1988) administered the MAS to classroom teachers of students who engaged in severe problem behavior including self-injury. The authors compared the outcomes from two teachers and then calculated correlation coefficients based on the results. These coefficients were calculated using the overall responses to the questions rather than on a question-by-question basis. The authors reported a high level of inter-rater reliability (e.g., correlation coefficients ranging from 0.62 to 0.90). Zarcone, Rodgers, Iwata, Rourke, and Dorsey (1991) conducted a replication of the study with both teachers and direct care staff of 55 individuals who engaged in self-injury. In addition to the overall correlation coefficient calculation, Zarcone et al. evaluated point-to-point correspondence between responses to specific questions. The authors reported low correlation coefficients for both reliability measures. In fact, only 15% of the sample had correlation coefficients above 0.80.

It is important to consider that low reliability scores do not necessarily reflect a failure of the assessment method. It is possible that the self-injury occurs under different circumstances for different people. Therefore, it is possible that two informants respond differently, but both are accurate. This might especially be the case when the assessment is administered in two different environments (e.g., school and home). It is equally possible that test-retest reliability is confounded by changes in behavioral function over time (Lerman, Iwata, Smith, Zarcone, & Vollmer, 1994). For example, it is possible that behavior that was once reinforced by access to attention is now reinforced by escape from instructional activity. Collectively, these considerations suggest that the reliability of indirect assessments may be improved by administering the assessment within a small time window, to individuals in the same environment who both have a lot of experience with the behavior.

Other studies have evaluated the validity of indirect assessments by comparing outcomes to the results from direct assessments (e.g., functional analyses) or treatment analyses (e.g.,

Matson, Bamburg, Cheery, & Paclawskyj, 1999). For example, a study by Arndorfer, Miltenberger, Woster, Rortvedt, and Gaffaney (1994) compared the results from structured interviews to analog functional assessments and found correspondence between the two assessment methods. Iwata, DeLeon, and Roscoe (2013) found that outcomes from the Functional Assessment Screening Tool (FAST) predicted the functional analysis condition with the highest rate of problem behavior in 63.8% of cases. Validity analyses of the MAS have produced mixed results. Durand and Crimmins compared the results from the MAS to analog functional assessments, using direct assessment procedures described by Carr and Durand (1985) as the point of comparison. The authors reported that the MAS accurately predicted the results from the functional analyses for eight out of eight participants. In contrast, a study by Crawford, Brockel, Schauss, and Miltenberger (1992) found poor validity between the MAS and both functional analyses and direct observations. The level of validity of indirect assessments may be related to the characteristics of the problem behavior. For example, Paclawskyj, Matson, Rush, Smalls, and Vollmer (2001) reported low validity scores between the QABF and analog functional analyses. However, the authors attributed the results in part to difficulties with the functional analysis methodology. That is, the problem behavior was low-frequency/high-intensity in nature and was not observed in the function analysis conditions. Although functional analysis is widely viewed as the "acid test" for behavioral function, it is not clear it is best suited as a point of comparison for low-rate behavior because the nonoccurrence of behavior during the functional analysis necessarily leads to a "no match" between the indirect and direct assessment.

To summarize, indirect assessments can provide useful information for subsequent direct assessments and for subsequent treatment recommendations. In addition, indirect assessments may be a useful option when the problem behavior is not conducive to direct assessment techniques, such as with extremely low-rate SIB or extremely dangerous forms of SIB. Numerous studies have examined the reliability and validity of indirect assessments, but further research is warranted to improve the utility of these assessments. More specifically, additional research may help to determine the conditions under which these assessments yield clear and accurate results. Finally, outcomes of indirect assessments should be viewed with caution due to the idiosyncrasies of subjective human report.

Descriptive Analysis

Descriptive analysis refers to the observation of behavior, usually during naturally occurring interactions (Bijou, Peterson, & Ault, 1968; Iwata, Kahng, Wallace, & Lindberg, 2000. Descriptive analyses are frequently used as one component of a comprehensive assessment of SIB and, in turn, as a basis for developing interventions to decrease SIB and to increase replacement behavior. This approach has been applied in a variety of settings including classrooms (e.g., Doggett, Edwards, Moore, Tingstrom, & Wilczynski, 2001; Ndoro, Hanley, Tiger, & Heal, 2006; Sasso et al., 1992; VanDerHeyden, Witt, & Gatti, 2001), residential settings (e.g., Lerman & Iwata, 1993; Mace & Lalli, 1991), and inpatient settings (e.g., Borrero, Vollmer, Borrero, & Bourret, 2005; Vollmer, Borrero, Wright, Van Camp, & Lalli, 2001). The descriptive analysis approach is used for a variety of response forms such as bizarre speech (Mace & Lalli, 1991), disruption, and aggression (e.g., Vollmer, Borrero, Wright, Van Camp, & Lalli, 2001), but the approach is applicable in the assessment of SIB. In this section, we will describe three commonly used approaches to descriptive analysis: direct observation, scatterplots, and antecedent-behavior-consequence (A-B-C) recording.

Direct Observation

One approach to descriptive analysis is to have the professional assessor directly observe behavior in the natural setting. One formal assessment tool that has been frequently used for this purpose is the Functional Assessment Observation (FAO) designed by O'Neill et al. (1997). When using the FAO, an observer collects data (using a "paper and pencil method") on various topographies of behavior, predictors of behavior (e.g., demands, difficult task, transitions, etc.), perceived functions of behavior (e.g., "get/obtain" and "escape/avoid" items or activities), and actual consequences for behavior. Subsequent analyses of data collected may provide information regarding the potential function of SIB and to assist with treatment recommendations. Of course, when collecting data based on naturalistic observations, a number of events typically occur at the same time, and it may be difficult to capture all of the events using a paper and pencil data collection method.

In recent years, much of the research on direct observation methods has involved continuous recording using computerized data collection programs, which allows a large number of events and behavior to be scored during the observation. The results of a direct observation with computerized data are often analyzed by calculating the number of events that occur antecedent and subsequent to the behavior assessed (e.g., Forman, Hall, & Oliver, 2002; Mace & Lalli, 1991; Ndoro, Hanley, Tiger, & Heal, 2006 & Oliver, Hall, & Nixon, 1999), with the most frequent antecedents and consequences considered as potential establishing operations and reinforcers. The general approach of using computerized assessment methodology is limited insofar as many practitioners do not have resources available for this purpose.

There are several potential advantages to using direct observation as an SIB assessment component. First, direct observation provides a means of obtaining a true baseline of SIB levels occurring in the natural environment. Having a true baseline should aid in subsequent decision-making about the efficacy or lack thereof of behavioral treatment or other forms of treatment (such as medical treatment). Second, direct observation may aid in developing operational definitions of the SIB. Third, idiosyncratic antecedent events or behavioral consequences might be identified. Fourth, direct observation may be practical in some settings where experimental manipulation of variables is not possible. For example, in some schools it is considered undesirable for a child to be pulled out of class for a lengthy assessment; yet, a descriptive analysis can occur in the classroom itself. A fifth potential advantage is that some severe forms of SIB cannot be allowed to occur in a functional analysis, especially if the functional analysis has a chance of temporarily increasing SIB rates. Although it might be argued that the same severe SIB should not be allowed to occur during direct observation either, an ethical argument can be made that the behavior does in fact occur already in the natural setting and a descriptive analysis can be kept very short if it is used mainly to capture baselines or to develop operational definitions.

If an eventual goal is to conduct a functional analysis of SIB, but SIB is extremely severe, a practitioner may wish to identify precursor behavior that is highly correlated with the occurrence of SIB. Descriptive analyses may be useful in identifying such precursors (Smith & Churchill, 2002). Recently Borrero and Borrero (2008) conducted descriptive analyses to identify precursors to more severe problem behavior and subsequently assessed both via functional analyses (Iwata, Dorsey, Slifer, Bauman, & Richman, 1982/1994). Results reported by Borrero and Borrero and Smith and Churchill showed that precursors to more severe problem behavior (e.g., vocalizations that reliably preceded SIB) were members of the same operant class as SIB (i.e., served the same operant function).

The principle limitation of a descriptive analysis in the form of direct observation (or any type of descriptive analysis for that matter) is that in the absence of experimental manipulation, functional relations between SIB and hypothesized variables cannot be confirmed. In fact, at times, correlations identified in a descriptive analysis are misleading. For example, St. Peter et al. (2005) showed via descriptive analysis that various forms of problem behavior were highly correlated with adult attention, but when a functional analysis was conducted, it was shown that adult attention did not reinforce the SIB. Thus, high positive correlations between SIB and consequent events do not equate to identification of a reinforcer. On the one hand, the severity of SIB makes it highly likely that care providers will in some way attend to the behavior (although the attention may be functionally irrelevant to the behavior). On the other hand, some SIB may only intermittently produce attention or other reinforcers (yielding a low correlation between SIB and the reinforcer), but such relations could represent lean variable ratio (VR) or variable interval (VI) schedules of reinforcement. For example, if a parent attends to SIB one out of every ten times it occurs on average, the behavior could be reinforced on a VR 10 schedule. Thus, like indirect assessments, descriptive analyses should be conducted in conjunction with functional analyses when possible to tease out correlation/causation distinctions (e.g., Arndorfer, Miltenberger, Woster, Rortvedt, & Gaffaney, 1994; Desrochers, Hile, & Williams-Mosely, 1997; Ellingson, Miltenberger, & Long, 1999).

It could be argued that, given the correlation/causation problem, why conduct a direct observation as a form of descriptive analysis at all? Why not skip directly to a functional analysis (to be described later in this chapter)? The answer is that the purpose of the direct observation would be to identify common situations in which the behavior occurs, to develop operational definitions, to gather baseline data, and so on (see advantages of direct observation). In addition, further utility of direct observation as a form of descriptive analysis will be discussed below. The purpose of the functional analysis would be to identify reinforcers maintaining behavior. It is important to note that direct observation may provide some hints about reinforcers maintaining behavior, but the true purpose of such an approach should be to gather the kinds of miscellaneous information about the environmental context that would not ordinarily emerge in a functional analysis. Thus, in our view, the purposes of a descriptive analysis and of a functional analysis are different.

If both a direct observation (as descriptive analysis) and a functional analysis are used to identify the operant function of behavior, the results of these methods too often do not match.

Thus, reinforcer identification via descriptive analysis is considered (at least by us) to be an inappropriate usage of the method. Whereas previously common usage of the descriptive analysis was as a prelude to a functional analysis (e.g., Lerman & Iwata, 1993; Mace & Lalli, 1991), a more recent usage of the direct observation during a descriptive analysis is just the opposite: to evaluate what reinforcement contingencies might look like in the natural environment once reinforcers have already been identified via functional analysis. In short, data obtained via direct observation can provide a means to quantify details of naturally occurring social interactions that might strengthen SIB. For example, descriptive data may be evaluated to compare probabilities during naturally occurring interactions (e.g., the probability of attention given SIB versus the overall probability of attention, Vollmer, Borrero, Wright, Van Camp, & Lalli, 2001) or to evaluate dynamic moment-to-moment changes in the probability of various environment-behavior relations via lag sequential analysis (e.g., Emerson, Thompson, Reeves, & Henderson, 1995; Samaha, Vollmer, Borrero, Sloman, & St. Peter, 2009).

Descriptive data may also be used to identify parameters of reinforcement for both SIB and replacement behavior, including the rate, duration, probability, quality, and delay to reinforcement (e.g., Borrero, Vollmer, Borrero, & Bourret, 2005). Conceivably such information could be critical to obtain as a baseline from which to compare the effects of care provider training. For example, in some cases, SIB must be reinforced (such as when a care provider must block attention-maintained SIB). As a result, the probability of attention following SIB may be very close to 1.0, but the care provider could improve the relative parameters of reinforcement for replacement behavior. Table 2 shows hypothetical data on reinforcement parameters for SIB reinforced by attention. The left two columns show the reinforcement parameters for SIB and replacement behavior prior to training, and the right two columns show the reinforcement parameters after training.

Hypothetical data on reinforcement parameters for SIB reinforced by attention. The left two

Table 2 Example of reinforcement paramenters assessment outcome

Reinforcement parameter	SIB	Replacement behavior	SIB	Replacement behavior
Rate	0.95 per min	0.12 per min	0.3 per min	0.95 per min
Duration	30 s	3 s	5 s	40 s
Probability	1.0	0.1	0.2	0.99
Delay	0 s	20 s	45 s	0 s

columns show the reinforcement parameters for SIB and replacement behavior prior to training, and the right two columns show the reinforcement parameters after training.

Scatterplot

At times, it is either inconvenient or not possible for a professional psychologist or behavior analyst to directly observe SIB. In such cases, care providers such as staff, parents, and teachers are asked to collect data, usually in some simplified and manageable format that would not require extensive training or time consumption. One example is the scatterplot technique. Touchette, MacDonald, and Langer (1985) used a scatterplot to estimate the frequency of problem behavior across days and weeks to identify patterns in responding. The scatterplot method usually involves a grid data sheet that allows for the recording of data in specified time intervals (e.g., 30-min intervals through school hours) that correspond to the individual's daily schedule. Typically, the frequency of behavior is scored as either "no occurrence" (or leaving the box blank), "low-rate responding" (e.g., drawing stripes in the box), or "high-rate responding" (e.g., filling in the box). Prior to completing the scatterplot, low- and high-rate responding must be defined on an individual basis. Figure 1 shows an example of a scatterplot data sheet.

After the scatterplot is completed, it may be possible to see patterns in responding, such as behavior occurring at a certain time of day or during a specific activity. In fact, Touchette, MacDonald, and Langer (1985) used the scatterplot to identify times of day associated with SIB and aggression and then made changes in the programmed schedule for participants, resulting in a decrease in problem behavior. Although it was not highlighted by Touchette et al., another potential advantage of a scatterplot is that it yields a visual display to estimate the occurrence of behavior both before and after the initiation of SIB treatment. Thus, advantages of the scatterplot method include ease of implementation, possible identification of SIB allocation by time of day or activity, and possible use as an estimate of baseline SIB occurrences.

Despite the possible advantages, there are some limitations to the scatterplot to consider. First, just as with any descriptive analysis method, only behavior-environment correlations can be obtained (rather than cause-effect relations). Second, while it may be fairly simple to complete the grid, the method may not be sensitive to changes in high-rate SIB. For example, if during baseline high-rate SIB occurs 20 or more times during a 30-min interval, the scatterplot might look the same following treatment even when a 50% reduction in behavior is obtained. Third, although identification of temporal patterns is a common usage of scatterplots, clear outcomes may be relatively rare. Kahng et al. (1998) evaluated completed scatterplots for 15 individuals (those individuals for whom acceptable reliability data were obtained) and found that out of the 15 scatterplots, no reliable temporal patterns of responding were identified via visual analysis.

A-B-C Recording

The A-B-C method is another relatively simple approach that is most often conducted by care providers, after a modicum of training, in the natural environment. The A-B-C method involves recording potential antecedents to and consequences of

Name __Client C__   Month __March__

☐ No responses   ▥ 1-5 responses   ▪ 5+ responses

Response __self-injury__

[Scatterplot table showing 30-min intervals from 9:00-5:30 across dates 1-19 with varying patterns indicating frequency of self-injury]

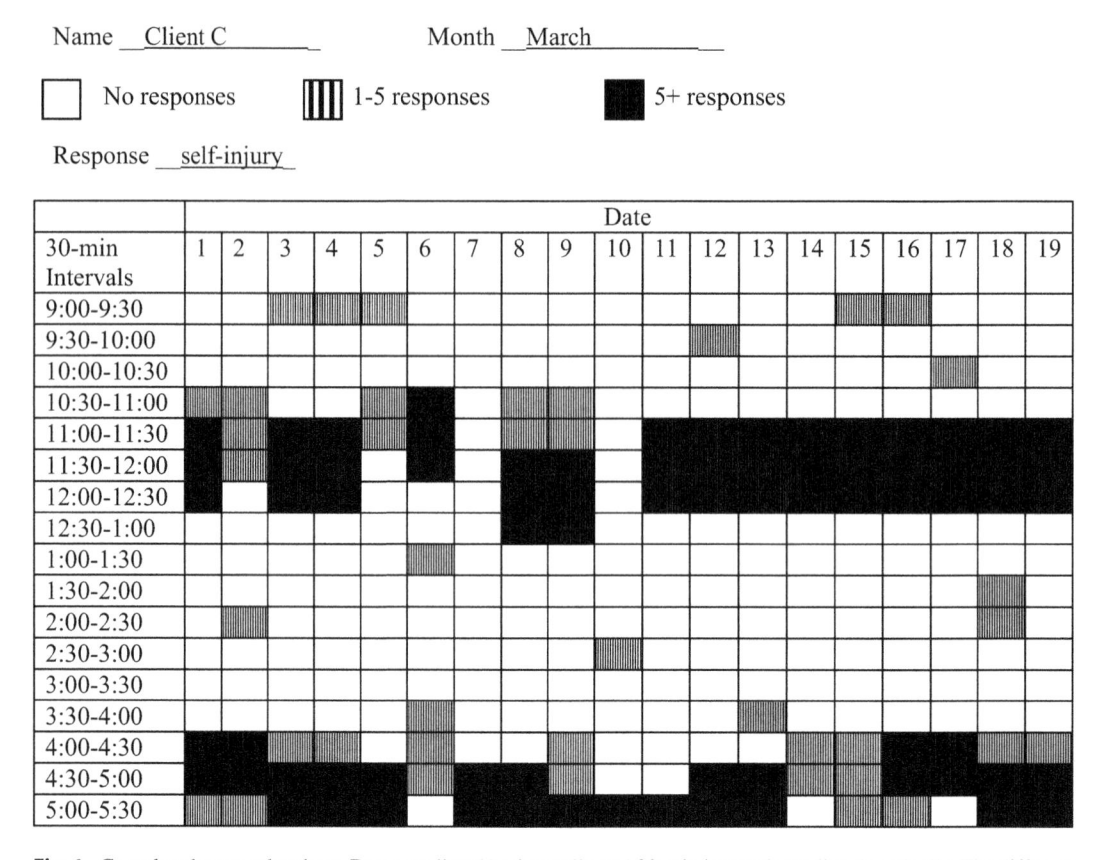

Fig. 1 Completed scatterplot sheet. Dates are listed horizontally and 30-min intervals are listed vertically. The different patterns denote different frequencies of self-injury for the particular interval

behavior, as suggested by Skinner's three-term contingency (Skinner, 1953). Simple A-B-C data sheets typically use narrative recording, and include a definition of the behavior, and columns where the observer should record what happened before and after the behavior. The space for recording antecedents and consequences can be left open ended (see Fig. 2) or might contain multiple options in order to focus the responses of the observer (see Fig. 3).

The primary advantage of the A-B-C method is the ease of implementation. A second advantage is that if behavior is low rate, a professional observer is not likely to see the behavior. Thus, having a care provider record instances of behavior allows the professional to obtain some level of information in the absence of direct observation. The potential disadvantages include possible problems with data reliability (given that observers are not professionally trained observers) and possible problems with the type of information reported. Although very little research has been conducted using parents and staff as observers, our experience has been that a wide range of descriptions are recorded on A-B-C sheets, and those descriptions are not always technically sound and do not always represent observable environmental events.

Functional Analysis

The term functional analysis as it relates to SIB assessment refers to specific procedures to identify relationships between antecedent and consequent events and behavior. Functional analysis differs from other forms of behavioral assessment in that it not only involves direct observation and

Instructions: When an instance of SIB occurs, record the activity/event that occurred prior to the behavior, and the activity/event that occurred following the behavior.

Date and Time SIB occurred	Description of SIB	What occurred before SIB?	What occurred after SIB?	Additional Comments

Fig. 2 An example of a simple A-B-C recording sheet

repeated measurement of behavior but also involves an experimental manipulation of environmental variables. That is, antecedent events (e.g., restriction of preferred items, presentation of demands) are controlled, and consequent events (e.g., delivery of preferred items, termination of demands) are provided contingent upon problem behavior in order to test hypotheses about the operant function of behavior. Functional analyses have been conducted for almost every type of SIB that has been reported in the literature, including head banging (Iwata, Pace, Cowdery, & Miltenberger, 1994), hand mouthing or biting (Goh et al., 1995), scratching (Cowdery, Iwata, & Pace, 1990), pica (Piazza, Hanley, & Fisher, 1996), and eye poking (Lalli, Livezey, & Kates, 1996), among many others.

The presentation of potential reinforcing events for SIB may seem counterintuitive upon initial consideration for assessment and treatment purposes. Why would the professional want to make the behavior worse? A medical analogy that helps make sense of the assessment logic is to consider the purpose of an allergy test: the allergist intentionally exposes the patient to hypothesized allergens and then evaluates the response to those hypothesized allergens. Analogously, in the assessment of SIB, a functional analysis is conducted as a means of exposing an individual, albeit temporarily, to possible environmental factors causing SIB. The functional analysis approach is considered the best practice for identifying environmental variables affecting problem behavior, at least when

Date and Time	Description of SIB	What occurred before SIB? (please check)	What occurred after the SIB? (please check)	Additional Comments
		__ Instructions __ Item Removed __ No Attention __ Close Proximity __ Diverted Attention __ No Specific Event __ Other	__ Instructions ended __ Instructions cont. __ Reprimand __ Medical Attention __ No Attention __ Item Presented __ No Specific Event __ Other	
		__ Instructions __ Item Removed __ No Attention __ Close Proximity __ Diverted Attention __ No Specific Event __ Other	__ Instructions ended __ Instructions cont. __ Reprimand __ Medical Attention __ No Attention __ Item Presented __ No Specific Event __ Other	
		__ Instructions __ Item Removed __ No Attention __ Close Proximity __ Diverted Attention __ No Specific Event __ Other	__ Instructions ended __ Instructions cont. __ Reprimand __ Medical Attention __ No Attention __ Item Presented __ No Specific Event __ Other	
		__ Instructions __ Item Removed __ No Attention __ Close Proximity __ Diverted Attention __ No Specific Event __ Other	__ Instructions ended __ Instructions cont. __ Reprimand __ Medical Attention __ No Attention __ Item Presented __ No Specific Event __ Other	

Fig. 3 An example of an A-B-C recording sheet with multiple options for antecedent and consequent events

behavior occurs at a high enough rate to be observed during relatively short-duration sessions and when an individual is not placed in immediate and severe danger (Hanley, Iwata, & McCord, 2003).

Typically, a functional analysis includes conditions to serve as analogs for typical situations in the individual's natural environment. Thus, the individual is not being exposed to situations he or she does not already experience on a day-to-day basis. A study conducted by Kahng et al. (2015) demonstrated that individuals with SIB were only slightly more likely to sustain an injury during a functional analysis when compared to typical daily activities. Functional analyses may lead to effective interventions because the treatment can be based on known functional properties of the SIB rather than being based on a priori assumptions, potentially spurious correlations (St. Peter et al., 2005), or verbal report. A complete functional analysis of behavior may also prevent the implementation of treatments that are contraindicated to the function of problem behavior (e.g., Iwata et al., 1994). For example, time-out might actually reinforce escape-maintained SIB.

Because SIB is such a dangerous behavior disorder, several considerations must be addressed before conducting functional analyses. For example, if there is risk of immediate tissue damage or trauma, medical personnel should be consulted. Medical personnel can help evaluate whether the SIB is amenable to a functional analysis and also help to determine appropriate session termination criteria if the SIB becomes too severe (Iwata et al., 1982/1994). There may be cases when the characteristics of the behavior (e.g., frequency or topography) are determined to be inappropriate for a functional analysis. For example, the behavior may occur at low rates (e.g., once per day) or the behavior may be too dangerous (e.g., pica with sharp metallic objects) to expose to a functional analysis. For these cases, other assessment methods (e.g., indirect assessments) or variations of traditional functional analyses may be more appropriate.

Although the functional analysis of SIB has been a hallmark of behavior analysis for many years (e.g., Lovaas & Simmons, 1969), Iwata et al. (1982/1994) presented the first empirical demonstration of functional analysis methodology designed specifically as an assessment method. Iwata et al. conducted functional analyses for nine children who engaged in SIB. The assessment results pointed to clear variables maintaining SIB for six of the nine participants. The methodology described by Iwata et al. has served as the standard model for a majority of subsequent functional analysis studies and clinical applications. Functional analyses are commonly conducted in highly controlled settings, such as inpatient hospital settings, so that all relevant environmental variables (e.g., delivery of attention) can be regulated. However, functional analyses have also been conducted in other environments such as an outpatient clinic, the client's home, or in a school (e.g., Bloom, Iwata, Fritz, Roscoe, & Carreau, 2011; Northup et al., 1994).

Most functional analyses include three test conditions and one control condition. The purpose of the control condition is to evaluate the effects of an environment in which little SIB is expected to occur (Iwata et al., 1982/1994). In the control condition, the client is typically given free access to preferred items, and the therapist delivers attention on a time-based schedule. Additionally, no demands are placed on the client. The purpose of two of the test conditions is to evaluate the sensitivity of SIB to common socially mediated consequences such as positive reinforcement (such as adult attention or contingent access to preferred tangible items) and negative reinforcement (such as escape from instructional activity or self-care routines). There is also usually a test condition for automatically reinforced behavior or behavior that occurs in the absence of socially medicated consequences (e.g., the client is left alone in a room in order to evaluate whether the behavior persists in the absence of socially mediated consequences.) Each session (whether test or control) typically lasts 5 to 15 minutes. The presentation of conditions is usually alternated randomly in a multielement experimental design (Sidman, 1960). However, other design variations have been used including the repeated measurement of SIB in reversal designs (e.g., Vollmer, Iwata, Duncan, & Lerman, 1993b) and alternation of one test and control condition at a time (pairwise design; Iwata, Duncan, Zarcone, Lerman, & Shore, 1994).

In most functional analysis conditions, the consequence is provided for each occurrence of problem behavior (a continuous reinforcement schedule, or CRF). For example, in the "attention" condition (described below), the adult therapist provides a reprimand, comfort statement, or some other form of attention every time SIB occurs. Some researchers have argued that CRF leads to better discrimination of test conditions and therefore yields clear assessment results (Iwata, Vollmer, & Zarcone, 1990). However, some researchers have used intermittent reinforcement schedules in order to more closely mimic consequences as they are delivered in the natural environment (e.g., Lalli & Casey, 1996). Whatever the reinforcement schedule, a common feature of functional analyses is that data are collected on the rates of SIB for the purposes of comparison in each of the conditions. The response patterns in each of the test conditions are then compared to the control condition. A higher rate of responding in a particular test condition indicates a possible source of reinforcement. Some of the most frequently used functional analysis conditions are described below.

Care provider attention has been shown to be one of the most common consequences for problematic behavior, including SIB (e.g., Thompson & Iwata, 2001). In the attention condition, the client has access to preferred items or activities, and the therapist engages in work or other activities away from the client. Some variations of this condition involve a "diverted" attention component in which the therapist attends to other individuals in the environment, and not the client. When an instance of SIB occurs, the therapist turns toward the client and provides brief attention. Higher rates of self-injury in the attention condition relative to the control condition would suggest that SIB is reinforced by attention. The upper panel of Fig. 4 shows hypothetical results of a functional analysis showing reinforcement via attention.

An attempt should be made to match the type of attention delivered in the functional analysis to the type of attention commonly provided in the client's natural environment. For example, some care providers are more likely to reprimand SIB, whereas other care providers are more likely to provide comfort or soothing conversation after SIB. Some studies have shown that the form of attention may influence the reinforcing value of attention as reinforcement for problem behavior (e.g., Fisher, Ninness, Piazza, & Owen-DeSchryver, 1996; Piazza et al., 1999). For example, Piazza et al. found that for some participants, verbal reprimands were actually more potent reinforcers than praise statements. Thus, consideration of the form of attention should be addressed prior to implementing a social positive reinforcement test condition.

Another form of social positive reinforcement is the delivery of preferred toys, food, or activities. In natural interactions, these items are sometimes given to clients after SIB as a means to distract or appease the client, but the result is an inadvertent reinforcement effect. The test condition for this type of reinforcement is sometimes called the "tangible" condition. In the tangible condition, the therapist provides attention to the client, but access to highly preferred items or activities is restricted. When SIB occurs, the therapist allows access to the items for a short period of time. Higher rates of SIB in the tangible condition, relative to the control condition, would suggest that SIB is reinforced by access to tangible items. The second panel of Fig. 4 shows hypothetical results for behavior reinforced by tangibles.

The tangible condition is typically included in the functional analysis if other assessments (e.g., caregiver interviews, direct observations) have determined that access to tangibles is a common consequence for the problem behavior. Otherwise, one concern is that the inclusion of tangible condition may lead to a false-positive functional analysis outcome (e.g., Shirley, Iwata, & Kahng, 1999). For example, Shirley et al. conducted functional analyses of hand mouthing for one participant and found that elevated rates of hand mouthing occurred across two test conditions, including the tangible condition. However, direct observations in the participant's natural environment showed that presentation of preferred items never followed hand mouthing. However, it is important to note that there may be some utility to including a tangible condition even if that is not how SIB is currently maintained for a given individual: that is, it could be argued that SIB is at least sensitive to tangible reinforcement and, therefore, clear recommendations could be made to avoid contingent delivery of tangibles as a consequence to SIB.

Escape from demands (e.g., academic tasks, self-care routines, chores) is another common consequence for SIB. In fact, Thompson and Iwata (2001) evaluated common consequences for various topographies of problem behavior and found that escape from demands was the most common consequence for SIB among adults with developmental disabilities living in a residential facility. To improve the validity of the functional analysis outcomes, the demand context should be similar to demands that the individual experiences in the natural environment. The type of demand presented may affect the functional analysis outcomes. For example, a client may readily

Behavioral Assessment of Self-Injury

Fig. 4 Hypothetical functional analysis outcomes. For all of the panels, the attention condition is represented by the open circles, the tangible condition is represented by the open squares, the escape condition is represented by the closed squares, the alone condition is represented by the open triangles, and the play condition is represented by the closed circles. (Upper panel) Functional analysis outcome for self-injury maintained by access to attention. (Upper middle panel) Functional analysis outcomes for self-injury maintained by access to tangibles. (Lower middle panel) Functional analysis outcome for self-injury maintained by escape from demands. (Lower panel) Functional analysis outcome for self-injury maintained by automatic reinforcement

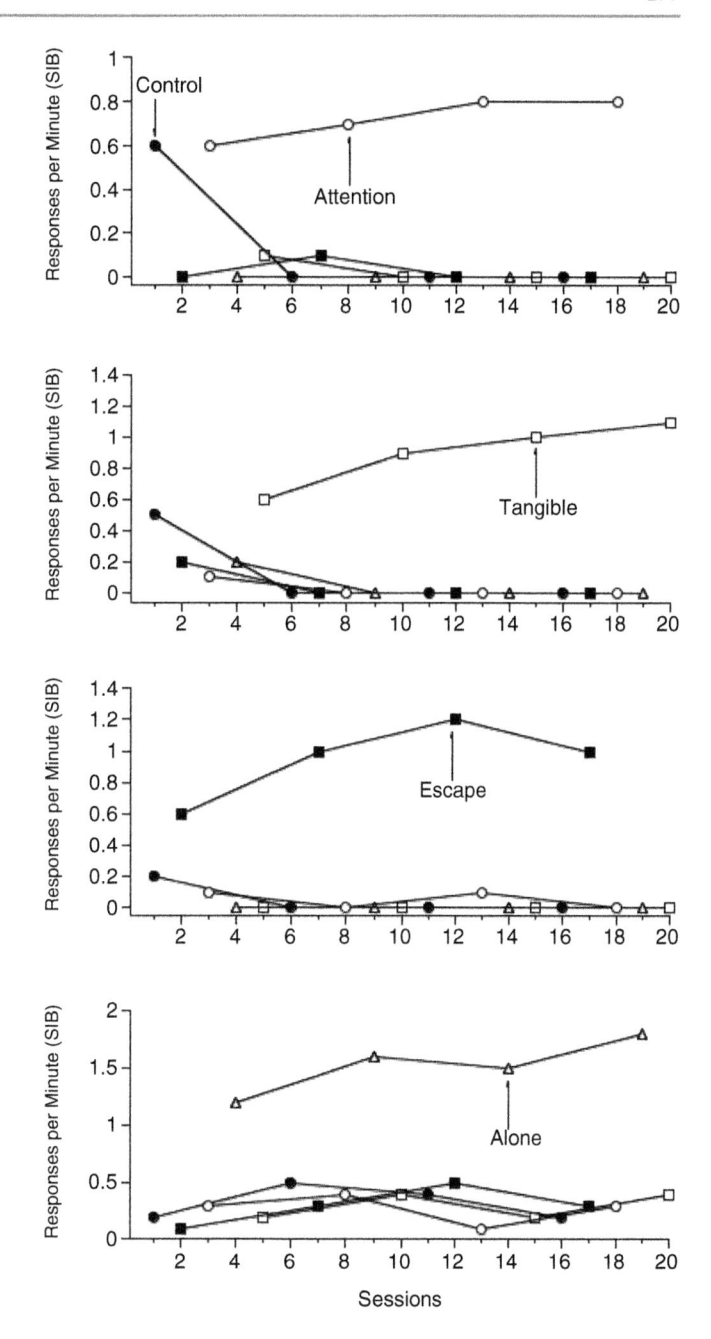

comply with academic tasks but may engage in SIB during self-care tasks. Using only academic tasks in the escape condition of the functional analysis would yield inaccurate results (i.e., a false negative).

In the escape condition (also called the "demand" condition), the therapist presents demands to the client using a three-step prompting sequence. The prompting sequence first begins with a verbal instruction. If the client does not comply within a specified time period (usually 5 or 10 s), the therapist performs a model or demonstration of the correct response. If the client again does not comply within a specified time period, the therapist physically guides him or her to comply. If compliance occurs at any point in the sequence, the therapist provides brief praise and then restarts the prompting sequence. This sequence continues unless the client engages in SIB. If SIB occurs, the therapist turns away from the client and provides a brief break from the instructional activities. Higher rates of responding in the escape condition relative to the control condition would suggest that SIB is reinforced by escape from demands. The third panel of Fig. 4 shows hypothetical results for SIB reinforced by escape.

The most common type of social negative reinforcement is escape from demands or instructional activities. However, in some cases, the mere proximity of another person may evoke self-injury. A variation of the escape condition, known as "social escape," has also been conducted in functional analyses (e.g., Iwata, Pace, Cowdery, & Miltenberger, 1994). In this condition, the therapist is in close proximity to the client and may provide attention. If SIB occurs, the therapist moves away from the client for a brief period of time. Higher rates in the social escape condition relative to the control condition indicate that behavior is reinforced by escape or avoidance of close social or physical proximity.

In some cases SIB may persist in the absence or independent of social consequences. This type of reinforcement has been referred to as automatic reinforcement because the behavior produces its own reinforcement in the form of sensory stimulation or pain attenuation. The meaning of "automatic" is simply to imply that no social mediation is responsible for reinforcement of the behavior; it is not an explanation of the actual source of reinforcement. An epidemiological study by Iwata et al. (1994) showed that over 25% of 152 participants' SIB was maintained by automatic reinforcement. An alone or no consequence condition is typically used to test if behavior is automatically reinforced. In these conditions, the client is either left alone in a room and observed through a one-way mirror or remains in the room with a therapist who provides no programmed consequences for SIB. Higher rates in the alone or no consequence condition relative to the control condition suggest that behavior is maintained by automatic reinforcement.

If there is reason to suspect that an individual's SIB is likely maintained by automatic reinforcement, repeated alone or no consequence sessions can be used as a screening tool prior to a functional analysis. Querim et al. (2013) conducted 5-min alone (no consequence) probe sessions prior to a functional analysis for 30 cases and found strong correspondence between the screening assessment and functional analysis outcomes. In other words, the screening was able to predict whether the individual's problem behavior was maintained by automatic reinforcement or socially mediated reinforcement. Undifferentiated responding, or responding that is high in all conditions including the control condition, may also suggest that behavior is maintained by automatic reinforcement, especially if the SIB does not extinguish following repeated alone or no consequence sessions (e.g., Vollmer, Marcus, Ringdahl, & Roane, 1995). The lower panel of Fig. 4 shows hypothetical results for SIB maintained by automatic reinforcement.

Hagopian, Rooker, and Zarcone (2015) proposed a model for classifying automatically reinforced SIB into three subtypes based on patterns of responding in a multielement functional analysis in conjunction with the presence or absence of self-restraint. The authors suggest that this subtype classification system could be useful to practitioners because of its ability to predict treatment outcomes. At the heart of this model is the notion that differentiated responding in an FA can be used as an indicator of behavioral sensitivity to environmental manipulations.

Subtype 1 is characterized by low levels of SIB in the play condition and high levels in the no interaction or alone conditions. When SIB is suppressed in the play condition, it suggests that alternative reinforcers have the potential to compete with the automatic reinforcement produced by SIB. Hagopian et al. hypothesized that the defining feature of Subtype 1 (sensitivity to environmental stimulation) suggests that this Subtype might be comparable to socially reinforced SIB and therefore might respond similarly to reinforcement-based treatments. Subtype 2 is characterized by high and undifferentiated levels of SIB across all conditions. When SIB is high in the play condition (as well as other conditions), it suggests that alternative reinforcers are not likely to compete with SIB. Subtype 3 is indicated by the presence of self-restraint during at least 25% of intervals for three alone sessions, and SIB is found to be automatically reinforced. The authors hypothesized that individuals with Subtypes 2 and 3 would be considerably more resistant to treatment and require more intrusive interventions than Subtype 1.

Results suggested that, consistent with the author's hypotheses, subtype classification was predictive of responsiveness or resistance to first-line, less intensive treatments. Individuals with Subtype 1 required less intensive interventions than individuals with Subtypes 2 and 3. Reinforcement as a sole intervention was only effective with individuals with Subtype 1. Individuals with Subtype 2 displayed more resistance to treatment and were the only participants that required treatments containing more than two components. Although conclusions about treatment outcomes for Subtype 3 were limited due to small sample size, this was the only group for whom restraint was necessary. Overall, these results suggest that the model outlined by Hagopian et al. could be helpful to practitioners because subtype classification could help guide the development of successful behavioral treatments for individuals with automatically reinforced SIB.

Carr and Durand (1985) presented another variation of functional analysis methodology with four children who engaged in problem behavior, including SIB, in a school setting. Only antecedent events (i.e., presentation of attention and demands) were manipulated, and no consequent events were programmed. Two experimental conditions and one control condition were included. One experimental condition evaluated the effects of low rates of antecedent teacher attention on problem behavior. Higher rates in this condition relative to the control condition suggested that behavior was sensitive to access to attention (i.e., the participants were motivated to increase attention levels under conditions of low attention). The other test condition evaluated the effects of presenting difficult demands on problem behavior. Higher rates in this condition relative to the control condition suggested behavior was sensitive to escape from demands (i.e., the participants were motivated to decrease demand difficulty under conditions of high demand). Results from Carr and Durand showed this method produced clear results for all four participants. In addition, treatments based on the results of the functional analysis were presented and showed decreases in disruptive behavior for all participants.

Carr and Durand's variation of functional analysis may have advantages over traditional functional analyses because no programmed consequences are delivered, so problem behavior is not intentionally reinforced. However, there may be some limitations to this methodology. First, because consequent events are not manipulated, there is no empirical demonstration of cause-and-effect relationships between reinforcement and behavior. Second, it is possible that behavior would extinguish or stop occurring during the sessions without the presentation of maintaining consequent events (i.e., reinforcers). Third, the antecedent manipulations may not be noticeable enough to produce differences across conditions. That is, this method requires the participant to be sensitive to slight changes such as delivery of attention once every 10 s in the control condition compared to delivery of attention once every 30 s in the attention condition (Fischer, Iwata, & Worsdell, 1997). Finally, this antecedent type of functional analysis fails to test for other possible sources of reinforcement such as access to preferred items or activities and automatic reinforcement.

Overall, a clear advantage of functional analysis as an SIB assessment is that functional relations between the behavior and environment are demonstrated. This is an advantage over descriptive analyses, where only correlations can be identified and it is an advantage over verbal reports and checklists because it is based on experimental logic and direct behavioral observation. Despite the utility of functional analyses, several potential limitations have been reported. One putative limitation of functional analysis methodology is the time required to complete the assessment. In some settings, time constraints may preclude a thorough functional analysis. However, some studies have evaluated the efficacy of brief functional analyses (e.g., Cooper et al., 1992; Cooper, Wacker, Sasso, Reimers, & Donn, 1990; Derby et al., 1992; Harding, Wacker, Cooper, Millard, & Jensen-Kovalan, 1994; Northup et al., 1991). For example, Northup et al. (1991) conducted brief functional analyses in an outpatient clinic setting with three individuals who engaged in aggressive behavior. In some cases, the time to conduct the assessment was limited to 90 minutes. The assessments involved one to two brief 10-minute exposures to functional analysis conditions similar to Iwata et al. (1994). For some participants, responding was differentially higher in the test conditions than the control condition. Additionally, implementation of a treatment resulted in high rates of appropriate behavior and low rates of problem behavior. Derby et al. (1992) conducted a large-scale study to evaluate the efficacy of brief functional analyses. Results from 79 brief functional analyses were summarized and showed that only 63% of the participants engaged in the problem behavior during the functional analysis. Maintaining variables were identified for 74% of the participants who did exhibit problem behavior during the brief assessment. Thus, brief functional analyses may only be effective for a limited number of individuals. In addition, data analysis techniques such as minute-by-minute evaluations can reduce the assessment duration in some cases (e.g., Vollmer, Marcus, Ringdahl, & Roane, 1995).

A second potential limitation of functional analysis is that it may be inappropriate for some types of behavior. For instance, the topography of SIB may be too severe to expose to functional analysis conditions. However, in these cases, it may be possible to identify precursor behavior (i.e., behavior that reliably precedes the self-injury) and conduct functional analyses of these responses. For example, Smith and Churchill (2002) conducted functional analyses of both SIB and precursor behavior for four participants and showed that the function of SIB could be inferred by conducting functional analyses of precursor behavior. Another modification that can be made if the topography of SIB is severe is to conduct a latency functional analysis. In a latency functional analysis, the session is terminated after the first instance of SIB. Short response latencies to SIB in a given test condition suggest a potential function. Thomason-Sassi, Iwata, Neidert, and Roscoe (2011) compared latency to rate measures during functional analyses and found that both measures produced similar outcomes with respect to identifying function. Functional analyses may also be inappropriate for behavior that occurs infrequently (e.g., once per day). However, varying the duration or structure of conditions of the functional analysis may better accommodate low-rate behavior. For example, it may be possible to identify specific times of the day that the behavior occurs and then conduct the functional analysis during these times. Furthermore, the time allotment for each condition can be increased from the typical 10 to 15 minutes to longer time periods (e.g., 1 to 2 hours) to adequately assess the behavior. Kahng, Abt, and Schonbachler (2001) reported the successful assessment and treatment of low-rate behavior using extended-time functional analysis methods for one participant in a hospital inpatient setting.

Another potential limitation is when functional analyses result in undifferentiated response patterns. This may occur for several reasons: the SIB may be automatically reinforced, the SIB may be multiply controlled (i.e., reinforced by more than one general type of consequence), the SIB might be maintained by an idiosyncratic reinforcer, the individual may not be discriminating the test conditions, or there may be carry over effects from one test condition to another. Although problematic, the issue of undifferentiated outcomes can be resolved in some cases, depending on the reason for the undifferentiated outcome. For example, undifferentiated results produced by automatic reinforcement can be identified by running numerous consecutive alone sessions to see if SIB extinguishes (e.g., Ellingson et al., 2000). Undifferentiated results produced by multiple control can be identified by sequentially implementing treatments to address one hypothesized operant function and then another (Smith, Iwata, Vollmer, & Zarcone, 1993). Undifferentiated outcomes produced by a failure to present the idiosyncratic antecedent and consequence events that occasion problem behavior can be remedied by identifying those events and modifying the functional analysis to include them. Roscoe, Schlichenmeyer, and Dube (2015) proposed a systematic method for developing modified functional analysis conditions following an inconclusive functional analysis. They used an indirect assessment (questionnaire) in isolation or in combination with a descriptive assessment to identify events to test in the modified functional analysis. The proposed method produced conclusive outcomes for five out of six subjects. Undifferentiated outcomes produced by discrimination failures can be overcome by enhancing (distinguishing) stimulus features of the test conditions, such as therapist, therapist clothing color, and so on (Conners et al., 2000). Undifferentiated results produced by carry-over effects from one condition to another can be identified by carefully evaluating within-session response patterns (Vollmer, Iwata, Duncan, & Lerman, 1993a). For example, Vollmer et al. found that sessions following attention sessions produced an apparent extinction burst of SIB that yielded similar overall session means but distinct response patterns that pointed to attention as a source of reinforcement.

Thus, functional analysis is a robust method for assessing SIB. In addition, the use of functional analysis techniques has resulted in the development of effective, function-based treatments. The results from several studies show that functional analysis methodology can be adapted for special situations in which traditional functional analysis methods either cannot be conducted or somehow produce unclear results. Nonetheless, more research on functional analysis is needed. Some of the most obvious assessment-related research questions remain unanswered as of this writing. For example: Does a functional analysis lead to overall better treatment effects than would have occurred if a reasonably educated professional implemented intervention after a modicum of direct observation?

Response Products

When assessing SIB through direct observation and functional analysis methods, results are presented using rate or interval recording methods. It is also sometimes useful to assess response severity or intensity and its corresponding response products (Marholin & Steinman, 1977). Response products involve measuring the outcome of a response rather than the rate of the response itself (Miltenberger, 2001). By definition, SIB suggests that physical damage has been caused by the response (Iwata et al., 1990). The type of injury caused by the response may differ depending on the topography of the response (e.g., self-biting, hitting head on a hard surface, skin-picking).

The principal advantage of an evaluation of SIB response products comes when assessing a response for which rate of responding does not indicate the level of damage caused by SIB. For example, if an individual hits his or her head on a hard surface, low-rate responding may still be problematic if such SIB causes substantial physical harm. A second advantage is that a baseline response product (injury) measurement provides a point of comparison when a goal of a SIB intervention is not merely to reduce SIB but to reduce its associated sequelae (i.e., injury itself). A third potential advantage of SIB response product measurement is that, in some cases, responses may only occur covertly (e.g., Grace, Thompson, & Fisher, 1996; Rapp, Miltenberger, Galensky, Ellingson, & Long, 1999); that is, responses occur either when the individual is alone or when the individual cannot be observed. Thus, response products of SIB may be the only evidence that the response has occurred and assessments of physical damage may be the only source of information regarding the severity and occurrence of a response. Although self-cutting displayed by otherwise typically developing adolescents is not a focus of this chapter, such SIB typically occurs covertly and might only be assessed via response products. Assessing response products for self-cutting therefore represents a promising future application.

Research on SIB response products has provided useful tools for the assessment of SIB severity (e.g., Iwata, Pace, Kissel, Nau, & Farber, 1990; Wilson, Iwata, & Bloom, 2012), including during SIB treatment (e.g., Carr & McDowell, 1980; Grace, Thompson, & Fisher, 1996). Iwata et al. developed the Self-Injury Trauma (SIT) scale to classify and quantify damage resulting from various topographies of SIB, including the location, number, severity, and type of injury. The researchers developed the scale to provide objective measurements of these variables and experimentally validated the reliability of 50 completed scales by assessing interobserver agreement (IOA) for all variables. Results showed that IOA calculated for the SIT scale was always above 89%, and, for some variables, including location of injuries, type of injuries, and severity of injuries, the overall agreement was at least 94%. Advantages of this instrument include the objective nature of the scale and its applicability to assess various aspects of injury. Disadvantages of the instrument include the lack of rate measures and difficulty in assessing internal injuries. Thus, as recommended by Iwata et al., the instrument should be used in conjunction with direct observations of the behavior and other medical evaluations.

Grace, Thompson, and Fisher (1996) conducted an assessment and treatment of severe SIB exhibited by an adult diagnosed with developmental disabilities with SIB response products serving as a dependent variable. The participant often engaged in SIB (i.e., skin picking, head banging, and inserting objects in his nose and ears), which was rarely observed. However, the SIB response products *were* observed (i.e., bleeding, objects observed in his nose and ears). In the study, nurses completed physical exams and documented existing physical injuries, as well as new ones. One specific dependent measure was the percentage of exams with new injuries. A subsequent treatment analysis was conducted and resulted in a decrease in the occurrence of new injuries.

Chapman, Fisher, Piazza, and Kurtz (1993) have applied a relatively novel approach to the use of response products, as applied to a particularly challenging form of self-injury. As a component of this study, Chapman et al. applied blue residue to pill bottles (containing colored placebos). In conjunction with direct observation, the researchers assessed pill bottle manipulation (correlated with pill ingestion) based on blue residue that appeared on the participant's hands and clothing. A treatment that involved differential reinforcement and ultimate elimination of the blue residue successfully reduced self-injury.

More recently, Wilson, Iwata, and Bloom (2012) used a computerized measurement of wound surface areas (WSA) to assess SIB. They compared the computerized method of measurement of WSA, using digital photographs, to the transparency method of measurement and found that the results were similar for both methods. Then the researchers compared the computerized measurement method to direct observation to determine if both methods were successful in identifying changes in the levels of SIB during assessment and treatment conditions. Results showed that both methods indicated changes in the levels of SIB and suggested that the computerized method for measuring response products may not only enhance the results of direct observation but may be used as a primary dependent variable for SIB.

As mentioned previously, there are some limitations to using response products as the dependent variable when assessing SIB. Perhaps, the most apparent limitation associated with using permanent products (alone) is the extent to which the "cause" of the injury can be adequately inferred. For example, an individual with an extensive history of self-injury may present with bruising as result of a fall or as a result of self-injury. Thus, interpretations based on response products should be interpreted cautiously and preferably should be used in conjunction with direct observation when possible. While it is important and often necessary to determine the extent of the physical damage caused by SIB, response products do not provide any information regarding the rate of self-injury and may not identify particular situations or conditions under which self-injury occurs. An additional limitation pointed out by Iwata et al. (1990) suggests that the SIT and similar methods merely provide a physical description of the injury on the surface of the skin and do not measure internal injuries. Additional medical assessments may be indicated to provide such information, such as X-rays, CT scans, ultrasounds, etc.

Protective Equipment

Protective equipment (helmets, gloves, mechanical restraints, etc.) is sometimes used to protect individuals who exhibit dangerous and severe SIB from injury. With some individuals, protective equipment might be worn continuously or for a majority of the day. For other individuals, protective equipment might only be applied following instances of SIB or as a crisis intervention. This practice should be regarded with caution, however, because some research has suggested that contingent application of protective equipment can sometimes function as positive reinforcement for SIB (e.g., Favell, McGimsey, & Jones, 1978).

Research suggests that there are advantages and disadvantages of using protective equipment during functional analyses. One disadvantage of using protective equipment during functional analyses is that protective equipment may suppress or eliminate SIB altogether, making it challenging to identify the function of SIB (Borrero, Vollmer, Wright, Lerman, & Kelley, 2002; Le & Smith, 2002). Despite these findings, there are some advantages of using protective equipment during functional analyses. First, the likelihood of an individual injuring themselves during the course of the assessment might be lower than if the individual's protective equipment was removed. Second, in some cases, protective equipment may help to reveal a socially mediated reinforcer maintaining SIB that is otherwise obscured. Kuhn and Triggs (2009) conducted an initial functional analysis with a young girl who exhibited severe head-directed SIB. SIB was high across all conditions of the functional analysis, suggesting either that her SIB was maintained by automatic reinforcement or multiply controlled. They conducted a second functional analysis in which the girl wore a helmet with a face shield. The authors hypothesized that the helmet served to mitigate the sensory stimulation produced by her SIB. In other words, the automatic reinforcement produced by her head-directed SIB was blocked by the helmet. This modification revealed that her SIB was also maintained by socially mediated positive reinforcement in the form of access to adult attention. Without the inclusion of protective equipment, the attention function would have gone undetected.

In addition to helmets, arm splints are another form of mechanical restraint that are used to protect individuals from the harmful effects of head-directed SIB. Although rigid arm splints are an effective short-term intervention because they prevent the occurrence of SIB altogether, they often prevent the individual from engaging in adaptive behaviors such as self-care or vocational tasks. Fisher, Piazza, Bowman, Hanley, and Adelinis (1997) described a variation of arm splints that were designed to allow care providers or therapists to manipulate the flexibility of the splints by adding or removing metal rods from the splints. Fisher et al. and other clinical researchers have described a procedure called "restraint fading" in which the flexibility of arm splints is systemically increased as long as SIB remains low. It is hypothesized that SIB remains low during this process because the arm splints acquire stimulus control over SIB despite the fact that the splints become increasingly flexible (Fisher, Piazza, Bowman, Hanley, & Adelinis, 1997). Despite the documented effectiveness of restraint fading, it can be time-consuming.

Wallace, Iwata, Zhou, and Goff (1999) outlined a rapid restraint analysis (RRA) aimed at identifying the optimal level of splint flexion for two individuals whose SIB warranted the use of arm splints. During the RRA, rates of SIB and adaptive behavior (eating or drinking) were measured during different conditions. In the baseline condition, the individual wore no splints. In the test conditions, the individual wore arm splints with different levels of flexibility, ranging from empty splints to rigid splints. The optimal level of splint flexion was described as the level with the best ratio of SIB to adaptive behavior (i.e., SIB was low and adaptive behavior was high).

Deshais, Fisher, Hausman, and Kahng (2015) reported RRA results and post-RRA outcomes for ten individuals with SIB. RRAs were conducted during the course of an inpatient admission to identify the optimal level of splint flexion for each individual. This level of flexion was then employed during all waking hours on the inpatient unit, and daily rates of SIB were monitored until the individuals were discharged from the inpatient unit. Overall, eight of the ten individuals were discharged from the inpatient unit wearing splints at the RRA level or at a more flexible level. Two of the ten individuals were discharged wearing splints less flexible than the RRA level. For six individuals, the RRA eliminated the need for restraint fading, and for two individuals, the RRA might have helped to identify a starting point for restraint fading that is less restrictive than rigid splints (thus avoiding unnecessary fading steps). This study demonstrated that the RRA can be used to quickly identify an appropriate level of arm splint flexion and might help save time by eliminating the need for restraint fading for some individuals. Post-RRA outcomes from the natural environment suggested that the RRA might be a useful clinical tool in the assessment of SIB.

In a departure from prior literature, DeRosa, Roane, Wilson, Novak, and Silkowski (2015) used a variety of adaptive tasks during RRAs rather than a single adaptive task with the aim of determining whether different activities required different levels of flexion. Each level of splint flexion was employed across a variety of adaptive tasks such as card touches, tracing, and receptive picture identification. Data were collected on SIB and the percentage of compliance with task instructions. Results suggested that for both individuals, different levels of flexion were optimal in different contexts.

These findings on the RRA suggest some important clinical implications for individuals with severe SIB. First, the RRA is an assessment that can quickly and effectively identify an appropriate level of arm splint flexion (one that suppresses SIB and still allows for adaptive behavior) for individuals who exhibit SIB. Second, for most individuals, the results of the RRA can be extrapolated to the natural environment. Third, the RRA has the potential to eliminate the need for restraint fading altogether or can help to circumvent fading steps for some individuals. Finally, for some individuals, it might be prudent to evaluate different levels of splint flexion across a variety of contexts (meals, skill acquisition programs, leisure time). Taken together, the RRA is an efficient assessment tool that has the potential to help clinicians identify the optimal level of arm splint flexion for individuals with severe SIB.

Conclusions

Self-injury is a complex and severe behavior disorder displayed by individuals with developmental disabilities. A large body of research suggests that SIB is learned (operant) behavior sometimes reinforced by other people and sometimes reinforced automatically. The purpose of a behavioral assessment is to identify where and when the SIB is most likely and least likely to occur and to identify possible sources of reinforcement for the behavior. Assessment methods include indirect techniques such as checklists and questionnaires, descriptive analysis, functional analysis, and response product measurement. Although each assessment type has its own set of strengths and limitations, some combination of assessment components is usually recommended, and rarely should any single assessment type be used in isolation.

An idealized behavioral assessment of SIB would include first a set of interviews with relevant care providers, second direct observation by a professional coupled with simple data collection by care providers, third a functional analysis of hypothesized sources of reinforcement, and fourth an evaluation of response products (injury) caused by the behavior. In addition, variables such as self-restraint and other forms of restraint should be considered. Collectively, the information obtained would serve as an empirical basis to address perceptions of relevant care providers, idiosyncrasies of the SIB in the natural environment, cause-and-effect relations, and the extent of tissue damage caused by the behavior.

References

Achenbach, T. M. (1991). *Manual for the Child Behavior Checklist/4–18 and 1991 Profile*. Burlington, VT, USA: University of Vermont, Department of Psychiatry.

Aman, M. G., Singh, N. N., Stewart, A. W., & Field, C. J. (1985). The aberrant behavior checklist: A behavior rating scale for the assessment of treatment effects. *American Journal of Mental Deficiency, 89*, 485–491.

Arndorfer, R. E., Miltenberger, R. G., Woster, S. H., Rortvedt, A. K., & Gaffaney, T. (1994). Home-based descriptive and experimental analysis of problem behaviors in children. *Topics in Early Childhood Special Education, 14*, 64–87.

Bijou, S. W., Peterson, R. F., & Ault, M. H. (1968). A method to integrate descriptive and experimental field studies at the levels of data and empirical concepts. *Journal of Applied Behavior Analysis, 1*, 175–191.

Bloom, S. E., Iwata, B. A., Fritz, J. N., Roscoe, E. M., & Carreau, A. B. (2011). Classroom application of a trial-based functional analysis. *Journal of Applied Behavior Analysis, 44*, 19–31.

Borrero, C. S. W., & Borrero, J. C. (2008). Descriptive and experimental analyses of potential precursors to problem behavior. *Journal of Applied Behavior Analysis, 41*, 83–96.

Borrero, C. S. W., Vollmer, T. R., Borrero, J. C., & Bourret, J. (2005). A method of evaluating parameters of reinforcement during parent-child interactions. *Research in Developmental Disabilities, 26*, 577–592.

Borrero, J. C., Vollmer, T. R., Wright, C. S., Lerman, D. C., & Kelley, M. E. (2002). Further evaluation of the role of protective equipment in the functional analysis of self-injurious behavior. *Journal of Applied Behavior Analysis, 35*, 69–72.

Carr, E. G. (1977). The motivation of self-injurious behavior: A review of some hypotheses. *Psychological Bulletin, 84*, 800–816.

Carr, E. G., & Durand, V. M. (1985). Reducing problem behavior through functional communication training. *Journal of Applied Behavior Analysis, 18*, 111–126.

Carr, E. G., & McDowell, J. J. (1980). Social control of self-injurious behavior of organicetiology. *Behavior Therapy, 11*, 402–409.

Chapman, S., Fisher, W., Piazza, C. C., & Kurtz, P. F. (1993). Functional assessment and treatment of life-threatening drug ingestion in a dually diagnosed youth. *Journal of Applied Behavior Analysis, 26*, 255–256.

Conners, J., Iwata, B. A., Kahng, S., Hanley, G. P., Worsdell, A. S., & Thompson, R. H. (2000). Differential responding in the presence and absence of discriminative stimuli during multielement functional analyses. *Journal of Applied Behavior Analysis, 33*, 299–308.

Cooper, L., Wacker, D., Sasso, G., Reimers, T., & Donn, L. (1990). Using parents as therapists to assess the appropriate behavior of their children: Application to a tertiary diagnostic clinic. *Journal of Applied Behavior Analysis, 23*, 285–296.

Cooper, L. J., Wacker, D. P., Thursby, D., Plagmann, L. A., Harding, J., Millard, T., & Derby, M. (1992). Analysis of the effects of task preferences, task demands, and adult attention on child behavior in outpatient and classroom settings. *Journal of Applied Behavior Analysis, 25*, 823–840.

Cowdery, G. E., Iwata, B. A., & Pace, G. M. (1990). Effects and side effects of DRO as treatment for self-injurious behavior. *Journal of Applied Behavior Analysis, 23*, 497–506.

Crawford, J., Brockel, B., Schauss, S., & Miltenberger, R. G. (1992). A comparison of methods for the functional assessment of stereotypic behavior. *Journal of the Association for Persons with Severe Handicaps, 17*, 77–86.

Derby, K. M., Wacker, D. P., Sasso, G., Steege, M., Northup, J., Cigrand, K., & Asmus, J. (1992). Brief functional assessments techniques to evaluate aberrant behavior in an outpatient setting: A summary of 79 cases. *Journal of Applied Behavior Analysis, 25*, 713–721.

DeRosa, N. M., Roane, H. S., Wilson, J. L., Novak, M. D., & Silkowski, E. L. (2015). Effects of arm-splint rigidity on self-injury and adaptive behavior. *Journal of Applied Behavior Analysis, 48*, 860–864.

Deshais, M. A., Fisher, A. B., Hausman, N. L., & Kahng, S. (2015). Further investigation of a rapid restraint analysis. *Journal of Applied Behavior Analysis, 48*, 845–859.

Desrochers, M. N., Hile, M. G., & Williams-Mosely, T. L. (1997). Survey of functional assessment procedures used with individuals who display mental retardation and severe problem behaviors. *American Journal on Mental Retardation, 101*, 535–546.

Doggett, A. R., Edwards, R. P., Moore, J. W., Tingstrom, D. H., & Wilczynski, S. M. (2001). An approach to functional assessment in general education classroom settings. *School Psychology Review, 30*, 313–328.

Durand, V. M., & Crimmins, D. B. (1988). Identifying the variables maintaining self-injurious behavior. *Journal of Autism and Developmental Disorders, 18*, 99–117.

Ellingson, S. A., Miltenberger, R. G., & Long, E. S. (1999). A survey of the use of functional assessment procedures in agencies serving individuals with developmental disabilities. *Behavioral Interventions, 14*, 187–198.

Ellingson, S. A., Miltenberger, R. G., Stricker, J. M., Garlinghouse, M. A., Roberts, J., Galensky, T. L., & Rapp, J. T. (2000). Analysis and treatment of finger sucking. *Journal of Applied Behavior Analysis, 33*, 41–52.

Emerson, E., Thompson, S., Reeves, D., & Henderson, D. (1995). Descriptive analysis of multiple response topographies of challenging behavior across two settings. *Research in Developmental Disabilities, 16*, 301–329.

Favell, J. E., McGimsey, J. F., & Jones, M. L. (1978). The use of physical restraint in the treatment of self-injury and as positive reinforcement. *Journal of Applied Behavior Analysis, 11*, 225–241.

Fischer, S. M., Iwata, B. A., & Worsdell, A. S. (1997). Attention as an establishing operation and as reinforcement during functional analyses. *Journal of Applied Behavior Analysis, 30*, 335–338.

Fisher, W. W., Bowman, L. G., Thompson, R. H., Contrucci, S. A., Burd, L., & Alon, G. (1998). Reductions in self-injury produced by transcutaneous electrical nerve stimulation. *Journal of Applied Behavior Analysis, 31*, 493–496.

Fisher, W. W., & Iwata, B. A. (1996). On the function of self-restraint and its relationship to self-injury. *Journal of Applied Behavior Analysis, 29*, 93–98.

Fisher, W. W., Ninness, H. A. C., Piazza, C. C., & Owen-DeSchryver, J. S. (1996). On the reinforcing effects of the content of verbal attention. *Journal of Applied Behavior Analysis, 29*, 235–238.

Fisher, W. W., Piazza, C. C., Bowman, L. G., Hanley, G. P., & Adelinis, J. D. (1997). Direct and collateral effects of restraints and restraint fading. *Journal of Applied Behavior Analysis, 30*, 105–120.

Forman, D., Hall, S., & Oliver, C. (2002). Descriptive analysis of self-injurious behavior and self-restraint. *Journal of Applied Research in Intellectual Disabilities, 15*, 1–7.

Goh, H., Iwata, B. A., Shore, B. A., DeLeon, I. G., Lerman, D. C., Ulrich, S. M., & Smith, R. G. (1995). An analysis of the reinforcing properties of hand mouthing. *Journal of Applied Behavior Analysis, 28*, 269–283.

Grace, N. C., Thompson, R., & Fisher, W. W. (1996). The treatment of covert self-injury through contingencies on response products. *Journal of Applied Behavior Analysis, 29*, 239–242.

Hagopian, L. P., Rooker, G. W., & Zarcone, J. R. (2015). Delineating subtypes of self-injurious behavior maintained by automatic reinforcement. *Journal of Applied Behavior Analysis, 48*, 523–543.

Hanley, G. P., Iwata, B. A., & McCord, B. E. (2003). Functional analysis of problem behavior: A review. *Journal of Applied Behavior Analysis, 36*, 147–185.

Harding, J., Wacker, D. P., Cooper, L. J., Millard, T., & Jensen-Kovalan, P. (1994). Brief hierarchical assessment of potential treatment components with children in an outpatient clinic. *Journal of Applied Behavior Analysis, 27*, 291–300.

Hutchinson, R. R. (1977). By-products of aversive control. In W. K. Honig & Staddon (Eds.), *Handbook of operant behavior* (pp. 415–431). Englewood Cliffs, NJ, USA: Prentice Hall.

Iwata, B., & DeLeon, I. (1996). The functional analysis screening tool. In *The Florida center on self-injury*. Gainesville, FL: University of Florida.

Iwata, B. A., DeLeon, I. G., & Roscoe, E. M. (2013). Reliability and validity of the functional analysis screening tool. *Journal of Applied Behavior Analysis, 46*, 271–284.

Iwata, B. A., Dorsey, M. F., Slifer, K. J., Bauman, K. E., & Richman, G. S. (1994). Toward a functional analysis of self-injury. *Journal of Applied Behavior Analysis, 197-209*, 27 Reprinted from *Analysis and Intervention in Developmental Disabilities, 2*, 3-20, 1982.

Iwata, B. A., Duncan, B. A., Zarcone, J. R., Lerman, D. C., & Shore, B. A. (1994). A sequential, test-control methodology for conducting functional analyses of self-injurious behavior. *Behavior Modification, 18*, 289–306.

Iwata, B. A., Kahng, S., Wallace, M. D., & Lindberg, J. S. (2000). The functional analysis model of behavioral assessment. In J. Austin & J. E. Carr (Eds.), *Handbook of applied behavior analysis* (pp. 61–89). Reno, NV: Context Press.

Iwata, B. A., Pace, G. M., Cowdery, G. E., & Miltenberger, R. G. (1994). What makes extinction work: An analysis of procedural form and function. *Journal of Applied Behavior Analysis, 27*, 131–144.

Iwata, B. A., Pace, G. M., Dorsey, M. F., Zarcone, J. R., Vollmer, T. R., Smith, R. G., et al. (1994). The functions of self-injurious behavior: An experimental-epidemiological analysis. *Journal of Applied Behavior Analysis, 27*, 215–240.

Iwata, B. A., Pace, G. M., Kalsher, M. J., Cowdery, G. E., & Cataldo, M. F. (1990). Experimental analysis and extinction of self-injurious escape behavior. *Journal of Applied Behavior Analysis, 23*, 11–27.

Iwata, B. A., Pace, G. M., Kissel, R. C., Nau, P. A., & Farber, J. M. (1990). The self-injury trauma (SIT) scale: A method for quantifying surface tissue damage caused by self-injurious behavior. *Journal of Applied Behavior Analysis, 23*, 99–110.

Iwata, B. A., Vollmer, T. R., & Zarcone, J. R. (1990). The experimental (functional) analysis of behavior disorders: Methodology, applications, and limitations. In A. C. Repp & N. N. Singh (Eds.), *Perspectives on the use of non-aversive and aversive interventions for persons with developmental disabilities* (pp. 301–330). Sycamore, IL, USA: Sycamore Publishing.

Kahng, S., Abt, K. A., & Schonbachler, H. E. (2001). Assessment and treatment of low-rate high-intensity problem behavior. *Journal of Applied Behavior Analysis, 34*, 225–228.

Kahng, S., Hausman, N. L., Fisher, A. B., Donaldson, J. M., Cox, J. R., Lugo, M., & Wiskow, K. M. (2015). The safety of functional analyses of self-injurious behavior. *Journal of Applied Behavior Analysis, 48*, 107–114.

Kahng, S. W., Iwata, B. A., Fischer, S. M., Page, T. J., Treadwell, K. R. H., Williams, D. E., et al. (1998). Temporal distributions of problem behavior based on scatter plot analysis. *Journal of Applied Behavior Analysis, 31*, 593–604.

Kuhn, S. A. C., & Triggs, M. (2009). Analysis of social variables when an initial functional analysis indicates automatic reinforcement as the maintaining variable for self-injurious behavior. *Journal of Applied Behavior Analysis, 42,* 679–683.

Lalli, J. S., & Casey, S. D. (1996). Treatment of multiply controlled problem behavior. *Journal of Applied Behavior Analysis, 29,* 391–396.

Lalli, J. S., Livezey, K., & Kates, K. (1996). Functional analysis and treatment of eye poking with response blocking. *Journal of Applied Behavior Analysis, 29,* 129–132.

Le, D. D., & Smith, R. G. (2002). Functional analysis of self-injury with and without protective equipment. *Journal of Developmental and Physical Disabilities, 14,* 277–290.

Lerman, D. C., & Iwata, B. A. (1993). Descriptive and experimental analysis of variables maintaining self-injurious behavior. *Journal of Applied Behavior Analysis, 26,* 293–319.

Lerman, D. C., Iwata, B. A., Smith, R. G., Zarcone, J. R., & Vollmer, T. R. (1994). Transfer of behavioral function as a contributing factor in treatment relapse. *Journal of Applied Behavior Analysis, 27,* 357–370.

Lesch, M., & Nyhan, W. L. (1964). A familial disorder of uric acid metabolism and central nervous system function. *American Journal of Medicine, 36,* 561–570.

Lewis, T. J., Scott, T. M., & Sugai, G. (1994). The problem behavior questionnaire: A teacher-based instrument to develop functional hypotheses of problem behavior in general education classrooms. *Diagnostique, 19,* 103–115.

Lovaas, I., Newsom, C., & Hickman, C. (1987). Self-stimulatory behavior and perceptual reinforcement. *Journal of Applied Behavior Analysis, 20,* 45–68.

Lovaas, O. I., & Simmons, J. Q. (1969). Manipulation of self-destruction in three retarded children. *Journal of Applied Behavior Analysis, 2,* 143–157.

Mace, F. C., & Lalli, J. S. (1991). Linking descriptive and experimental analyses in the treatment of bizarre speech. *Journal of Applied Behavior Analysis, 24,* 553–562.

Marcus, B. A., & Vollmer, T. R. (1996). Combining noncontingent reinforcement and differential reinforcement schedules as treatment for aberrant behavior. *Journal of Applied Behavior Analysis, 29,* 43–51.

Marholin, D., & Steinman, W. M. (1977). Stimulus control in the classroom as a function of the behavior reinforced. *Journal of Applied Behavior Analysis, 10,* 465–478.

Matson, J. L., Bamburg, J. W., Cheery, K. E., & Paclawskyj, T. R. (1999). A validity study on the questions about behavioral function (QABF) scale: Predicting treatment success for self-injury, aggression, and stereotypies. *Research in Developmental Disabilities, 20,* 163–175.

Matson, J. L., Kuhn, D. E., Dixon, D. R., Mayville, S. B., Laud, R. B., Cooper, C. L., et al. (2003). The development and factor structure of the functional assessment for multiple causality (FACT). *Research in Developmental Disabilities, 24,* 485–495.

Matson, J. L., & Vollmer, T. R. (1995). *User's guide: Questions about behavioral function (QABF).* Baton Rouge, LA, USA: Disability Consultants, LLC.

Matson, J. (ed). (2009). *Assessing childhood psychopathology and developmental disabilities.* pp. 341–369. New York, NY: Spring Science+Business Media.

Miltenberger, R. G. (2001). *Behavior modification: Principles and procedures.* Belmont, CA, USA: Wadsworth.

Ndoro, V. W., Hanley, G. P., Tiger, J. H., & Heal, N. A. (2006). A descriptive assessment of instruction-based interactions in the preschool classroom. *Journal of Applied Behavior Analysis, 39,* 79–90.

Northup, J., Wacker, D., Sasso, G., Steege, M., Cigrand, K., Cook, J., & DeRaad, A. (1991). A brief functional analysis of aggressive and alternative behavior in an outclinic setting. *Journal of Applied Behavior Analysis, 24,* 509–522.

Northup, J., Wacker, D. P., Berg, W. K., Kelly, L., Sasso, G., & DeRaad, A. (1994). The treatment of severe behavior problems in school settings using a technical assistance model. *Journal of Applied Behavior Analysis, 27,* 33–48.

Oliver, C., Hall, S., & Nixon, J. (1999). A molecular to molar analysis of communicative and problem behavior. *Research in Developmental Disabilities, 20,* 197–213.

O'Neill, R. E., Horner, R. H., Albin, R. W., Sprague, J. R., Storey, K., & Newton, J. S. (1997). *Functional assessment and program development for problem behavior: A practical handbook* (2nd ed.). Pacific Grove, CA, USA: Brooks.

Paclawskyj, T. R., Matson, J. L., Rush, K. S., Smalls, Y., & Vollmer, T. R. (2001). The validity of the questions about behavioral function (QABF). *Journal of Intellectual Disabilities, 45,* 484–494.

Piazza, C. C., Bowman, L. G., Contrucci, S. A., Delia, M. D., Adelinis, J. D., & Goh, H. (1999). An evaluation of the properties of attention as reinforcement for destructive and appropriate behavior. *Journal of Applied Behavior Analysis, 32,* 437–449.

Piazza, C. C., Hanley, G. P., & Fisher, W. W. (1996). Functional analysis and treatment of cigarette pica. *Journal of Applied Behavior Analysis, 29,* 437–449.

Querim, A. C., Iwata, B. A., Roscoe, E. M., Schlichenmeyer, K. J., Ortega, J. V., & Hurl, K. E. (2013). Functional analysis screening for problem behavior maintained by automatic reinforcement. *Journal of Applied Behavior Analysis, 46,* 47–60.

Rapp, J. T., Miltenberger, R. G., Galensky, T. L., Ellingson, S. A., & Long, E. S. (1999). A functional analysis of hair pulling. *Journal of Applied Behavior Analysis, 32,* 329–337.

Rojahn, J., Matson, J. L., Lott, D., Esbensen, A. J., & Smalls, Y. (2001). The behavior problems inventory: An instrument for the assessment of self-injury, stereotyped behavior, and aggression/destruction in individuals with developmental disabilities. *Journal of Autism and Developmental Disorders, 6,* 577–588.

Rooker, G. W., & Roscoe, E. M. (2005). Functional analysis of self-injurious behavior and its relation to self-restraint. *Journal of Applied Behavior Analysis, 38*, 537–542.

Roscoe, E. M., Schlichenmeyer, K. J., & Dube, W. V. (2015). Functional analysis of problem behavior: A systematic approach for identifying idiosyncratic variables. *Journal of Applied Behavior Analysis, 48*, 289–314.

Sandman, C. A., Datta, P. C., Barron, J., Hoehler, F. K., Williams, C., & Swanson, J. M. (1983). Naloxone attenuates self-abusive behavior in developmentally disabled clients. *Applied Research in Mental Retardation, 4*, 5–11.

Sasso, G. M., Reimers, T. M., Cooper, L. J., Wacker, D., Berg, W., Steege, M., et al. (1992). Use of descriptive and experimental analyses to identify the functional properties of aberrant behavior in school settings. *Journal of Applied Behavior Analysis, 25*, 809–821.

Scheithauer, M., O'Connor, J., & Toby, L. M. (2015). Assessment of self-restraint using a functional analysis of self-injury. *Journal of Applied Behavior Analysis, 48*, 907–911.

Shirley, M. J., Iwata, B. A., & Kahng, S. (1999). False-positive maintenance of self-injurious behavior by access to tangible reinforcers. *Journal of Applied Behavior Analysis, 32*, 201–204.

Sidman, M. (1960). *Tactics of scientific research*. New York: Basic Books.

Skinner, B. F. (1953). *Science and human behavior*. New York: The Macmillan Company.

Sloman, K. N., Vollmer, T. R., Cotnoir, N. M., Borrero, C. S. W., Borrero, J. C., Samaha, A. L., et al. (2005). Descriptive analysis of caregiver reprimands. *Journal of Applied Behavior Analysis, 38*, 373–383.

Smith, R. G., & Churchill, R. M. (2002). Identification of environmental determinants of behavior disorders through functional analysis of precursor behaviors. *Journal of Applied Behavior Analysis, 35*, 125–136.

Smith, R. G., Iwata, B. A., Vollmer, T. R., & Pace, G. M. (1992). On the relationship between self-injurious behavior and self-restraint. *Journal of Applied Behavior Analysis, 25*, 433–445.

Smith, R. G., Iwata, B. A., Vollmer, T. R., & Zarcone, J. R. (1993). Experimental analysis and treatment of multiply controlled self-injury. *Journal of Applied Behavior Analysis, 26*, 183–196.

St. Peter, C. C., Vollmer, T. R., Bourret, J. C., Borrero, C. S. W., Sloman, K. N., & Rapp, J. T. (2005). On the role of attention in naturally occurring matching relations. *Journal of Applied Behavior Analysis, 38*, 429–443.

Steege, M. W., Wacker, D. P., Cigrand, K. C., Berg, W. K., Novak, C. G., Reimers, T. M., ... DeRaad, A. (1990). Use of negative reinforcement in the treatment of self-injurious behavior. *Journal of Applied Behavior Analysis, 23*, 459–467.

Thomason-Sassi, J. L., Iwata, B. A., Neidert, P. L., & Roscoe, E. M. (2011). Response latency as an index of response strength during functional analyses of problem behavior. *Journal of Applied Behavior Analysis, 44*, 51–67.

Thompson, R. H., & Iwata, B. A. (2001). A descriptive analysis of social consequences following problem behavior. *Journal of Applied Behavior Analysis, 34*, 169–178.

Touchette, P. E., MacDonald, R. F., & Langer, S. N. (1985). A scatter plot for identifying stimulus control of problem behavior. *Journal of Applied Behavior Analysis, 18*, 343–351.

Van Houten, R., & Rolider, A. (1991). Research in applied behavior analysis. In J. L. Matson & J. A. Mulick (Eds.), *Handbook of mental retardation* (2nd ed.). New York: Pergamon Press.

VanDerHeyden, A. M., Witt, J. C., & Gatti, S. (2001). Descriptive assessment method to reduce overall disruptive behavior in a preschool classroom. *School Psychology Review, 30*, 548–567.

Vollmer, T. R., Borrero, J. C., Wright, C. S., Van Camp, C., & Lalli, J. S. (2001). Identifying possible contingencies during descriptive analyses of severe behavior disorders. *Journal of Applied Behavior Analysis, 34*, 269–287.

Vollmer, T. R., Iwata, B. A., Duncan, B. A., & Lerman, D. C. (1993a). Within-session patterns of self-injury as indicators of behavioral function. *Research in Developmental Disabilities, 14*, 479–492.

Vollmer, T. R., Iwata, B. A., Duncan, B. A., & Lerman, D. C. (1993b). Extensions of multielement functional analyses using reversal-type designs. *Journal of Developmental and Physical Disabilities, 5*, 311–325.

Vollmer, T. R., Marcus, B. A., & Ringdahl, J. E. (1995). Noncontingent escape as treatment for self-injurious behavior maintained by negative reinforcement. *Journal of Applied Behavior Analysis, 28*, 15–26.

Vollmer, T. R., Marcus, B. A., Ringdahl, J. E., & Roane, H. S. (1995). Progressing from brief to extended experimental analyses in the evaluation of aberrant behavior. *Journal of Applied Behavior Analysis, 28*, 561–576.

Vollmer, T. R., Sloman, K. N., & Borrero, C. S. W. (2009). Behavioral assessment of self-injury. In J. Matson (ed). *Assessing childhood psychopathology and developmental disabilities*. pp. 341–369. New York, NY: Spring Science+Business Media.

Wallace, M. D., Iwata, B. A., Zhou, L., & Goff, G. A. (1999). Rapid assessment of the effects of restraint on self-injury and adaptive behavior. *Journal of Applied Behavior Analysis, 32*, 525–528.

Weiseler, N. A., Hanson, R. H., Chamberlain, T. R., & Thompson, T. (1985). Functional taxonomy of stereotypic and self-injurious behavior. *Mental Retardation, 23*, 230–234.

Wilson, D. M., Iwata, B. A., & Bloom, S. E. (2012). Evaluation of a computer-assisted technique for measuring wound severity. *Journal of Applied Behavior Analysis, 45*, 797–808.

Zarcone, J. R., Rodgers, T. A., Iwata, B. A., Rourke, D. A., & Dorsey, M. F. (1991). Reliability analysis of the motivation assessment scale: A failure to replicate. *Research in Developmental Disabilities, 12*, 349–360.

Assessment of Pica

Abigail Issarraras and Johnny L. Matson

Introduction

Pica is the consumption of nonnutritive, nonfood items. In some cultures, it is a culturally sanctioned and religious behavior with long tradition. However, in children and adolescents with developmental disabilities, it is a common self-injurious behavior that requires additional attention and treatment (Barrett, 2008). Self-injurious behavior refers to the deliberate infliction of harm to the body, and it can include behaviors such as head-banging, self-scratching, and self-biting, among others (Barrett, 2008). Due to the potentially serious damage to the digestive system following consumption of nonfood items, researchers have classified pica as self-injurious behavior in the developmental disabilities population (Call, Simmons, Lomas Meyers, & Alvarez, 2015; Williams & McAdam, 2012). In fact, pica might be the most dangerous form of self-injurious behavior, as just one ingestion of a lethal, poisonous, or sharp object can cause severe injury, require extensive surgery, involve additional medical complications, and in the worst cases, even death of the individual (Williams, Kirkpatrick-Sanchez, Enzinna, Dunn, & Borden-Karasack, 2009).

The preferred item for ingestion varies by individual. McAdam, Breibord, Levine, and Williams (2012) have proposed six classes of these pica items based on the material consumed; several terms are a combination of the type of item's prefix and the suffix "phagy" which denotes the consumption of a specific item. The first class of pica items include those of biologic secretions, including coprophagia (consumption of feces), emetophagia (consumption of vomit), and mucophagia (consumption of mucous). The second class of pica items includes those of biologic solids, such as trichophagia (consumption of hair) and onychophagia (consumption of fingernails). In the third class, items may include chemical consumption such as plumbophagia (consumption of lead chips). The fourth class refers to food items, though as will be discussed, these would not warrant a diagnosis of pica. The fifth class refers to organic materials; these include amylophagia (consumption of laundry starch), geophagia (consumption of dirt, sand, clay), and foliophagia (consumption of grass, leaves). The final and perhaps most immediately dangerous class includes physically damaging pica items such as hyalophagia (consumption of glass), tobaccophagia (consumption of cigarette buds), and acuphagia (consumption of sharp items). Though this list is extensive, pica items may not be limited to those described previously (C. R. Johnson, 1990). Additionally, the use of these groups and terminologies is not consistently applied in research or clinical settings.

Failure to assess for and diagnose pica is not only highly dangerous and potentially fatal to the client but also bars them from opportunities to receive evidence-based treatment to specifically address the pica. Behavioral interventions have been shown to reduce pica behavior up to 90% (Hagopian, Rooker, & Rolider, 2011). Unfortunately, for many clinicians and parents, pica is not always considered a medically urgent or a pressing concern (McAdam, Breibord, Levine, & Williams, 2012; McAlpine & Singh, 1986; Sturmey & Williams, 2016); clinicians are indebted to their clients to seriously consider the consequences should the pica go untreated. Though review of recent medical records (e.g., recently conducted X-rays, a series of intestinal surgeries to remove blocked items) may be sufficient to inform a diagnosis in some cases, clinicians must also be aware of other methods to assess for this behavior. Thus, the focus of this chapter is on the assessment of clinical forms of pica among individuals with developmental disabilities. First, a discussion of culturally normative forms of pica will be discussed, as it is important to understand how the clinical severity of pica in individuals with developmental disabilities differs from nonclinical populations. This will be followed by a brief history of pica, the changes made to diagnostic criteria in the *Diagnostic and Statistical Manual of Mental Disorders,* and estimates of prevalence of pica (American Psychiatric Association, 2013). A discussion of methods for assessing pica will then be followed by a discussion of both important considerations for assessing pica in individuals with developmental disabilities and directions for future research.

Culturally Normative Forms of Pica

Though pica featured historically as a symptom of various medical conditions, pica behaviors have also held cultural significance in different locations and across different cultures. For example, Young (2010) described several instances when pica was a socially accepted behavior. In times of great famine and lack of resources, many people turn to eat earth and clay out of necessity (Sturmey & Williams, 2016; Young, 2010); this behavior still occurs in countries such as Haiti, where access to nutritional and filling foods requires some citizens to consume the earth rather than starve. This practice was also reported in children and pregnant woman in areas of Africa (Nchito, Geissler, Mubila, Friis, & Olsen, 2004). Sturmey and Williams (2016) also describe certain religious practices where eating sacred earth holds a special significance for the group.

In populations with developmental disabilities, pica shares some similarities, yet is also markedly different than in nonclinical populations. Regarding culturally significant pica, the social reinforcement for following the types of cultural customs described previously (e.g., eating sacred earth) is markedly different than the reinforcement experienced by individuals with developmental disabilities who engage in pica. Though both populations may appear "obsessed" with the pica item and find it powerfully reinforcing, as Young (2010) states, the intense craving for the pica substance is notably absent in the cultural practices. That is, the "obsession" with the pica item has nothing to do with any physical properties or tastes of the item itself, but rather, the cultural and social significance of the pica item for the cultural practice. Although the strong preference for a specific pica item can vary greatly (e.g., hair, strings, cigarettes, paper, dirt, feces) for both clinical and nonclinical populations, functional analyses typically indicate that in individuals with developmental disabilities, pica behavior is not associated with any social consequences or normative behavior (Piazza, Hanley, & Fisher, 1996; Sturmey & Williams, 2016). In the absence of social reinforcement for the pica behavior, individuals with developmental disabilities are actually often subject to immediate and unpleasant consequences (e.g., physical restraints, choking, injury) following their pica behavior.

An additional normative form of pica occurs in pregnant woman across cultures; this form of pica has been largely documented throughout history (Johnson & Gretton, 2017). Researchers estimate that the worldwide prevalence of pica during pregnancy is 27.8% (Fawcett, Fawcett, & Mazmanian, 2016). This study by Fawcett, Fawcett, and Mazmanian (2016) found that prevalence of pica increased in pregnant women as educational attainment decreased and as the prevalence of anemia increased. In pregnant women, pica has also been associated with deficiencies in zinc, iron, calcium, thiamine, and vitamin C (Johnson & Gretton, 2017; Upadhyaya & Sharma, 2012). Similarly, researchers have also found elevated prevalence rates of pica in individuals who are frequent blood donors, which is also thought to be related to an iron deficiency (Chansky et al., 2017). Both of these forms of pica differ from pica behavior in individuals with developmental disabilities, as there is no association with any known nutrient deficiencies in most cases.

The culturally normative forms of pica discussed previously should be easily differentiated by experienced clinicians from the clinical form of pica in individuals with developmental disabilities. However, it may be more difficult to differentiate pica behavior from the normative mouthing period of development that children experience, which occurs in estimates of 10–32% of children aged 1–6 (Motta & Basile, 1998; Rose, Porcelli, & Neale, 2000). As Barrett (2008) discusses, prior to age 2, many toddlers explore their environments by putting nonfood objects in their mouths, which can lead to accidental and intentional ingestions of the objects. Should the individual persist in this behavior beyond the age of 2, with no accompanying decrease in the frequency of the pica behavior, then an evaluation for developmental disabilities is warranted, as this could be a sign of clinical forms of pica, intellectual disability, autism, and other developmental issues (Barrett, 2008). Because it is difficult to differentiate age-appropriate mouthing and exploration and pica before the age of 2, the APA recommends waiting until the child is over 2 years of age before making an official diagnosis of pica (American Psychiatric Association, 2013).

History of Pica

Pica has been recorded extensively throughout history, with the earliest reports of the disorder made 2000 years ago by the philosopher Hippocrates (Johnson & Gretton, 2017). Historically, the focus on unusual eating behaviors was on pregnant women, who often had intense cravings for unusual foods, and children, who frequently mouthed and ingested nonfood objects (Johnson, 1990; Parry-Jones & Parry-Jones, 1992). Interestingly, pica was not thought of as a separate diagnostic category until well into the mid-twentieth century. It had previously been associated with other illnesses and conditions, such as anemia, intellectual disability, and pregnancy, and it was not thought to warrant its own clinical attention.

The etymology of the word "pica" indicates that it was once the medieval Latin word for "magpie" (Cone Jr., 1969). The magpie is a bird that many claimed would "peck at or crave everything," including edible and nonedible items such as clay (Parry-Jones & Parry-Jones, 1992). Though for centuries pica was described as a symptom of other medical conditions, such as pregnancy, anemia, intellectual disability, and others (Parry-Jones & Parry-Jones, 1992), the shift toward an association with mental health problems began in the late nineteenth century. This was due to the publication of the publication of the *Diagnostic and Statistical Manual of Mental Disorders*, 3rd Edition (*DSM*-III; American Psychiatric Association, 1980), which classified pica as a separate disorder in 1980.

Diagnostic Criteria

Diagnosis of pica can be made using the *Diagnostic and Statistical Manual of Mental Disorders* (*DSM*-5; American Psychiatric Association, 2013). Clinicians should not confuse pica with other disorders in the *DSM*-5 or other behaviors, which may have a similar form or function. A common confusion occurs in differentiating from hand mouthing or chronic mouthing of other objects. This behavior looks similar to those exhibited by individuals with pica, and researchers have found that chronic mouthing of objects is a nonsocial behavior, likely to be automatically, positively reinforced (Hartmann, Becker, Hampton, & Bryant-Waugh, 2012; Piazza et al., 1996; Sturmey & Williams, 2016). Similar analyses of pica behavior have demonstrated that the same automatic reinforcement is present. Additionally, as Hartman and colleagues (2012) report, pica may resemble behaviors associated with or overlap with symptoms of avoidant/restrictive food intake disorder (ARFD). However, the restricted interests in ARFD involve actual food items.

Pica was first described in the third edition of the *DSM* (*DSM*-III; American Psychiatric Association, 1980) under the category of Infancy, Childhood, or Adolescence Disorders. It was reportedly a rare disorder, with age of onset usually from 12 to 24 months. The essential feature in the *DSM*-III was "persistent eating of a nonnutritive substance" for at least 1 month with no aversion to food. In the *DSM*-III, pica could not be diagnosed in the presence of another disorder such as infantile autism, schizophrenia, or physical disorders. The *DSM*-IV (American Psychiatric Association, 2000) kept the diagnosis of pica in the category of disorders usually first diagnosed in infancy, childhood, or adolescence. Similar to criteria in the *DSM*-III, to receive a diagnosis of pica, the individual must engage in persistent eating of the nonnutritive substances for at least 1 month. Additionally, the *DSM*-IV stated that the consumption of nonnutritive substances must be inappropriate to the developmental level and not part of a culturally sanctioned practice.

In the *DSM*-5, pica has been moved to the section entitled "Feeding and Eating Disorders" (American Psychiatric Association, 2013). A notable change in this edition emphasizes that the disorder can occur across development, not limited to childhood. Under the new DSM-5 criteria, pica can now be diagnosed in adulthood as well. Criteria for the diagnosis of pica in the DSM-5 now specify that, for at least 1 month, the individual engages in persistent eating "nonnutritive, nonfood substances." This change was intended to guide clinicians in differentiating behaviors that warrant the label of pica from those behaviors that are culturally supported or developmentally normative. A common example is in the excessive consumption of diet soda; though the item is nonnutritive, it is still a food item and thus would not qualify an individual to receive a diagnosis of pica (Hartmann et al., 2012; Sturmey & Williams, 2016). The DSM-5 also recommends a minimum age of 2 years to ensure that developmentally appropriate mouthing behaviors are not confused with pica behaviors as well. Finally, the DSM-5 recommended that pica be diagnosed comorbid to autism spectrum disorders (ASD), intellectual disability (ID), and other mental disorders only if the severity/frequency of the pica behavior warrants its own independent, clinical attention.

Prevalence Rates

The prevalence of pica in the general population remains unclear. This could be due to the stigma an individual experiences regarding their consumption of these nonfood items, hindering them from seeking out treatment services. As stated previously, prevalence of pica in pregnant women has been estimated to be 27.8%, and the prevalence among children ages 1–6 is estimated to be between 10 and 32% (Barrett, 2008; Fawcett et al., 2016; Motta & Basile, 1998). Estimating the prevalence of pica in clinical populations has proven to be equally difficult, though the reasons for this may be different.

Per the DSM-5, prevalence estimates of pica are difficult to ascertain, as pica is commonly underreported or missed by clinicians (American Psychiatric Association, 2013; Rose et al., 2000). Pica is commonly comorbid with autism spectrum disorder (ASD) and intellectual disability (ID), and it is less commonly comorbid with schizophrenia and obsessive-compulsive disorder (OCD; APA, 2013). One study by Kinnell (1985) found that 60% of the those with ASD ($N = 70$) engaged in pica while only 4% of individuals with Down syndrome (*N* = 70) engaged in pica. Tracy et al. (1996) found that of 400 patients diagnosed with schizophrenia, only 4% displayed pica. Among individuals with ID, several factors, including genetic conditions and the environment where data was collected, have been associated with higher prevalence of pica. For example, individuals with profound ID are most likely to engage in pica, as prevalence among individuals with ID appears to increase with severity of ID (Ali, 2001; American Psychiatric Association, 2013). Additionally, although pica is not commonly reported among individuals with ID living in the community, higher rates of pica (i.e., an estimated 5.7–25.8%) have been found among individuals with ID living in clinics and institutions (Ashworth, Hirdes, & Martin, 2009; Danford & Huber, 1982). In a sample of individuals with cri du chat syndrome, a rare genetic condition that results in ID, about 27% of the sample (*N* = 66) also displayed pica (Sturmey & Williams, 2016).

Researchers have found that prevalence of pica is also associated with the severity of comorbid ID and impairments in social skills (Matson & Bamburg, 1999; Matson, Hattier, & Turygin, 2012; Sturmey & Williams, 2016; Tewari, Krishnan, Valsalan, & Roy, 1995). Additionally, Matson, Hattier, and Turygin (2012) found that in individuals with ID alone (*N* = 22), with ID and ASD (*N* = 22), and with ID, ASD, and pica (*N* = 15), the pica behavior was highly associated with other self-injurious behaviors, such as hand-biting, head-banging, and hair pulling, rather than stereotypical behaviors (e.g., repetitive hand flapping, finger flicking) or aggressive/destructive behaviors (e.g., hitting, kicking, scratching others). This study also reported similar results when they compared the social skills among the three groups (Matson et al., 2012). Results indicated that the group with ID, ASD, and pica had fewest positive and most negative social skills and behaviors, supporting the claim that pica tends to be more common in those individuals with ID and/or ASD with more severe disabilities (Ali, 2001; Matson et al., 2012; Sturmey & Williams, 2016).

Assessment

Assessing for pica is different from other assessments in that no screen or measure currently exists to specifically identify the issue. Most often, clinicians must ask parents a variety of questions to understand the frequency and severity of the child's pica. Some questions that should always be asked if concerns related to pica are present include: how often does the individual attempt to eat the nonfood item (e.g., daily, at least once a week, at least once a month, etc.)? Is the child limited to the one nonfood item or does the child attempt to ingest a variety of nonfood items? Has the child successfully ingested a nonfood item recently or ever in their lifetime? How do parents or caregivers typically respond to this behavior? Does the child persist in the attempt to ingest the nonfood item after the parent or caregiver has redirected the child? All of these questions are important for understanding not only whether the child would meet criteria for a pica diagnosis, but these questions would also be helpful in initial steps of treatment planning.

Should parents not report the pica behavior immediately, then other signs and symptoms may alert the clinician to probe further. For example, if the child is known to have a developmental disability and frequently suffers from stomach aches, constipation, or chronic abdominal pain, then further observation and investigation into the probability of discreet ingestion of the nonfood items should be considered (Barrett, 2008). Parents or caregivers may feel embarrassed or ashamed, depending on the nature of the nonfood item their child prefers, and so they may be more reluctant to disclose this information in the assessment. Building strong clinical rapport and trust in the clinicians' ability to help the family is crucial so that parents disclose the most accurate information regarding the difficulties their child is currently experiencing.

Assessment of pica can be difficult when the behavior occurs at very low rates. A child may quickly ingest a life-threatening item and thus professionals must proceed carefully in their assessments to ensure a comprehensive evaluation of the issue. For individuals with developmental disabilities, pica-related deaths are not uncommon (Decker, 1993; Foxx & Livesay, 1984; McLoughlin, 1988; Williams & McAdam, 2012). Though a universal method for diagnosing or screening for pica does not exist, clinicians may examine medical records, directly observe the child, or ask parents to conduct stool checks. Determining whether the pica behavior has occurred previously, whether it occurred on more than one occasion, and the severity of the situation should be top priorities for any clinician assessing for pica. Additionally, clinicians may also need to recommend additional medical testing depending on the nature of the pica item; if parents or caregivers report that the individual regularly ingests possibly toxic items, such as paint chips, chemicals, or cigarette butts, then the clinician should direct the family to obtain lab tests of the child's lead levels and other toxins (Mishori & McHale, 2014). This would prevent further, possibly life-threatening infections and illness as well (e.g., lead poisoning, parasitic infections, etc.).

Behavioral interventions are the most commonly accessed treatment for treating pica; meta-analyses have found that comprehensive behavioral interventions are well-established and have been highly effective in treating pica, and several studies have found a greater than 90% reduction of pica (Call et al., 2015; Hagopian et al., 2011). A behavior plan also helps to ensure the reduction of the use of temporary restraints, protections, etc. (Sturmey, 2015). Methods of behavioral and functional assessment are described below, in addition to brief descriptions of measures that can be administered during diagnostic assessments to screen for pica behaviors.

Behavioral Assessment

Behaviorism is the theoretical basis used to identify the environmental variables resulting in the pica behavior in order to understand and change the behavior. Cooper, Heron, and Heward (2007) offer a thorough review of the concepts of applied behavior analysis, including those used in the following descriptions. ABA is extremely useful in clinical populations such as ASD, ID, and others (Sturmey, 2007).When conducting a behavioral assessment of pica, the antecedent behavior (e.g., scavenging for the desired food item) and the desired adaptive behavior (e.g., eating appropriate food items) must also be considered besides the target behavior (pica). A stimulus preference assessment of food items should also be conducted to reinforce appropriate behaviors efficiently in treatment. Data on the frequency of the behavior should also be taken regularly, as pica is a brief, discrete behavior that may not be observed every day. If the clinician is having difficulties observing the behavior, then other methods exist to elicit the pica behavior.

Matson, Belva, Hattier, and Matson (2011) described an approach, known as "baiting," that is largely unique to pica assessment; this involved placing placebo pica items in plain sight of the individual, therefore "baiting" them to engage in the behavior. In addition to the nonfood pica items, a variety of edible items should also be in the individual's view. This approach was used by Donnelly and Olczak (1990) for treatment of cigarette pica. The "bogus" cigarette butts in this intervention allowed the therapist to directly observe the behavior without the obvious safety issues of ingesting cigarettes (e.g., toxicity, gagging, nausea). In this approach, the assessment of potential pica behavior can occur as intervention on also occurs.

Clinicians may also choose to conduct a functional behavioral assessment (FBA), which is an extremely valuable tool in changing undesired behaviors. The FBA, or the process of gathering and interpreting data related to the function of a problem behavior, provides information about what reinforcers to change to reduce pica behavior through an individualized treatment (O'Neill et al., 1997) . There are many studies which have demonstrated FBAs as effective in identifying the reinforcers that maintain challenging behavior such as pica, and thus special education laws not require functional assessments when challenging behaviors are present (Sturmey & Williams, 2016; Turnbull, 2005).

Functional assessments of pica should aim to identify consequences for both pica and the appropriate behavior (Piazza et al., 1996; Sturmey, 2007). A full description of the behaviors and factors leading to pica or attempted pica is also necessary. In a similar vein, a full description of the appropriate behavior following the pica should be presented as well; this may include eating of appropriate food items or disposing of nonfood items in the trash. An important consideration when conducting an FBA for pica is to consider whether the pica behavior occurs at a frequency high enough to even permit a functional assessment. This important limitation may draw clinicians to briefer, indirect methods of assessment, as those described below.

Individual Assessment Measures

Beyond functional analysis of the behavior, several measures exist as efficient and appropriate tools for assessing for pica and other challenging behaviors in individuals with developmental disabilities. Often the time required to conduct a full functional analysis is not feasible for clinicians, or the pica behavior does not occur at high enough rates for the clinicians to properly conduct the full functional assessment. The measures described below offer quicker methods of assessing for a variety of behavior problems, including pica.

QABF
The Questions About Behavioral Function (QABF; Paclawskyj, Matson, Rush, Smalls, & Vollmer, 2000) is a 25 item questionnaire that asks raters to determine how often the client engages in the behavior in the situation described. Samples of items include "engages in the behavior because there is nothing else to do," "engages in the behavior when asked to do something," and "engages in the behavior to try to get people to leave him alone." The QABF aids clinicians in quickly determining the function of the target behavior. Based on ratings, the behavior is hypothesized to serve primary functions of attention, escape, nonsocial, physical, or access to tangibles.

Though not used to probe for or identify any behaviors specifically, a clinician can use this tool once parent report or other questionnaires have confirmed that there are concerns related to pica. The use of this instrument would aid clinicians in understanding the function of the pica behavior in the individual. Studies have found average scores on assessments of function of pica using the QABF are often nonsocial, which are similar to various functional analyses of pica (Applegate, Matson, & Cherry, 1999; Matson & Bamburg, 1999; Wasano, Borrero, & Kohn, 2009).

STEP
The Screening Tool of Feeding Problems (STEP; Matson & Kuhn, 2001) screens for a variety of feeding problems in five categories, including aspiration risk, selectivity, skills, food refusal-related behavior problems, and nutrition-related behavior problems. A total of 23 items assess the frequency and severity of these problems. Parents rate items such as "he/she chokes on food" or "he/she spits out their food before swallowing." For each item, parents answer how often the behavior has occurred in the last month (i.e., 0 – Not at all/Not a problem; 1 – Between 1 and 10 times; or 2 – More than 10 times) and how serious the behavior has been during the last month (i.e., 0 – Caused no harm/problems; 1 – Caused minimal harm/problems; or 2 – Caused serious injury/problems).

The STEP was not designed to identify or diagnose pica specifically but rather is a broad screen for feeding problems. An item that may be associated with pica is "he/she eats or attempts to eat items that are not food," which would prompt clinicians to probe for additional information should a parent or guardian endorse this item for their child. Though not sufficient for a diagnosis of pica without follow-up with parents, the STEP could prove very useful to clinicians, as parents can fill out this measure on their own and fairly quickly (about 10–15 min).

ASD-CC
The Autism Spectrum Disorder – Diagnostic for Children and Autism Spectrum Disorder -

Comorbid for Children Scale (ASD-DC; ASD-CC; Matson & Wilkins, 2008) are used to obtain a measure of ASD symptom severity and comorbid conditions. As individuals with ASD are at higher risk for engaging in pica, having a screen for the pica behavior in ASD diagnostic measures could be especially useful for clinicians. The ASD-CC contains 39 items that screen for many comorbid conditions for individuals with ASD. These include depression, specific phobia, eating difficulties, conduct disorder, and attention-deficit/hyperactivity disorder (ADHD). Raters are asked to answer each item as to whether recently it has not been a problem, been a mild problem, or a severe problem.

The ASD-CC is an informant-based measure where the clinician reads each of the items out loud to the informant. Though not specifically assessing for pica, clinicians may consider further assessment were a parent to endorse the item "eats things that are not meant to be eaten (e.g., paint chips, dirt, hair, cloth, etc.)" during the administration of this measure. The ASD-CC offers the additional flexibility for the clinician to stop administering items to follow up with more questions immediately once the pica item was endorsed. The clinician should ensure to probe further for what types of items are ingested by the child, whether the child has successfully swallowed the item, the frequency in which the child attempts to engage in the behavior, and whether any serious medical consequences have ever occurred.

BPI

The Behavior Problems Inventory (BPI; Rojahn et al., 2012), originally appearing in German, used to only measure self-injury in the developmental disabilities population. The BPI now screens for a behavior problems in individuals with developmental disabilities in three categories: self-injurious behavior (SIB), stereotypic behavior items, and aggressive/destructive behavior. The total BPI consists of 52 items, but a short form of 30 items (BPI-S) also exists. Both forms are available for immediate download online, as well as many translations of the measure (e.g., Spanish, Arabic, Chinese, Italian, French, etc.). Parents rate both the frequency (i.e., never, monthly, weekly, daily, or hourly) and the severity (i.e., mild, moderate, or severe) of the behavior. Items related to pica are included within the SIB section. Item 7 asks specifically about pica and thus would prompt further investigation should a parent endorse this item.

Conners CBRS

The Conners Comprehensive Behavior Rating Scales (CBRS; Conners, 2008) are designed to assess for a variety of clinical problems in order to diagnose and treat children and adolescents. To assess for pica, clinicians can choose to administer the Parent or Self-Report form of the CBRS, as these forms include a subscale of pica specifically. The Conners CBRS-Parent can be used with children ages 6–18; the Conners CBRS-Self-Report is suitable for children ages 8–18. Response options to each item across each form are as follows: 0 = Not true at all (Never, Seldom), 1 = Just a little true (Occasionally), 2 = Pretty much true (Often, Quite a bit), and 3 = Very much true (Very often, Very frequently). Clinicians should be aware that these scales are not solely assessing for pica or challenging behaviors, and thus the forms are lengthy (i.e., 203 items in the CBRS-Parent and 179 items in the CBRS-Self-Report); the estimated time of completion for both the Parent and Self-Report form is 20 min. An additional strength of the CBRS is the availability of a Spanish edition of the scales, which would assist clinicians in diagnosing and monitoring a variety of issues, including pica, in children from Spanish-speaking families.

Assessment of Severity

Regarding the severity of pica, one study by Williams developed a 5-point Severity Index for Pica that could prove clinically useful (Sturmey & Williams, 2016). The index has not been systematically evaluated, but can be an important step during the assessment process for determining the risk to the individual's safety. The index, developed by Don E. Williams, Ph.D., BCBA-D, is presented below:

1. *Mild*: Mouths objects and has swallowed small pieces of paper or strings without and passed with no difficulty known.
2. *Moderate*: Mouths objects and has swallowed small pieces of paper or strings or other items considered non-dangerous in small amounts. Has experienced one or two incidents of choking and coughing up items.
3. *Severe*: Mouths objects and has swallowed small pieces of paper or strings or other items considered non-dangerous in small amounts. Has experienced one or two incidents of choking and coughing up items. Has also had X-rays to rule out pica on more than one occasion.
4. *Dangerous*: Ingests foreign object during probes at least weekly. History shows several X-rays and documented ingestion of foreign objects considered dangerous (screws, bolts, jewelry, metal coins).
5. *Life-threatening*: Has had one or more surgeries for the removal of foreign objects and continues to engage in pica at least once every 30–90 days during probes.

As state previously, this scale has not been evaluated; however, the clinical utility could prove useful for communication among clinicians about the severity of the individuals' behavior. Future research into methods of categorizing the severity of pica behavior in individuals with developmental disabilities would have clinical utility as well as introduce new ways of investigating differences in groups of individuals diagnosed with pica.

Discussion

Assessment of pica should be a top priority for clinicians in order to recommend the best course of treatment moving forward. On some occasions, pica may be assessed as a low-risk behavior managed through a behavior support plan, supervision, and redirection. For individuals with developmental disabilities, there are additional risks that can result from overlooked pica behavior that can have serious consequences. Though this self-injurious behavior may not occur at as high rates as others (e.g., head-banging, biting), for some individuals with developmental disabilities, the risk to that individual's safety is still a cause for concern. These include risk of infection, transmission of diseases such as HIV or hepatitis, choking, objects lodged in the gastrointestinal tub, surgeries to remove blockage, and severe damage to the gastrointestinal system that can result in injury and even death (Sturmey & Williams, 2016; Tewari et al., 1995).

Assessing for pica in individuals with disabilities also requires the important consideration of several ethical issues. First, the client's dignity should always be upheld during assessment of pica and in planning treatment. The Association for Behavior Analysis states that a clinician's responsibility is to ensure their client's right to effective treatment (Association for Behavior Analysis, 1989). For clinicians working with individuals with developmental disabilities, this means upholding that their clients have the right to services whose goal is the individual's personal welfare and the right to the most effective interventions available. This can be complicated when a parent's or inexperienced caregiver's immediate response to the pica behavior may be movement restriction or a physical restraint to prevent short-term harm to the individual. For example, in a report by Williams, Kirkpatrick-Sanchez, Enzinna, Dunn, and Borden-Karasack (2009), individuals who engaged in pica were applied with protective equipment (e.g., mittens, split jackets, helmets with plastic mouth covers, etc.) to prevent further ingestion of nonfood items. Physical restraints can be traumatic experiences for the individual being restrained, and so clinicians should work to decrease the use of physical restraints as much as possible (Sturmey, 2015).

Ensuring that families of individuals with developmental disabilities not only recognize the importance of treating the pica behavior but also follow through with any treatment recommendations is critical to ensure the wellbeing of the individual. Future research should seek to understand factors that contribute to the high rates of underreported pica, which is known to occur in populations with developmental disabilities. Developing quicker screening practices to identify pica is also of importance for not only psychologists but pediatricians, nurses, therapists, and other professionals who routinely assess children. Differentiating pica in its clinical form in very young children (under 5 years) from typical mouthing and exploration behaviors is also critical, and, thus, a reliable and valid screen for these problems should also be appropriate to the individual's developmental level. As discussed before, the etiology of pica and its' developmental progression is not well understood, and so future research should also seek to investigate these issues as well. Perhaps most importantly, researchers should work to gather the most accurate estimates of the prevalence of pica in the developmental disabilities population compared to children without any known psychological disorders or developmental delays.

Conclusion

Pica, the consumption of nonfood, nonnutritive substances, varies in the frequency and severity of the behavior, as well as type of item consumed (e.g., dirt, hair, paper, string, etc.). Though pica does occur in typically developing populations, including pregnant women and, in some cultures, for religious beliefs, clinical attention is warranted especially in developmental disabilities populations due to high possibility of injury or even death. Higher prevalence rates of pica have been found in individuals with severe and profound intellectual disabilities, in those with accompanying social impairments, and in individuals with ASD.

Though no direct screener or measure currently assess for pica specifically, clinicians have a few measures based on parent report that could assist in directing their clinical attention to this issue should parents endorse specific items on those measures. Researchers must continue to investigate and understand the etiological theories leading to pica, such as what behaviors typically precede pica in specific populations, what factors put an individual at greater risk for developing pica, and what maintains the behavior. Additionally, having better prevalence estimates of pica in individuals with developmental disabilities who are not institutionalized should be a priority for researchers, as well as understanding the progression of pica from a developmental standpoint. For clinicians, it is essential to routinely screen for pica in order to assess, prevent, and implement treatment procedures as soon as possible to avoid serious medical consequences.

References

Ali, Z. (2001). Pica in people with intellectual disability: A literature review of etiology, epidemiology, and complications. *Journal of Intellectual & Developmental Disability, 26*, 205–215.

American Psychiatric Association. (1980). *DSM-III: Diagnostic and statistical manual of psychiatric disorders*. Washington, DC: American Psychiatric Association.

American Psychiatric Association. (2000). *Diagnostic and statistical manual of mental disorders: DSM-IV-TR*. Washington, DC: American Psychiatric Association.

American Psychiatric Association. (2013). *Diagnostic and statistical manual of mental disorders* (5th ed.). Washington, DC: American Psychiatric Association.

Applegate, H., Matson, J. L., & Cherry, K. E. (1999). An evaluation of functional variables affecting severe problem behaviors in adults with mental retardation by using the questions about behavioral function scale (QABF). *Research in Developmental Disabilities, 20*, 229–237.

Ashworth, M., Hirdes, J. P., & Martin, L. (2009). The social and recreational characteristics of adults with intellectual disability and pica living in institutions. *Research in Developmental Disabilities, 30*, 512–520.

Association for Behavior Analysis. (1989). *The right to effective behavioral treatment*. Retrieved from www.abainternational.org/ABA/statements/treatment.asp.

Barrett, R. P. (2008). Atypical behaviors: Self-injury and pica. In M. Wolraich, D. D. Drotar, P. H. Dworkin, & E. C. Perrin (Eds.), *Developmental and behavioral pediatrics: Evidence and practice*. Philadelphia: Elsevier.

Call, N. A., Simmons, C. A., Lomas Meyers, J. E., & Alvarez, J. P. (2015). Clinical outcomes of behavioral treatments for pica in children with developmental disabilities. *Journal of Autism and Developmental Disorders, 45*, 2105–2114.

Chansky, M. C., King, M. R., Bialkowski, W., Bryant, B. J., Kiss, J. E., D'Andrea, P., & Mast, A. E. (2017). Qualitative assessment of pica experienced by frequent blood donors. *Transfusion, 57*(4), 946–951.

Cone, T. E., Jr. (1969). The origin of the word PICA. *Pediatrics, 44*, 548.

Conners, C. K. (2008). *Conners comprehensive behavior rating scales manual*. North Tonawanda, NY: Multi-Health Systems Inc.

Cooper, J. ., Heron, T. E., & Heward, W. L. (2007). *Applied behavior analysis* (2nd ed.). Upper Saddle River, NJ: Pearson.

Danford, D. E., & Huber, A. E. (1982). Pica among mentally retarded adults. *American Journal of Mental Deficiency, 87*, 141–146.

Decker, C. J. (1993). Pica in the mentally handicapped: A 15-year surgical perspective. *Canadian Journal of Surgery, 36*, 551–554.

Donnelly, D. R., & Olczak, P. V. (1990). The effect on differential reinforcement of incompatible behaviors (DRI) on pica for cigarettes in persons with intellectual disability. *Behavior Modification, 14*, 81–96.

Fawcett, E. J., Fawcett, J. M., & Mazmanian, D. (2016). A meta-analysis of the worldwide prevalence of pica during pregnancy and the postpartum period. *International Journal of Gynecology & Obsterics, 133*(3), 277–283.

Foxx, R. M., & Livesay, J. (1984). Maintenance of response suppression following overcorrection: A 10-year retrospective examination of eight cases. *Analysis and Intervention in Developmental Disabilities, 4*, 65–70.

Hagopian, L. P., Rooker, G. W., & Rolider, N. U. (2011). Identifying empirically supported treatments for pica in individuals with intellectual disabilities. *Research in Developmental Disabilities, 32*(6), 2114–2120. https://doi.org/10.1016/j.ridd.2011.07.042

Hartmann, A. S., Becker, A. E., Hampton, C., & Bryant-Waugh, R. (2012). Pica and rumination disorder in DSM-5. *Psychiatric Annals, 42*, 426–430.

Johnson, C. R. (1990). Pica. In H. K. Walker, W. D. Hall, & J. W. Hurst (Eds.), *Clinical methods: The history, physical, and laboratory examinations* (3rd ed., pp. 709–710). Boston, MA: Butterworth Publishers.

Johnson, D., & Gretton, K. (2017). Pica during pregnancy. *International Journal of Childbirth Education, 32*(1), 45–47.

Kinnell, H. G. (1985). Pica as a feature of autism. *The British Journal of Psychiatry, 147*, 80–82.

Matson, J. L., & Bamburg, J. W. (1999). A descriptive study of pica behavior in persons with mental retardation. *Journal of Developmental and Physical Disabilities, 11*, 353–361.

Matson, J. L., Belva, B., Hattier, M. A., & Matson, M. L. (2011). Pica in persons with developmental disabilities: Characteristics, diagnosis, and assessment. *Research in Autism Spectrum Disorders, 5*, 1459–1464.

Matson, J. L., & Kuhn, D. E. (2001). Identifying feeding problems in mentally retarded persons: Development and reliability of the screening tool for feeding problems (STEP). *Research in Developmental Disabilities, 22*, 165–172.

Matson, J. L., Hattier, M. A., & Turygin, N. (2012). An evaluation of social skills in adults with pica, autism spectrum disorders, and intellectual disability. *Journal of Developmental and Physical Disabilities, 24*(5), 505–514. https://doi.org/10.1007/s10882-012-9286-0

Matson, J. L., & Wilkins, J. (2008). Reliability of the autism spectrum disorders-comorbid for children (ASD-CC). *Journal of Developmental and Physical Disabilities, 20*(4), 327–336. https://doi.org/10.1007/s10882-008-9100-1

McAdam, D. B., Breibord, J., Levine, M., & Williams, D. E. (2012). Pica. In P. Sturmey & M. Hersen (Eds.), *Handbook of evidence-based practice in clinical psychology, Child and adolescent disorders* (Vol. 1, pp. 303–321). New York: Wiley.

McAlpine, C., & Singh, N. N. (1986). Pica in institutionalized mentally retarded persons. *Journal of Mental Deficiency Research, 30*, 171–178.

McLoughlin, I. J. (1988). Pica as a cause of death in three mentally handicapped men. *The British Journal of Psychiatry, 152*, 842–845.

Mishori, R., & McHale, C. (2014). Pica: An age-old eating disorder that's often missed. *The Journal of Family Practice, 63*(7), 1–4.

Motta, R. W., & Basile, D. (1998). Pica. In L. Phelps (Ed.), *Health related disorders in children and adolescents* (pp. 524–527). Washington, DC: American Psychological Association.

Nchito, M., Geissler, P. W., Mubila, L., Friis, H., & Olsen, A. (2004). Effects of iron and multimicro-nutrient supplementation on geophagy: A two-by-two factorial study among Zambian school children in Lusaka. *Transactions of the Royal Society of Tropical Medicine and Hygiene, 98*, 218–227.

O'Neill, R. E., Horner, R. H., Albin, R. W., Sprague, J. R., Storey, K., & Newton, J. S. (1997). *Functional assessment and program development for problem behavior*. Pacific Grove, CA: Cole Publishing.

Paclawskyj, T. R., Matson, J. L., Rush, K. S., Smalls, Y., & Vollmer, T. R. (2000). Questions about behavioral function (QABF): A behavioral checklist for functional assessment of aberrant behavior. *Research in Developmental Disabilities, 21*(3), 223–229. https://doi.org/10.1016/S0891-4222(00)00036-6

Parry-Jones, B., & Parry-Jones, W. L. (1992). Pica: Symptom or eating disorder? A historical assessment. *British Journal of Psychiatry, 160*, 341–354.

Piazza, C. C., Hanley, G. P., & Fisher, W. W. (1996). Functional analysis and treatment of cigarette pica. *Journal of Applied Behavior Analysis, 29*, 437–450.

Rojahn, J., Rowe, E. W., Sharber, A. C., Hastings, R., Matson, J. L., Didden, R., & Dumont, E. L. M. (2012). The behavior problems inventory-short form for individuals with intellectual disabilities: Part I: Development and provisional clinical reference data: Behavior problems inventory-S: Part I. *Journal of Intellectual Disability Research, 56*(5), 527–545. https://doi.org/10.1111/j.1365-2788.2011.01507.x

Rose, E. A., Porcelli, J. H., & Neale, A. V. (2000). Pica: Common, but commonly missed. *Journal of the American Board of Family Practice, 13*(5), 353–358.

Sturmey, P. (2007). *Functional analysis in clinical treatment*. New York: Academic Press.

Sturmey, P. (2015). *Reducing restraint and restrictive behavior management practices*. Cham: Springer International Publishing Retrieved from http://libezp.lib.lsu.edu/login?url=http://search.ebscohost.com/login.aspx?direct=true&db=psyh&AN=2015-34061-000&site=ehost-live&scope=site

Sturmey, P., & Williams, D. E. (2016). *Pica in individuals with developmental disabilities*. Cham: Springer International Publishing.

Tewari, S., Krishnan, V. H. R., Valsalan, V. C., & Roy, A. (1995). Pica in learning disability hospital: A clinical survey. *British Journal of Developmental Disability, 41*, 13–22.

Tracy, J. I., de Leon, J., Qureshi, G., McCann, E. M., McGrory, A., & Josiassen, R. C. (1996). Repetitive behaviors in schizophrenia: A single disturbance of discrete symptoms? *Schizophrenia Research, 20*, 221–229.

Turnbull, H. R. (2005). Individuals with disabilities education act reauthorization: Accountability and personal responsibility. *Remedial and Special Education, 26*, 320–326.

Upadhyaya, S., & Sharma, A. (2012). Onset of obsessive compulsive disorder in pregnancy with pica as the sole manifestation. *Indian Journal of Psychological Medicine, 34*(3), 276–278.

Wasano, L. C., Borrero, J. C., & Kohn, C. S. (2009). Brief report: A comparison of indirect versus experimental strategies for the assessment of pica. *Journal of Autism and Developmental Disorders, 39*, 1582–1586.

Williams, D. E., Kirkpatrick-Sanchez, S., Enzinna, C., Dunn, J., & Borden-Karasack, D. (2009). The clinical management and prevention of pica: A retrospective follow up of 41 individuals with intellectual disabilities and pica. *Journal of Applied Research in Intellectual Disabilities, 22*, 210–215.

Williams, D. E., & McAdam, D. (2012). Assessment, behavioral treatment, and prevention of pica: Clinical guidelines and recommendations for practitioners. *Research in Developmental Disabilities, 33*, 2050–2057.

Young, S. L. (2010). Pica in pregnancy: New ideas about an old condition. *Annual Review of Nutrition, 30*, 403–422.

Social Skills

Elizabeth K. Wilson, Kaitlin A. Cassidy, Delaney J. Darragh, and Jacob L. DeBoer

Social skills are specific behaviors, within specific situations, that bring about judgments from others as to whether or not the individual performing these behaviors is competent or incompetent in accomplishing a given social task (Gresham, 2016). Although important throughout an individual's lifespan, proficient social skills are paramount to various aspects of childhood development. Social skills facilitate the learning of new information and the formation of peer and adult relationships. An individual's social skills, or lack thereof, can influence numerous short- and long-term outcomes for children as they transition into adolescence and ultimately adulthood.

Social skills deficits can have major ramifications for a child's development, in the short term and long term. Short-term outcomes that are of great social importance include peer rejection and/or acceptance, the ability to maintain friendships, academic achievement, judgments of social competence from teachers and parents, consistent school attendance, and number of school disciplinary referrals. Low scores on any of these outcomes in childhood predict adjustment difficulties in adolescence and early adulthood (Gresham, 2016).

Children's social competence in early childhood has been tied to both social and academic outcomes throughout a person's lifespan (Frey, Elliot, & Gresham, 2011). A child that possesses adequate social skills is more likely to succeed academically, go on to higher education, have lasting relationships, and sustain employment. Poor social skills can lead to higher school dropout rates, juvenile delinquency, adult mental instability, and higher incarceration rates (Gresham, 2016). Therefore, an individual's social skills proficiency level contributes significantly to both short-term and long-term outcomes.

Social skills are context-based, social constructs that are situation and audience specific. For example, some behaviors in a classroom that a student sees as appropriate may be seen in a different light from the perspective of the teacher. *Teacher-preferred social skills* are those behaviors exhibited by the students which comply with the classroom instructional environment the teacher has required (Hersh & Walker, 1983). Examples of these skills are compliance with teacher instruction, completing school work independently, following classroom rules, and not getting up without permission from the teacher. *Peer-preferred social skills* are those behaviors exhibited by the students that promote friendships, escalate social status, and maintain

E. K. Wilson (✉) · K. A. Cassidy · D. J. Darragh
J. L. DeBoer
Department of Psychology, Lousiana State University, Baton Rouge, LA, USA
e-mail: Ewils24@lsu.edu

social connections. These peer-preferred behaviors include both verbal and nonverbal communication between peers, the displaying of positive attitudes toward one another, and sometimes direct disobedience to authority. A classic, school setting example of *teacher-preferred social skills* vs. *peer-preferred social skills* is when the teacher would expect the students to be silently completing a task, whereas students would expect their peers to talk and interact with them during recess. Another way in which social skills are context based is the difference of skills preferred in different environments. For instance, certain social behaviors expected at school, such as raising hand to speak and staying in seat, may seem out of place in a home environment.

A *social skills deficit* is defined as a discrepancy between the current skill level and desired skill level of performance (Bergan & Kratochwill, 1990). This discrepancy can be due to an acquisition or performance deficit. The Collaborative for Academic, Social, and Emotional Learning (CASEL, 2015) model focuses on these two types of deficits. *Acquisition deficits* are defined as the absence of knowledge about how to perform a certain social skill or not understanding when it is the socially appropriate setting or situation in which to perform that certain skill. These deficits are often referred to as "can't do" problems, as the child is unable to perform the skill and it is not a matter of choice. *Performance deficits* are defined as the failure to perform a certain social skill, even though the child has the physical capability and is aware of how and when to perform that skill appropriately. These deficits are often referred to as "won't do" problems, as the child is refusing to perform a skill that he knows how to do.

These skill discrepancies can also be influenced by a behavioral excess. Gresham, Van, and Cook (2006) describe *behavioral excesses* as competing problem behaviors that are socially reinforced that can cause a deficit or delay in social skills. Therefore, because the child is engaging in the behavioral excess, they cannot simultaneously engage in the appropriate social skill, as these two behaviors are in competition. These behavioral excesses can be externalizing behaviors (i.e., aggression, disruptive behaviors in the classroom, or defiance) or internalizing symptoms (i.e., social withdrawal, panic attacks, or depression).

Types of Social Skills Tests

Various types of decisions can be determined via the assessment process (i.e., screening decisions, identification decisions, intervention decisions, or progress-monitoring decisions). Depending on the decision type that is being sought, different types of assessment tests may be selected. For instance, a *screening test* assesses for indicators of a potential presence of a precise problem or disease. A *diagnostic assessment test* examines more thoroughly for the definitive presence of a problem or disease. A *monitoring test* tracks the progress of a problem or disease.

Screeners

Universal screeners are defined as the utilization of concise measures across a population to identify individuals whom are at risk for or whom have a current deficiency within a specific skill set (Jenkins, Hudson, & Johnson, 2007). Universal screeners that focus on social skills can be used to identify specific children with deficiencies in that area or children at risk for developing significant social skills deficits. This allows for early identification of social skills deficits, which can lead to better outcomes in intervention and treatment. The later a child is introduced to effective social skills interventions, the more resistant their inappropriate social behaviors will be to change (Bierman & Greenberg, 1996).

The ultimate goal of universal screeners is to flag children with social skills deficits or excesses, who require a more comprehensive and specialized diagnostic assessment to determine an appropriate intervention. In order to effectively achieve this goal, the screener must have reliable and valid cutoff scores, which accurately indicate which children require further assessment and which do not. Screener decisions should have high sensitivity and specificity. The probabilities representing sensitivity and specificity of assessments should meet or exceed .80 (Carran & Scott, 1992). *Sensitivity* of a screener is the probability of a true positive, or in other words, those who screened positive for deficits actually have those deficits. False positives are when those who screened positive for deficits do not actually have those deficits. *Specificity* of a screener is the probability of a true negative, or when those screened negative for deficits truly do not possess those deficits. False negatives are when those screened negative for deficits actually do have those deficits. False negatives are the least advantageous, because the consequences of not receiving further assessments or critical interventions when they are warranted are grander than receiving unnecessary assessments or noncritical interventions (Lane, Oakes, Manzies, & Germer, 2014).

Screeners assessing social skills among children are utilized in both schools and clinic settings. While schools and clinics may use the same screeners, why and when these screeners are given may differ between the two settings. Within psychological clinics or service centers, screeners with social skills components are often given during the initial intake procedures to determine the direction or need for a diagnostic assessment. These screeners are universal in that they may be given to all children that seek services at the clinic, though they do not reach as wide of a population that school settings could potentially access.

Within schools, a *multi-tiered system of supports* (MTSS) model is often utilized to systematically assess all students. MTSS is a problem-solving approach which uses tiers to identify at-risk students and implement appropriate interventions that are specifically geared toward those students. The *problem-solving approach* refers to a logical method for identifying problem behaviors and resolving those behaviors in congruence with promoting well-being behaviors. Within the social skills context, the problem behaviors would refer to social skills deficits, while the well-being behaviors would refer to maintaining an appropriate understanding and use of social skills in comparison to what is expected at a certain child's developmental age. Within the MTSS model, the assessments and interventions intensify as students are moved up from the first to last tier. All students begin in the first tier where they receive universal screeners and services, and those identified as needing more individualized or intensive instruction in a specific skill are moved up to a more intensive and student-specific tier.

Under the MTSS framework, universal screeners should be given to students within the first tier to aide with the identifying component of this problem-solving approach. The students' scores on the screeners may then be compared to their peers within the school as well as normative samples. The results from these screeners can be used as tools for identifying children that need a more intensive diagnostic assessment, as well as for informing what possible deficiencies may need to be more heavily focused on within that assessment. Education policy makers and educators are beginning to implement screeners within schools more routinely; however, it is still a relatively new approach to identifying students, so there may be issues with underidentification of students (Glover & Albers, 2007).

It is often recommended that these screeners are conducted consistently throughout a school year and there should be screeners for elementary, middle school, and high school students, in order to maximize opportunities for identifying children who are at risk for behavioral concerns at different developmental stages (Lane, Oakes, & Menzies, 2010). Clinics only supply screeners to children who seek out services at the clinic and often supply screeners only once during the initial intake procedure. Therefore, in order to properly identify at-risk children in need of these services, there is clearly a need for schools to implement routine screeners.

Assessment

Social skills assessments differ from social skills screeners as the goal of assessment is to use an efficient and effective method to diagnose and classify the problem, as well as inform intervention or treatment to optimize the social emotional competencies of the targeted child. Those who were identified by the screener require comprehensive assessments such as diagnostic tests to identify the presence of a problem. The diagnostic assessments are conducted to examine these flagged children more thoroughly to further assess if the irregularities found within the screener are inconsequential or if symptoms of a social skills deficit are significantly interfering with the child's everyday functioning. Diagnostic assessments are used to label the presenting maladaptive symptoms, so that there can be clear communication between medical professionals when discussing the treatment of the child.

To inform more intensive, specialized treatments as opposed to merely diagnosing the problem, schools and behaviorally based clinics often conduct *functional behavioral assessments* (FBAs). An FBA is a systematic process used to identify events in the environment such as antecedents (i.e., occurrences that happen before the behavior) and consequences (i.e., events that happen after the behavior) that reinforce and maintain the behavior. Knowing the circumstances surrounding the behavior helps to determine the possible intervention strategies that best target the function of the behavior that is maintaining the specific social skills deficit or behavioral excess exhibited in the specific child (Cooper, Heron, & Heward, 2007). The *function of the behavior* refers to the purpose that the behavior is serving for that particular child, whether it be positively or negatively reinforcing. In the case of social skills, if a child engages in disruptive classroom behavior, such as talking out of turn, and receives peer attention for this inappropriate behavior, that child could be positively reinforced by receiving the desired peer attention. In contrast, if the child displays disruptive classroom behavior by throwing a tantrum when he or she should be completing a class project, this inappropriate behavior could be negatively reinforced because the child is successfully avoiding the project. Knowing the function of a behavior helps a professional determine what aspect(s) of the child's environment to target when creating an intervention, because sometimes two different children can display the same inappropriate social behaviors for different reasons.

Assessment instruments are also used as a tool to monitor and measure a child's progress throughout problem-specific interventions by aiding in collecting reliable and valid data. This system is referred to as *progress monitoring* and is defined as the best practice in assessing behavioral performance and evaluating the effectiveness an intervention has in improving the target behavior (Sprague, Cook, Browning-Wright, & Sadler, 2008). Measures used as progress-monitoring tools must be reliable and valid, as well as sensitive to small changes in behavior. Professionals monitor the progress of social skills proficiency throughout behavioral interventions; the frequency is dependent upon intensity of behavior.

Types of Measures

Measures used to evaluate social skills can be used as screeners, diagnostic assessments, and progress-monitoring tools across various settings. These measures can be either indirect or direct procedures for assessing a child's current level of social skills. Indirect measures are removed in time and place from the occurrence of the behavior and require the informant to rely on memory or perception of the child's social skills. Direct measures require the informant to observe the child, preferably in the most naturalistic setting, and report on behavior during the observation or immediately after the observation. Four types of measures have been commonly used in the field to assess social skills at all levels of assessment and across settings: behavior rating skills, systematic direct observations, direct behavior ratings, and role-play assessments. The differences, similarities, advantages, and disadvantages of these four methods will be discussed in the following sections.

Behavior Rating Scales

Behavior rating scales are indirect assessments which ask informants (i.e., self, parent, teacher, etc.)

to rate the frequency or intensity of specific behaviors based on their perception of and experience with an individual in question, over a given period of time (Campbell & Hammond, 2014). The items posed within behavior rating scales are structured on an item response scale, where the informant is told how to interpret the rating scale (e.g., a scale of 1–4, where 1 equals never occurs and 4 equals always occurs) and then rates the individual accordingly. Behavior rating scales can be used for multiple purposes such as screening, informing identification and classification decisions, planning treatment, and monitoring progress.

Depending on the purpose of utilization, a narrowband or broadband behavior rating scale would be preferred. *Broadband* behavior rating scales are designed to formulate a comprehensive profile of an individual. Other scales are *narrowband*, which are designed to assess more specific behaviors or diagnoses in question. For example, if a clinician were using a behavior rating scale for progress-monitoring purposes, they may use a narrowband scale to track the progress of specifically targeted behaviors within the intervention. A clinician may be able to make progress-monitoring or intervention decisions with raw scores of a behavior rating scale. However, to make diagnostic decisions, behavior rating scales' raw scores can have criterion cutoffs or be transformed into T scores for normative scoring. *Criterion scoring* is when there is an established standard that determines whether the individual passes the assessment. For instance, a grade-level curriculum-based measure may have a criterion score of 80, meaning all individuals must receive above an 80 to be considered at grade level, regardless of how their peers perform on the measure. *Normative scoring* for behavior rating scales are often the raw scores transformed into a T score scale. This scale is determined by how the population did on the measure rather than a specific cutoff point. This allows clinicians to interpret the individual's score and determine whether the score falls within the clinical, subclinical, at-risk, or typical range.

There are several advantages to behavior rating scales. For instance, these scales are inexpensive, in that they often require no training time, often take 5–10 min to complete, and do not require a professional to be present. Additionally, these scales allow for data collection of low incident but severe behaviors (i.e., violent behavior, tantrums) that may not be captured in a direct observation. Further, the structured format allows for a more systematic review of data than an unstructured interview would allow. Many behavior rating scales allow for multiple perspectives by having student, teacher, and parent versions of the forms. These forms give insight into an individual's behaviors as well as to the informants' perceptions of the individual. While this can be an advantage, the informants' biases can also hinder the ability to objectively assess the results. Informant discrepancies are common among different informants ratings of social, emotional, or behavior problems of children (Achenbach, McConaughy, & Howell, 1987). Bias of response can be attributed to halo effects, leniency or severity, or central tendency effects. *Halo effects* occur when an informant overgeneralizes an individual's negative or positive characteristics as an overall positive or negative manner. *Leniency* or *severity* is the tendency of a rater to be too critical or generous in their ratings of all students. *Central tendency effect* is the tendency to avoid the endpoints of the scale and rate individuals near the midpoints of the scale. These biases can impact interpretation accuracy of behavior rating scales.

The Social Skills Improvement System-Social Emotional Learning (SSIS-SEL) The SSIS-SEL offers a multi-informant series of behavior rating scales for teachers, parents, and students (Gresham et al., 2017). Teachers and parents can rate students, 3–18 years old, by denoting the frequency with which the child in question has exhibited each skill, within the last 2 months on a 4-point scale of *Never, Seldom, Often,* and *Almost Always*. Students, ages 8–18, can complete the self-report version by indicating how true a statement describing a skill proficiency or deficit is for them, on a 4-point scale of Not True, a Little True, a Lot True, and Very True. Each form version includes items for each of the five SEL competency domains identified by the CASEL model: self-awareness, self-management, social awareness, relationship skills, and responsible decision-making. The SSIS-SEL rating forms were designed for assessment content to be in alignment with the intervention content; therefore, it ensures the measure is an appropriate tool for assessment testing that ultimately leads to intervention decision-making and progress monitoring of the implemented intervention. Further, there is a ten-item core SEL scale (one self-awareness item, four self-management items, one social awareness item, three relationship skills items, and one responsible decision-making item) embedded within the overall measure to be used as a brief, norm-referenced screening and/or progress-monitoring scale for the SSIS-SEL classroom intervention program (CIP). The SSIS-SEL rating forms were normed on a nationwide representative sample of 4700 children who were assessed at 115 sites in 36 different states (Gresham et al., 2017). The SSIS-SEL has been found to be psychometrically reliable and valid. Specifically, internal consistency of scores have been found to be within an acceptable range (Cronbach's alpha = .70–.97; Gresham & Elliott, 2017a, b). The SSIS-SEL has been found to have high concurrent validity to other measures assessing social skills such as the Behavioral and Emotional Screening System (BESS) discussed below (Gresham & Elliott, 2017a, Gresham & Elliott, 2017b).

The Social, Academic, and Emotional Behavior Risk Screener (SAEBRS) The SAEBRS is a 19-item teacher rating scale designed to assess a wide range of constructs (i.e., social, academic, and emotional behaviors) via a concise number of items (Kilgus, Chafouleas, Riley-Tillman, & von der Embse, 2014). The SAEBRS provides a total behavior score that is made up of three subscales: social behavior (SB; six items), academic behavior (AB; six items), and emotional behavior (EB; seven items). All items on the SAEBRS direct teachers to indicate the frequency in which a student has exhibited the described behaviors within the previous month, utilizing a four-point rating scale (0 = *never*; 1 = *sometimes*; 2 = *often*; and 3 = *almost always*). The SAEBRS utilizes cut scores within each of the four scales as indicators for screening decisions. Higher scores are indicative of higher proficiency of social skills; therefore, if a student falls below the specified cut score, they are considered at risk for problems within that scale construct. Cut scores (SB ≤ 12, AB ≤9, EB ≤ 17, TB ≤ 36) for elementary and middle school students have been found with acceptably high levels of sensitivity (.79–.97) and specificity (.65–.93; Kilgus, Wesley, von der Embse, & Taylor, 2016). The SAEBRS is constructed to be contextually relevant (DiPerna, 2006; Kilgus et al., 2016), time-efficient, and technically adequate across the K–12 grade-level spectrum (Kilgus, Chafouleas, & Riley-Tillman, 2013; Kilgus et al., 2016). The SAEBRS has been found to be psychometrically reliable and valid. Specifically, internal consistency of scores has been found to be within an acceptable range (Cronbach's alpha = .79–.94; Kilgus et al., 2016). Further strong concurrent validity and diagnostic accuracy were established relative to previous forms of the SSIS (Kilgus et al., 2016) and the BESS (r = .72–.94; Kamphaus & Reynolds, 2007), which will be discussed below.

The BASC-3 Behavioral and Emotional Screening System (BESS) The BESS is a brief behavior rating scale that measures behavioral and emotional strengths and weaknesses of youth 2–19 years old (Kamphaus & Reynolds, 2015). This measure is utilized by clinicians, school psychologists, and researchers to assess behavioral and emotional disorders that are connected to adjustment problems. Similar to the SSIS-SEL, there are teacher, parent, and student self-report versions of the assessment, which can be used individually or in combination to screen, assess, or progress monitor a wide variety of behavioral and emotional strengths and weaknesses: internalizing problems, externalizing problems, school problems, and adaptive skills. The student form is available for students grades 3–12, and there is a Spanish version available for the parent and student self-report forms.

All three versions have 25–30 items and take about 5–10 min to administer. The BASC-3 BESS is a norm-referenced tool with T scores (M = 50; SD = 10), percentile ranks, and cutoff points (i.e., *normal*, *elevated*, and *extremely elevated*) that aid in determining a youth's level of risk. The BESS has yielded high internal consistency (Cronanbach's alpha = .92–.96; Kamphaus & Reynolds, 2007) and concurrently valid in comparison to the SIBS, SEBS, SAEBRS, and SSIS-SEL (Hartman, Gresham, & Byrd, 2017; Kamphaus & Reynolds, 2007; Gresham & Elliott, 2017a).

Student Internalizing Behavior Screener (SIBS) The SIBS is a brief seven-item screener that assesses for internalizing behavior problems, such as anxiety, bullying victimization, isolation or rejection by peers, excessive time spent with adults rather than peers, withdrawal, sadness, and somatic complaints (Cook et al., 2011). Similar to the abovementioned scales, the SIBS directs teachers to rate the frequency in which a student exhibits the described behaviors based on a four-point rating scale (0 = never, 1 = seldom, 2 = sometimes, 3 = frequently). The sum score of the assessment is used to screen for internalizing problems. Lower scores are indicative of more appropriate internalizing behaviors. A cut score of ≥8 (sensitivity = .86 and specificity = .99) is suggested for determining an excess of internalizing behaviors at the elementary level (Cook et al. 2011). The SIBS has yielded acceptable internal consistency reliability among past studies, with a Cronbach's alpha value of .82 (Kilgus et al., 2016) and high criterion validity (Cook et al., 2011) compared to similar measures, such as the Student Risk Screening Scale (SRSS; Drummond, 1994).

Student Externalizing Behavior Screener (SEBS) Similar to the SIBS, the SEBS is a brief seven-item screening instrument and uses the same four-point response scale (see above); however the SEBS measures external behavior problems rather than internal (Cook et al., 2011). These external behaviors include defiance toward adults, fights with peers, bullies others, easily angered, lies to avoid consequences, disrupts class instruction, and has difficulty sitting still. The SEBS has yielded acceptable internal consistency reliability among past studies, with a Cronbach's alpha value of .82 (Cook, 2012). Similar to the SIBS, the SEBS has been found to have high criterion validity compared to the SRSS (Cook, 2012).

Systematic Direct Observations (SDOs)

SDOs have long been regarded as the best measure of social skills because they provide a direct measure of an individual's behavior in a natural setting (e.g., classroom, home, or free play settings). SDOs can be used to assess an individual's behavior before, during, and after an intervention or treatment has been established. They are used to measure different dimensions of behavior such as frequency/rate, temporality (i.e., duration, response latency, interresponse time), temporal locus, and permanent products (Cooper et al., 2007). SDOs can be completed by single or multiple observers at one time, can target a single behavior (e.g., eye contact) or a class of behaviors (e.g., prosocial behaviors), and can be useful for multiple purposes during the assessment process such as diagnosis, treatment planning, and progress monitoring.

SDOs quantify behaviors through standard systems for coding the occurrence and nonoccurrence of operationally defined target behaviors and can employ these procedures across observers and settings. Target behaviors are usually observed during specified intervals of time using certain types of SDO methods, such as whole-interval recording, momentary time sampling, and partial-interval recording, dependent upon the type of behavior.

Whole-interval recording is used when observing behaviors that are expected to occur for long durations (i.e., academic or positive social engagement); therefore, the behavior must be observed during the entire interval in order to be coded as "occurred." *Momentary time sampling* is used when observing high-frequency behaviors that are difficult to count; therefore, the observer will be alerted to attend to the individual at the start of every interval (e.g., every 10 or 15 s), and if the individual is exhibiting the behavior, it is coded as "occurred" (Volpe, McConaughy, & Hintze, 2009). *Partial-interval recording* is used when observing brief, frequent, and often problematic behaviors (e.g., out of seat, talking out, working quietly at desk); therefore, if the behavior is observed at any time during the interval, which is usually 10–15 s long, it is coded as "occurred." Social skills are usually recorded using partial-interval recording time sampling methods as prosocial behaviors are often what are being coded for. *Prosocial behaviors* are defined as "behaviors that are directed toward other people that involve effective communication skills, cooperative acts, self-control in difficult situations, and empathetic or supportive responses to others who experience a problem" (Gresham & Elliott, 2008). To get a reliable sample of an individual's prosocial behavior, a 15-min, partial-interval recording SDO will include 60, 15-s intervals. The score is then expressed as the percentage of the 60 intervals in which the behavior occurred.

SDOs have many advantages, such as their sensitivity to short-term changes in social behavior specifically; however, they do have unique disadvantages. SDOs require a high amount of training and effort from observers. There is also little guidance on the most reliable and dependable amount or duration of observations that provides an accurate representation of a child's behavior. Additionally, as with any direct observation method, reactivity of the individual being observed can interfere with the accuracy of the measure (Merrell, 2008).

Direct Behavior Ratings (DBRs)

DBRs are one of the most commonly used methods of social skills assessment. DBRs, which consist of a direct observation of behavior followed by a brief rating, were created with the intent to standardize informal behavior ratings that had long been used in school-based assessments and combine the most useful features of other commonly used measures, such as systematic direct observations. DBRs combine the direct, repeatable, and flexible features of behavior rating scales with the efficient, broad, and cross-context usability of behavior rating scales. Preferably, DBRs are to be used in a naturalistic setting such as a classroom, playground, or home interaction.

Typically, a DBR consists of an objectively defined target behavior definition and a rating scale based on a predetermined coding system. Although a rating system does give way to subjectivity of the rater, training and tightly defined scales can limit this subjectiveness. The independent observer evaluates the child and then immediately uses the scale to record the desired information about the child's target behavior. The main advantage to DBRs is the temporal proximity of the observer's rating to the actual behavior, which allows for the measure to be sensitive to small, yet relevant, changes in the child's behavior. DBR can include one target behavior to be rated or multiple target behaviors to be rated, making it even more versatile. Chafouleas, Riley-Tillman, and Christ (2009) proposed three unique characteristics that define DBRs as a unique behavior assessment method: (1) behavior rating occurs immediately after the observation period, (2) rater is a person who has firsthand experience with the child during the observation period (e.g., guardian, teacher, doctor), and (3) minimal inference is required to discern the target behavior because it is predetermined and operationally defined before the observation.

DBRs are not defined by a specific measure or cluster of behaviors, but can be adapted to assess a variety of behaviors. It is a relatively new concept in the field as it is a hybrid assessment tool that is practical, time-efficient, repeatable, and capable of detecting small changes in behavior. For example, when used to assess social skills, a multi-item DBR (DBR-MIS) might be created by the school psychologist in a public school to be used by the teacher as a progress-monitoring tool to track a specific student's behavior in the classroom. When used as a social skills assessment tool, the DBR should have predetermined, operationally defined target behaviors that the teacher will be able to clearly identify and rate accordingly. The DBR should specify certain time frames in which the informant will observe the behavior and consequently rate the behavior immediately. Within the context of social skills, the target behaviors could be things such as makes developmentally appropriate eye contact with peers, stays within an appropriate distance of peers during peer interaction, and stays on topic when conversing with peers.

Role-Play Assessment

A common way to assess social skills as well as monitor an individual's progress during treatment or intervention is with role-play exercises. There have been quantitative assessments created to measure social skills using role-play techniques. For example, the *Social Skills Performance Assessment* (SSPA; Patterson, Moscona, McKibbin, Davidson, & Jeste, 2001) is a performance-based measure that assesses the social skills of adults with autism spectrum disorder (ASD). The SSPA successfully discriminates between individuals with ASD and those without ASD by focusing on the verbal and nonverbal skills needed in two different interaction tasks. Another quantitative assessment using role-play is the *Contextual Assessment of Social Skills* (CASS; Ratto, Turner-Brown, Rupp, Mesibov, & Penn, 2011). This is a measure of children's social skills in an everyday simulated setting, in which individuals are observed having a conversation with a confederate, who demonstrates different levels of interest in the conversation. The child or adolescent must adjust to the change in conversation or social context (Verhoeven, Smeekens, & Didden, 2013).

More often, role-play assessments serve as a more qualitative way of gathering information about how an individual is functioning socially within a certain context. During the course of a social skills intervention, role-play is usually used as a progress-monitoring tool by the clinician to determine how well the individual is learning a certain skill. For example, the clinician may ask the child to role-play a scenario in which he or she is having a conversation with a same-aged peer about a certain topic and to stay on that topic for a predetermined amount of time. In this role-play situation, the clinician can assess for both developmentally and situationally appropriate, verbal and nonverbal social skills. Nonverbal social skills include appropriate eye contact and facial expression, level of positive emotion and level of interest expressed using body language, frequency and quality of gestures, intensity and frequency of body movement, degree of tension or relaxation in posture, and amount of personal space given. Verbal social skills include vocal expressiveness and appropriate vocal intonation, appropriate questions asked to engage in conversation with another person, ability to stay on topic in conversation, and level of comfort and balance of conversation in an interaction with another person (Ratto et al., 2011).

Role-play assessments do not always focus on the back and forth of conversation. The context could be different social settings or scenes, such as a positive social interactions including offering help to, making requests of, and giving compliments to others. There could also be negative social interactions such as responding to negative provocation and refusing an unreasonable request (Kazdin, Matson, & Esveldt-Dawson, 1984).

Considerations and Implications

Informed consent is required of the parent, meaning that the entire assessment process has been explained and parents have given written permission that the clinician may assess their child. Assent is also required from the child, where the clinician explicitly explains the procedures of assessment to the child using developmentally appropriate language. The child has to agree to continue with the process before the clinician can do any assessments. Similarly, schools need consent from parents to screen, assess, or implement interventions with students (Bailey & Burch, 2011).

When choosing a social skills measure, anything from the informant to the setting can affect the validity of the measurement and should be taken into account during the selection process. Relying on one informant rather than another or integrating information put forth by multiple informants can consist of differing perspectives regarding whether a child possesses particular skills deficits. Since parents and teachers interact with the same child in different contexts, those environments could influence their perspective of a child's social skills proficiency, especially if assessing a context-driven behavior. *Context-driven behavior* is specific to a certain environment and can also be referred to as setting discrepancies (De Los Reyes & Kazdin, 2005). Ideally, as children develop, they will learn to adapt their behavior to fit appropriately within specific environments; therefore, social skills should be assessed among various settings and from various informant accounts.

The selection of the assessment measure is often heavily influenced by feasibility, contextual appropriateness, technical adequacy, and resources available, especially in schools. Oftentimes, a clinician will conduct a full psychological evaluation on a specific child with a portion of the data collected focusing on the assessment of social skills. This will usually consist of behavior rating scales, as these types of measures allow for multiple perspectives to be represented among different informant point of views. Within a school setting, an SDO may be conducted provided the time and resources are available. Alternatively, a DBR can be used, which any school staff can easily be trained to adequately complete.

Universal screeners for behavioral problems have only recently begun to be utilized within school settings. Therefore, the issue of underidentification of behavioral problems among children, including social skills deficits, should be addressed within schools by administering screeners more widely and routinely.

Summary and Conclusion

Proficient social skills are critical to many aspects of childhood development. Social skills facilitate the learning of new information and the formation of relationships. A significant deficiency in a child's social skills can lead to numerous short- and long-term outcomes. The more concerning negative outcomes include increased chance of school dropout, increased chance of juvenile delinquency, and increased mental instability.

Previous research has demonstrated the importance of identifying possible social skill deficiencies early in order to provide the child with the appropriate intervention. Within a multi-tiered system of supports (MTSS), the process encompasses initially screening the whole population to identify individuals who display limited social skills relative to his or her peers. Possible screening assessments include the BESS and the SAEBRS. The results from the screener are then used to identify children who need a more intensive diagnostic assessment.

Children who require additional assessments are then administered behavior rating scales that can be either broadband or narrowband measures. These behavior rating scales are used to determine whether or not the social skill deficiencies identified by the screener are significantly interfering with the child's everyday functioning or if the deficits are inconsequential.

Broadband measures provide a comprehensive profile of the child, measuring areas other than just social skills, whereas narrowband measures are specific to the social skill that would be targeted during the intervention process. For the purpose of progress monitoring, narrowband measures are considered to be more appropriate because they are intended to address the specific behaviors of concern. An example of a broadband behavior rating scale is the SSIS-SEL. The SIBS and the SEBS are considered narrowband measures that address only internalizing behaviors or externalizing behaviors, respectively.

If further assessment is needed, a systematic direct observation (SDO) or a functional behavioral assessment (FBA) can be conducted. Both SDOs and FBAs are advantageous in that they occur in the child's natural environment and are more sensitive to short-term changes in behavior, whereas behavior rating scales are completed in hindsight of behaviors occurrence. That being said, because SDOs and FBAs are extremely labor intensive and require highly trained observers, they are typically reserved for children with significant behavioral concerns that are being moved beyond the universal tier. An alternative to SDOs and FBAs is using direct behavior ratings (DBRs), which have become one of the most commonly used methods of social skills assessment. Relative to SDOs and FBAs, DBRs are less time-consuming, require less training to be administered, and can also be administered in the child's naturalistic setting.

An additional way to assess social skills is within a role-play setting. Relative to the more structured methods above, role-play assessments normally occur within a counseling or one-on-one setting. They are typically administered outside of the classroom and are more qualitative in nature. That being said, there have been quantitative measures developed for role-play assessment which include the Social Skills Performance Assessment (SSPA) and the Contextual Assessment of Social Skills (CASS).

This book chapter is not intended to be an exhaustive list of all possible ways to assess social skills. Instead, it presents the more well-known, researched measures currently and widely available. Similar to most other areas of assessment, the assessment of social skills should encompass a wide-range of considerations including, but not limited to, cultural norms, professional experience, and resources available. By first acknowledging these factors, the practitioner can then proceed onto determining the assessment most appropriate for his or her given situation.

References

Achenbach, T. M., McConaughy, S. H., & Howell, C. T. (1987). Child/adolescent behavioral and emotional problems: Implications of cross-informant correlations for situational specificity. *Psychological Bulletin, 101*, 213–223.

Bailey, J., & Burch, M. (2011). *Ethics for behavior analysts* (2nd Expanded Ed., p. 203). New York: Taylor and Francis Group, LLC.

Bergan, J., & Kratochwill, T. (1990). *Behavioral consultation and therapy*. New York: Plenum.

Bierman, K., & Greenberg, M. (1996). Social skills training in the Fast Track program. In R. Peters & R. McMahon (Eds.), *Preventing childhood disorders, substance abuse, and delinquency* (pp. 65–89). Thousand Oaks, CA: Sage.

Campbell, J. M., & Hammond, R. K. (2014). Best practices in rating scale assessment of children's behavior. In A. Thomas & P. Harrison (Eds.), *Best practices in school psychology, VI* (pp. 287–304). Bethesda, MD: National Association of School Psychologists.

Carran, D. T., & Scott, K. G. (1992). Risk assessment in preschool children: Research implications for the early detection of educational handicaps. *Topics in Early Childhood Special Education, 12*, 196–211.

Chafouleas, S. M., Riley-Tillman, T. C., & Christ, T. J. (2009). Direct behavior rating (DBR): An emerging method for assessing social behavior within a tiered intervention system. *Assessment for Effective Intervention, 34*(4), 195–200.

Collaborative for Academic, Social, and Emotional Learning. (2015). *District guide to systemic social and emotional learning*. Chicago: Author.

Cook, C. R. (2012). The student externalizing behavior screener. Unpublished document, University of Washington.

Cook, C. R., Rasetshwane, K. B., Truelson, E., Grant, S., Dart, E. H., Collins, T. A., & Sprague, J. (2011). Development and validation of the Student Internalizing Behavior Screener: Examination of reliability, validity, and classification accuracy. *Assessment for Effective Intervention, 36*, 71–79. https://doi.org/10.1177/1534508410390486

Cooper, J., Heron, T., & Heward, W. (2007). *Applied behavior analysis* (2nd ed.). Upper Saddle River, NJ: Prentice-Hall.

De Los Reyes, A., & Kazdin, A. E. (2005). Informant discrepancies in the assessment of childhood psychopathology: A critical review, theoretical framework, and recommendations for further study. *Psychological Bulletin, 131*(4), 483–509. https://doi.org/10.1037/0033-2909.131.4.483

DiPerna, J. C. (2006). Academic enablers and student achievement: Implications for assessment and intervention services in the schools. *Psychology in the Schools, 43*, 7–17.

Drummond, T. (1994). *The Student Risk Screening Scale (SRSS)*. Grants Pass, OR: Oregon Social Learning Center.

Frey, J. R., Elliot, S. N., & Gresham, F. M. (2011). Preschoolers' social skills: Advances in assessment for intervention using social behavior ratings. *School Mental Health, 3*, 179–190. https://doi.org/10.1007/s12310-011-9060-y

Glover, T. A., & Albers, C. A. (2007). Considerations for evaluating universal screening instruments. *Journal of School Psychology, 45*, 117–135. https://doi.org/10.1016/j.jsp.2006.05.005

Gresham, F. M. (2016). *Social skills for children and youth: Evidence-based practices in assessment and intervention*. New York: Guilford Press.

Gresham, F. M., & Elliott, S. N. (2008). *Social skills improvement system: Rating scales manual*. Minneapolis, MN: Pearson Assessments.

Gresham, F. M., & Elliott, S. N. (2017a). *Social skills improvement system social emotional learning edition rating forms*. Minneapolis, MN: Pearson Assessments.

Gresham, F. M., & Elliott, S. N. (2017b). *Social skills improvement system social emotional learning edition manual*. Minneapolis, MN: Pearson Assessments.

Gresham, F. M., Elliott, S. N., Metallo, S., Byrd, S., Wilson, E., & Cassidy, K. (2017). Cross-informant agreement of children's social-emotional skills: An investigation of ratings by teachers, parents, and students from a nationally representative sample. *Psychol Schs. 2018, 55*, 208–223 https://doi.org/10.1002/pits.22101

Gresham, F. M., Van, M., & Cook, C. R. (2006). Social skills training for teaching replacement behaviors: Remediation of acquisition deficits for at-risk children. *Behavioral Disorders, 30*, 32–46.

Hersh, R. H., & Walker, H. M. (1983). Great expectations: Making schools effective for all students. *Policy Studies Review, 2*(1), 147–188.

Hartman, K., Gresham, F. M., Byrd, S. (2017). Student internalizing and externalizing behavior screeners: Evidence for reliability, validity, and usability in elementary schools. *Behavioral Disorders, 42*(3), 108–118.

Jenkins, J. R., Hudson, R. F., & Johnson, E. S. (2007). Screening for at-risk readers in a response to intervention framework. *School Psychology Review, 36*, 582–600.

Kamphaus, R., & Reynolds, C. (2015). *BASC-3 Behavioral and emotional screening system*. Minneapolis, MN: Pearson Assessments.

Kazdin, A., Matson, J., & Esveldt-Dawson, K. (1984). The relationship of role play assessment of children's social skills to multiple measures of social competence. *Behavior, Research, and Therapy, 22*(2), 129–139.

Kilgus, S. P., Chafouleas, S. M., & Riley-Tillman, T. C. (2013). Development and initial validation of the Social and Academic Behavior Risk Screener for elementary grades. *School Psychology Quarterly, 28*, 210–226.

Kilgus, S. P., Chafouleas, S. M., Riley-Tillman, T. C., & von der Embse, N. P. (2014). *Social, Academic, and Emotional Behavior Risk Screener (SAEBRS)*. Minneapolis, MN: Theodore J. Christ & Colleagues.

Kilgus, S. P., Wesley, S. A., von der Embse, N. P., & Taylor, C. N. (2016). Technical adequacy of the social, academic, and emotional behavior risk screener in an elementary sample. *Assessment for Effective Intervention, 42*(1), 46–59.

Kamphaus, R. W., Reynolds, C. R. (2007). BASC-2 behavioral and emotional screening system manual. Bloomington, MN: Pearson. Google Scholar

Lane, K., Oakes, W., & Menzies, H. (2010). Systematic screenings to prevent the development of learning and behavior problems: Considerations for practitioners, researchers, and policy makers. *Journal of Disability Policy Studies, 21*(3), 160–172.

Lane, K., Oakes, W., Menzies, H., & Germer, K. (2014). Screening and identification approaches for detecting students at risk. In H. M. Walker & F. M. Gresham (Eds.), *Handbook of evidence-based practices for emotional and behavior disorders: Applications in schools* (pp. 129–151). New York: Guilford Press.

Merrell, K. W. (2008). Direct behavioral observation. In K. W. Merrell (Ed.), *Behavioral, social, and emotional assessment of children and adolescents* (3rd ed., pp. 63–95). New York: Lawrence Erlbaum.

Patterson, T. L., Moscona, S., McKibbin, C. L., Davidson, K., & Jeste, D. V. (2001). Social skills performance assessment among older patients with schizophrenia. *Schizophrenia Research, 48*(2–3), 351–360.

Ratto, A., Turner-Brown, L., Rupp, B., Mesibov, G., & Penn, D. (2011). Development of the contextual assessment of social skills (CASS): A role play measure of social skills for individuals with high functioning autism. *Journal of Autism and Developmental Disorders, 41*, 1277–1286.

Sprague, J., Cook, C., Browning-Wright, D., & Sadler, C. (2008). *RTI and behavior: A guide to integrating behavioral and academic supports*. Horsham, PA: LRP Publications.

Verhoeven, E. W. M., Smeekens, I., & Didden, R. (2013). Brief report: Suitability of the social skills performance assessment (SSPA) for the assessment of social skills in adults with autism spectrum disorders. *Journal of Autism and Developmental Disorders, 43*, 2990–2996. https://doi.org/10.1007/s10803-013-1843-6

Volpe, R. J., McConaughy, S. H., & Hintze, J. M. (2009). Generalizability of classroom behavior problem and on-task scores from the direct observation form. *School Psychology Review, 38*(3), 382–401.

Communication Disorders

W. Jason Peters and Johnny L. Matson

Introduction

Communicative competence, according to Light and McNaughton (2014), rests upon three fundamental constructs. The first, functionality of communication, refers to the successful engagement in communication skills necessary to meet the demands of one's environment. Adequacy of communication, the second construct, refers to attaining a sufficient level of communicative skills so as to meet environmental demands. The third and final fundamental construct, sufficient knowledge, judgment, and skills, refers to having an adequate level of skills necessary to meet communicative demands. Alternatively, others have described communication as a broad area that refers to the ability to convey or understand ideas, information, beliefs, or emotions through various forms of expression including verbally, nonverbally, receptively, or expressively between individuals or to a group or community (Beighley, Matson, Rieske, Konst, & Tureck, 2014; Feldman, 2005). According to Eriksson, Hartelius, and Saldert (2016), factors that influence communication include characteristics of the communicative participants (e.g., age, sex), goals of the communicative participants, attitudes, emotions, as well as the relationship between communicative participants.

Communication disorders are often characterized by delays in speech, hearing, or language (Gregg, 2017). Researchers estimate that the prevalence of speech and language delay is approximately 5–6% (Law, Boyle, Harris, Harkness, & Nye, 2000). Additionally, these types of delays, especially delays in expressive language, are often among the primary concerns parents present with when seeking a developmental assessment for their child (Rescorla & Alley, 2001; Rescorla, Ratner, Jusczyk, & Jusczyk, 2005). Children with language or communication disorders account for a significant percentage of the children seen by speech-language pathologists (SLP) in school settings as part of their caseload (Caesar & Kohler, 2009). Additionally, interventions targeting the concerns these children present with, sometimes referred to as specific language impairment (SLI), are among some of the most frequent types of interventions SLPs administer. According to Bishop (1998), a child is diagnosed with SLI when they have significant difficulties in regard to mastering language and there is no known reason. Additionally, children with SLI, with their primary difficulty being language delay, may not be identified until they are 3 or 4 years of age (Rescorla et al., 2005). Taken together, this suggests that the appropriate assessment and

W. J. Peters (✉) · J. L. Matson
Department of Psychology, Louisiana State University, Baton Rouge, LA, USA
e-mail: wpeter7@lsu.edu

diagnosis of communication skills and disorders is particularly important among children.

At present, there are four main communication disorders that affect children according to the *Diagnostic and Statistical Manual of Mental Disorders* (DSM-5) including language disorder, speech sound disorder, childhood-onset fluency disorder (stuttering), and social (pragmatic) communication disorder (American Psychiatric Association, 2013). Diagnoses are based on difficulties with language or speech production and use, as well as the absence of any known cause (e.g., medical). A common criterion between all four is age of onset, where symptoms must be present in the early developmental period. The main differences between the four communication disorders is in the primary difficulty the child may be experiencing. For example, a diagnosis of language disorder requires that an individual demonstrates difficulties in the acquisition and use of language. Alternatively, the main difficulty in speech sound disorder is concerned with the production of intelligible speech. The only communication disorder currently listed in the DSM-5 that does not apply only to children is adult-onset fluency disorder (stuttering), where onset of symptoms occurs in adulthood as opposed to the early developmental period (APA, 2013).

With publication of the DSM-5 came many changes. Relevant to communication disorders was the introduction of social (pragmatic) communication disorder (SPCD; APA, 2013). SPCD is characterized by impairments in both verbal and nonverbal communication resulting in difficulties using communication for social purposes, following narrative or conversational conventions, inferring what is not explicitly stated, and adapting communication to the current context (Mandy, Wang, Lee, & Skuse, 2017). According to Brukner-Wertman, Laor, and Golan (2016), SPCD and autism spectrum disorder (ASD), another change made to the DSM, significantly overlap as both disorders are characterized by impairments in social communication. ASD is differentiated from SPCD based on the presence of restricted and repetitive behaviors (RRB; APA, 2013).

However, some researchers have suggested that the two conditions are not, in fact, separate disorders. For example, evidence presented by Mandy et al. (2017) suggests that SPCD is not qualitatively distinct from ASD. Additionally, some have concerns regarding the distinction made between the two diagnoses as they argue it forces a categorical view of what many agree is a spectrum with potentially dependent social communication and RRB phenotypes (Brukner-Wertman et al., 2016). Although difficult, some researchers have demonstrated the ability to differentiate SPCD from ASD and other communication difficulties using very strictly defined criteria (Gibson, Adams, Lockton, & Green, 2013; Taylor & Whitehouse, 2016). Overall, it appears that SPCD may best be conceptualized as a dimensional symptom profile potentially present across various neurodevelopmental disorders (Norbury, 2014).

Associated Characteristics and Difficulties

Children with communication disorders experience a variety of accompanying difficulties. For example, children with communication disorders may engage in fewer positive social interactions as well as converse with peers less often when compared with typically developing children; however, both groups of children are equally accepted among peers according to peer sociometric ratings (Guralnick, Connor, Hammond, Gottman, & Kinnish, 1996). One noteworthy aspect of children with communication difficulties is that of stuttering. According to Bakhtiar, Seifpanahi, Ansari, Ghanadzade, and Packman (2010), stuttering appears early on life, typically in early childhood. Additionally, onset of stuttering most often occurs between the ages of 2 and 5, with approximately 90% of cases beginning prior to the age of 5 (Cavenagh, Costelloe, Davis, & Howell, 2015). Unless adequate treatment is received or a child recovers naturally, emotional, social, and mental health outcomes later in life can be negatively affected (Craig, Blumgart, & Tran, 2009; Craig & Tran,

2006; Iverach et al., 2016; McAllister, 2016). For example, according to Adriaensens, Beyers, and Struyf (2015), adolescents' evaluations of global self-esteem and social competence are negatively influenced by stuttering severity, indicating that adolescents who experience more severe levels of stuttering evaluate their self-esteem and social competence as lower.

Other researchers have established among adolescents who stutter the negative impact their stuttering has on their perceived communicative competence, their experience of bullying or teasing from peers who do not stutter, as well as heightened communication apprehension (Erickson & Block, 2013). Further, families of children and adolescents who stutter also report experiencing difficulties including high levels of family conflict, emotional strain, as well as difficulty managing their child's frustrations. In regard to perceived social competence, however, Hertsberg and Zebrowski (2016) demonstrated no differences between children who stutter and those who don't. Further difficulties are evident for children who stutter in regard to executive functioning as parents of preschool children who stutter rate their children lower on measures of working memory and overall executive functioning skills than parents of children who do not stutter (Ntourou, Anderson, & Wagovich, 2018). Taken together, it is evident that stuttering has a wide-ranging impact across a number of domains.

The presence of stuttering is relatively common in children, with an estimated incidence of approximately 5% among preschoolers (Cavenagh et al., 2015; Månsson, 2000). According to Cavenagh et al. (2015), gender is a risk factor in the development of stuttering as boys are affected more often than girls; however, they generally experience onset later. Additionally, there appears to be a familial risk involved in the development of stuttering, where previous researchers have established that a family history of stuttering is present in a significant percentage of individuals who stutter compared with individuals who do not stutter (Cavenagh et al., 2015; Choi et al., 2018).

Another important aspect to consider in regard to the assessment of communication difficulties is bilingualism as not much is known regarding typical development of expressive language among bilingual individuals (Patterson, 1998). According to Boerma and Blom (2017), bilingualism is an important and complicating factor to consider in the assessment of communication difficulties. For example, bilingual children may score significantly lower than monolingual children when being tested in one language. As a result, it may be important to test bilingual children in both languages as the presence of a language impairment will impact both of the child's spoken languages. Therefore, it is recommended that a bilingual child suspected of having a language impairment be tested in both languages. However, according to Paradis, Emmerzael, and Duncan (2010), gathering information on both languages can be challenging, especially for English language learners as it can be difficult to observe or assess their primary language, highlighting the importance of having widely used and well-validated measures translated into other languages. Fortunately, clinicians, SLPs, and other examiners can follow guidelines provided by Pieretti and Roseberry-McKibbin (2016) in assessing English language learners that provide research-based recommendations regarding the pre-evaluation process, dynamic assessment procedures, assessment of information-processing, as well as language sampling.

Challenging behavior is another difficulty that has been associated with communication disorders. According to Gregg (2017), children with communication disorders may become frustrated and may use challenging behaviors, such as aggression, to express those frustrations. Children with communication disorders, such as speech sound disorder, may also experience difficulties with speech perception. For example, Hearnshaw, Baker, and Munro (2018) provided evidence that children with speech sound disorder demonstrated poorer perceptual accuracy on tasks of lexical and phonetic judgment than did typically developing peers suggesting that they perceive speech less accurately.

In addition to the difficulties described above, individuals with communication disorders also experience high rates of mental health issues and psychiatric disorders (Lewis et al., 2016). For example, stuttering in childhood is associated with increased risk for anxiety disorders such as social anxiety disorder or generalized anxiety disorder (Iverach et al., 2016). Additional researchers suggest an association between attention-deficit/hyperactivity disorder (ADHD) and stuttering, where children with ADHD produce significantly more stuttering behaviors when compared to a control group (Lee, Sim, Lee, & Choi, 2017). Further, children with comorbid communication and psychiatric disorders demonstrate significantly worse functioning later in life (Stivanin, de Oliveira, dos Santos, dos Santos, & Scivoletto, 2016). Overall, when assessing for the presence of a communication disorder, there are a number of associated characteristics, difficulties, and comorbidities that the clinician needs to account for so as to accurately and appropriately assess a child presenting with communication or language concerns.

Assessment Methods and Tools

Conducting a comprehensive assessment of an individual's communication can be a complex process. According to guidelines provided by the American Speech-Language-Hearing Association, a comprehensive speech-language assessment includes several components such as a review of case history; client and family interview; a review of cognitive, visual, motor, and auditory status; measures (standardized or non-standardized) of speech and language; as well as identification and follow-up on effective intervention strategies (Association, 2004). Within the last few decades, a number of assessment methods and tools have been developed to assess for the presence and describe the characteristics of various communication problems that can assist in the evaluation and diagnosis of a communication disorder. There exists a significant literature regarding communication and communication disorders, and these assessment methods and tools have been an important part of that research literature. The following sections describe and review several of these methods and tools.

Clinical Evaluation of Language Fundamentals

The *Clinical Evaluation of Language Fundamentals*, now in its fifth edition (CELF-5; Wiig, Secord, & Semel, 2013), is a test battery used to measure and assess changes in language and communication, including oral and written language in addition to nonverbal communication skills. It can also be used to determine the presence of and diagnose a language disorder as well as describe the nature of the disorder. The CELF-5 is designed to be used with individuals between 5 and 21 years of age and helps to identify an individual's strengths and weaknesses in language, provide intervention or treatment strategies, determine service eligibility, as well as measure intervention efficacy. Additionally, it can be used within a number of contexts including educational, clinical, and research settings. The measure is composed of 16 subtests that are age-specific, meaning that some subtests are intended for use only with younger children (i.e., 5–8 years of age) while others are meant for other age groups (i.e., 9–21 years of age). Twelve of those subtests are combined to create a Core Language Score as well as 5 indices measuring receptive language, expressive language, language content, language structure, and language memory (Wiig et al., 2013). All subtests, with the exception of structured writing, are comprised of between 16 and 50 items or statements that are scored as either a 1 (correct) or 0 (incorrect). However, two subtests, formulated sentences and recalling sentences, are scored on a three-point and four-point Likert-type scale, respectively.

The first subtest, the Observation Rating Scale, is recommended by the authors of the measure to be used first for the purpose of identifying areas of concern and can be used with individuals of all ages for which the measure was intended (Wiig et al., 2013). Other relevant subtests can then be administered to determine and evaluate the existence and nature of a communication or language deficit. This flexible administration allows for the evaluation of specific language skills relevant to the individual, or the CELF can be used as a battery for a comprehensive language assessment. The CELF-5 is one of the most widely used measures for assessing language and communication. According to a survey conducted by Caesar and Kohler (2009), the CELF was reported to be the most frequently used measure among school-based SLPs as a formal, standardized procedure that is part of their assessment process.

Psychometric evidence regarding the CELF-5 indicates acceptable to excellent split-half reliability for all age groups as well as good internal consistency (Wiig et al., 2013). Other analyses of test-retest and interrater reliability indicate acceptable to excellent reliabilities for all subtests across age groups. According to the manual, the CELF-5 demonstrates adequate to excellent concurrent validity with a previous version of the CELF, as well as with the Peabody Picture Vocabulary Test-Fourth Edition (PPVT-4; Dunn & Dunn, 2007). The CELF has been used by researchers to compare the language skills of children in clinical settings including those with SLI and ASD (Lloyd, Paintin, & Botting, 2006), Rolandic epilepsy (Overvliet et al., 2013), as well as individuals with traumatic brain injury (Turkstra, 1999), demonstrating its use across a number of clinical populations.

Children's Communication Checklist: Second Edition

The Children's Communication Checklist-Second Edition (CCC-2; Bishop, 2006) is a parent- or caregiver-completed checklist for use with children aged between 4 years and 16 years, 11 months. Additionally, it is intended to be used for children with normal hearing and who speak English as their primary language. The CCC-2 is used to identify pragmatic language impairment, screen receptive and expressive language skills, and assist in screening for ASD. The original version of the CCC-2 was developed in the United Kingdom and has since been modified for use in the United States through spelling and phrasing changes. Additionally, the original CCC used teachers or speech-language professionals as respondents and was developed to identify patterns of language difficulties of children already diagnosed with a language impairment (Bishop, 1998). The US version of the CCC-2 is comprised of 70 items divided into 10 separate 7-item scales (Bishop, 2006). Each scale measures a separate aspect of language or communication in addition to characteristics related to ASD. The first four scales, labeled A through D, assess aspects of language associated with specific impairments including speech, syntax, semantics, and coherence. The second set of four scales, labeled E through H, evaluate pragmatic impairments such as initiation, scripted language, context, and nonverbal communication. Lastly, the final two scales, labeled I and J, assess non-language behaviors associated with ASD (i.e., social relations, interests). Of the seven items on each scale, five are intended to measure difficulties in communication while two are intended to measure strengths. In the structure of the checklist, communication difficulties are evaluated prior to strengths.

Research on the CCC-2 has demonstrated good psychometric properties including good to excellent test-retest reliability, as well as strong internal consistency (Bishop, 2006). Additional research has demonstrated good construct validity indicating that the CCC-2 may be helpful in evaluating children with communication and pragmatic language difficulties; however, there are concerns as to how well it evaluates those difficulties among a normal population (i.e., no diagnosed language impairment; Ketelaars, Cuperus, van Daal, Jansonius, & Verhoeven, 2009; Laws & Bishop, 2004). Further, the CCC has been translated into and validated in several languages including Thai (Chuthapisith, Taycharpipranai, Roongpraiwan, & Ruangdaraganon, 2014), Serbian (Glumbić & Brojčin, 2012), Dutch (Geurts, 2007; Ketelaars et al., 2009), Norwegian (Helland, Biringer, Helland, & Heimann, 2009), and Quebec French (Vézina, Samson-Morasse, Gauthier-Desgagné, Fossard, & Sylvestre, 2011). The CCC-2 has been used to examine pragmatic language impairments in a number of clinical populations including individuals with Williams syndrome (Hoffmann, Martens, Fox, Rabidoux, &

Andridge, 2013), ADHD (Bignell & Cain, 2007; Grzadzinski et al., 2011; Timler, 2014; Vaisanen, Loukusa, Yliherva, & Moilanen, 2014), and ASD (Grzadzinski et al., 2011; Volden & Phillips, 2010; Whitehouse, Barry, & Bishop, 2008) indicating its usefulness in identifying communication impairments across a number of individuals who present with various communication difficulties.

Language Development Survey

The Language Development Survey (LDS; Rescorla, 1989) is a parent report measure designed to screen the expressive vocabulary and word combinations of toddlers between the ages of 18 and 35 months to identify early language delay. It is comprised of 310 words arranged both alphabetically and according to 14 semantic categories (e.g., foods, action words, animals, etc.). According to the test author, the LDS can be administered in about 10 min, and parents are asked to identify words on the checklist that their child spontaneously uses (Rescorla, 1989; Rescorla & Alley, 2001). The LDS is also used to identify if the child being assessed has begun combining words to form phrases or sentences, and parents are asked to provide up to five examples of these phrases. Each word endorsed by the parents is scored as a 1. Additionally, the parents can endorse up to five words spontaneously used by their child not listed on the LDS to create a maximum score of 315. For the purposes of identifying language delay, the test author recommends using a cutoff of 50 words for toddlers aged 24 months (Rescorla, 1989).

Psychometric analyses of the LDS have indicated excellent internal consistency and test-retest reliability (Rescorla, 1989; Rescorla & Alley, 2001). Convergent validity with other measures of object/picture naming has also been established as indicated by correlations between total vocabulary identified by the LDS and total number of named objects and pictures (Rescorla, 1989; Rescorla, Hadicke-Wiley, & Escarce, 1993). Concurrent validity with the MacArthur-Bates Communicative Development Inventory: Words and Sentences has also been established (Rescorla et al., 2005). As a screening instrument, the LDS has also demonstrated good sensitivity and specificity in identifying toddlers with language delay (Rescorla, 1989; Rescorla & Alley, 2001; Rescorla et al., 1993). Researchers have used the LDS to evaluate the prevalence of expressive language delay among toddlers, demonstrating prevalence rates between 10% and 20% (Klee et al., 1998; Rescorla, 1989; Rescorla & Alley, 2001). Additionally, the LDS has been used to identify language delay among preterm infants at age 18 months (Beaulieu-Poulin, Simard, Babakissa, Lefebvre, & Luu, 2016; Mossabeb, Wade, Abbasi, Finnegan, & Sivieri, 2012). The LDS has also been translated into several other languages including Spanish (Patterson, 1998), Greek (Papaeliou & Rescorla, 2011), Portuguese (Rescorla, Nyame, & Dias, 2016), Polish (Rescorla, Constants, Białecka-Pikul, Stępień-Nycz, & Ochał, 2017), Korean (Rescorla, Lee, Kim, & Oh, 2013), French (Beaulieu-Poulin et al., 2016), and Italian (Rescorla, Frigerio, Sali, Spataro, & Longobardi, 2014) and has been used to compare the language development of English-speaking children and children who speak other languages.

Macarthur-Bates Communicative Development Inventory

The Macarthur-Bates Communicative Development Inventory (CDI; Fenson et al., 1993) is a parent-report measure designed to elicit information about children's early language skills and social communication. The CDI exists in two separate forms, the infant and toddler forms, which evaluate the child's use of words and gestures and their use of words and sentences, respectively. The infant form, intended for children between 8 and 16 months of age, consists of two parts which elicit information through questioning and a 396-item checklist regarding a child's response to and use of words (Part 1) and a child's use of gestures (Part 2). The toddler form, otherwise known as the Macarthur-Bates Communicative Development Inventory: Words and Sentences (CDI:WS) evaluates the number and types of words present in a child's vocabulary as well as their use of syntactic forms and is intended for children between 16 and 30 months of age. The CDI:WS is comprised of 680 items divided into two separate sections. The first section of the CDI:WS, similar to the LDS, contains a list of words organized into semantic categories, and parents are asked to endorse which words their child produces. The second section assesses aspects related to the child's sentence production and use of grammar. One important and noteworthy feature of the CDI is that it evaluates the absence or delay of social communication behaviors such as imitation, declarative gestures, and functional and symbolic play, in addition to assessing early language development. According to the test authors, the CDI takes approximately 30 min to complete (Fenson et al., 1993). Additionally, the scoring for the CDI uses norms based on a sample of typically developing children.

In regard to the psychometric properties of the CDI, previous researchers have demonstrated good internal consistency, as well as good to excellent test-retest reliability (Fenson et al., 1994). Additionally, convergent validity with other language measures has also been demonstrated (Dale, 1991; Fenson et al., 1994; Heilmann, Weismer, Evans, & Hollar, 2005; Rescorla et al., 2005). Further, researchers have demonstrated that the CDI is valid for use among several clinical populations including individuals with ASD (Charman, Drew, Baird, & Baird, 2003; Luyster, Lopez, & Lord, 2007; Luyster, Qiu, Lopez, & Lord, 2007), very preterm infants (Foster-Cohen, Edgin, Champion, & Woodward, 2007), and children with cochlear implants (Thal, DesJardin, & Eisenberg, 2007). The potential of deriving a screening instrument based on the CDI has also been examined; however, analyses indicated that the screening version did not perform adequately (Westerlund, Berglund, & Eriksson, 2006). The CDI has also been translated into Spanish (Fenson, 2003) and Swedish (Berglund & Eriksson, 2000).

Test of Pragmatic Language: Second Edition

The Test of Pragmatic Language, Second Edition (TOPL-2; Phelps-Terasaki & Phelps-Gunn, 2007) is designed to provide an overall assessment of an individual's pragmatic language ability. The main version of the TOPL-2 is intended for use among children between the ages of 8 and 18; however, there is a second, shorter version available for use among children between the ages of 6 and 7. The TOPL-2 is comprised of 43 total items that measure several underlying areas of pragmatics such as physical context, topic, purpose, audience, abstractions, visual-gestural cues, and pragmatic evaluation. The shortened version of the TOPL-2 for younger children contains only the first 17 items. Scores for the TOPL-2 are standardized (i.e., mean of 100 and standard deviation of 15) where higher scores indicate better pragmatic abilities; however, separate scores are not provided for the underlying areas of pragmatics. During the TOPL-2, children are asked to give information about a particular story and its characters, many of which are presented in picture form, for the purpose of eliciting functional communicative interactions between the child and assessor. Scoring for the items on the TOPL-2 is dichotomous, meaning that they are scored as either correct or incorrect (Phelps-Terasaki & Phelps-Gunn, 2007).

According to the test manual, the TOPL-2 has adequate to good internal consistency, as well as excellent test-retest and interrater reliability (Phelps-Terasaki & Phelps-Gunn, 2007). Analyses of validity indicated that the TOPL-2 demonstrated adequate content, criterion, and construct validity. Overall, the TOPL and TOPL-2 have been used on a limited basis with the exception of studies that have used these measures to assess pragmatic language abilities in individuals with ASD (Volden, Coolican, Garon, White, & Bryson, 2009; Volden & Phillips, 2010; Young, Diehl, Morris, Hyman, & Bennetto, 2005) as well as individuals with Williams syndrome (Hoffmann et al., 2013).

Diagnostic Interview for Social and Communication Disorders

The Diagnostic Interview for Social and Communication Disorders (DISCO; Leekam, Libby, Wing, Gould, & Taylor, 2002) is a semi-structured interview schedule used in the assessment of information relevant to ASD. Information for the DISCO can be gathered from parents or caregivers and can be used to assess individuals of any age. Additionally, the DISCO elicits information not only on the core symptoms of autism (e.g., social and communication impairment) but also on a number of other domains including sensory symptoms, gross and fine motor skills, maladaptive behavior, and sleep difficulties, among others. Further, the DISCO scoring provides algorithms that can be used in the diagnosis of ASD according to criteria presented in either the DSM or the International Classification of Diseases. Lastly, this measure has a strong focus on the individual's development as it includes a detailed evaluation of their current level of development, as well as any developmental delays. Due to the broad nature of the information collected, the clinician can therefore use the DISCO to understand an individual's difficulties in communication, reciprocal social interaction, and repetitive behaviors against their own pattern of developmental skills and difficulties. According to the test authors, the DISCO can also elicit information on other related disorders, such as language or motor impairments, that can be further assessed if concerns are indicated (Leekam et al., 2002).

The DISCO interview schedule is composed of over 300 questions divided into eight separate sections and generally takes approximately 2–3 h to complete. The first section elicits identifying, family, and medical information, while the second section is focused on the early developmental period of infancy. The infancy section mainly focuses on gathering medical information relevant to a diagnosis of Rett's syndrome, as well as some questions regarding infant behaviors. The third section, the largest one on the DISCO, focuses on developmental skills and gathers information on a number of domains including gross motor skills, visuo-manual skills, independence, self-care, domestic skills, verbal and non-verbal communication, social play and leisure, social interaction with adults and peers, cognitive skills, pictures, reading, writing, and imagination. All items in this section are rated by the interviewer in regard to their current level, any delay in acquiring the relevant skills, and atypical behavior, both past and present, associated with the relevant skills. The remaining sections of the DISCO gather information regarding repetitive behaviors (Sect. 4; e.g., stereotypies, routines), emotions (Sect. 5; e.g., anxiety, mood), maladaptive behavior (Sect. 6; e.g., aggression, sleep disturbances), and other psychiatric concerns (Sect. 8; e.g., schizophrenia, eating disorders). The remaining section, Section 7, is used by the assessor to help guide them in determining their clinical judgment independent of the quantitative results already obtained. This section does not typically involve direct questioning and instead includes the assessor's judgments on the individual's skills based on an overview of the available information (Leekam et al., 2002).

Previous researchers have demonstrated that the DISCO has good to excellent interrater reliability (Leekam et al., 2002; Wing, Leekam, Libby, Gould, & Larcombe, 2002). Additionally, other researchers have established excellent criterion and convergent validity for the DISCO when compared with clinical diagnoses as well as the Autism Diagnostic Interview-Revised, Autism Diagnostic Observation Schedule, and Social Communication Questionnaire (Maljaars, Noens, Scholte, & van Berckelaer-Onnes, 2011; Nygren et al., 2009). The DISCO, which originated in the United Kingdom, has been translated into and validated in other languages including Dutch (Maljaars et al., 2011; van Berckelaer-Onnes, Noens, & Dijkxhoorn, 2008) and Swedish (Nygren et al., 2009). Researchers have also used the DISCO among individuals with various levels of intellectual disability, demonstrating its clinical use in this population (Maljaars et al., 2011). Lastly, other researchers have identified subsets of items on the DISCO that can be used to "signpost" (i.e., using an item set to guide clinicians in choosing an appropriate pathway to diagnosis) or to identify children who exhibit pathological demand avoidance (Carrington et al., 2015; O'Nions et al., 2016).

Social and Communication Disorders Checklist

The Social and Communication Disorders Checklist (SCDC; Skuse et al., 1997) is a parent or teacher questionnaire consisting of 12 items designed to measure traits of autism (e.g., social and communication impairment) in children and adolescents as they currently present. Items for the SCDC are scored on a three-point Likert-type scale (i.e., 2 = very true; 1 = quite true; and 0 = not true). Additionally, the items on the SCDC primarily evaluate the extent to which the individual being assessed has social difficulties. Examples of items include "does not realize when others are upset or angry," "behavior often disrupts normal family life," "difficult to reason with when upset," or "does not pick up on body language" (pg. 9; Skuse et al., 1997). Higher scores on the SCDC suggest greater difficulty in regard to perceiving others' moods or feelings, poor reciprocal social skills, and may also demonstrate poor communication skills on the part of the individual.

According to Skuse, Mandy, and Scourfield (2005), internal consistency and test-retest reliability for the SCDC is good to excellent. Additional analyses conducted by Skuse and colleagues indicated that the measure also demonstrates good concurrent, discriminant, and criterion validity. Further, as the SCDC is primarily used as a screening instrument, adequate sensitivity has been established; however, specificity for the instrument was demonstrated to be low (i.e., <0.70). Analyses in a separate study conducted by Skuse et al. (2009) using a larger, clinically diverse sample and a lower cutoff score yielded adequate sensitivity and specificity for the SCDC suggesting its validity in the screening of ASD. Further research by Bölte, Westerwald, Holtmann, Freitag, and Poustka (2011) supports the adequate sensitivity and specificity previously established. While intended primarily for use in assisting in the identification of ASD, the SCDC has also been used among individuals with learning disabilities; ADHD; speech, language, and communication needs; emotional and behavioral maladjustment; physical and sensory disabilities; pragmatic language impairment; Turner's syndrome; obsessive-compulsive disorder; and Tourette's syndrome (Skuse et al., 1997, 2009, 2005). The SCDC has also been translated into German (Bölte et al., 2011), Hindi, Bengali (Rudra et al., 2014), and Spanish (de la Osa, Granero, Penelo, & Ezpeleta, 2014).

Peabody Picture Vocabulary Test

The Peabody Picture Vocabulary Test, Fourth Edition (PPVT-4; Dunn & Dunn, 2007) is designed to assess an individual's receptive vocabulary. It is intended to evaluate the receptive vocabulary among individuals between the ages of 3 and 90 years. Currently, the PPVT-4 exists in two forms, Form A and Form B. Both forms of the PPVT-4 are comprised of 228 items, each of which contain four pictures. During administration of the PPVT-4, the examiner selects an appropriate start point based on the age of the examinee and verbally speaks a word within a prompt (e.g., "point to [word]"). The examinee is asked to point to the picture that corresponds to the spoken word and its meaning. Once the examinee understands the task, the prompt can be faded until only the stimulus word is spoken. The manual does provide alternative responding styles for individuals who may have a motor impairment and are unable to point as requested. Each item is scored as either correct or incorrect, and the total number of correct items is summed to create a raw score. Raw scores are then converted to standard scores to allow for comparison of the examinee's performance to previously established norms (e.g., age or grade equivalents). The PPVT-4 is individually administered and untimed, although it takes approximately 15–20 min to administer. According to the manual, the PPVT-4 has several areas of application such as screening verbal development, measuring response to vocabulary instruction, and assisting in the diagnosis of reading difficulties or the detection of language impairments, among others (Dunn & Dunn, 2007).

Psychometric analyses of the PPVT-4 have indicated good to excellent internal consistency, alternate form reliability, as well as test-retest reliability (Dunn & Dunn, 2007). Additional analyses demonstrated that the PPVT-4 correlates well with other measures of oral language and expressive vocabulary indicating good criterion validity. Further, the PPVT-4 demonstrates good content validity as all items on the measure were pulled from recent editions of *Webster's New Collegiate Dictionary* and the *Merriam-Webster's Collegiate Dictionary*. According to the test authors, the PPVT-4 can be used across various clinical populations including individuals with ASD, individuals with cerebral palsy, or individuals with moderate visual disabilities (e.g., color blindness; Dunn & Dunn, 2007). Additionally, the PPVT-4 is among the instruments most frequently used by SLPs to assist in the diagnosis of SLI in clinical practice (Eickhoff, Betz, & Ristow, 2010). Previous versions of the PPVT have also been translated into other languages including French (Dunn, Theriault-Whalen, & Dunn, 1993) and Spanish (Dunn, Padilla, Lugo, & Dunn, 1986).

Test of Childhood Stuttering

The Test of Childhood Stuttering (TOCS; Gillam, Logan, & Pearson, 2009) is an individually administered assessment of speech fluency. It is intended to be used in children between the ages of 4 and 12 years. Additionally, it is designed to identify children who stutter, to determine the severity of their stuttering, to document and evaluate changes in their stuttering over time, and to facilitate research on stuttering among children. The TOCS is divided into three separate components including a standardized Speech Fluency Measure, Observation Rating Scales, and Supplemental Clinical Assessment Activities. Within the Speech Fluency Measure, the child is asked to complete four tasks such as rapid picture naming, modeled sentences, structured conversation, and narration. In rapid picture naming, the child is shown a series of pictures and is asked to name those pictures as rapidly as possible. For modeled sentences, the child is shown two pictures. The examiner then models a sentence using the first, while the child is asked to produce a sentence using the second picture and the same syntactic structure as the examiner. During structured conversation, the child being assessed is asked questions about a series of pictures so as to assess stuttering in the context of a dialogue. Lastly, for narration, the child is asked to tell a story based on the pictures used in structured conversation. The purpose of these tasks is to elicit speech samples so as to identify the presence of stuttering (Gillam et al., 2009).

The Observation Rating Scales are based on parent or caregiver report and allow for the examiner to evaluate parental concern in regard to the nature of their child's stuttering (Gillam et al., 2009). The Observation Rating Scales are comprised of two scales measuring the child's speech fluency as well as disfluency-related consequences. Additionally, they can be administered by either the examiner, the child's parents, or teacher. Data obtained from the Observation Rating Scales and Speech Fluency Measure are used to determine the severity of the child's stuttering. The Supplemental Clinical Assessment Activities include activities that provide additional analyses on the child's stuttering including speech rate analysis, repetition unit analysis, and speech naturalness analysis, among others. According to the manual, the TOCS provides raw scores, index scores, and percentile ranks, which are used to compare the child being assessed to standardization samples of typically developing children as well as children who stutter. Overall, the TOCS' Speech Fluency Measure and Observation Rating Scales take approximately 30 min combined to administer. According to the test authors, speech sample transcription can be time-consuming to complete, and the TOCS provides an efficient alternative (Gillam et al., 2009).

Psychometric evidence regarding the TOCS indicates that it has adequate to excellent internal consistency, as well as good test-retest reliability (Gillam et al., 2009). Additionally, the examiner's manual provides adequate evidence of content, criterion, concurrent, and construct validity for both the Speech Fluency Measure and Observational Rating Scale. It is important to note that independent analyses regarding the psychometric properties of the TOCS have been lacking as only one study has demonstrated the usefulness of the TOCS in documenting parental accuracy in perception of their child's stuttering (Tumanova, Choi, Conture, & Walden, 2018). Additionally, the TOCS has been translated and validated into Persian (Naderi, Shahbodaghi, Khatonabadi, Dadgar, & Jalaie, 2011).

Stuttering Severity Instrument

The *Stuttering Severity Instrument-Fourth Edition* (SSI-4; Riley & Bakker, 2009) is designed to evaluate the severity of an individual's stuttering by assessing the frequency and duration of stuttering, as well as physical concomitants (i.e., extraneous body movements and sounds). Frequency of stuttering is measured as the percent of syllables stuttered, and duration of stuttering is measured as the average of the three longest stuttering events. Either two conversational samples or one conversational sample and one reading sample, all between 150 to 500 syllables each, are recorded via video or audio. Video recording is necessary to score physical concomitants. Computer software is provided with the instrument to assist in collecting frequency and duration data; however, the manual does provide instructions for alternative methods of collecting this data (Riley & Bakker, 2009).

After watching all speaking samples, the examiner rates physical concomitants (e.g., facial grimaces, movements of the extremities, head movements, and distracting sounds) using a six-point, Likert-type scale ranging from 0 = none to 5 = severe and painful looking. The raw data for all three measured aspects of stuttering are converted to scale scores and then combined to create a total score. The total score is converted into a percentile rank which corresponds to one of five severity levels (i.e., very mild, mild, moderate, severe, very severe) indicating the overall severity of the individual's stuttering. After scoring the speaking samples, the examiner is then required to make a speech naturalness judgment using a nine-point scale ranging from 1 = highly natural sounding speech to 9 = highly unnatural sounding speech. Lastly, this new version of the SSI also includes a self-report measure, the Clinical Use of Self-Reports, that asks the individual being assessed to answer 13 questions regarding various components of stuttering (e.g., social, emotional, cognitive) when speaking to others in person or on the telephone using a similar nine-point scale. It is important to note that the SSI-4 is not intended to be used as a diagnostic instrument as it is only designed to provide a severity rating, not identify an individual as someone who stutters (Riley & Bakker, 2009).

Overall, psychometric evidence regarding the SSI-4 indicates poor to good intra-rater and inter-rater reliability, ranging between .50 and .88 for all components of the instrument (Riley & Bakker, 2009). These results are similar to reliability analyses of a previous version, as well as the current version, of the instrument (Davidow & Scott, 2017; Hall, Lynn, Altieri, Segers, & Conti, 1987). In regard to validity, adequate evidence is provided for both criterion and construct validity (Riley & Bakker, 2009). The SSI has also been translated into Persian (Bakhtiar et al., 2010).

Preschool Language Scale

The Preschool Language Scale, Fifth Edition (PLS-5; Zimmerman, Steiner, & Pond, 2011) is a comprehensive developmental language assessment intended for children from birth to age 7 years and 11 months. The purpose of the PLS-5 is to identify delays in both receptive and expressive language. It can also be used to assess an individual's relative strengths and weaknesses in language development, determine eligibility for interventions, as well as evaluate the efficacy of those interventions. The PLS-5 is comprised of two scales, the auditory comprehension (AC) scale and the expressive communication (EC) scale. On the AC scale, children are asked to point to items and follow directions. According to the test authors, the AC scale is designed to assess attention, semantics, and play. For the EC scale, children are asked to express quantity, name objects, and use sentence structures and particular grammatical markers. The EC scale is designed to evaluate social communication and vocabulary development. Both scales also measure gesture, language structure, and emergent literacy (Zimmerman et al., 2011).

All items on the PLS-5 are scored as either correct (1) or incorrect (0), with scoring criteria provided for each item (Zimmerman et al., 2011). For both the AC and EC scales, the PLS-5 provides norm-referenced scores. Additionally, a norm-referenced total score can also be calculated. In addition to the two main scales, the PLS-5 also includes three supplementary measures: Language Sample Checklist, Articulation Screener, and Home Communication Questionnaire. The Language Sample Checklist evaluates a child's spontaneous utterances, the Articulation Screener determines if additional evaluation of a child's articulation is necessary, and the Home Communication Questionnaire solicits information from the parents or caregivers regarding their child's communication skills. Overall, administration of the PLS-5 takes approximately 20–25 min but can take up to 50 min depending on the child's age (Zimmerman et al., 2011).

According to the test manual, the PLS-5 demonstrates good to excellent test-retest and interrater reliability across age groups (Zimmerman et al., 2011). Additionally, the measure demonstrates good to excellent internal consistency for both the AC and EC scales across children from the normative sample, as well as separate groups of children including those with language disorder and others with language delay. Further, both content and construct validity evidence are provided. Research using the PLS-5 is limited; however, it has been translated into Spanish, Mandarin (Ren, Rattanasone, Wyver, Hinton, & Demuth, 2016), and Turkish (Sahli & Belgin, 2017), and previous versions of the PLS have been used to evaluate language among preschoolers with ASD (Volden et al., 2011).

Dynamic Assessment

As an alternative to standardized testing methods, many clinicians have begun to use dynamic assessment procedures in the assessment of language and communication (Mann, Peña, & Morgan, 2014). According to McLaughlin and Cascella (2008), dynamic assessment is generally comprised of three parts including identifying a child's current skill level, attempting techniques to elicit a more advanced or novel skills, and assessing the benefits of those techniques. One noteworthy feature of dynamic assessment is that it is a useful tool in the assessment of individuals of varying cultural or linguistic backgrounds as it can help in reducing test bias these individuals may otherwise experience (Mann et al., 2014). Additionally, dynamic assessment is individualized in a way that many standardized tests based on static norms are not (Lidz, 1983). Dynamic assessment can also allow the clinician or assessor to identify supports necessary for an individual to engage in a new communication skill (McLaughlin & Cascella, 2008). While it is a relatively new procedure, some researchers have demonstrated the effectiveness of dynamic assessment procedures in the assessment and intervention of communication disorders in individuals who are deaf (Mann et al., 2014) as well as individuals with intellectual disability (McLaughlin & Cascella, 2008).

Conclusion

Communication skills refer to the ability to convey information or ideas through various means (e.g., verbally, nonverbally, etc.; Beighley et al., 2014; Feldman, 2005). Disorders of communication oftentimes come as a result of delays in speech, language, or hearing (Gregg, 2017). Individuals with poor communication skills and those who have been diagnosed with a communication disorder often experience poor outcomes in adolescence and adulthood such as reduced self-esteem, lower perception of social competence, poor social and emotional functioning, increased levels of anxiety, and overall reduced quality of life (Adriaensens et al., 2015; Craig et al., 2009; Craig & Tran, 2006; McAllister, 2016). Additionally, delays in communication are often among the primary reason parents seek evaluation (Rescorla & Alley, 2001; Rescorla et al., 2005), and children with communication difficulties or SLI account for a large percentage of the caseloads of SLPs (Caesar & Kohler, 2009). Taken together, this suggests that it is imperative that appropriate assessment methods and tools be used to identify and describe a child's communication difficulties so that accurate diagnoses can be made and appropriate interventions can be identified.

Currently, there are four communication disorders diagnoses according to the DSM-5 (i.e., language disorder, speech sound disorder, childhood-onset fluency disorder (stuttering), and social (pragmatic) communication disorder; APA, 2013). All of these diagnoses are characterized by impairments in communication development and production, as well as difficulty in engaging in expected communication in a variety of contexts with a subsequent impact on functioning. Communication impairments are also characteristic of other disorders (e.g., ASD), further indicating the importance of accurately assessing and describing the nature and characteristics of a child's communication difficulties, especially in the process of differential diagnosis.

This chapter describes and reviews a number of assessment methods and tools commonly used in the field to assess and diagnose communication difficulties and disorders. Many of the measures described are accompanied by a significant body of supporting literature (e.g., CELF-5, CCC-2, CDI, etc.) with supporting psychometric evidence indicating that these measures are reliable and valid tools for identifying and describing communication disorders in children. Additionally, many of these tools can also be used to identify targets for intervention, which is important to consider given the associated outcomes described above for those who don't receive adequate treatment.

References

Adriaensens, S., Beyers, W., & Struyf, E. (2015). Impact of stuttering severity on adolescents' domain-specific and general self-esteem through cognitive and emotional mediating processes. *Journal of Communication Disorders, 58*, 43–57 https://doi.org/10.1016/j.jcomdis.2015.10.003

American Psychiatric Association. (2013). *Diagnostic and statistical manual of mental disorders* (5th ed.). Washington, DC: American Psychiatric Association.

Association, A. S.-L.-H. (2004). Assessment and evaluation of speech-language disorders in schools. Retrieved 20 Feb 2018, from https://www.asha.org/SLP/Assessment-and-Evaluation-of-Speech-Language-Disorders-in-Schools/

Bakhtiar, M., Seifpanahi, S., Ansari, H., Ghanadzade, M., & Packman, A. (2010). Investigation of the reliability of the SSI-3 for preschool Persian-speaking children who stutter. *Journal of Fluency Disorders, 35*(2), 87–91 https://doi.org/10.1016/j.jfludis.2010.02.003

Beaulieu-Poulin, C., Simard, M.-N., Babakissa, H., Lefebvre, F., & Luu, T. M. (2016). Validity of the language development survey in infants born preterm. *Early Human Development, 98*, 11–16 https://doi.org/10.1016/j.earlhumdev.2016.06.003

Beighley, J. S., Matson, J. L., Rieske, R. D., Konst, M. J., & Tureck, K. (2014). Differences in communication skills in toddlers diagnosed with autism spectrum disorder according to the DSM-IV-TR and the DSM-5. *Research in Autism Spectrum Disorders, 8*(2), 74–81.

Berglund, E., & Eriksson, M. a. (2000). Communicative development in Swedish children 16-28 months old: The Swedish Early Communicative Development Inventory—Words and sentences. *Scandinavian Journal of Psychology, 41*(2), 133–144.

Bignell, S., & Cain, K. (2007). Pragmatic aspects of communication and language comprehension in groups of children differentiated by teacher ratings of inattention and hyperactivity. *British Journal of Developmental Psychology, 25*(4), 499–512.

Bishop, D. V. (1998). Development of the Children's Communication Checklist (CCC): A method for assessing qualitative aspects of communicative impairment in children. *The Journal of Child Psychology and Psychiatry and Allied Disciplines, 39*(6), 879–891.

Bishop, D. V. (2006). *CCC-2: Children's Communication Checklist-2 - U.S. Edition*. New York, NY: The Psychological Corporation.

Boerma, T., & Blom, E. (2017). Assessment of bilingual children: What if testing both languages is not possible? *Journal of Communication Disorders, 66*, 65–76 https://doi.org/10.1016/j.jcomdis.2017.04.001

Bölte, S., Westerwald, E., Holtmann, M., Freitag, C., & Poustka, F. (2011). Autistic traits and autism spectrum disorders: The clinical validity of two measures presuming a continuum of social communication skills.

Journal of Autism and Developmental Disorders, 41(1), 66–72.

Brukner-Wertman, Y., Laor, N., & Golan, O. (2016). Social (pragmatic) communication disorder and its relation to the autism spectrum: Dilemmas arising from the DSM-5 classification. *Journal of Autism and Developmental Disorders, 46*(8), 2821–2829 https://doi.org/10.1007/s10803-016-2814-5

Caesar, L. G., & Kohler, P. D. (2009). Tools clinicians use: A survey of language assessment procedures used by school-based speech-language pathologists. *Communication Disorders Quarterly, 30*(4), 226–236.

Carrington, S., Leekam, S., Kent, R., Maljaars, J., Gould, J., Wing, L., … Noens, I. (2015). Signposting for diagnosis of Autism Spectrum Disorder using the Diagnostic Interview for Social and Communication Disorders (DISCO). *Research in Autism Spectrum Disorders, 9*, 45–52 https://doi.org/10.1016/j.rasd.2014.10.003

Cavenagh, P., Costelloe, S., Davis, S., & Howell, P. (2015). Characteristics of young children close to the onset of stuttering. *Communication Disorders Quarterly, 36*(3), 162–171 https://doi.org/10.1177/1525740114549955

Charman, T., Drew, A., Baird, C., & Baird, G. (2003). Measuring early language development in preschool children with autism spectrum disorder using the MacArthur Communicative Development Inventory (Infant Form). *Journal of Child Language, 30*(1), 213–236.

Choi, D., Conture, E. G., Tumanova, V., Clark, C. E., Walden, T. A., & Jones, R. M. (2018). Young children's family history of stuttering and their articulation, language and attentional abilities: An exploratory study. *Journal of Communication Disorders, 71*, 22–36 https://doi.org/10.1016/j.jcomdis.2017.11.002

Chuthapisith, J., Taycharpipranai, P., Roongpraiwan, R., & Ruangdaraganon, N. (2014). Translation and validation of the Children's Communication Checklist to evaluate pragmatic language impairment in Thai children. *Pediatrics International, 56*(1), 31–34.

Craig, A., Blumgart, E., & Tran, Y. (2009). The impact of stuttering on the quality of life in adults who stutter. *Journal of Fluency Disorders, 34*(2), 61–71.

Craig, A., & Tran, Y. (2006). Chronic and social anxiety in people who stutter. *Advances in Psychiatric Treatment, 12*, 63–68.

de la Osa, N., Granero, R., Penelo, E., & Ezpeleta, L. (2014). Usefulness of the Social and Communication Disorders Checklist (SCDC) for the assessment of social cognition in preschoolers. *European Journal of Psychological Assessment, 30*(4), 296–303 https://doi.org/10.1027/1015-5759/a000193

Dale, P. S. (1991). The validity of a parent report measure of vocabulary and syntax at 24 months. *Journal of Speech, Language, and Hearing Research, 34*(3), 565–571.

Davidow, J. H., & Scott, K. A. (2017). Intrajudge and interjudge reliability of the Stuttering Severity Instrument–Fourth Edition. *American Journal of Speech-Language Pathology, 26*(4), 1105–1119.

Dunn, L. M., & Dunn, D. M. (2007). *PPVT-4: Peabody Picture Vocabulary Test.* Minneapolis, MN: Pearson Assessments.

Dunn, L. M., Padilla, E. R., Lugo, D. E., & Dunn, L. M. (1986). *Examiner's manual for the Test de vocabulario en Imagenes Peabody: Adaptiacion Hispanoamericana.* Circle Pines, MN: American Guidance Services.

Dunn, L. M., Theriault-Whalen, C. M., & Dunn, L. M. (1993). *Manual for échelle de vocabulaire en images Peabody.* Toronto, ON: Psycan.

Eickhoff, J., Betz, S. K., & Ristow, J. (2010). Clinical procedures used by speech-language pathologists to diagnose SLI. In *Symposium on Research in Child Language Disorders.* WI: Madison.

Erickson, S., & Block, S. (2013). The social and communication impact of stuttering on adolescents and their families. *Journal of Fluency Disorders, 38*(4), 311–324 https://doi.org/10.1016/j.jfludis.2013.09.003

Eriksson, K., Hartelius, L., & Saldert, C. (2016). Participant characteristics and observed support in conversations involving people with communication disorders. *International Journal of Speech-Language Pathology, 18*(5), 439–449.

Feldman, H. M. (2005). Evaluation and management of language and speech disorders in preschool children. *Pediatrics in Review, 26*(131), 40.

Fenson, L. (2003). *MacArthur Inventarios del Desarrollo de Habilidades Comunicativas: User's guide and technical manual.* Baltimore, MD: Brookes Pub.

Fenson, L., Dale, P., Reznick, S., Thal, D., Bates, E., Hartung, J., … Reilly, J. (1993). *MacArthur communicative developmental inventories.* Baltimore: Paul H. Brookes.

Fenson, L., Dale, P. S., Reznick, J. S., Bates, E., Thal, D. J., Pethick, S. J., … Stiles, J. (1994). Variability in early communicative development. *Monographs of the Society for Research in Child Development, 59*(5), 1–173 i–185.

Foster-Cohen, S., Edgin, J. O., Champion, P. R., & Woodward, L. J. (2007). Early delayed language development in very preterm infants: Evidence from the MacArthur-Bates CDI. *Journal of Child Language, 34*(3), 655–675.

Geurts, H. M. (2007). *Handleiding CCC-2-NL. Manual CCC-2-NL.* Amsterdam: Harcourt Test Publishers.

Gibson, J., Adams, C., Lockton, E., & Green, J. (2013). Social communication disorder outside autism? A diagnostic classification approach to delineating pragmatic language impairment, high functioning autism and specific language impairment. *Journal of Child Psychology & Psychiatry, 54*(11), 1186–1197 https://doi.org/10.1111/jcpp.12079

Gillam, R. B., Logan, K. J., & Pearson, N. A. (2009). *TOCS: Test of Childhood Stuttering.* Austin, TX: Pro-Ed.

Glumbić, N., & Brojčin, B. (2012). Factor structure of the Serbian version of the Children's Communication Checklist-2. *Research in Developmental Disabilities, 33*(5), 1352–1359.

Gregg, K. (2017). Communication disorders and challenging behaviors: Supporting children's functional communication goals in the classroom. *Early Childhood Education Journal, 45*(4), 445–452.

Grzadzinski, R., Di Martino, A., Brady, E., Mairena, M. A., O'Neale, M., Petkova, E., ... Castellanos, F. X. (2011). Examining autistic traits in children with ADHD: Does the autism spectrum extend to ADHD? *Journal of Autism and Developmental Disorders, 41*(9), 1178–1191.

Guralnick, M. J., Connor, R. T., Hammond, M. A., Gottman, J. M., & Kinnish, K. (1996). The peer relations of preschool children with communication disorders. *Child Development, 67*(2), 471–489.

Hall, D. E., Lynn, J. M., Altieri, J., Segers, V. D., & Conti, D. (1987). Inter-intrajudge reliability of the stuttering severity instrument. *Journal of Fluency Disorders, 12*(3), 167–173 https://doi.org/10.1016/0094-730X(87)90023-4

Hearnshaw, S., Baker, E., & Munro, N. (2018). The speech perception skills of children with and without speech sound disorder. *Journal of Communication Disorders, 71*, 61–71 https://doi.org/10.1016/j.jcomdis.2017.12.004

Heilmann, J., Weismer, S. E., Evans, J., & Hollar, C. (2005). Utility of the MacArthur—Bates Communicative Development Inventory in identifying language abilities of late-talking and typically developing toddlers. *American Journal of Speech-Language Pathology, 14*(1), 40–51.

Helland, W. A., Biringer, E. V. A., Helland, T., & Heimann, M. (2009). The usability of a Norwegian adaptation of the Children's Communication Checklist Second Edition (CCC-2) in differentiating between language impaired and non-language impaired 6-to 12-year-olds. *Scandinavian Journal of Psychology, 50*(3), 287–292.

Hertsberg, N., & Zebrowski, P. M. (2016). Self-perceived competence and social acceptance of young children who stutter: Initial findings. *Journal of Communication Disorders, 64*, 18–31 https://doi.org/10.1016/j.jcomdis.2016.08.004

Hoffmann, A., Martens, M. A., Fox, R., Rabidoux, P., & Andridge, R. (2013). Pragmatic language assessment in Williams syndrome: A comparison of the Test of Pragmatic Language—2 and the Children's Communication Checklist—2. *American Journal of Speech-Language Pathology, 22*(2), 198–204.

Iverach, L., Jones, M., McLellan, L. F., Lyneham, H. J., Menzies, R. G., Onslow, M., & Rapee, R. M. (2016). Prevalence of anxiety disorders among children who stutter. *Journal of Fluency Disorders, 49*, 13–28 https://doi.org/10.1016/j.jfludis.2016.07.002

Ketelaars, M. P., Cuperus, J. M., van Daal, J., Jansonius, K., & Verhoeven, L. (2009). Screening for pragmatic language impairment: The potential of the children's communication checklist. *Research in Developmental Disabilities, 30*(5), 952–960 https://doi.org/10.1016/j.ridd.2009.01.006

Klee, T., Carson, D. K., Gavin, W. J., Hall, L., Kent, A., & Reece, S. (1998). Concurrent and predictive validity of an early language screening program. *Journal of Speech, Language, and Hearing Research, 41*(3), 627–641.

Law, J., Boyle, J., Harris, F., Harkness, A., & Nye, C. (2000). Prevalence and natural history of primary speech and language delay: Findings from a systematic review of the literature. *International Journal of Language and Communication Disorders, 35*, 165–188.

Laws, G., & Bishop, D. V. (2004). Pragmatic language impairment and social deficits in Williams syndrome: A comparison with Down's syndrome and specific language impairment. *International Journal of Language & Communication Disorders, 39*(1), 45–64.

Lee, H., Sim, H., Lee, E., & Choi, D. (2017). Disfluency characteristics of children with attention-deficit/hyperactivity disorder symptoms. *Journal of Communication Disorders, 65*, 54–64 https://doi.org/10.1016/j.jcomdis.2016.12.001

Leekam, S. R., Libby, S. J., Wing, L., Gould, J., & Taylor, C. (2002). The diagnostic interview for social and communication disorders: Algorithms for ICD-10 childhood autism and Wing and Gould autistic spectrum disorder. *Journal of Child Psychology and Psychiatry, 43*(3), 327–342 https://doi.org/10.1111/1469-7610.00024

Lewis, B. A., Patton, E., Freebairn, L., Tag, J., Iyengar, S. K., Stein, C. M., & Taylor, H. G. (2016). Psychosocial co-morbidities in adolescents and adults with histories of communication disorders. *Journal of Communication Disorders, 61*, 60–70.

Lidz, C. S. (1983). Dynamic assessment and the preschool child. *Journal of Psychoeducational Assessment, 1*(1), 59–72.

Light, J., & McNaughton, D. (2014). Communicative competence for individuals who require augmentative and alternative communication: A new definition for a new era of communication? *Augmentative and Alternative Communication, 30*(1), 1–18 https://doi.org/10.3109/07434618.2014.885080

Lloyd, H., Paintin, K., & Botting, N. (2006). Performance of children with different types of communication impairment on the Clinical Evaluation of Language Fundamentals (CELF). *Child Language Teaching & Therapy, 22*(1), 47–67 https://doi.org/10.1191/0265659006ct297oa

Luyster, R., Lopez, K., & Lord, C. (2007). Characterizing communicative development in children referred for autism spectrum disorders using the MacArthur-Bates Communicative Development Inventory (CDI). *Journal of Child Language, 34*(3), 623–654.

Luyster, R., Qiu, S., Lopez, K., & Lord, C. (2007). Predicting outcomes of children referred for autism using the MacArthur–Bates Communicative Development Inventory. *Journal of Speech, Language, and Hearing Research, 50*(3), 667–681.

Maljaars, J., Noens, I., Scholte, E., & van Berckelaer-Onnes, I. (2011). Evaluation of the criterion and convergent validity of the Diagnostic Interview for Social and Communication Disorders in young and low-functioning children. *Autism, 16*(5), 487–497 https://doi.org/10.1177/1362361311402857

Mandy, W., Wang, A., Lee, I., & Skuse, D. (2017). Evaluating social (pragmatic) communication disorder. *Journal of Child Psychology and Psychiatry, 58*(10), 1166–1175 https://doi.org/10.1111/jcpp.12785

Mann, W., Peña, E. D., & Morgan, G. (2014). Exploring the use of dynamic language assessment with deaf children, who use American Sign Language: Two case studies. *Journal of Communication Disorders, 52*, 16–30 https://doi.org/10.1016/j.jcomdis.2014.05.002

Månsson, H. (2000). Childhood stuttering: Incidence and development. *Journal of Fluency Disorders, 25*(1), 47–57.

McAllister, J. (2016). Behavioural, emotional and social development of children who stutter. *Journal of Fluency Disorders, 50*, 23–32 https://doi.org/10.1016/j.jfludis.2016.09.003

McLaughlin, K., & Cascella, P. W. (2008). Eliciting a distal gesture via dynamic assessment among students with moderate to severe intellectual disability. *Communication Disorders Quarterly, 29*(2), 75–81.

Mossabeb, R., Wade, K. C., Abbasi, S., Finnegan, K., & Sivieri, E. (2012). Language development survey provides a useful screening tool for language delay in preterm infants. *Clinical Pediatrics, 51*(7), 638–644.

Naderi, S., Shahbodaghi, M., Khatonabadi, S. A., Dadgar, H., & Jalaie, S. (2011). Translation of the test of childhood stuttering into Persian and investigation of validity and reliability of the test. *Journal of Modern Rehabilitation, 5*(2), 29–34.

Norbury, C. F. (2014). Practitioner review: Social (pragmatic) communication disorder conceptualization, evidence and clinical implications. *Journal of Child Psychology and Psychiatry, 55*(3), 204–216.

Ntourou, K., Anderson, J. D., & Wagovich, S. A. (2018). Executive function and childhood stuttering: Parent ratings and evidence from a behavioral task. *Journal of Fluency Disorders, 56*, 18–32 https://doi.org/10.1016/j.jfludis.2017.12.001

Nygren, G., Hagberg, B., Billstedt, E., Skoglund, A., Gillberg, C., & Johansson, M. (2009). The Swedish version of the Diagnostic Interview for Social and Communication Disorders (DISCO-10). Psychometric properties. *Journal of Autism and Developmental Disorders, 39*(5), 730–741 https://doi.org/10.1007/s10803-008-0678-z

O'Nions, E., Gould, J., Christie, P., Gillberg, C., Viding, E., & Happé, F. (2016). Identifying features of "pathological demand avoidance" using the Diagnostic Interview for Social and Communication Disorders (DISCO). *European Child & Adolescent Psychiatry, 25*(4), 407–419.

Overvliet, G. M., Besseling, R. M., van der Kruijs, S. J., Vles, J. S., Backes, W. H., Hendriksen, J. G., … Aldenkamp, A. P. (2013). Clinical evaluation of language fundamentals in Rolandic epilepsy, an assessment with CELF-4. *European Journal of Paediatric Neurology, 17*(4), 390–396.

Papaeliou, C. F., & Rescorla, L. A. (2011). Vocabulary development in Greek children: A cross-linguistic comparison using the Language Development Survey. *Journal of Child Language, 38*(4), 861–887.

Paradis, J., Emmerzael, K., & Duncan, T. S. (2010). Assessment of English language learners: Using parent report on first language development. *Journal of Communication Disorders, 43*(6), 474–497 https://doi.org/10.1016/j.jcomdis.2010.01.002

Patterson, J. L. (1998). Expressive vocabulary development and word combinations of Spanish-English bilingual toddlers. *American Journal of Speech-Language Pathology, 7*(4), 46–56.

Phelps-Terasaki, D., & Phelps-Gunn, T. (2007). *Test of Pragmatic Language (TOPL-2)*. Austin, TX: Pro-Ed.

Pieretti, R. A., & Roseberry-McKibbin, C. (2016). Assessment and intervention for English language learners with primary language impairment: Research-based best practices. *Communication Disorders Quarterly, 37*(2), 117–128 https://doi.org/10.1177/1525740114566652

Ren, Y., Rattanasone, N. X., Wyver, S., Hinton, A., & Demuth, K. (2016). Interpretation of errors made by Mandarin-speaking children on the Preschool Language Scales--5th Edition Screening Test. *Australian Journal of Educational and Developmental Psychology, 15*, 24–34.

Rescorla, L. (1989). The Language Development Survey: A screening tool for delayed language in toddlers. *The Journal of Speech and Hearing Disorders, 54*(4), 587–599.

Rescorla, L., & Alley, A. (2001). Validation of the Language Development Survey (LDS): A parent report tool for identifying language delay in toddlers. *Journal of Speech, Language, and Hearing Research, 44*(2), 434–445.

Rescorla, L., Constants, H., Białecka-Pikul, M., Stępień-Nycz, M., & Ochał, A. (2017). Polish vocabulary development in 2-year-olds: Comparisons with english using the language development survey. *Journal of Speech, Language, and Hearing Research, 60*(4), 1029–1035 https://doi.org/10.1044/2016_JSLHR-L-15-0385

Rescorla, L., Frigerio, A., Sali, M. E., Spataro, P., & Longobardi, E. (2014). Typical and delayed lexical development in Italian. *Journal of Speech, Language, and Hearing Research, 57*(5), 1792–1803.

Rescorla, L., Hadicke-Wiley, M., & Escarce, E. (1993). Epidemiological investigation of expressive language delay at age two. *First Language, 13*(37), 5–22.

Rescorla, L., Lee, Y. M., Kim, Y. A., & Oh, K. Y. (2013). Examining noun bias in the lexical development of Korean toddlers. *Journal of Speech, Language, and Hearing Research, 56*, 735–747.

Rescorla, L., Nyame, J., & Dias, P. (2016). Vocabulary development in European Portuguese: A replication study using the Language Development Survey. *Journal of Speech, Language, and*

Hearing Research, 59(6), 1484–1490 https://doi.org/10.1044/2016_JSLHR-L-15-0294

Rescorla, L., Ratner, N. B., Jusczyk, P., & Jusczyk, A. M. (2005). Concurrent validity of the Language Development Survey: Associations with the MacArthur-Bates Communicative Development Inventories: Words and sentences. *American Journal of Speech-Language Pathology, 14*(2), 156–163.

Riley, G. D., & Bakker, K. (2009). *Stuttering Severity Instrument: SSI-4*. Austin, TX: Pro-Ed.

Rudra, A., Banerjee, S., Singhal, N., Barua, M., Mukerji, S., & Chakrabarti, B. (2014). Social and communication disorders checklist--Hindi and Bengali versions. *PsycTESTS*. https://doi.org/10.1037/t60152-000

Sahli, A. S., & Belgin, E. (2017). Adaptation, validity, and reliability of the Preschool Language Scale–Fifth Edition (PLS–5) in the Turkish context: The Turkish Preschool Language Scale-5 (TPLS–5). *International Journal of Pediatric Otorhinolaryngology, 98*, 143–149 https://doi.org/10.1016/j.ijporl.2017.05.003

Skuse, D. H., James, R. S., Bishop, D. V., Coppin, B., Dalton, P., Aamodt-Leeper, G., ... Jacobs, P. A. (1997). Evidence from Turner's syndrome of an imprinted X-linked locus affecting cognitive function. *Nature, 387*(6634), 705.

Skuse, D. H., Mandy, W., Steer, C., Miller, L. L., Goodman, R., Lawrence, K., ... Golding, J. (2009). Social communication competence and functional adaptation in a general population of children: Preliminary evidence for sex-by-verbal IQ differential risk. *Journal of the American Academy of Child & Adolescent Psychiatry, 48*(2), 128–137.

Skuse, D. H., Mandy, W. P., & Scourfield, J. (2005). Measuring autistic traits: Heritability, reliability and validity of the Social and Communication Disorders Checklist. *The British Journal of Psychiatry, 187*(6), 568–572.

Stivanin, L., de Oliveira, C. C., dos Santos, F. P., dos Santos, B., & Scivoletto, S. (2016). Co-occurrence of communication disorder and psychiatric disorders in maltreated children and adolescents: Relationship with global functioning. *Revista Brasileira de Psiquiatria, 38*(1), 39–45 https://doi.org/10.1590/1516-4446-2014-1564

Taylor, L. J., & Whitehouse, A. J. (2016). Autism spectrum disorder, language disorder, and social (pragmatic) communication disorder: Overlaps, distinguishing features, and clinical implications. *Australian Psychologist, 51*(4), 287–295.

Thal, D., DesJardin, J. L., & Eisenberg, L. S. (2007). Validity of the MacArthur–Bates Communicative Development Inventories for measuring language abilities in children with cochlear implants. *American Journal of Speech-Language Pathology, 16*(1), 54–64.

Timler, G. R. (2014). Use of the Children's communication Checklist—2 for classification of language impairment risk in young school-age children with attention-deficit/hyperactivity disorder. *American Journal of Speech-Language Pathology, 23*(1), 73–83.

Tumanova, V., Choi, D., Conture, E. G., & Walden, T. A. (2018). Expressed parental concern regarding childhood stuttering and the Test of Childhood Stuttering. *Journal of Communication Disorders* https://doi.org/10.1016/j.jcomdis.2018.01.002

Turkstra, L. S. (1999). Language testing in adolescents with brain injury: A consideration of the CELF-3. *Language, Speech, and Hearing Services in Schools, 30*(2), 132–140.

van Berckelaer-Onnes, I. A., Noens, I., & Dijkxhoorn, Y. (2008). *Diagnostic Interview for Social and Communication Disorders: Nederlandse Vertaling [Diagnostic Interview for Social and Communication Disorders: Dutch Translation]*. Leiden, Netherlands: Universiteit Leiden.

Vaisanen, R., Loukusa, S., Yliherva, A., & Moilanen, I. (2014). Language and pragmatic profile in children with ADHD measured by Children's Communication Checklist 2nd edition. *Logopedics, Phoniatrics, Vocology, 39*(4), 179–187.

Vézina, M., Samson-Morasse, C., Gauthier-Desgagné, J., Fossard, M., & Sylvestre, A. (2011). Développement de la version québécoise francophone du Children's Communication Checklist–2 (CCC-2). Traduction, adaptation et équivalence conceptuelle. *Revue Canadienne D'orthophonie et D'audiologie (RCOA), 35*(3), 244–253.

Volden, J., Coolican, J., Garon, N., White, J., & Bryson, S. (2009). Brief report: Pragmatic language in autism spectrum disorder: Relationships to measures of ability and disability. *Journal of Autism and Developmental Disorders, 39*(2), 388.

Volden, J., & Phillips, L. (2010). Measuring pragmatic language in speakers with autism spectrum disorders: Comparing the Children's Communication Checklist—2 and the Test of Pragmatic Language. *American Journal of Speech-Language Pathology, 19*(3), 204–212.

Volden, J., Smith, I. M., Szatmari, P., Bryson, S., Fombonne, E., Mirenda, P., ... Zwaigenbaum, L. (2011). Using the preschool language scale, to characterize language in preschoolers with autism spectrum disorders. *American Journal of Speech-Language Pathology, 20*(3), 200–208.

Westerlund, M., Berglund, E., & Eriksson, M. a. (2006). Can severely language delayed 3-year-olds be identified at 18 months? Evaluation of a screening version of the MacArthur–Bates Communicative Development Inventories. *Journal of Speech, Language, and Hearing Research, 49*(2), 237–247.

Whitehouse, A. J., Barry, J. G., & Bishop, D. V. (2008). Further defining the language impairment of autism: Is there a specific language impairment subtype? *Journal of Communication Disorders, 41*(4), 319–336.

Wiig, E. H., Secord, W. A., & Semel, E. (2013). *Clinical Evaluation of Language Fundamentals (CELF-5)*. Bloomington, MN: NCS Pearson.

Wing, L., Leekam, S. R., Libby, S. J., Gould, J., & Larcombe, M. (2002). The diagnostic interview for social and communication disorders: Background, inter-rater reliability and clinical use. *Journal of Child Psychology and Psychiatry, 43*(3), 307–325.

Young, E. C., Diehl, J. J., Morris, D., Hyman, S. L., & Bennetto, L. (2005). The use of two language tests to identify pragmatic language problems in children with autism spectrum disorders. *Language, Speech, and Hearing Services in Schools, 36*(1), 62–72.

Zimmerman, I. L., Steiner, V. G., & Pond, R. E. (2011). *Preschool language scale* (5th ed.) *PsycTESTS*. https://doi.org/10.1037/t15141-000

Sleep Disorders: Prevalence and Assessment in Childhood

Catherine Winsper

Introduction

Sleep is an essential biological function, which is integral to good health and quality of life (Mukherjee et al., 2015). It plays a major role in recovery, energy conservation, and survival and helps regulate vital functions such as metabolism and toxin removal (Cincin et al., 2015; Davies et al., 2014). Sleep is especially important for young children, directly impacting on brain maturation and emotional and cognitive development (Sadeh, Gruber, & Raviv, 2002; Winsper & Wolke, 2014). It is therefore not surprising that children require considerably more sleep than adults (Galland, Taylor, Elder, & Herbison, 2012).

Most children grow out of any sleeping difficulties by the time they reach elementary school. However, several of the major sleep disorders increase in severity with age. Approximately 30% of children in special education for learning, behavioural, or emotional problems have a sleep disorder, which directly impacts on their daytime functioning (Luginbuehl & Kohler, 2009). Research suggests that childhood emotional and behavioural problems would significantly improve (or even in some cases remit) if sleep disorders were corrected (Chervin & Guilleminault, 1996; Dahl, Holttum, & Trubnick, 1994). Many physical health risks, such as obesity, could also be avoided with improved detection and treatment of youth sleep problems (Chervin & Guilleminault, 1996; Tauman, 2008; US Department of Health, 1993).

The current chapter begins with a definition of childhood. Next, there is a description of the normative development of sleep across this period. Then, follows a discussion of the various sleep problems found in childhood, including details on prevalence and co-occurrence with major psychiatric disorders. The subsequent sections deal with the assessment of sleep problems in childhood, detailing the various approaches to assessing sleep, the contexts in which they would be used, and associated strengths and weaknesses. The chapter rounds off by drawing together the various threads of discussion and highlighting areas for future development. Please see Box 1 for a list of acronyms used throughout the chapter.

C. Winsper (✉)
University of Warwick, Coventry, UK
e-mail: C.Winsper@warwick.ac.uk

Box 1 Acronyms Used Throughout the Chapter

ADHD	Attention deficit hyperactivity disorder
BIC-C; BIC-LST; BIC-SOA	Behavioural insomnia in childhood – combined type, limit-setting type, and sleep-onset association type
BISQ	Brief Infant Sleep Questionnaire
BPD	Borderline personality disorder
CNS	Central nervous system
CSF	Cerebrospinal fluid
CSHQ	Children's Sleep Habit Questionnaire
DSM-IV	*Diagnostic and Statistical Manual of Mental Disorders*, Fourth Edition
EDS	Excessive daytime sleepiness
EEG	Electroencephalogram
EMG	Electromyography
EOG	Electro-oculogram
GAD	Generalised anxiety disorder
ICSD	International Classification of Sleep Disorders
MDD	Major depressive disorder
MSLT	Multiple sleep latency test
NREM	Non-rapid eye movement
OSA	Obstructive sleep apnoea
PLMS	Periodic limb movements in sleep
PSG	Polysomnography
REM	Rapid eye movement
RLS	Restless leg syndrome
SDB	Sleep-disordered breathing
SDIS-C	Sleep Disorders Inventory for Students – Children's Form
SDSC	Sleep Disturbance Scale for Children
SE	Sleep efficiency
SL	Sleep latency
SOL	Sleep-onset latency
SOREMP	Sleep-onset REM-sleep periods
SRBD	Sleep-related breathing disorders
SWS	Slow-wave sleep
TST	Total sleep time
UARS	Upper airway resistance syndrome
WASO	Wake after sleep onset

Definitions of Childhood

Definitions of childhood vary and may refer to chronological age or biological development. The World Health Organization (WHO) defines a child as a person who is 19 years of age or younger. Within these parameters, an individual between the ages of 10 and 19 years is classed an adolescent (http://www.who.int/hiv/pub/guidelines/arv2013/intro/keyterms/en/). Infancy and toddlerhood refer to very early childhood, most often the period between birth and 3 years (https://www.cdc.gov/parents/infants/milestones.html). This chapter incorporates the broader definition of childhood, i.e. 0–19 years, and will cover the literature on sleep problems during infancy, childhood, and adolescence.

Normative Sleep Patterns Across Childhood

Sleep may be distinguished from wakefulness according to several physiological changes including cardiovascular and brain wave activity, posture, mobility, response to stimulation, level of alertness, eyelid movement, respiration, and body temperature. Sleep comprises alternating patterns of rapid eye movement (REM) or "active sleep" and non-rapid eye movement (NREM) or "quiet sleep". NREM sleep is further divided into three stages with increasing levels of depth. Stage three, the deepest, is referred to as delta or slow-wave sleep (SWS) (Gregory & Sadeh, 2016).

Sleep-wake patterns change dramatically during early childhood (Gregory & Sadeh, 2016). Newborns do not have an established circadian rhythm (i.e. 24-h sleep-wake cycle). Instead, their sleep is distributed throughout the day and night to accommodate frequent feeds (Galland et al., 2012). At approximately 3 months of age, circadian regulatory mechanisms become stronger and infant sleep becomes more nocturnal (Sheldon, 2002). This process is called "settling", and most infants learn to sleep throughout the night with little disruption (Hoban, 2010). Failure to achieve this developmental milestone, however, is associated with excessive and extended night waking (Hysing et al., 2014).

Daily sleep duration declines further during the toddler and preschool years. At 1 year of age, average daily sleep duration is 13.9 h. This decreases to 11.4 h at 5 years of age (Iglowstein, Jenni, Molinari, & Largo, 2003). Quantitative changes are accompanied by qualitative changes in sleep architecture. In early infancy, REM sleep constitutes approximately 50% of total sleep time. This declines to approximately 20% by age 5 (Hoban, 2010), which is a similar to the proportion exhibited by older children and adults (Anders & Guilleminault, 1975).

Decreases in sleep duration slow down throughout the school-age and adolescent years (Gregory & Sadeh, 2016). Average daily sleep duration declines from 11 h at age 6–10 h at age 9. There is a further decrease to 9 h at age 13 (Hoban, 2010). By age 16 years, adolescents sleep approximately 8 h (Iglowstein et al., 2003). This decline is paralleled by a delay in sleep-onset time, which starts in the preschool years and begins to accelerate in adolescence (Carskadon, Vieira, & Acebo, 1993).

One final developmental trend involves the localisation, distribution, and coherence of brain activity during sleep. There is a maturational shift of slow-wave activity from posterior to anterior brain regions, an increase in the coherence of EEG (electroencephalogram) activity in both left and right hemispheres, and a decrease in NREM slow-wave activity. These patterns likely reflect changes in brain organisation and synaptic pruning, which occur during adolescent development (Gregory & Sadeh, 2016). Having described normative sleep development throughout childhood, the next section deals with sleep problems and disorders that can be identified during this period.

Sleep Disorders During Childhood

Sleep is a vulnerable state that can be affected by medical, physiological, environmental, and psychological factors (Gregory & Sadeh, 2016). It is therefore not surprising that sleep problems are common throughout childhood and adolescence, affecting approximately 30–40% of youth at some point during development (Baweja, Calhoun, & Singareddy, 2013).

The classification of sleep problems in childhood is challenging. There is a wide range of sleep behaviours between "normal" and "pathologic", and definitions can be subjective. Indeed, a plethora of different sleep indices are evident within the research literature. Some researchers use a priori definitions of disturbed sleep, some rely on comparisons with normative populations, some define specific sleep behaviours (e.g. self-soothing), and others base their definition on subjective parental report (Owens, 2007). Large epidemiological studies tend to rely on one of two relatively general questions, such as "Do you have trouble falling asleep" or "Do you have problems staying asleep?" (Wong & Brower, 2012). Clinically speaking, there are several classification systems which are applicable to sleep problems in child populations. Among them are the International Classification of Sleep Disorders (ICSD) and the Diagnostic and Statistical Manual (DSM) of Mental Disorders. The ICSD-3rd edition delineates six main categories: insomnia, sleep-related breathing disorders (SRBD), central disorders of hypersomnolence (i.e. excessive sleepiness), circadian rhythm sleep-wake disorders, parasomnias, and sleep-related movement disorders (American Academy of Sleep Medicine, 2014). Of note, some of the disorders listed in the ICSD are almost exclusively found in children (e.g. behavioural insomnia of childhood), while others include diagnostic criteria for both adults and children (e.g. psychophysiologic insomnia). These latter groupings may not adequately capture features unique to paediatric populations, including developmentally specific manifestations or impacts on the caregiver (Owens, 2007).

For the remainder of this section, childhood sleep disorders will be grouped into the two broad categories of dyssomnias and parasomnias. Dyssomnias describe a difficulty in getting to sleep, remaining asleep, or excessive sleepiness. Parasomnias refer to abnormal behaviours, emotions, perceptions, or dreams that occur during or after sleep initiation (Mindell, 1993). Below follows a description of the main dyssomnias and parasomnias, including characteristic features, prevalence across development, and diagnosis. A discussion of the causes and treatment of these disorders is beyond the scope of this chapter. The interested reader is directed towards Baweja et al. (2013) for a comprehensive review.

The Dyssomnias

Insomnia

Insomnia is defined as a difficulty in initiating or maintaining sleep and/or a feeling of unrest after sleep with associated impairment in social, academic, or occupational functioning. The two most common forms of childhood insomnia are *behavioural*, which is more common in young children, and *psychophysiologic*, which is more common in adolescents (Baweja et al., 2013).

Behavioural Insomnia

Behavioural insomnia describes a difficulty in falling asleep or staying asleep. These symptoms are often referred to as sleep-onset or sleep-maintenance difficulties in the research literature (Baweja et al., 2013; Lereya, Winsper, Tang, & Wolke, 2017). The International Classification of Sleep Disorders (ICSD) delineates three types of behavioural insomnia: the sleep-onset association (BIC-SOA) type, the limit-setting type (BIC-LST), and the combined type (BIC-C), i.e. the co-occurrence of both BIC-SOA and BIC-LST (American Academy of Sleep Medicine, 2014).

Young children with BIC-SOA are unable to self-soothe to sleep at bedtime or during the night. According to the ICSD, there are four diagnostic criteria: (1) prolonged sleep onset, (2) demanding sleep-onset conditions, (3) significant delay in sleep onset in the absence of these conditions, and (4) caregiver intervention is required to help the child return to sleep. Because the skill of self-soothing is co-learned (with the caregiver) during the first few months of life (Goodlin-Jones, Burnham, Gaylor, & Anders, 2001), a diagnosis of BIC-SOA is not normally given before 6 months of age (Owens & Mindell, 2011).

BIC-LST is characterised by noncompliant behaviours at bedtime, including bed refusals, verbal protests, and repeated demands. BIC-LST is more common in children who are of preschool age or older and can result from insufficient limit setting and a lack of routine at bedtime (Hoban, 2010). Diagnostic criteria include (1) trouble initiating or maintaining sleep, (2) stalling or refusing to go to sleep at bedtime or after waking, and (3) a lack of sufficient limit setting from caregivers (American Academy of Sleep Medicine, 2005).

The Prevalence of Behavioural Insomnia

A degree of night-time waking is normal in young children, especially during infancy when one could expect, on average, two awakenings per night (Sadeh, Lavie, Scher, Tirosh, & Epstein, 1991). Around 25–50% of infants and toddlers (over 6 months of age) will experience a problematic level of night waking (Owens & Mindell, 2011). Bedtime resistance is less common in this age group affecting approximately 10–15% of toddlers, though definitive rates for night waking versus bedtime resistance are difficult to establish as many studies conflate these two problems during assessment (Owens & Mindell, 2011).

Difficulties in falling asleep and night waking remain common throughout early to middle childhood, affecting approximately 15–30% of preschoolers (Kerr & Jowett, 1994; Mindell, Meltzer, Carskadon, & Chervin, 2009). In a sample of 494 children aged 4–11 years, 37% were described by a parent as having a significant sleep problem in at least one domain; bedtime resistance (15.1%) was the most common problem (Owens, Spirito, McGuinn, & Nobile, 2000). In another study, this time an anonymous survey of parents of 987 children aged 5–12 years, bedtime resistance was again the most prevalent problem affecting 27% of children (Blader, Koplewicz, Abikoff, & Foley, 1997).

Psychophysiologic Insomnia

Psychophysiologic insomnia is characterised by excessive worry about sleep and the daytime consequences of not getting enough sleep, along with an increase in anxiety as bedtime approaches (Baweja et al., 2013). Psychophysiologic insomnia usually presents in older children and adolescents (American Academy of Sleep Medicine, 2005). It is often underpinned by predisposing factors (e.g. medical or psychiatric conditions) and can be perpetuated by caffeine or technology use, maladaptive sleep cognitions, or poor sleep habits (Owens & Mindell, 2011).

A diagnosis of insomnia according to the Diagnostic Statistical Manual (DSM) of Mental Disorders and the International Classification of Sleep Disorders (ICSD) requires that the individual experiences a difficulty in initiating/maintaining sleep, waking too early, and/or non-restorative sleep. The sleep difficulty should be related to daytime impairment and be present for at least one month (American Academy of Sleep Medicine, 2005; American Psychiatric Association, 2013).

Prevalence of Insomnia in Older Children and Adolescents
The sleep changes (e.g. sleep/wake cycle, circadian rhythm) accompanying pubertal development, in addition to the social and emotional demands of this period, make adolescence a time of heightened risk for psychophysiologic insomnia (Johnson, Roth, Schultz, & Breslau, 2006). Studies report a wide variety of prevalence estimates, ranging from 7% to 40%. In an epidemiological study of 1014 randomly selected adolescents aged 13–16 years, Johnson et al. (2006) estimated a lifetime prevalence of 11% for DSM-IV-defined insomnia; 88% of adolescents with a history of insomnia reported current insomnia, indicating that these symptoms are chronic for many youths. In a more recent study of 384 Australian adolescents aged 13–18 years, Dohnt, Gradisar, and Short (2012) reported largely similar findings though there were variations in prevalence according to the diagnostic tool. According to ICSD-II diagnosis, 10.9% of adolescents were classified as having general insomnia, while 7.8% were classified as having primary insomnia according to DSM-IV criteria. Only 3.4% were classified as having ICSD-II psychophysiological insomnia. A much higher proportion of adolescents (i.e. 34.6%) in this study reported (sub-diagnostic) insomnia symptoms.

Narcolepsy
Narcolepsy is a chronic neurological disorder characterised by excessive daytime sleepiness, sleep paralysis, cataplexy (sudden loss of skeletal muscle tone in response to emotional triggers), and sleep-related hallucinations. These four symptoms form the classic tetrad of narcolepsy (Peterson & Husain, 2008) and result from impaired arousal mechanisms and the intrusion of REM sleep onto wakefulness (Kotagal & Pianosi, 2006). Narcolepsy is relatively uncommon, affecting approximately 0.02–0.05% of individuals in Western countries (Peterson & Husain, 2008; Stores, Montgomery, & Wiggs, 2006). Age of onset of narcolepsy can vary, though symptoms often emerge between 10 and 15 years of age (Challamel et al., 1994; Kotagal, 1996). In a study of two large populations of patients in France and Quebec, Dauvilliers et al. (2001) reported a bimodal distribution of age of onset; the first peak occurred at 14.7 years and the second at 35 years.

Paediatric narcolepsy is a serious disorder. It is associated with lifelong disruptions across academic, work, and leisure domains. It is also associated with behavioural and personality changes (Nevsimalova, 2014). The exact prevalence of childhood narcolepsy is not firmly established due to a lack of studies and heterogeneity across diagnostic criteria (Nevsimalova, 2014; Peterson & Husain, 2008). The estimated incidence (i.e. occurrence of new cases) in a paediatric referral clinic in China was low (0.04%), with a male to female ratio of three to one (Han et al., 2001).

Due to its variable phenotype (i.e. observable characteristics), narcolepsy is under-recognised and often diagnosed very late, e.g. up to a decade after the onset of symptoms (Peterson & Husain, 2008). Childhood symptoms may differ markedly from adult symptoms, which can lead to misdiagnosis. This is unfortunate as early identification and treatment can greatly improve the quality of life of patients, especially as more treatment options become available (Nevsimalova, 2014).

Diagnosing Paediatric Narcolepsy
To be diagnosed with narcolepsy, the DSM-5 (the most recent version of the Diagnostic and Statistical Manual) requires that the patient exhibits excessive daytime sleepiness (EDS) in association with one of the following: (1) cataplexy, (2) CSF (cerebrospinal) hypocretin

deficiency, (3) REM-sleep latency ≤15 min on nocturnal polysomnography (PSG), or (4) mean sleep latency ≤8 min on multiple sleep latency testing (MSLT) with ≥2 sleep-onset REM-sleep periods (SOREMPs). The ICSD-3 criteria require EDS in addition to (1) cataplexy and either positive MSLT/PSG findings or CSF hypocretin deficiency; (2) MSLT criteria as delineated in the DSM-5, except that a SOREMP on PSG may count as one of the SOREMPs required on MSLT; and (3) for narcolepsy type 1, there should be the presence of cataplexy or documented CSF hypocretin deficiency, and for narcolepsy type 2, there is no cataplexy and normal or undocumented CSF hypocretin levels (Ruoff & Rye, 2016).

Sleep-Disordered Breathing

Sleep-disordered breathing (SDB) in childhood covers a wide spectrum of disorders of increasing severity including primary snoring, upper airway resistance syndrome (UARS), obstructive sleep apnoea (OSA), and obstructive hypoventilation (apnoea, oxygen desaturation, plus hypercarbia) (Baweja et al., 2013). SDB results from a structurally narrow airway in combination with a reduction in neuromuscular tone and increased airway collapsibility. Presentation of childhood SDB varies by age and can range from snoring and frequent arousals to enuresis (bed wetting) and hyperactivity. If left untreated, SDB can lead to complications including learning difficulties, memory loss, hypertension, depression, and poor growth (Sinha & Guilleminault, 2010).

Obstructive sleep apnoea (OSA) is characterised by prolonged partial upper airway obstruction, intermittent complete (obstructive apnoea) or partial (hypopnoea) obstruction, or both prolonged and intermittent obstruction that disrupts ventilation during sleep, normal sleep patterns, or both (Sinha & Guilleminault, 2010). The most common causes of childhood OSA are adenotonsillar hypertrophy, craniofacial anomalies, and neuromuscular disorders (Kotagal & Pianosi, 2006). The ICSD defines apnoea as a cessation of airflow over two or more respiratory cycles (American Academy of Sleep Medicine, 2005). The definition of hypopnoea is more variable, though many agree that a reduction in airflow of at least 30% is required (with or without arousal) and oxygen desaturation of 3–4%. The mildest form of OSA-UARS has more subtle indications (as measured objectively with PSG), with an increased effort in breathing often leading to an arousal (Sinha & Guilleminault, 2010).

Prevalence of SDB

As with narcolepsy, the prevalence of SDB is difficult to ascertain, as definitions vary and the childhood condition was only recently recognised. In a meta-analysis, the prevalence of parent-reported snoring (the least severe manifestation of SDB) was 7.5%, while the prevalence of OSA (diagnosed with varying criteria) was 1–4% (Lumeng & Chervin, 2008).

Delayed Sleep Phase Syndrome

Delayed sleep phase syndrome (DSPS) is a circadian rhythm sleep disorder, involving a significant delay in the cycle of sleep and wakefulness in a person's 24-h day (Winsper, Tang, et al., 2017). Patients with DSPS can initiate and maintain sleep on their delayed schedule, i.e. they show relatively normal sleep quantity and quality (Kotagal & Pianosi, 2006). Problems arise when they attempt to synchronise their schedules with the demands of society, because their sleep cycle is out of phase with usual work or school demands. Potential consequences of DSPS include sleep loss, disturbed sleep, excessive daytime sleepiness, and impaired waking function (Crowley, Acebo, & Carskadon, 2007). DSPS is more common in adolescents and young adults, particularly males (Kotagal & Pianosi, 2006). Hormones are believed to play a role in triggering the syndrome (Garcia & Applebee, 2013), as are the social and academic demands of this period (Baweja et al., 2013). Thus, DSPS may represent an extreme manifestation of the homeostatic and circadian changes experienced in adolescence (Crowley et al., 2007).

The ICSD (American Academy of Sleep Medicine, 2005) lists DSPS under the umbrella category of circadian rhythm sleep disorders and delineates three general criteria: (1) a persistent pattern of sleep disturbance resulting from a mismatch between endogenous rhythm and external factors, (2) sleep disruption which leads to insomnia and/or excessive daytime sleepiness, and (3) impaired social and occupational functioning associated with the sleep disturbance. The diagnosis of DSPS should be differentiated from school avoidance, which is often found in adolescents with delinquent and antisocial behaviour. Sleep logs and wrist actigraphy (see later sections) may be helpful in establishing the diagnosis (Kotagal & Pianosi, 2006).

Prevalence of DSPS
As with other sleep disorders, prevalence estimates for DSPS vary widely (Crowley et al., 2007). In a large sample of adolescents, the rate of DSM-IV circadian disorders was only 0.4% (Ohayon, Roberts, Zulley, Smirne, & Priest, 2000). Similar prevalence rates have been reported in studies from Japan (0.4%) and Norway (0.17%) (Garcia, Rosen, & Mahowald, 2001). However, other studies indicate higher prevalence of 7–16% (American Academy of Sleep Medicine, 2005; American Psychiatric Association, 2001), and a meta-analysis of 41 studies found that adolescent sleep is typified by late bed and waking-up times (Gradisar, Gardner, & Dohnt, 2011).

Sleep-Related Movement Disorders
Restless leg syndrome (RLS), also known as Willis-Ekbom disease, is a common neurological disorder (Pereira Jr, Pradella-Hallinan, & Alves, 2014). RLS is characterised by insomnia due to a "creepy or crawling" feeling, which is accompanied by an urge to move the limbs (Kotagal & Pianosi, 2006). Patients with RLS may experience daytime sleepiness, fatigue, and inattentiveness. RLS is diagnosed by the following criteria: (1) symptoms occur when the patient is at rest; (2) symptoms cause an impetus to move the legs; (3) the patient experiences relief during movement; and (4) the condition only occurs at night or is worse at night (Pereira et al., 2014). In many patients with RLS, polysomnography assessments will reveal periodic limb movements (i.e. intermittent and repetitive movements) in sleep (PLMS) (Baweja et al., 2013).

Prevalence of RLS
In population-based studies of children and adolescents in the United Kingdom, the United States, and Turkey, the prevalence of RLS ranges from 2% to 4% (Picchietti et al., 2007; Turkdogan, Bekiroglu, & Zaimoglu, 2011; Yilmaz, Kilincaslan, Aydin, & Kor, 2011).

The Parasomnias

Parasomnias are recurrent episodes of behaviour, experiences, or physiological changes that intrude on sleep (American Academy of Sleep Medicine, 2005). After insomnia and nocturnal awakenings, they are the most common sleep disorders in children. Most parasomnias occur in otherwise healthy children and tend to remit by adolescence. Thus, they are often viewed as transient disruptive phenomena rather than medical conditions (Laberge, Tremblay, Vitaro, & Montplaisir, 2000). When parasomnias occur frequently, however, they can impact on sleep continuity and reduce its restorative effects, leading to daytime fatigue and somnolence, i.e. sleepiness (Laberge et al., 2000). Parasomnia episodes can occur during various stages of sleep and tend to be grouped into non-REM and REM parasomnias (Baweja et al., 2013). These will be discussed in turn.

Non-REM Parasomnias
Non-REM (NREM) parasomnias occur during N3 stage (i.e. deep or delta-wave) sleep and are thus common during the first third of the night when N3 sleep is most abundant. NREM parasomnias include night terrors, sleepwalking, confusional arousals, somniloquy (sleep talking), and nocturnal enuresis (Baweja et al., 2013).

Somniloquy is the most common parasomnia (Laberge et al., 2000). In a population survey of 2,022 school children aged 3–10 years, over half demonstrated somniloquy at least once a year (Reimão & Lefévre, 1980). Confusional arousals are more common in toddlers, while sleepwalking and night terrors increase during the first decade of life. Frequent sleepwalking affects approximately 2–3% of children, though up to

40% will exhibit at least one episode (Klackenberg, 1982; Laberge et al., 2000).

Night terrors are described as an arousal response associated with feelings of fear, a loud piercing scream, and an autonomic activation. There are large disparities in reported prevalence rates of night terrors. In a study of 6–12-year-olds, 6.2% experienced at least one night terror episode per year (Vela-Bueno, 1985). In a more recent study, Laberge et al. (2000) reported a higher overall prevalence of 17.3% in children aged 3–13 years. Variations in prevalence likely reflect differences in definitions, sampling methodologies, and time spans, and the conflation of night terrors and nightmares, especially in the retrospective literature.

Nocturnal enuresis is common in children aged 6–12 years. According to the ICSD, nocturnal enuresis is present if a child over 5 years of age wets the bed more than twice weekly (American Academy of Sleep Medicine, 2005). Primary enuresis (i.e. the child has never been persistently dry at night) is associated with a family history of the problem, developmental lag, or lower bladder capacity. Secondary enuresis (a recurrence of bed wetting following a year or more of bladder control) is more likely to be associated with emotional distress or an underlying medical condition (Robson, 2008). Nocturnal enuresis becomes less common with advancing age. It affects approximately 15% of 3–10-year-olds and only 2% of 13-year-olds (Laberge et al., 2000).

REM Parasomnias

REM parasomnias typically occur during the early hours of the morning when REM sleep is more abundant (Kotagal, 2009). REM-sleep behaviour disorder is characterised by motoric re-enactment of dreams due to a failure to inhibit skeletal muscle activity (via the nucleus reticularis gigantocellularis). REM-sleep behaviour has been associated with narcolepsy, brain stem tumour, autism spectrum disorder, and the use of selective serotonin reuptake inhibitors (Baweja et al., 2013).

Nightmares occur during REM sleep and are thought to result from waking up during a frightening dream. Nightmares are distinguished from night terrors as the child fully awakens, responds to consolation from the parent, and has a recollection of dream content. Nightmares during childhood are relatively common. They affect over half of school-aged children occasionally, though only 3% frequently (Smedje, Broman, & Hetta, 1999). Persistent nightmares may signal an underlying psychological problem or future psychopathology (Lereya et al., 2017).

Sleep in Children with Psychiatric Disorders

Considering the importance of sleep to brain development and information processing, it is unsurprising that insufficient sleep is linked to compromised cognitive, emotional, and behavioural regulation throughout childhood (Winsper & Wolke, 2014). The relationships between sleep problems and psychiatric disturbances in childhood are complex, but very relevant for clinicians (Baweja et al., 2013). The DSM-5 lists sleep disturbances among the criteria for a number of psychiatric disorders, e.g. depression and bipolar disorder (American Psychiatric Association, 2013). An understanding of co-occurring sleep and psychiatric difficulties may help elucidate the progression of symptoms, aid in early identification and prevention, and inform nosology, i.e. the classification of disorders (Gregory & Sadeh, 2012).

Sleep and Depression

Several reviews have examined associations between sleep and depression in children and adolescents. The interested reader is directed towards Lofthouse, Gilchrist, and Splaingard (2009) for a more detailed discussion. Children with depression symptoms (or major depressive disorder, MDD) often experience sleep problems, including insomnia, nightmares (Liu et al., 2007; Sivertsen, Harvey, Lundervold, & Hysing, 2014), and OSA (Yilmaz, Sedky, & Bennett, 2013). Sleep problems can be a marker of more severe depression and importantly signal an increased risk of suicidality (Liu & Buysse, 2006; Winsper & Tang, 2014).

While cross-sectional studies indicate increased likelihood of sleep problems in youths with depression, prospective studies are needed to understand potential aetiological associations (i.e. do sleep problems lead to depression or does depression lead to sleep problems)?

Several studies report predictive associations between sleep problems and subsequent depression (Gregory, Rijsdijk, Lau, Dahl, & Eley, 2009; Roane & Taylor, 2008; Roberts & Duong, 2013). Greene, Gregory, Fone, and White (2015), for example, found that 5-year-old children with parent-reported severe sleep problems were at significantly increased risk of depression 30 years later, even after controlling for several important confounders. There is also evidence that depression symptoms may predict later sleep problems. Roberts and Duong (2013) reported a reciprocal relationship between insomnia and depression among adolescents (i.e. they found that baseline insomnia increased subsequent risk of major depression and, conversely, that depression increased risk of subsequent insomnia).

Overall, the weight of evidence appears to indicate that sleep disturbances predict depression rather than vice versa (Alvaro, Roberts, & Harris, 2013; Lovato & Gradisar, 2014).

For a discussion of potential mechanisms underpinning these complex associations, see Gregory and Sadeh (2016).

Sleep and Anxiety

Anxiety is associated with a range of sleep disturbances in childhood. Approximately 80–90% of anxious youth have at least one sleep-related problem. The most common of which include feeling fatigued, insomnia, nightmares, and a refusal to sleep alone (Peterman, Carper, & Kendall, 2015).

Objective measures (i.e. polysomnography) indicate that children with anxiety disorders experience less slow-wave sleep (SWS) and wake more during the night than those with MDD or no psychiatric disorder (Forbes et al., 2008). Some studies suggest nuanced associations depending on subtype of anxiety. Alfano, Reynolds, Scott, Dahl, and Mellman (2013) found that children with generalised anxiety disorder (GAD) had longer sleep-onset latency (SOL) and reduced REM latency compared to controls. Chase and Pincus (2011) reported specific associations between separation anxiety disorder and nightmares and children walking and talking in their sleep and between social phobia and fatigue.

As observed in the depression literature, it appears that sleep problems in childhood may predict later anxiety (Jansen et al., 2011; Shanahan, Copeland, Angold, Bondy, & Costello, 2014). Again, there is some evidence for bidirectional associations (Shanahan et al., 2014), though sleep disturbance may be more likely to predict anxiety symptoms than vice versa (Jansen et al., 2011).

Sleep and Bipolar Disorder

Disturbed sleep is a feature of both manic (e.g. decreased sleep requirement) and depressive (e.g. insomnia or hypersomnia) episodes in bipolar disorder (American Psychiatric Association, 2013). Meta-analyses indicate a decreased need for sleep in paediatric populations with mania (Kowatch, Youngstrom, Danielyan, & Findling, 2005). Other studies demonstrate links between early-onset bipolar disorder and insomnia symptoms (Faedda, Baldessarini, Glovinsky, & Austin, 2004; Lofthouse, Fristad, Splaingard, & Kelleher, 2007). Further (though preliminary) evidence indicates that youth with bipolar disorder may also be more likely to experience parasomnias and enuresis (Gregory & Sadeh, 2016).

It is suggested that sleep disturbance may be a prodrome for early-onset bipolar disorder (Faedda et al., 2004; Lunsford-Avery, Judd, Axelson, & Miklowitz, 2012), though the mechanisms via which sleep impacts on symptom development are presently unknown (Gregory & Sadeh, 2016).

Sleep and Psychosis

The majority of research on associations between sleep and psychotic (or schizophrenic spectrum) disorders has focused on adults (Gregory & Sadeh, 2016). Nevertheless, there is growing interest in sleep-psychosis associations in young people, reflecting an awareness of the high prevalence of psychotic symptoms in early life (Poulton et al., 2000; Singh, Winsper, Wolke, & Bryson, 2014).

Concurrent associations between psychotic symptoms and sleep disturbances (e.g. insomnia, excessive daytime sleepiness, and cataplexy) have been reported in adolescent populations (Lee, Cho, Cho, Jang, & Kim, 2012). There is also evidence of prospective associations. In a large UK community study of over 4, 000 children, previous nightmares and sleep terrors predicted psychotic symptoms at 12 (Fisher et al., 2014) and 18 years (Thompson et al., 2015). In a study of high-risk adolescents and young adults, sleep disturbances were found to predict first episode psychosis (Ruhrmann et al., 2010). This prospective evidence supports that sleep could play a role (or is a prodromal symptom) in the development of psychosis (Gregory & Sadeh, 2016).

Sleep and Borderline Personality Disorder

Although disturbed sleep is not listed as one of the DSM diagnostic criteria for borderline personality disorder (BPD), associations between BPD and a variety of sleep problems are commonly reported in the adult literature (Winsper, Tang, et al., 2017). Studies of children and adolescents are sparse due to historical controversy regarding the BPD diagnosis in younger populations (Winsper, Lereya, et al., 2016). Nevertheless, a small number of studies support that youngsters with BPD may suffer from sleep disturbances.

In a very recent community study, Lereya et al. (2017) found that chronic nightmares in childhood predicted BPD symptoms in early adolescence and also mediated (i.e. partly explained) associations between abuse, harsh parenting, and subsequent BPD. Dagan, Stein, Steinbock, Yovel, and Hallis (1998) found that adolescents with BPD were more susceptible to DSPS. Finally, Huỳnh, Guilé, Breton, and Godbout (2016) found that adolescents with BPD experienced wider sleep variability between weekdays and weekends and hypothesised that sleep-wake pattern disruptions could contribute to BPD symptoms in adolescents. In view of the strong and complex associations between BPD, suicidality, and sleep (Balestrieri et al., 2006; Winsper & Tang, 2014), this area merits future research and clinical attention.

Sleep and Attention-Deficit Hyperactivity Disorder

Approximately 25–30% of children and adolescents with attention-deficit hyperactivity disorder (ADHD) have sleep problems (Weiss & Salpekar, 2010). Children with ADHD are more likely to sleep poorly and be diagnosed with OSA and PLMS (Cortese, Faraone, Konofal, & Lecendreux, 2009; Sedky, Bennett, & Carvalho, 2014). Meta-analytic studies indicate that children with ADHD have lower sleep efficiency, more sleep stage shifts, and a higher apnoea-hypopnea index (Cortese et al., 2009; Sadeh, Pergamin, & Bar-Haim, 2006). Parents of children with ADHD commonly report bedtime struggles, delayed sleep onset, increased night waking, restless sleep, and reduced sleep duration. As observed in the anxiety literature, sleep associations may vary according to subtypes of ADHD. Mayes, Calhoun, Bixler, Vgontzas, et al. (2009), for example, found that sleep problems were associated with ADHD combined type, but not ADHD inattentive type.

Prospective associations between sleep and ADHD are reported (Scott et al., 2013), again suggesting that sleep disturbance may play an aetiological role in the development of psychopathology (Gregory & Sadeh, 2016). Conversely, ADHD may contribute to sleep problems, e.g. psychostimulants used to treat ADHD may contribute to insomnia symptoms (Cohen-Zion & Ancoli-Israel, 2004).

Sleep and Autism

Sleep problems (according to parental report) occur in over half of autistic children (Mayes, Calhoun, Bixler, & Vgontzas, 2009). In comparison to healthy controls, children with autism have more trouble falling asleep, wake more during the night, wake earlier in the morning, sleep less, sleep talk-and-walk more during sleep, have more nightmares, and wet the bed more often (Krakowiak, Goodlin-Jones, Hertz-Picciotto, Croen, & Hansen, 2008; Mayes, Calhoun, Bixler, & Vgontzas, 2009). A recent meta-analysis of objective assessments (including actigraphy and polysomnography) confirmed that children with autism spectrum disorders have small but discernible differences across sleep parameters, including less TST, longer SL periods, and decreased SE. These findings are notable as poor sleep in autism can intensify symptoms and reduce daytime cognitive and adaptive functioning (Schreck, Mulick, & Smith, 2004; Taylor, Schreck, & Mulick, 2012).

Sleep in Mental Retardation and Neurologic Conditions

Parent-reported sleep problems are approximately 2–4 times more common in children with mental retardation in comparison to healthy children (Quine, 1991). Children with Down syndrome demonstrate less REM sleep and increased occurrence of SDB (de Miguel-Díez, Villa-Asensi, & Alvarez-Sala, 2003; Diomedi et al., 1999). Both subjective and objective measures indicate a high frequency of sleep problems in children with epilepsy and cerebral palsy (Quine, 1991), traumatic brain injury (Bandla & Splaingard, 2004), chromosomal disorders, brain malformations (Grigg-Damberger, 2004), and brain damage (Halpern & Baumeister, 1995).

Sleep in Children with Medical Disorders

The respiratory, cardiovascular, and gastrointestinal systems undergo significant physiological changes during sleep (Bandla & Splaingard, 2004). Hence, disturbed sleep can lead to an increased risk of diabetes, hypertension, and changes in immune response, among other problems (Bixler et al., 2008; Gottlieb et al., 2005). Equally, medical conditions can impact on sleep. Obese children and those with progressive neuromuscular disease, scoliosis, and craniofacial abnormalities are at increased risk of developing SRBDs and nocturnal hypoventilation (Bandla & Splaingard, 2004). Children with asthma have reduced mean sleep time and increased number (and duration) of nocturnal awakenings (Sadeh, Horowitz, Wolach-Benodis, & Wolach, 1998). Young children with gastroesophageal reflux may have trouble initiating sleep, increased nocturnal awakenings, and excessive daytime sleepiness (Ghaem et al., 1998).

In a cross-sectional study of 700 young children, insomnia symptoms were significantly associated with gastrointestinal regurgitation and headaches after controlling for socio-economic status and a range of mental health problems (e.g. ADHD, learning disorder). Overall, findings underline the importance of routinely inquiring about sleeping difficulties when children present to primary care with medical issues (Singareddy et al., 2009). Considering the high levels of co-occurrence between medical problems, psychiatric disorders, and disturbed sleep (Dixon-Gordon, Whalen, Layden, & Chapman, 2015), future studies should examine the synergistic processes which maintain this triad of problems (Winsper & Tang, 2014).

Assessing Sleep Problems in Childhood

By now it should be evident that sleep is a complex phenomenon, which can be examined on various levels including brain activity (e.g. EEG), behaviour (e.g. lack of movement), and subjective report (e.g. sleep diary). Furthermore, there are numerous elements of sleep to consider such as duration, sleep stage, distribution throughout the day, and quality (Sadeh, 2015). In reflection of this complexity, many types of assessment tool have been developed. These can be broadly categorised into objective and subjective measures.

Objective tools include polysomnography (PSG), videosomnography, actigraphy, smartphone applications, and direct observation. Subjective measures include sleep diaries and questionnaires (Gregory & Sadeh, 2016; Sadeh, 2015). Below follows a description of each method (see Table 1 for a summary comparison of these methods).

Polysomnography

Polysomnography (PSG) is considered the "gold standard" of sleep assessment in adults (Thoman & Acebo, 1995). While it is also highly rated for use in child populations, it is not suitable for very young children (see later discussion).

Table 1 A summary of objective and subjective methodologies for assessing sleep in childhood

Assessment method	Description	Sleep parameters assessed	Strengths	Weaknesses
Polysomnography (PSG)	Collects data via sensors attached to the skin. Usually lab based, but ambulatory PSG also available	Brain activity Sleep architecture Sleep stages Sleep quality Arousals Breathing patterns Oxygen saturation Eye and leg movements	Provides rich data which can aid in the diagnosis of a range of disorders, e.g. OSA, REM parasomnias, narcolepsy, REM-sleep disorders, insomnia Researcher has considerable control over conditions	Expensive Usual unnatural environment Intrusive Labour-intensive scoring Difficult to perform in young children and those with certain disorders, e.g. autism Less informative for behavioural insomnia Some data parameters have insufficient reliability and validity
Videosomnography	Records night-time sleep via a camera (s) installed in the child's bedroom	Specific behaviours (e.g. waking, night terrors) Caregivers' intervention	Relatively nonintrusive, so usually well tolerated by child Records sleep in child's natural environment	Relatively time intensive as requires installation, visual inspection, and scoring May be security and privacy concerns Recording may miss some sleep patterns if the child's position obscures view
Direct observational assessment	Conducted by trained observers who complete real-time scoring of sleep and wakefulness states	Alert Non-alert waking Fuss or cry Drowse Daze or sleep-wake transition Active sleep Quiet sleep Active-quiet transition sleep	Has been described as gold standard measure for very young children May be done in the child's natural environment Provides rich information on sleep and wake patterns	Very labour intensive Usually limited to a few hours Only applicable for infants and very young children May interfere with family routines and threaten privacy

(continued)

Table 1 (continued)

Assessment method	Description	Sleep parameters assessed	Strengths	Weaknesses
Actigraphy	Watch-like device which continuously monitors body movements	Information on sleep-wake patterns	Can distinguish between sleep- disturbed and control infants Ideal for assessment of sleep schedule disorders as enables continuous monitoring for prolonged periods Allows assessment in child's natural environment	Only measures activity, i.e. no direct data on sleep stages, etc. Less clinical utility in assessing sleep onset Not tolerated by all children Logistical costs are relatively high Artefacts related to external motion and device removal can threaten validity
Smartphone applications	Use high-quality sensors (which detect movement and sound) to draw inferences about sleep	Sleep apnoea	Relatively new, promising assessment tool for medical problems including sleep	Lack of validation studies due to novelty
Sleep diaries/logs	Chart filled in daily by parent or child (if older) over several weeks Typically competed in the morning for the previous night	Sleep-onset latency (SOL) Wake after sleep onset (WASO)	Cost effective Can be reliable Useful for assessment and treatment monitoring Provides quantitative data on sleep patterns and trends May provide more accurate data on some sleep parameters (e.g. duration) in comparison to questionnaires	Can place considerable burden on parents which can lead to compliance issues Response bias Parents may not be aware of all their child's sleep behaviours
Questionnaires	Often administered in large epidemiological studies to parents or (older) children Used as a screening tool in clinical settings	A wide range of sleep problems (see Tables 2 and 3 for more details)	Cost effective Questionnaires developed for a wide range of sleep parameters Subjective reports may provide unique additional (to objective measures) information	Response bias Compliance issues Not all questionnaires are well validated

PSG is usually conducted in the laboratory over one or two nights, though portable devices are also available. PSG collects data via sensors attached to the skin. The child is required to tolerate these sensors for the duration of the study (Gregory & Sadeh, 2016). The most common features recorded with PSG include behaviour, respiration, eye movements (EOG), brain electrical activity (EEG), muscle tone (EMG) or motor activity, and heart rate (ECG). Thoman and Acebo (1995) discuss these parameters in detail.

Standardised methods have been developed for scoring polysomnography data collected from infants and children (Iber, Ancoli-Israel, Chesson, & Quan, 2007; Thoman & Acebo, 1995). These can vary according to developmental stage. Once infants reach 4 months of age, EEG signals become more differentiated and contain landmarks similar to those observed in adults. At this point, the researcher may use criteria adapted from adult standards (Thoman & Acebo, 1995). Guidelines also exist for the coding of specific sleep phenomena, e.g. arousals, leg movements (American Sleep Disorders Association, 1992), and for the use of PSG in clinical practice (Kushida et al., 2005).

There are several advantages to assessing sleep with PSG. First, it provides the most detailed information on sleep-related features. This rich data is invaluable for clinical research and can aid in the diagnosis of a range of sleep disorders including sleep apnoea, periodic movements in sleep, parasomnias, seizures, narcolepsy, REM-sleep disorders, and insomnia (Sadeh, 2015). Second, it can also be used to assess daytime sleepiness through the multiple sleep latency test (MSLT). The MSLT is designed to give individuals several opportunities (i.e. four or five planned nap opportunities) to fall asleep throughout the day. PSG can then be used to measure latency to sleep onset (Kotagal & Pianosi, 2006). Third, detailed PSG recordings can be fully stored to facilitate complex computations such as spectral analysis of density and localisation of EEG frequencies and cyclic alternating patterns. Such analyses can provide important information on sleep instability (Parrino, Ferri, Bruni, & Terzano, 2012). Finally, as PSG is usually conducted in the lab, it gives the researcher a great degree of control over conditions (Sadeh, 2015).

While PSG is often considered the most reliable method of studying sleep, there are some limitations associated with its use, especially in younger children (Thoman & Acebo, 1995). First, PSG requires that infants and young children are attached to sensors and must sleep under unnatural conditions. Children (particularly those with special needs or autism) can be sensitive to changes in normal sleep conditions, potentially leading to the collection of unrepresentative data (Sitnick, Goodlin-Jones, & Anders, 2008). Second, PSG is expensive and inconvenient, which usually limits the assessment period to just one or two nights. This can further compromise the representativeness of the data. Third, young children, and especially infants, often sleep at unexpected times (e.g. sporadically throughout the day). PSG would miss these unexpected sleep episodes (Sadeh, 2015).

Videosomnography

Video recordings are a commonly used assessment method in child development research. In videosomnography, one or more video cameras are installed in the child's bedroom to record (and later examine) night-time sleep patterns and any associated parental interventions (Sadeh, 2015). Less formally, home videos may be used to document parent-reported sleep episodes (e.g. night terrors) for later clinical evaluation (Sadeh, 2015). Videosomnography can provide information on sleep-wake states, percentage of time spent sleeping, and wake after sleep onset (WASO) (Hodge, Parnell, Hoffman, & Sweeney, 2012). Video studies have helped illuminate night-time sleep-wake patterns and the development of self-soothing skills in very young children (Anders, Halpern, & Hua, 1992; Burnham, Goodlin-Jones, Gaylor, & Anders, 2002).

The main advantage of videosomnography is that it facilitates the direct assessment of sleep in the child's natural environment (Sadeh, 2015). Further, in comparison to more intrusive methods such as PSG, videosomnography is well tolerated by children, including sensitive groups such as those with autism (Hodge et al., 2012; Sitnick et al., 2008).

This approach also has limitations. First, home installation is required, which can involve safety and privacy issues. Second, the video cameras can only detect movement in a predetermined location (Hodge et al., 2012). Thus, interruptions in data collection may occur due to unfortunate positioning of the camera or the child's movements during the night (Sadeh, 2015). Finally, videotaping relies on parents remembering to activate the equipment prior to sleep onset (Sitnick et al., 2008).

There is some evidence for the validity of videosomnography in assessing child sleep. Sitnick et al. (2008) compared data from videosomnography and actigraphy assessments across several sleep domains (i.e. sleep latency, total sleep time, and WASO) in school-aged children. They considered videosomnography to be the benchmark against which to assess the accuracy of actigraphy. While overall agreement between the two assessment tools was good (94%), actigraphy had poor agreement for detecting night awakenings in comparison to the video observations. The authors concluded that differences across the two methods were due to the methodological limitations associated with actigraphy (Hodge et al., 2012) – more on this later. Anders and Sostek (1976) confirmed the validity of videosomnography for infants at 2 and 8 weeks of age by comparing video recordings to polygraphic measures. They reported an interrater reliability (i.e. agreement between raters) of 0.92 for the video recordings. The overall product-moment correlation between polygraphic and video measures was a respectable 0.79. In a later study, Thoman, Ingersoll, and Acebo (1991) reported significant observer and measurement reliability when comparing the derived sleep states from video recordings to behavioural observations.

Direct Behavioural Observation

Direct behavioural observation is most commonly used for assessing the sleep patterns of infants. In fact, it is often considered the "gold standard" of sleep assessment for very young children. In the earliest months of life, sleep cannot be delineated from EEG patterns alone. These states, however, may be reliably distinguished behaviourally. For this reason, behavioural observations are often used as an adjunct to PSG recordings during early infancy (Thoman & Acebo, 1995).

During behavioural observation, trained researchers complete a real-time scoring of sleep and wakefulness states over a designated period. Observation usually takes place in the child's home or a nursery setting (Sadeh, 2015). The following eight states have been derived from direct observations: (1) alert, (2) non-alert waking, (3) fuss or cry, (4) drowse, (5) daze or sleep-wake transition, (6) active sleep, (7) quiet sleep, and (8) active-quiet transition sleep (Thoman, 1990). A good level of reliability has been reported for these sleep-wake states in infants (including premature) and young children (Sadeh, 2015; Thoman & Acebo, 1995). In addition, they have demonstrated predictive validity (e.g. inconsistent states predict later mental disabilities) in several studies (Sadeh, 2015; Thoman, 1990; Thoman & Acebo, 1995).

One key advantage of behavioural observations is that they record waking (in addition to sleeping) states (Thoman & Acebo, 1995). Waking and sleeping comprise a system of interrelated state behaviours serving several important functions. Therefore, an understanding of these states can provide key information on central nervous system (CNS) regulatory controls (Thoman, 1990). Another benefit of direct observations is that they are minimally intrusive and can be conducted in the child's own home (Thoman & Acebo, 1995).

This approach does have some drawbacks. First, it is labour intensive. Assessment can be limited by human resources, such as observer attentiveness and endurance, and the availability of sequential observers. Second, direct observations are difficult to conduct throughout the night, though they may be facilitated with the use of a dim light (Thoman & Acebo, 1995). Further, observation can be complemented with the simultaneous recording of respiration using a pressure-sensitive pad (Sadeh, 2015).

Actigraphy

Actigraphy utilises a wristwatch-like device to continuously monitor body movements over extended periods. These small devices can be attached to the ankles of infants and toddlers and the wrists of older children and enable monitoring in the child's natural environment (Sadeh, 2015). Based on the pattern and intensity of the movements recorded by actigraphy, a computer analysis provides information on sleep-wake states, e.g. data on the total amount of sleep time and distribution of sleep episodes (Hodge et al., 2012).

Actigraphy data is ideal for the visual analysis of activity levels, which may be used to evaluate treatment efficacy or corroborate parental report of child sleep (Meltzer, Montgomery-Downs, Insana, & Walsh, 2012). As actigraphy facilitates continual monitoring over extended periods, it may be particularly useful for assessing insomnia and circadian rhythm disorders (Kotagal & Pianosi, 2006). It is also used to monitor sleep during naturalistic studies of sleep restriction or other imposed demands (Fallone, Seifer, Acebo, & Carskadon, 2002). The American Academy of Sleep Medicine practice parameters state that actigraphy is indicated for delineating sleep patterns in infants and children when traditional sleep monitoring by PSG is difficult to perform or interpret (Morgenthaler et al., 2006).

The data collected from actigraphy can be translated into validated sleep measures. Nevertheless, it is cautioned that actigraphy sleep estimates should only be used when recording device and sleep measure (e.g. TST) are established as valid in comparison to a gold standard assessment such as PSG or direct observation. In relation to actigraphy measures, researchers define *sensitivity* as the proportion of sleep epochs (e.g. 30-second duration of sleep with a sleep stage designation) accurately scored as sleep according to both PSG and actigraphy. *Specificity* refers to the proportion of PSG-scored wake epochs accurately identified as wake by actigraphy (Meltzer et al., 2012). Studies in infant, preschool, and adolescent samples tend to report high sensitivity and low specificity. In a relatively recent review of 228 studies, over half of the reported specificities were below 60% (Meltzer et al., 2012).

The main advantages of actigraphy are that it can be used in the child's natural environment, it is less invasive than PSG, and it is very easy to use and relatively cost-effective (Thoman & Acebo, 1995). Another benefit is that it permits continuous, prolonged recordings which are not restricted to one location or sleeping position (Thoman & Acebo, 1995).

There are also disadvantages associated with this approach. First, artefacts, which can result from externally induced movement (e.g. mother rocking her baby during sleep), present a major threat to the validity of actigraphy data (see above comments on specificity). These artefacts can cause confusion between sleep and waking states and should thus be removed during a monitoring period prior to the automatic sleep-wake scoring. Sleep diaries can be an especially useful tool for identifying potential artefacts (Sadeh, 2015). Second, although relatively un-intrusive, some children are unable to tolerate actigraphy devices (Hodge et al., 2012), especially those with learning difficulties or autism (Hering, Epstein, Elroy, Iancu, & Zelnik, 1999; Sadeh et al., 1991).

Smartphone Applications

Smartphones are powerful tools, offering both computational and communication opportunities. These have been leveraged for the benefit of healthcare (Behar, Roebuck, Domingos, Gederi, & Clifford, 2013) and may be especially useful for younger populations who commonly use this technology (Seko, Kidd, Wiljer, & McKenzie, 2014).

There are two sensors on mobile phones that are relevant to the assessment of sleep disorders: actigraphy and audio (Behar et al., 2013). Actigraphy measures have already been discussed in some detail. Audio measures, which to date have been underused, can provide information about respiratory activity during sleep. This information can be useful in determining whether a subject has sleep apnoea (Pevernagie, Aarts, & De Meyer, 2010). A number of smartphone applications for sleep disorders have appeared over recent years, though there is currently a lack of scientific evidence for their validity (Behar et al., 2013).

Sleep Diaries

Sleep diaries are commonly used in research on infants and children. Parents are asked to report daily on their child's sleep patterns, though older children may complete the diary for themselves. Typical sleep parameters recorded include bed and waking times, time to sleep onset, night waking, subsequent returns to sleep, and daytime napping (Hodge et al., 2012). Sleep diaries can be a cost-effective and reliable alternative to objective methods and an important baseline tool for the healthcare professional (Werner, Molinari, Guyer, & Jenni, 2008). There are numerous sleep diaries available (see, e.g. http://yoursleep.aasmnet.org/pdf/sleepdiary.pdf), which vary in format and can provide valuable longitudinal data (Badin, Haddad, & Shatkin, 2016).

It is usually suggested that at least 14 days of recording are needed to ensure the validity of diary data (Stores, 2001). This may place a considerable burden on parents and potentially lead to compliance issues (see disadvantages). Diary data appears to be relatively reliable for sleeping schedules (Sadeh, 2015), but less so for sleep quality (Tikotzky & Sadeh, 2001). There is also evidence for the reliability of self-report diaries in high school children (Gaina, Sekine, Chen, Hamanishi, & Kagamimori, 2004).

Advantages of sleep diaries include their cost-effectiveness, ease of use, and ability to measure a wide variety of sleep parameters (Sadeh, 2015). Downsides include potential response bias, compliance issues, and subject burden (Sadeh, 2015).

Sleep Questionnaires

The evaluation of sleep in epidemiological studies is a challenge. Questionnaires offer a cost-effective way of obtaining extensive information about sleep in larger samples. Nevertheless, only a few (of the many available) questionnaires have been fully validated and standardised using appropriate psychometric criteria (see Spruyt and Gozal (2011) for an extensive review of published and unpublished instruments). The below tables present a summary comparison of the items assessed and psychometric properties of some common sleep questionnaires for infants (Table 2) and children and adolescents (Table 3).

As outlined in the tables, there are a wealth of sleep questionnaires, many of which have been assessed for reliability and (to a lesser extent) validity. Most scales demonstrate at least adequate test-retest reliability and/or internal consistency. Test-retest reliability measures the extent to which a tool produces consistent results across time (assessed with a correlation coefficient); internal consistency measures the strength of relationship between individual items within the same scale (assessed with Cronbach's alpha: α). Thresholds for these two indices are usually set at acceptable (≥ 0.7), good (≥ 0.8), and excellent (≥ 0.9).

Generally, questionnaires have not fared quite as well in terms of construct (i.e. convergent and discriminative) validity, which describes the extent to which they accurately measure the sleep characteristics they are designed to measure. Further validity studies are needed as reliability can only tell us that a tool is measuring something consistently; it cannot provide information on what the tool is actually measuring (Spruyt & Gozal, 2011). See Table 1 for an overview of the advantages and disadvantages associated with sleep questionnaires.

The Assessment of Child Sleep Problems in Primary Care

Questionnaires may be used in clinical settings to screen for sleep problems (Luginbuehl & Kohler, 2009). In view of the strong link between disordered sleep and medical problems, the clinician should also conduct a physical exam to rule out any potential physical causes. A discussion with parents regarding the sleep environment, any bedtime routines, parental responses during night waking, and morning and daytime functioning is also warranted (Honaker & Meltzer, 2014).

While paediatricians generally report regularly "screening" for sleep disorders in younger children, they will often only ask a single question about the child's sleep patterns or parental concerns. A relatively recent survey indicated that paediatrician knowledge regarding sleep disorders, and in particular the less common ones (e.g. narcolepsy, OSA), is limited and that few paediatricians have ever received formal training on sleep disorders (Faruqui, Khubchandani, Price, Bolyard, & Reddy, 2011). These gaps in knowledge and confidence may explain the low rates of screening and management of sleep disorders in primary care. See Honaker and Meltzer (2016) for an in-depth review on sleep-related practices in paediatric primary care settings.

Table 2 Comparison of commonly used sleep assessment questionnaires for infants

Name of tool	Main sleep problems assessed	Applicable ages	Completed by	Validated against	Psychometric properties
Brief Infant Sleep Questionnaire (BISQ) Sadeh (2004)	**13 items** including sleep duration; night waking; sleep-onset time; location of sleep; preferred body position	Infants	Parent	Sleep diary; actigraphy	Test-retest reliability $r = 0.82–0.95$ Correlations with other sleep measures (convergent validity): $r = 0.23–0.83$ Good discriminative validity: 85% correct classifications
Infant Sleep Questionnaire (ISQ) Morrell (1999a)	**10 items** including settling; night waking; parent views on problem	Young infants	Parent	Sleep diary	Test-retest reliability $r = 0.92$ Good concurrent validity: sensitivity = 89.5%; specificity = 96.7% compared to diary cutoff scores
Maternal Cognitions about Infant Sleep Questionnaire (MCISQ) Morrell (1999b)	**20 items** including limit setting; anger; doubt; feeding; safety	Infants	Parent	Research criteria; sleep diaries	Test-retest reliability $r = 0.81$ Internal consistency: $\alpha = 0.80–0.84$ Adequate construct validity (i.e. identify extreme groups): for setting limits, anger, doubt, and total scale scores Convergent validity (whole scale): $r = 0.48$
Parental Interactive Bedtime Behaviour Scale (PIBBS) Morrell and Cortina-Borja (2002)	**19 items** including active and passive physical comforting; encouraging infant autonomy; movement; social comforting	Infants	Parent	Richman's sleep diary	Internal consistency: $\alpha = 0.71$ Construct validity: significant difference in PIBBS scores between non-sleep and sleep problem groups Convergent validity (for diary total score and PIBBS subscales): $r = 0.08–0.73$
Sleep and Settle Questionnaire (SSQ) Matthey (2001)	**34 items** including sleep patterns; settle time; duration of crying; waking temperament; confidence getting baby back to sleep	Young infants	Parent	Edinburgh Postnatal Depression Scale	Test-retest reliability low to moderate Convergent validity: significant correlations between maternal mood and unsettled infant behaviour: $r = 0.46–0.51$

Test-retest reliability: the degree to which test results are consistent over time and is measured with a reliability coefficient; internal consistency: correlations between items within a scale and is usually measured with Cronbach's alpha (α); construct validity: degree to which a questionnaire measures what it is supposed to be measuring and includes convergent (the extent to which measures that should be related are related in reality) and discriminant (tests whether measures that should *not* be related are in reality *not* related) validity

Table 3 Comparison of commonly used sleep assessment questionnaires for children and adolescents

Name of tool	Main sleep problems assessed	Applicable ages	Completed by	Validated against	Psychometric properties
Adolescent Sleep Wake Scale (ASWS) LeBourgeois, Giannotti, Cortesi, Wolfson, and Harsh (2005)	28 items including going to bed; falling asleep; maintaining sleep; reinitiating sleep; wakefulness	Adolescents	Self	N/A	Internal consistency $\alpha = 0.80$–0.86
Bedtime Routines Questionnaire (BRQ) Henderson and Jordan (2010)	31 items including weekday and weeknight bedtime routines	Preschool and early school age	Parent	Child Routines Questionnaire; Children's Sleep Hygiene Scale; Children's Sleep Wake Scale	Internal consistency: $\alpha = 0.88$ Convergent validity $r = 0.36$–0.51
Children's Sleep Status Questionnaire (CSSQ) XiaoNa et al. (2009)	47 items including bedtime routines; sleep patterns; sleep disorders; sleep habits	Children	Parent	N/A	Test-retest reliability $r = 0.74$–0.94
Children's Sleep Habit Questionnaire (CSHQ) Owens, Spirito, and McGuinn (2000)	45 items including bedtime behaviour; sleep onset; sleep duration; sleep anxiety; sleep-disordered breathing; parasomnias; daytime sleepiness	School-aged children	Parent	Clinical diagnosis of sleep disorder	Test-retest reliability $r = 0.62$–0.79 Internal consistency $\alpha = 0.68$–0.78 Good discriminative validity: CSHQ scores correctly identified 80% of clinical group
Insomnia Scale (IS) Abdel-Khalek (2004)	12 items including difficulties sleeping; interrupted sleep; tired on waking; consequences of sleep problems	Older adolescents	Self	Arabic sleep disorders scale & the Sleep Questionnaire	Test-retest reliability (total scale) $r = 0.81$–0.83 Internal consistency $\alpha = 0.84$–0.87 Good convergent validity $r = 0.76$–0.94
Obstructive Sleep Disorders 6-Survey (OSD-6) de Serres et al. (2000)	6 items including physical suffering; sleep disturbance; speech/swallowing difficulties; emotional distress; caregiver concern	Young children to adolescents	Parent	Clinician estimate	Test-retest reliability $r = 0.69$–0.86 Internal consistency: $\alpha = 0.80$ Convergent validity $r = 0.36$
Paediatric Sleep Questionnaire (PSQ) Chervin, Hedger, Dillon, and Pituch (2000)	22 items including snoring; stop breathing during sleep; restless sleep; unrefreshed after sleep	Children and adolescents	Parent	Polysomnograph-confirmed SRBD	Test-retest reliability $r = 0.66$–0.92 Internal consistency $\alpha = 0.66$–0.89 Good discriminate validity: total score correctly identified 85–86.4% of SRBD

(continued)

Table 3 (continued)

Name of tool	Main sleep problems assessed	Applicable ages	Completed by	Validated against	Psychometric properties
Paediatric Daytime Sleepiness Scale (PDSS) Drake, Nickel, and Burduvali (2003)	**8 items** including daily sleep patterns; daytime sleepiness	School-aged children	Self	Negative school outcomes	Internal consistency $\alpha = 0.80$ Construct validity: predicted lower achievement; less school enjoyment; more illness
Sleep Disorders Inventory for Students (SDIS-Child & SDIS-Adolescent) Luginbuehl, Bradley-Klug, Ferron, Anderson, and Benbadis (2008)	**43 items** including OSAS; PLMD; NARC; DSPS	Child/adolescent version	School psychologists/parents	Polysomnography Respiratory distress index (RDI); sleep specialist's diagnosis	Test-retest reliability $r = 0.97/0.86$ Internal consistency $\alpha = 0.91/0.92$ Concurrent validity with PSG & RDI: OSAS scale $r = 0.33$ and 0.57; snore scale $r = 0.43$ and 0.64 Discriminative validity: positive predictive power = 0.54–0.86; negative predictive power = 0.84–1.0
Sleep Disturbance Scale for Children (SDSC) Bruni et al. (1996)	**27 items** including all major sleep disorders	Children and adolescents	Parent	Against clinical diagnosis	Test-retest reliability $r = 0.71$ Internal consistency $\alpha = 0.71$–0.79 Good diagnostic accuracy: correct 89.1% of sleep disordered individuals
School Sleep Habits Survey (SSHS) Wolfson et al. (2003)	**63 items** including school and weekend night sleep time; bedtime and rise times; typical daytime functioning	Adolescents	Self	Sleep diary; actigraphy	Internal consistency $\alpha = 0.75$ Concurrent validity (diary) $r = 0.38$–0.76 Concurrent validity (actigraphy) $r = 0.31$–0.77
Tayside Children's Sleep Questionnaire McGreavey, Donnan, Pagliari, and Sullivan (2005)	**10 items** including problems with initiating or maintaining sleep and parental interventions	Young children	Parent	Case notes and mothers' reports of known cases	Internal consistency $\alpha = 0.85$ Good discriminate validity: for all cases mother's own accounts of their children's sleep patterns corroborate questionnaire results

Test-retest reliability refers to the degree to which test results are consistent over time and is measured with a reliability coefficient; internal consistency represents the correlations between items within a scale and is usually measured with Cronbach's alpha (α); construct validity is the degree to which a questionnaire measures what it is supposed to be measuring and includes convergent (the extent to which measures that should be related are related in reality) and discriminant (tests whether measures that should *not* be related are in reality *not* related) validity

Conclusions

Sleep is very complex. It can vary from one night to the next, and the ways in which it can be disrupted are multifaceted and dynamic. Sleep patterns are continually changing across the lifespan and are affected by chronological age, physiologic age, and a range of other factors including psychiatric and medical comorbidities (Ohayon, Carskadon, Guilleminault, & Vitiello, 2004). All these elements make the assessment of sleep a challenge.

Different aspects of sleep are suited to different assessment methods. While each approach has its limitations and advantages, the choice of methodology will depend on specific assessment goals, age of the child, and availability of equipment and specialist knowledge (Sadeh, 2015). Many researchers (and some clinicians) use questionnaires or daily logs as the most readily accessible instrument. While these tools are often considered "second best", they can provide important unique information on sleep duration, sleep schedule, and sleep-related behaviour (Gregory & Sadeh, 2016). If a deeper understanding of sleep quality or architecture is needed, more sophisticated methods such as PSG can be utilised (Sadeh, 2015).

Sleep disorders are common in children and adolescents. They can have a large impact on quality of life and may contribute to the development of a wide range of mental (and physical) health problems (Behar et al., 2013). With the increasing use of technology in young populations, sleep problems look set to rise further (Calamaro, Mason, & Ratcliffe, 2009). This highlights the importance of effective screening and intervention programmes for sleep disorders in youth. Research indicates that childhood sleep problems are not being regularly identified in primary care. Future research is needed to develop and disseminate validated tools to aid clinicians in the management of paediatric sleep problems (Honaker & Meltzer, 2016).

References

Abdel-Khalek, A. M. (2004). Prevalence of reported insomnia and its consequences in a survey of 5,044 adolescents in Kuwait. *Sleep, 27*(4), 726–731.

Alfano, C. A., Reynolds, K., Scott, N., Dahl, R. E., & Mellman, T. A. (2013). Polysomnographic sleep patterns of non-depressed, non-medicated children with generalized anxiety disorder. *Journal of Affective Disorders, 147*(1), 379–384.

Alvaro, P. K., Roberts, R. M., & Harris, J. K. (2013). A systematic review assessing bidirectionality between sleep disturbances, anxiety, and depression. *Sleep, 36*(7), 1059–1068.

American Academy of Sleep Medicine. (2005). *The international classification of sleep disorders: Diagnostic and coding manual*. Westchester, IL: American Academy of Sleep Medicine.

American Academy of Sleep Medicine. (2014). *International classification of sleep disorders* (3rd ed.). Darien, IL: American Academy of Sleep Medicine.

American Psychiatric Association. (2001). *Diagnostic statistical manual of mental disorders* (4th ed.). Washington, DC: American Psychiatric Association.

American Psychiatric Association. (2013). *Diagnostic statistical manual of mental disorders* (5th ed.). Washington, DC: American Psychiatric Association.

American Sleep Disorders Association. (1992). Scoring rules and examples. A preliminary report from the sleep disorders atlas task force of the American Sleep Disorders Association. *Sleep, 15*(2), 173–184.

Anders, T. F., & Guilleminault, C. (1975). The pathophysiology of sleep disorders in pediatrics. Part I. Sleep in infancy. *Advances in Pediatrics, 22*, 137–150.

Anders, T. F., Halpern, L. F., & Hua, J. (1992). Sleeping through the night: A developmental perspective. *Pediatrics, 90*(4), 554–560.

Anders, T. F., & Sostek, A. M. (1976). The use of time lapse video recording of sleep-wake behavior in human infants. *Psychophysiology, 13*(2), 155–158.

Badin, E., Haddad, C., & Shatkin, J. P. (2016). Insomnia: The sleeping giant of pediatric public health. *Current Psychiatry Reports, 18*(5), 1–8.

Balestrieri, M., Rucci, P., Sbrana, A., Ravani, L., Benvenuti, A., Gonnelli, C., … Cassano, G. B. (2006). Lifetime rhythmicity and mania as correlates of suicidal ideation and attempts in mood disorders. *Comprehensive Psychiatry, 47*(5), 334–341.

Bandla, H., & Splaingard, M. (2004). Sleep problems in children with common medical disorders. *Pediatric Clinics of North America, 51*(1), 203–227.

Baweja, R., Calhoun, S., & Singareddy, R. (2013). Sleep problems in children. *Minerva Pediatrica, 65*(5), 457–472.

Behar, J., Roebuck, A., Domingos, J. S., Gederi, E., & Clifford, G. D. (2013). A review of current sleep screening applications for smartphones. *Physiological Measurement, 34*(7), R29.

Bixler, E. O., Vgontzas, A. N., Lin, H.-M., Liao, D., Calhoun, S., Fedok, F., ... Graff, G. (2008). Blood pressure associated with sleep-disordered breathing in a population sample of children. *Hypertension, 52*(5), 841–846.

Blader, J. C., Koplewicz, H. S., Abikoff, H., & Foley, C. (1997). Sleep problems of elementary school children: A community survey. *Archives of Pediatrics & Adolescent Medicine, 151*(5), 473–480.

Bruni, O., Ottaviano, S., Guidetti, V., Romoli, M., Innocenzi, M., Cortesi, F., & Giannotti, F. (1996). The Sleep Disturbance Scale for Children (SDSC) Construction and validation of an instrument to evaluate sleep disturbances in childhood and adolescence. *Journal of Sleep Research, 5*(4), 251–261.

Burnham, M. M., Goodlin-Jones, B. L., Gaylor, E. E., & Anders, T. F. (2002). Nighttime sleep-wake patterns and self-soothing from birth to one year of age: A longitudinal intervention study. *Journal of Child Psychology and Psychiatry, 43*(6), 713–725.

Calamaro, C. J., Mason, T. B., & Ratcliffe, S. J. (2009). Adolescents living the 24/7 lifestyle: Effects of caffeine and technology on sleep duration and daytime functioning. *Pediatrics, 123*(6), e1005–e1010.

Carskadon, M. A., Vieira, C., & Acebo, C. (1993). Association between puberty and delayed phase preference. *Sleep-New York, 16*, 258–258.

Challamel, M.-J., Mazzola, M.-E., Nevsimalova, S., Cannard, C., Louis, J., & Revol, M. (1994). Narcolepsy in children. *Sleep, 17*(8 Suppl), S17–S20.

Chase, R. M., & Pincus, D. B. (2011). Sleep-related problems in children and adolescents with anxiety disorders. *Behavioral Sleep Medicine, 9*(4), 224–236.

Chervin, R. D., & Guilleminault, C. (1996). Obstructive sleep apnea and related disorders. *Neurologic Clinics, 14*(3), 583–609.

Chervin, R. D., Hedger, K., Dillon, J. E., & Pituch, K. J. (2000). Pediatric sleep questionnaire (PSQ): Validity and reliability of scales for sleep-disordered breathing, snoring, sleepiness, and behavioral problems. *Sleep Medicine, 1*(1), 21–32.

Cincin, A., Sari, I., Oğuz, M., Sert, S., Bozbay, M., Ataş, H., ... Basaran, Y. (2015). Effect of acute sleep deprivation on heart rate recovery in healthy young adults. *Sleep and Breathing, 19*(2), 631–636.

Cohen-Zion, M., & Ancoli-Israel, S. (2004). Sleep in children with attention-deficit hyperactivity disorder (ADHD): A review of naturalistic and stimulant intervention studies. *Sleep Medicine Reviews, 8*(5), 379–402.

Cortese, S., Faraone, S. V., Konofal, E., & Lecendreux, M. (2009). Sleep in children with attention-deficit/hyperactivity disorder: Meta-analysis of subjective and objective studies. *Journal of the American Academy of Child & Adolescent Psychiatry, 48*(9), 894–908.

Crowley, S., Acebo, C., & Carskadon, M. (2007). Sleep, circadian rhythms, and delayed phase in adolescence. *Sleep Medicine, 8*(6), 602.

Dagan, Y., Stein, D., Steinbock, M., Yovel, I., & Hallis, D. (1998). Frequency of delayed sleep phase syndrome among hospitalized adolescent psychiatric patients. *Journal of Psychosomatic Research, 45*(1), 15–20.

Dahl, R. E., Holttum, J., & Trubnick, L. (1994). A clinical picture of child and adolescent narcolepsy. *Journal of the American Academy of Child & Adolescent Psychiatry, 33*(6), 834–841.

Dauvilliers, Y., Montplaisir, J., Molinari, N., Carlander, B., Ondze, B., Besset, A., & Billiard, M. (2001). Age at onset of narcolepsy in two large populations of patients in France and Quebec. *Neurology, 57*(11), 2029–2033.

Davies, S. K., Ang, J. E., Revell, V. L., Holmes, B., Mann, A., Robertson, F. P., ... Kayser, M. (2014). Effect of sleep deprivation on the human metabolome. *Proceedings of the National Academy of Sciences, 111*(29), 10761–10766.

de Miguel-Díez, J., Villa-Asensi, J. R., & Alvarez-Sala, J. L. (2003). Prevalence of sleep-disordered breathing in children with Down syndrome: Polygraphic findings in 108 children. *Sleep, 26*(8), 1006–1009.

de Serres, L. M., Derkay, C., Astley, S., Deyo, R. A., Rosenfeld, R. M., & Gates, G. A. (2000). Measuring quality of life in children with obstructive sleep disorders. *Archives of Otolaryngology–Head & Neck Surgery, 126*(12), 1423–1429.

Diomedi, M., Curatolo, P., Scalise, A., Placidi, F., Caretto, F., & Gigli, G. L. (1999). Sleep abnormalities in mentally retarded autistic subjects: Down's syndrome with mental retardation and normal subjects. *Brain and Development, 21*(8), 548–553.

Dixon-Gordon, K. L., Whalen, D. J., Layden, B. K., & Chapman, A. L. (2015). A systematic review of personality disorders and health outcomes. *Canadian Psychology/Psychologie Canadienne, 56*(2), 168.

Dohnt, H., Gradisar, M., & Short, M. A. (2012). *Insomnia and its symptoms in adolescents: Comparing DSM-IV and ICSD-II diagnostic criteria*. American Academy of Sleep Medicine.

Drake, C., Nickel, C., & Burduvali, E. (2003). The pediatric daytime sleepiness scale (PDSS): Sleep habits and school outcomes in middle-school children. *Sleep, 26*(4), 455–458.

Faedda, G. L., Baldessarini, R. J., Glovinsky, I. P., & Austin, N. B. (2004). Pediatric bipolar disorder: Phenomenology and course of illness. *Bipolar Disorders, 6*(4), 305–313.

Fallone, G., Seifer, R., Acebo, C., & Carskadon, M. A. (2002). How well do school-aged children comply with imposed sleep schedules at home? *Sleep, 25*(7), 739–745.

Faruqui, F., Khubchandani, J., Price, J. H., Bolyard, D., & Reddy, R. (2011). Sleep disorders in children: A national assessment of primary care pediatrician practices and perceptions. *Pediatrics, 128*, peds. 2011-0344.

Fisher, H. L., Lereya, S. T., Thompson, A., Lewis, G., Zammit, S., & Wolke, D. (2014). Childhood parasomnias and psychotic experiences at age 12 years in a United Kingdom birth cohort. *Sleep, 37*(3), 475–482.

Forbes, E. E., Bertocci, M. A., Gregory, A. M., Ryan, N. D., Axelson, D. A., Birmaher, B., & Dahl, R. E. (2008). Objective sleep in pediatric anxiety disorders and major depressive disorder. *Journal of the American Academy of Child & Adolescent Psychiatry, 47*(2), 148–155.

Gaina, A., Sekine, M., Chen, X., Hamanishi, S., & Kagamimori, S. (2004). Validity of child sleep diary questionnaire among junior high school children. *Journal of Epidemiology, 14*(1), 1–4.

Galland, B. C., Taylor, B. J., Elder, D. E., & Herbison, P. (2012). Normal sleep patterns in infants and children: A systematic review of observational studies. *Sleep Medicine Reviews, 16*(3), 213–222.

Garcia, J., & Applebee, G. (2013). Delayed sleep phase syndrome in adolescents. In *Sleep disorders in women* (pp. 75–83). New York: Springer.

Garcia, J., Rosen, G., & Mahowald, M. (2001). *Circadian rhythms and circadian rhythm disorders in children and adolescents*. Paper presented at the Seminars in Pediatric Neurology.

Ghaem, M., Armstrong, K., Trocki, O., Cleghorn, G., Patrick, M., & Shepherd, R. (1998). The sleep patterns of infants and young children with gastro-oesophageal reflux. *Journal of Paediatrics and Child Health, 34*(2), 160–163.

Goodlin-Jones, B. L., Burnham, M. M., Gaylor, E. E., & Anders, T. F. (2001). Night waking, sleep-wake organization, and self-soothing in the first year of life. *Journal of Developmental and Behavioral Pediatrics: JDBP, 22*(4), 226.

Gottlieb, D. J., Punjabi, N. M., Newman, A. B., Resnick, H. E., Redline, S., Baldwin, C. M., & Nieto, F. J. (2005). Association of sleep time with diabetes mellitus and impaired glucose tolerance. *Archives of Internal Medicine, 165*(8), 863–867.

Gradisar, M., Gardner, G., & Dohnt, H. (2011). Recent worldwide sleep patterns and problems during adolescence: A review and meta-analysis of age, region, and sleep. *Sleep Medicine, 12*(2), 110–118.

Greene, G., Gregory, A. M., Fone, D., & White, J. (2015). Childhood sleeping difficulties and depression in adulthood: The 1970 British Cohort Study. *Journal of Sleep Research, 24*(1), 19–23.

Gregory, A. M., Rijsdijk, F. V., Lau, J., Dahl, R. E., & Eley, T. C. (2009). The direction of longitudinal associations between sleep problems and depression symptoms: A study of twins aged 8 and 10 years. *Sleep, 32*(2), 189–199.

Gregory, A. M., & Sadeh, A. (2012). Sleep, emotional and behavioral difficulties in children and adolescents. *Sleep Medicine Reviews, 16*(2), 129–136.

Gregory, A. M., & Sadeh, A. (2016). Annual research review: Sleep problems in childhood psychiatric disorders–a review of the latest science. *Journal of Child Psychology and Psychiatry, 57*(3), 296–317.

Grigg-Damberger, M. (2004). Neurologic disorders masquerading as pediatric sleep problems. *Pediatric Clinics of North America, 51*(1), 89–115.

Halpern, L. F., & Baumeister, A. A. (1995). Infant sleep-wake characteristics: Relation to neurological status and the prediction of developmental outcome. *Developmental Review, 15*(3), 255–291.

Han, F., Chen, E., Wei, H., Dong, X., He, Q., Ding, D., & Strohl, K. P. (2001). Childhood narcolepsy in North China. *Sleep, 24*(3), 321–324.

Henderson, J. A., & Jordan, S. S. (2010). Development and preliminary evaluation of the Bedtime Routines Questionnaire. *Journal of Psychopathology and Behavioral Assessment, 32*(2), 271–280.

Hering, E., Epstein, R., Elroy, S., Iancu, D. R., & Zelnik, N. (1999). Sleep patterns in autistic children. *Journal of Autism and Developmental Disorders, 29*(2), 143–147.

Hoban, T. F. (2010). Sleep disorders in children. *Annals of the New York Academy of Sciences, 1184*(1), 1–14.

Hodge, D., Parnell, A., Hoffman, C. D., & Sweeney, D. P. (2012). Methods for assessing sleep in children with autism spectrum disorders: A review. *Research in Autism Spectrum Disorders, 6*(4), 1337–1344.

Honaker, S. M., & Meltzer, L. J. (2014). Bedtime problems and night wakings in young children: An update of the evidence. *Paediatric Respiratory Reviews, 15*(4), 333–339.

Honaker, S. M., & Meltzer, L. J. (2016). Sleep in pediatric primary care: A review of the literature. *Sleep Medicine Reviews, 25*, 31–39.

Huỳnh, C., Guilé, J.-M., Breton, J.-J., & Godbout, R. (2016). Sleep-wake patterns of adolescents with borderline personality disorder and bipolar disorder. *Child Psychiatry & Human Development, 47*(2), 202–214.

Hysing, M., Harvey, A. G., Torgersen, L., Ystrom, E., Reichborn-Kjennerud, T., & Sivertsen, B. (2014). Trajectories and predictors of nocturnal awakenings and sleep duration in infants. *Journal of Developmental & Behavioral Pediatrics, 35*(5), 309–316.

Iber, C., Ancoli-Israel, S., Chesson, A., & Quan, S. F. (2007). *The AASM manual for the scoring of sleep and associated events: Rules, terminology and technical specifications* (Vol. 1). Westchester, IL: American Academy of Sleep Medicine.

Iglowstein, I., Jenni, O. G., Molinari, L., & Largo, R. H. (2003). Sleep duration from infancy to adolescence: Reference values and generational trends. *Pediatrics, 111*(2), 302–307.

Jansen, P. W., Saridjan, N. S., Hofman, A., Jaddoe, V. W., Verhulst, F. C., & Tiemeier, H. (2011). Does disturbed sleeping precede symptoms of anxiety or depression in toddlers? The generation R study. *Psychosomatic Medicine, 73*(3), 242–249.

Johnson, E., Roth, T., Schultz, L., & Breslau, N. (2006). Epidemiology of DSM-IV insomnia in adolescence: Lifetime prevalence, chronicity, and an emergent gender difference. *Pediatrics, 117*(2), e247–e256.

Kerr, S., & Jowett, S. (1994). Sleep problems in preschool children: A review of the literature. *Child: Care, Health and Development, 20*(6), 379–391.

Klackenberg, G. (1982). Somnambulism in childhood-prevalence, course and behavioral correlations. *Acta Paediatrica, 71*(3), 495–499.

Kotagal, S. (1996). *Narcolepsy in children*. Paper presented at the seminars in pediatric neurology.

Kotagal, S. (2009). Parasomnias in childhood. *Sleep Medicine Reviews, 13*(2), 157–168.

Kotagal, S., & Pianosi, P. (2006). Sleep disorders in children and adolescents. *BMJ: British Medical Journal, 332*(7545), 828.

Kowatch, R. A., Youngstrom, E. A., Danielyan, A., & Findling, R. L. (2005). Review and meta-analysis of the phenomenology and clinical characteristics of mania in children and adolescents. *Bipolar Disorders, 7*(6), 483–496.

Krakowiak, P., Goodlin-Jones, B., Hertz-Picciotto, I., Croen, L. A., & Hansen, R. L. (2008). Sleep problems in children with autism spectrum disorders, developmental delays, and typical development: A population-based study. *Journal of Sleep Research, 17*(2), 197–206.

Kushida, C. A., Littner, M. R., Morgenthaler, T., Alessi, C. A., Bailey, D., Coleman, J., Jr., et al. (2005). Practice parameters for the indications for polysomnography and related procedures: An update for 2005. *Sleep, 28*(4), 499–521.

Laberge, L., Tremblay, R. E., Vitaro, F., & Montplaisir, J. (2000). Development of parasomnias from childhood to early adolescence. *Pediatrics, 106*(1), 67–74.

LeBourgeois, M. K., Giannotti, F., Cortesi, F., Wolfson, A. R., & Harsh, J. (2005). The relationship between reported sleep quality and sleep hygiene in Italian and American adolescents. *Pediatrics, 115*(Supplement 1), 257–265.

Lee, Y. J., Cho, S.-J., Cho, I. H., Jang, J. H., & Kim, S. J. (2012). The relationship between psychotic-like experiences and sleep disturbances in adolescents. *Sleep Medicine, 13*(8), 1021–1027.

Lereya, S. T., Winsper, C., Tang, N. K., & Wolke, D. (2017). Sleep problems in childhood and borderline personality disorder symptoms in early adolescence. *Journal of Abnormal Child Psychology, 45*(1), 193–206.

Liu, X., & Buysse, D. J. (2006). Sleep and youth suicidal behavior: A neglected field. *Current Opinion in Psychiatry, 19*(3), 288–293.

Liu, X., Buysse, D. J., Gentzler, A. L., Kiss, E., Mayer, L., Kapornai, K., ... Kovacs, M. (2007). Insomnia and hypersomnia associated with depressive phenomenology and comorbidity in childhood depression. *Sleep, 30*(1), 83–90.

Lofthouse, N., Fristad, M., Splaingard, M., & Kelleher, K. (2007). Parent and child reports of sleep problems associated with early-onset bipolar spectrum disorders. *Journal of Family Psychology, 21*(1), 114.

Lofthouse, N., Gilchrist, R., & Splaingard, M. (2009). Mood-related sleep problems in children and adolescents. *Child and Adolescent Psychiatric Clinics of North America, 18*(4), 893–916.

Lovato, N., & Gradisar, M. (2014). A meta-analysis and model of the relationship between sleep and depression in adolescents: Recommendations for future research and clinical practice. *Sleep Medicine Reviews, 18*(6), 521–529.

Luginbuehl, M., Bradley-Klug, K. L., Ferron, J., Anderson, W. M., & Benbadis, S. R. (2008). Pediatric sleep disorders: Validation of the sleep disorders inventory for students. *School Psychology Review, 37*(3), 409.

Luginbuehl, M., & Kohler, W. C. (2009). Screening and evaluation of sleep disorders in children and adolescents. *Child and Adolescent Psychiatric Clinics of North America, 18*(4), 825–838.

Lumeng, J. C., & Chervin, R. D. (2008). Epidemiology of pediatric obstructive sleep apnea. *Proceedings of the American Thoracic Society, 5*(2), 242–252.

Lunsford-Avery, J. R., Judd, C. M., Axelson, D. A., & Miklowitz, D. J. (2012). Sleep impairment, mood symptoms, and psychosocial functioning in adolescent bipolar disorder. *Psychiatry Research, 200*(2), 265–271.

Matthey, S. (2001). The sleep and settle questionnaire for parents of infants: Psychometric properties. *Journal of Paediatrics and Child Health, 37*(5), 470–475.

Mayes, S. D., Calhoun, S., Bixler, E. O., & Vgontzas, A. N. (2009). Sleep problems in children with autism, ADHD, anxiety, depression, acquired brain injury, and typical development. *Sleep Medicine Clinics, 4*(1), 19–25.

Mayes, S. D., Calhoun, S. L., Bixler, E. O., Vgontzas, A. N., Mahr, F., Hillwig-Garcia, J., ... Parvin, M. (2009). ADHD subtypes and comorbid anxiety, depression, and oppositional-defiant disorder: Differences in sleep problems. *Journal of Pediatric Psychology, 34*(3), 328–337.

McGreavey, J., Donnan, P., Pagliari, H., & Sullivan, F. (2005). The Tayside children's sleep questionnaire: A simple tool to evaluate sleep problems in young children. *Child: Care, Health and Development, 31*(5), 539–544.

Meltzer, L. J., Montgomery-Downs, H. E., Insana, S. P., & Walsh, C. M. (2012). Use of actigraphy for assessment in pediatric sleep research. *Sleep Medicine Reviews, 16*(5), 463–475.

Mindell, J. A. (1993). Sleep disorders in children. *Health Psychology, 12*(2), 151.

Mindell, J. A., Meltzer, L. J., Carskadon, M. A., & Chervin, R. D. (2009). Developmental aspects of sleep hygiene: Findings from the 2004 National Sleep Foundation Sleep in America Poll. *Sleep Medicine, 10*(7), 771–779.

Morgenthaler, T. I., Owens, J., Alessi, C., Boehlecke, B., Brown, T. M., Coleman, J., ... Pancer, J. (2006). Practice parameters for behavioral treatment of bedtime problems and night wakings in infants and young children. *Sleep-New York Then Westchester, 29*(10), 1277.

Morrell, J. (1999a). The infant sleep questionnaire: A new tool to assess infant sleep problems for clinical and research purposes. *Child Psychology and Psychiatry Review, 4*(01), 20–26.

Morrell, J. (1999b). The role of maternal cognitions in infant sleep problems as assessed by a new instrument, the maternal cognitions about infant sleep questionnaire. *Journal of Child Psychology and Psychiatry, 40*(2), 247–258.

Morrell, J., & Cortina-Borja, M. (2002). The developmental change in strategies parents employ to settle young children to sleep, and their relationship to infant sleeping problems, as assessed by a new questionnaire: The Parental Interactive Bedtime Behaviour Scale. *Infant and Child Development, 11*(1), 17–41.

Mukherjee, S., Patel, S. R., Kales, S. N., Ayas, N. T., Strohl, K. P., Gozal, D., & Malhotra, A. (2015). An official American Thoracic Society statement: The importance of healthy sleep. Recommendations and future priorities. *American Journal of Respiratory and Critical Care Medicine, 191*(12), 1450–1458.

Nevsimalova, S. (2014). The diagnosis and treatment of pediatric narcolepsy. *Current Neurology and Neuroscience Reports, 14*(8), 1–10.

Ohayon, M. M., Carskadon, M. A., Guilleminault, C., & Vitiello, M. V. (2004). Meta-analysis of quantitative sleep parameters from childhood to old age in healthy individuals: Developing normative sleep values across the human lifespan. *Sleep-New York Then Westchester, 27*, 1255–1274.

Ohayon, M. M., Roberts, R. E., Zulley, J., Smirne, S., & Priest, R. G. (2000). Prevalence and patterns of problematic sleep among older adolescents. *Journal of the American Academy of Child & Adolescent Psychiatry, 39*(12), 1549–1556.

Owens, J. (2007). Classification and epidemiology of childhood sleep disorders. *Sleep Medicine Clinics, 2*(3), 353–361.

Owens, J., & Mindell, J. A. (2011). Pediatric insomnia. *Pediatric Clinics of North America, 58*(3), 555–569.

Owens, J., Spirito, A., & McGuinn, M. (2000). The Children's Sleep Habits Questionnaire (CSHQ): Psychometric properties of a survey instrument for school-aged children. *Sleep-New York, 23*(8), 1043–1052.

Owens, J., Spirito, A., McGuinn, M., & Nobile, C. (2000). Sleep habits and sleep disturbance in elementary school-aged children. *Journal of Developmental & Behavioral Pediatrics, 21*(1), 27–36.

Parrino, L., Ferri, R., Bruni, O., & Terzano, M. G. (2012). Cyclic alternating pattern (CAP): The marker of sleep instability. *Sleep Medicine Reviews, 16*(1), 27–45.

Pereira, J. C., Jr., Pradella-Hallinan, M., & Alves, R. C. (2014). Childhood restless legs syndrome. *Medical Express, 1*(3), 116–122.

Peterman, J. S., Carper, M. M., & Kendall, P. C. (2015). Anxiety disorders and comorbid sleep problems in school-aged youth: Review and future research directions. *Child Psychiatry & Human Development, 46*(3), 376–392.

Peterson, P. C., & Husain, A. M. (2008). Pediatric narcolepsy. *Brain and Development, 30*(10), 609–623.

Pevernagie, D., Aarts, R. M., & De Meyer, M. (2010). The acoustics of snoring. *Sleep Medicine Reviews, 14*(2), 131–144.

Picchietti, D., Allen, R. P., Walters, A. S., Davidson, J. E., Myers, A., & Ferini-Strambi, L. (2007). Restless legs syndrome: Prevalence and impact in children and adolescents—The Peds REST study. *Pediatrics, 120*(2), 253–266.

Poulton, R., Caspi, A., Moffitt, T. E., Cannon, M., Murray, R., & Harrington, H. (2000). Children's self-reported psychotic symptoms and adult schizophreniform disorder: A 15-year longitudinal study. *Archives of General Psychiatry, 57*(11), 1053–1058.

Quine, L. (1991). Sleep problems in children with mental handicap. *Journal of Intellectual Disability Research, 35*(4), 269–290.

Reimão, R. N., & Lefévre, A. B. (1980). Prevalence of sleep-talking in childhood. *Brain and Development, 2*(4), 353–357.

Roane, B. M., & Taylor, D. J. (2008). Adolescent insomnia as a risk factor for early adult depression and substance abuse. *Sleep, 31*(10), 1351–1356.

Roberts, R. E., & Duong, H. T. (2013). Depression and insomnia among adolescents: A prospective perspective. *Journal of Affective Disorders, 148*(1), 66–71.

Robson, W. L. M. (2008). Current management of nocturnal enuresis. *Current Opinion in Urology, 18*(4), 425–430.

Ruhrmann, S., Schultze-Lutter, F., Salokangas, R. K., Heinimaa, M., Linszen, D., Dingemans, P., … Heinz, A. (2010). Prediction of psychosis in adolescents and young adults at high risk: Results from the prospective European prediction of psychosis study. *Archives of General Psychiatry, 67*(3), 241–251.

Ruoff, C., & Rye, D. (2016). The ICSD-3 and DSM-5 guidelines for diagnosing narcolepsy: Clinical relevance and practicality. *Current Medical Research and Opinion, 32*(10), 1611–1622.

Sadeh, A. (2004). A brief screening questionnaire for infant sleep problems: Validation and findings for an Internet sample. *Pediatrics, 113*(6), e570.

Sadeh, A. (2015). III. Sleep assessment methods. *Monographs of the Society for Research in Child Development, 80*(1), 33–48.

Sadeh, A., Gruber, R., & Raviv, A. (2002). Sleep, neurobehavioral functioning, and behavior problems in school-age children. *Child Development, 73*(2), 405–417.

Sadeh, A., Horowitz, I., Wolach-Benodis, L., & Wolach, B. (1998). Sleep and pulmonary function in children with well-controlled, stable asthma. *Sleep, 21*(4), 379–385.

Sadeh, A., Lavie, P., Scher, A., Tirosh, E., & Epstein, R. (1991). Actigraphic home-monitoring sleep-disturbed and control infants and young children: A new method for pediatric assessment of sleep-wake patterns. *Pediatrics, 87*(4), 494–499.

Sadeh, A., Pergamin, L., & Bar-Haim, Y. (2006). Sleep in children with attention-deficit hyperactivity disorder:

A meta-analysis of polysomnographic studies. *Sleep Medicine Reviews, 10*(6), 381–398.

Schreck, K. A., Mulick, J. A., & Smith, A. F. (2004). Sleep problems as possible predictors of intensified symptoms of autism. *Research in Developmental Disabilities, 25*(1), 57–66.

Scott, N., Blair, P. S., Emond, A. M., Fleming, P. J., Humphreys, J. S., Henderson, J., & Gringras, P. (2013). Sleep patterns in children with ADHD: A population-based cohort study from birth to 11 years. *Journal of Sleep Research, 22*(2), 121–128.

Sedky, K., Bennett, D. S., & Carvalho, K. S. (2014). Attention deficit hyperactivity disorder and sleep disordered breathing in pediatric populations: A meta-analysis. *Sleep Medicine Reviews, 18*(4), 349–356.

Seko, Y., Kidd, S., Wiljer, D., & McKenzie, K. (2014). Youth mental health interventions via mobile phones: A scoping review. *Cyberpsychology, Behavior, and Social Networking, 17*(9), 591–602.

Shanahan, L., Copeland, W. E., Angold, A., Bondy, C. L., & Costello, E. J. (2014). Sleep problems predict and are predicted by generalized anxiety/depression and oppositional defiant disorder. *Journal of the American Academy of Child & Adolescent Psychiatry, 53*(5), 550–558.

Sheldon, S. H. (2002). Sleep in infants and children. *Sleep: A comprehensive handbook*, 507–510.

Singareddy, R., Moole, S., Calhoun, S., Vocalan, P., Tsaousso-glou, M., Vgontzas, A., & Bixler, E. (2009). Medical complaints are more com-mon in young school-aged children with parent reported insomnia symptoms. *Journal of Clinical Sleep Medicine, 5*(6), 549–553.

Singh, S. P., Winsper, C., Wolke, D., & Bryson, A. (2014). School mobility and prospective pathways to psychotic-like symptoms in early adolescence: A prospective birth cohort study. *Journal of the American Academy of Child & Adolescent Psychiatry, 53*(5), 518–527. e511.

Sinha, D., & Guilleminault, C. (2010). Sleep disordered breathing in children. *Indian Journal of Medical Research, 131*, 311–320.

Sitnick, S. L., Goodlin-Jones, B. L., & Anders, T. F. (2008). The use of actigraphy to study sleep disorders in preschoolers: Some concerns about detection of nighttime awakenings. *Sleep-New York Then Westchester, 31*(3), 395.

Sivertsen, B., Harvey, A. G., Lundervold, A. J., & Hysing, M. (2014). Sleep problems and depression in adolescence: Results from a large population-based study of Norwegian adolescents aged 16–18 years. *European Child & Adolescent Psychiatry, 23*(8), 681–689.

Smedje, H., Broman, J. E., & Hetta, J. (1999). Parents' reports of disturbed sleep in 5–7-year-old Swedish children. *Acta Paediatrica, 88*(8), 858–865.

Spruyt, K., & Gozal, D. (2011). Pediatric sleep questionnaires as diagnostic or epidemiological tools: A review of currently available instruments. *Sleep Medicine Reviews, 15*(1), 19–32.

Stores, G. (2001). *Sleep-wake function in children with neurodevelopmental and psychiatric disorders*. Paper presented at the seminars in pediatric neurology.

Stores, G., Montgomery, P., & Wiggs, L. (2006). The psychosocial problems of children with narcolepsy and those with excessive daytime sleepiness of uncertain origin. *Pediatrics, 118*(4), e1116–e1123.

Tauman, R. (2008). Sleep and obesity in children. In *Sleep and psychiatric disorders in children and adolescents* (pp. 383–405). New York, NY: Informa Health Care.

Taylor, M. A., Schreck, K. A., & Mulick, J. A. (2012). Sleep disruption as a correlate to cognitive and adaptive behavior problems in autism spectrum disorders. *Research in Developmental Disabilities, 33*(5), 1408–1417.

Thoman, E. B. (1990). Sleeping and waking states in infants: A functional perspective. *Neuroscience & Biobehavioral Reviews, 14*(1), 93–107.

Thoman, E. B., & Acebo, C. (1995). Monitoring of sleep in neonates and young children. In *Principles and practice of sleep medicine in the child* (pp. 55–68). Philadelphia, PA: WB Saunders.

Thoman, E. B., Ingersoll, E. W., & Acebo, C. (1991). Premature infants seek rhythmic stimulation, and the experience facilitates neurobehavioral development. *Journal of Developmental & Behavioral Pediatrics, 12*(1), 11–18.

Thompson, A., Lereya, S. T., Lewis, G., Zammit, S., Fisher, H. L., & Wolke, D. (2015). Childhood sleep disturbance and risk of psychotic experiences at 18: UK birth cohort. *The British Journal of Psychiatry*, bjp. bp. 113.144089.

Tikotzky, L., & Sadeh, A. (2001). Sleep patterns and sleep disruptions in kindergarten children. *Journal of Clinical Child Psychology, 30*(4), 581–591.

Turkdogan, D., Bekiroglu, N., & Zaimoglu, S. (2011). A prevalence study of restless legs syndrome in Turkish children and adolescents. *Sleep Medicine, 12*(4), 315–321.

US Department of Health. (1993). *Wake up America national sleep alert*.

Vela-Bueno, A. (1985). Prevalence of night terrors and nightmares in elementary school children: A pilot study. *Research Communications in Psychology, Psychiatry & Behavior, 10*, 177–188.

Weiss, M. D., & Salpekar, J. (2010). Sleep problems in the child with attention-deficit hyperactivity disorder. *CNS Drugs, 24*(10), 811–828.

Werner, H., Molinari, L., Guyer, C., & Jenni, O. G. (2008). Agreement rates between actigraphy, diary, and questionnaire for children's sleep patterns. *Archives of Pediatrics & Adolescent Medicine, 162*(4), 350–358.

Winsper, C., Lereya, S. T., Marwaha, S., Thompson, A., Eyden, J., & Singh, S. P. (2016). The aetiological and psychopathological validity of borderline personality disorder in youth: A systematic review and meta-analysis. *Clinical Psychology Review, 44*, 13–24.

Winsper, C., & Tang, N. K. (2014). Linkages between insomnia and suicidality: Prospective associations, high-risk subgroups and possible psychological mechanisms. *International Review of Psychiatry, 26*(2), 189–204.

Winsper, C., Tang, N. K., Marwaha, S., Lereya, S. T., Gibbs, M., Thompson, A., & Singh, S. P. (2017). The sleep phenotype of Borderline Personality Disorder: A systematic review and meta-analysis. *Neuroscience & Biobehavioral Reviews 73*, 48–67.

Winsper, C., & Wolke, D. (2014). Infant and toddler crying, sleeping and feeding problems and trajectories of dysregulated behavior across childhood. *Journal of Abnormal Child Psychology, 42*(5), 831–843.

Wolfson, A. R., Carskadon, M. A., Acebo, C., Seifer, R., Fallone, G., Labyak, S. E., & Martin, J. L. (2003). Evidence for the validity of a sleep habits survey for adolescents. *Sleep-New York Then Westchester, 26*(2), 213–217.

Wong, M. M., & Brower, K. J. (2012). The prospective relationship between sleep problems and suicidal behavior in the National Longitudinal Study of Adolescent Health. *Journal of Psychiatric Research, 46*(7), 953–959.

XiaoNa, H., HuiShan, W., JingXiong, J., YuYan, M., Lin, A., & XiCheng, L. (2009). The epidemiology of sleep and its disorder in Chinese children aged 0-5 years. *Biological Rhythm Research, 40*(5), 399–411.

Yilmaz, E., Sedky, K., & Bennett, D. S. (2013). The relationship between depressive symptoms and obstructive sleep apnea in pediatric populations: A meta-analysis. *Journal of Clinical Sleep Medicine, 9*(11), 1213–1220.

Yilmaz, K., Kilincaslan, A., Aydin, N., & Kor, D. (2011). Prevalence and correlates of restless legs syndrome in adolescents. *Developmental Medicine & Child Neurology, 53*(1), 40–47.

Pain

Soeun Lee, Lara M. Genik, and C. Meghan McMurtry

Overview

Pediatric pain has not always been well understood. Dating back to the times of Ancient Greece, there were common misunderstandings regarding how infants and children experienced and expressed pain (Unruh & McGrath, 2013). For example, it was commonly believed that children did not feel pain in the same way as adults, and there was difficulty in judging how to tell when a child was in pain (Unruh & McGrath, 2013). Even as recently as the last quarter century, misconceptions regarding children's pain led to undertreatment; compared to adult patients, it was common for children who underwent major surgeries to be withheld pain-relieving medication (Schechter, Allen, & Hanson, 1986), and infants were often withheld anesthesia during surgery (Unruh & McGrath, 2013). Over the past few decades, relevant research has flourished, increasing understanding of how children experience and express pain.

To lay the groundwork for evidence-based pain assessment, this chapter will provide a brief overview of the current understanding of pediatric pain and frameworks used to describe the development and maintenance of pain in youth (i.e., children and adolescents). Assessment considerations, such as development, family, and gender, will be reviewed next. An overview of selected assessment measures that have demonstrated good psychometric properties for use in typically developing youth with acute and chronic pain will be provided; finally, pain assessment in youth with developmental disabilities will be explored, including an illustrative case example. Measures reviewed in all sections are presented in Table 1. As pain assessment in infants is beyond the current scope, the reader is directed to a review by Franck, Greenberg, and Stevens (2000), as well as "neonatal and infant pain assessment" in the *Oxford Textbook of Paediatric Pain* (Lee & Stevens, 2013).

S. Lee · L. M. Genik
Department of Psychology, University of Guelph, Guelph, ON, Canada

C. M. McMurtry (✉)
Department of Psychology, University of Guelph, Guelph, ON, Canada

Pediatric Chronic Pain Program, McMaster Children's Hospital, Hamilton, ON, Canada

Department of Paediatrics, Western University, London, ON, Canada

Children's Health Research Institute, London, ON, Canada
e-mail: cmcmurtr@uoguelph.ca

Biopsychosocial Model of Pain

The International Association for the Study of Pain's (IASP) official definition of pain is "an unpleasant sensory and emotional experience

Table 1 Assessment domains, measure names, appropriate age ranges, pain type, recommendations, and accessibility

Assessment domain	Measure	Age range	Acute pain	Chronic pain	Highly recommended	Availability
Pain intensity	Pieces of Hurt/Poker Chip Tool	3–18	✓	?	✓ (Recommended for 3–5 for acute pain)	Instructions as per Hester, 1979; tool can be constructed with own materials
	Faces Pain Scale – Revised (FPS-R)	4–19	✓	✓^	✓ (Recommended for 5–12 for acute pain)	www.iasp-pain.org/FPSR
	Numerical Rating Scale (NRS)	8 and older	✓	✓	✓ (Recommended for 8 and older for acute or chronic pain)	Free for use from the PROMIS® registry at: www.healthmeasures.net/search-view-measures
	The Oucher	3–12	✓	✓^		www.oucher.org/order.html
	Wong-Baker FACES Pain Scale	3 and older	✓	✓^		Free for research and clinical use with permission wongbakerfaces.org/types-of-access/
	Visual Analogue Scales (VAS)	8 and older	✓	✓		For an example, see page 3 at: www.painedu.org/Downloads/NIPC/Pain%20Assessment%20Scales.pdf
Pain location	Adolescent Pediatric Pain Tool (APPT)	2 and older	✓	?		www.allcare.org/CancerPain-and-SymptomManagement/comfort/cfm3/appt.pdf
	Eland Color Tool	4–10	✓	?		Unknown. Contact authors. Some copies available on web but unknown copyright.
Fear of pain	Children's Fear Scale (CFS)	5 and older	✓	?		www.uoguelph.ca/pphc/childrens-fear-scale
	Fear of Pain Questionnaire (FOPQ)	8–17	N/A	✓		With permission from the author: med.stanford.edu/bpplab/measures.html
Functional disability	Functional Disability Inventory (FDI)	8–17	N/A	✓	✓	www.childrenshospital.vanderbilt.org/uploads/documents/FDI_Manual.pdf
	Pediatric Quality of Life Inventory (PedsQL)	2–18	N/A	✓		Free for non-funded research. Various licensing fees depending on study funding and use may apply. For further instructions, see: eprovide.mapi-trust.org/instruments/pediatric-quality-of-life-inventory

Sleep	Children's Sleep Habits Questionnaire (CSHQ)	4–10	N/A	✓	Unknown. Contact authors. Some copies available on web but unknown copyright.
	Children's Report of Sleep Patterns (CRSP)	8–12	N/A	✓	Unknown. Contact authors. Some copies available on web but unknown copyright.
	Adolescent Sleep-Wake Scale (ASWS)	12–18	N/A	✓	Unknown. Contact authors. Some copies available on web but unknown copyright.
Psychosocial factors	Pain Catastrophizing Scale (PCS)	8–18	N/A	✓	www.midss.org/content/pain-catastrophizing-scale-child-version-and-parent-version
	Adult Responses to Children's Symptoms (ARCS)	8–18	N/A	✓	Available for use with permission from the authors.
	Chronic Pain Acceptance Questionnaire for Adolescents (CPAQ-A)	10–18	N/A	✓	Available for use with permission from the authors.
	Child Self-Efficacy Scale (CSE)	8–18	N/A	✓	Unknown. Contact authors. Some copies available on web but unknown copyright.
	Youth Life Orientation Test (YLOT)	8–12	N/A	✓	Unknown. Contact authors. Some copies available on web but unknown copyright.
Youth with developmental disabilities	Non-communicating Children's Pain Checklist – Postoperative Version (NCCPC-PV)	3–18	✓	?	pediatric-pain.ca/resources/our-measures/
	Revised Face, Leg, Activity, Cry, and Consolability (r-FLACC) scale	4–21	✓	?	Unknown. Contact authors. Some copies available on web but unknown copyright
	Individualized Numeric Rating Scale (INRS)	3 and older	✓	?	www.marthaaqcurley.com/inrs.html
	Pediatric Pain Profile (PPP)	1–18	✓	?	www.ppprofile.org.uk/ppptooldownload.php?s=209

✓ = established psychometrics in given population/context; ✓^ = established psychometrics in disease-related pain but not necessarily chronic pain, has been recommended in a previous systematic review for disease-related pain (Stinson, Kavanagh, Yamada, Gill, & Stevens, 2006); ? = unknown psychometrics; N/A = not applicable in context.

associated with actual or potential tissue damage, or described in terms of such damage" (Merskey & Bogduk, 1994, pp. 210). This definition asserts that although pain often has a related physical cause, pain itself is a subjective experience and "a psychological state" that can extend beyond direct tissue damage (Merskey & Bogduk, 1994). Therefore, pain is much more than the biomedical conceptualization of a simple relation between a noxious stimulus and an internal experience of pain. In 1965, Melzack and Wall challenged the prevailing biomedical model and proposed the gate control theory, which was revolutionary to the conceptualization of pain (Gatchel, Peng, Peters, Fuchs, & Turk, 2007; Melzack & Wall, 1965). The gate control theory posits that pain is *perceived* as a function of information traveling through the spinal cord and to the brain via nociceptive (i.e., pain transmitting) or non-nociceptive (e.g., transmitting touch, pressure, and vibrations) nerve fibers in a "bottom-up process." Therefore, nociception does not always evoke a pain sensation, which can be dependent on numerous other factors. These factors could include "top-down" processes, such as the individual's emotions, thoughts, and mental states (Melzack & Wall, 1965).

The gate control theory helped to redefine pain as a subjective experience to noxious stimuli. In line with this theory, the biopsychosocial model of pain considers physical and psychosocial factors to be related, dynamic processes that continuously impact upon (and themselves are impacted by) an individual's pain. The biopsychosocial approach to pain represents the complex interrelations among the biological (e.g., genetics, sex), psychological (e.g., fear, anxiety, depression), and social (e.g., parental responses, social support) factors that are related to pain experience (internal subjective experience) and pain expression (observable response) (Turk & Monarch, 2002). Therefore, adequate pain management cannot be achieved by treating physiologic pathology alone (if present) but must also consider relevant emotional and cognitive factors. For example, emotional stress could impact an individual's reporting of symptoms and response to treatment, thus making it an important consideration in assessment, diagnosis, and treatment (Gatchel et al., 2007); conversely, ongoing pain could result in considerable stress.

Acute Pain

Pain is common throughout childhood and can take many forms, including acute and chronic. Acute pain can be the result of tissue damage, injury, postoperative pain, or medical procedures such as needle pokes (McGrath et al., 2008). Pain from medical procedures, such as vaccinations, is common throughout childhood – young children have typically received over a dozen vaccinations by the time they are 6 years of age (Public Health Agency of Canada). Furthermore, children with chronic illnesses, such as cancer or diabetes, are subject to even more painful procedures (e.g., bone marrow aspirations, lumbar punctures, insulin injections; Hockenberry et al., 2011; Stevens et al., 2011). Unmanaged procedural pain and fear can have both short- and long-term consequences including longer procedure times, negative memories, greater distress at future procedures, and delays or avoidance in seeking healthcare (McMurtry et al., 2015; Noel, Chambers, McGrath, Klein, & Stewart, 2012; Taddio et al., 2012; Taddio, Katz, Illersich, & Koren, 1997). These consequences can impact both children and their caregivers. Subsequent avoidance of preventative medical procedures could increase risk of adverse health outcomes and potentially increase economic burden in the long run (Hamilton, 1995; McMurtry et al., 2015; McMurtry et al., 2016).

The precise mechanisms by which acute pain in children transitions to chronic pain are unknown but may include differences in pain processing, psychological factors, poor sleep, and age (Holley, Wilson, & Palermo, 2017; McKillop & Banez, 2016). The pediatric fear-avoidance model proposes a process by which acute experiences of pain can become chronic and persistent in youth (Asmundson, Noel, Petter, & Parkerson, 2012). According to this model, a youth experiences an injury or illness that produces an acute experience of pain. Youth who perceive and appraise this pain as unpleasant, but attribute a low fear response to the pain, proceed on a path of healing and recovery. In contrast, youth who appraise their pain with fear and anxiety based on predisposing characteristics (such as familial beliefs about pain/parental modeling, heightened anxiety sensitivity), and their current psychological state, develop a fear of pain and pain-related anxiety which serve to perpetuate pain (Asmundson et al., 2012).

Chronic Pain

Chronic pain is defined as recurrent and/or persistent pain that lasts for longer than 3 months (Task Force on Taxonomy of the IASP, 2012) or beyond normal time for tissue healing (Treede et al., 2015). Chronic pain can be a persistent symptom from an acute injury, accompany a chronic disease, or originate from no known cause (Liossi & Howard, 2016). Contrary to acute pains, which are seen as adaptive responses that serve to protect from dangerous stimuli, chronic pain is intrusive and maladaptive and can interfere with many areas of health and functioning. Chronic pain in youth is associated with a host of negative concomitant consequences, including mood disruption (Asmundson et al., 2012; King et al., 2011), fewer peer relationships (Forgeron et al., 2010), lower school attendance (Dick & Pillai Riddell, 2010), and sleep disturbances (Palermo et al., 2005), signifying many potential avenues for decreased quality of life.

Some of the most common pediatric chronic pains include headaches, abdominal pain, back pain, and musculoskeletal pain (King et al., 2011). Median prevalence rates for chronic pain in youth range from 11% to 38%, with approximately 5% of those youth experiencing moderate to severe chronic pains that are accompanied by functional impairments (i.e., pain-related activity limitations) and lower quality of life (Claar & Walker, 2006; Huguet & Miró, 2008; King et al., 2011). Furthermore, chronic pain is a costly health concern. Total estimated costs for chronic pain healthcare in adults are $6 billion per year in Canada (Lynch, 2011) and over $260 billion per year in the United States (Gaskin & Richard, 2012). Total financial cost (including days of work missed) is estimated to be over $560 billion per year in the United States, making chronic pain more economically burdensome than heart disease, cancer, and diabetes (Gaskin & Richard, 2012). Less is known about the economic cost of pediatric chronic pain. One study from the United States estimated that the total cost to society for adolescents with moderate to severe chronic pains was over $19.5 billion a year (Groenewald, Essner, Wright, Fesinmeyer, & Palermo, 2014). Prevalence rates for pediatric chronic pain appear to increase with age (King et al., 2011); youth who have chronic pain also have an increased risk of experiencing chronic pain and its related functional impairments into adulthood (Lynch, 2011; Walker, Dengler-Crish, Rippel, & Bruehl, 2010). Therefore, economic costs related to pediatric pain may be compounded as youth transition into adulthood. In sum, pediatric chronic pain is both a prevalent health and economic concern that requires proper assessment, diagnosis, and treatment.

Pediatric Pain Assessment

Pain assessment serves several functions aside from diagnosis. These include identifying relations between pain and other variables (e.g., sleep, mood, etc.), as well as guiding intervention (Blount & Loiselle, 2009; McGrath et al., 2008). Consistent with the biopsychosocial model, using a multimodal assessment strategy can help identify all of the potential biological, psychological, and social contributors that may cause, exacerbate, or perpetuate a child's pain (Liossi & Howard, 2016). The Pediatric Initiative on Methods, Measurement, and Pain Assessment in Clinical Trials (PedIMMPACT) identified core domains that should be assessed in addition to pain intensity in both acute and chronic pediatric pain contexts. Core outcome domains to be considered in acute pain include pain intensity, symptoms and adverse events, physical recovery, emotional response, economic factors, and satisfaction with treatment (McGrath et al., 2008). For chronic pain, the domains are similar with additional consideration of sleep and role functioning. Further, "physical functioning" and "emotional functioning" replace "physical recovery" and "emotional response" to highlight the long-term trajectories these factors have in chronic pain contexts (McGrath et al., 2008).

Assessment Considerations: Format, Development, Family, and Gender

Assessment of pediatric pain can include behavioral (i.e., observational), self-report, or physiological (e.g., heart rate variability) measures. Since pain is a subjective experience, self-report has been emphasized for pediatric pain assessment (Twycross, Voepel-Lewis, Vincent, Franck, & von Baeyer, 2015). Self-reports are low in cost and efficient for gathering information. However, they also require a level of cognitive development (e.g., ability to seriate, sufficient receptive language) to accurately understand and respond, and most self-report measures have an age range beyond which the tool is not valid for use. For example, young children under the age of 6 years have considerable difficulty in using a self-report tool for pain (Stanford, Chambers, & Craig, 2006). Notably, 3- and 4-year-olds (and some 5-year-olds) may use the extreme ends of self-report measures of pain intensity, making their use in this age range potentially problematic (von Baeyer et al., 2017). A recent systematic review recommended that scales with fewer response options are needed for preschool-aged children (von Baeyer et al., 2017). In addition to self-report, additional assessment strategies (e.g., parent-proxy reports, medical history, and responses to previous treatments) should be considered when formulating a treatment plan (Twycross et al., 2015; Vetter, Bridgewater, Ascherman, Madan-Swain, & McGwin, 2014).

As foreshadowed above, a developmental perspective must be adopted when considering the cognitive demands of self-reporting pain. Both age and cognitive ability are important considerations, as some pain assessments may exceed a child's ability to accurately report their pain, leading to an over- or underestimation of the child's pain experience, and impact subsequent pain management strategies (Jaaniste, Noel, & von Baeyer, 2016). Further, there are developmental differences in the prevalence of pediatric pain; in general, chronic pain in youth increases with age, and is more common in females than males, especially after the onset of puberty (King et al., 2011; Liossi & Howard, 2016). Specific chronic pain presentations also appear to be developmentally influenced, with abdominal pain being more common in younger children, while prevalence rates for other pains increase with age (King et al., 2011).

Pediatric pain is a condition that is inherently linked to the family system. Family context considerations can be situated at multiple levels, including individual factors (e.g., parenting styles and responses), the parent-child relationship (e.g., quality of interactions), and overall family functioning (Palermo & Chambers, 2006). For example, during acutely painful medical procedures, parents have been found to be more accurate reporters of children's pain than physicians or nurses, although they generally underestimate their children's pain (Birnie, Boerner, & Chambers, 2013). Thus, parent-proxy reports of children's acute pain are an important source of complementary but not entirely overlapping information. Furthermore, there are complex, bidirectional relations between parental factors and the child's pain experience. For example, parental behaviors of reassurance and distraction have been found to differentially impact child pain experience during painful medical procedures. Parental reassurance appears to be interpreted by children as indicating parental fear and has been associated with increased child distress and fear; in contrast, distraction has been associated with increased child coping (McMurtry, McGrath, & Chambers, 2006; McMurtry, Chambers, McGrath, & Asp, 2010; Schechter et al., 2007).

Parents of youth with chronic pain have been found to report high levels of anxiety, depressive symptoms, and parenting stress (Palermo, Valrie, & Karlson, 2014). Moreover, in a bidirectional relation, this appears to vary with the child's level of pain intensity; mothers of children with more severe chronic pains were more likely to report social, relational, and financial stressors compared to mothers of children with less severe pains (Hunfeld et al., 2001). Similarly, greater psychological and emotional distress in mothers has been associated with higher child-reported pain intensity (Palermo & Eccleston, 2009). On a broader scale, poor family functioning – characterized by less family cohesion and organization, and greater conflict – is related to higher functional disability in children with chronic pain (Birnie et al., 2013; Lewandowski et al., 2010). Therefore, pediatric chronic pain assessment should include parent reports of children's symptoms but also information on the parents' own psychological functioning and beliefs about their child's pain.

Although research regarding parental influences on children's pain has primarily been limited to mothers, fathers' roles are also important to consider (Birnie et al., 2013). For example, fathers have shown higher agreement with child ratings of pain and may be more accurate reporters in comparison to mothers (Moon et al., 2008). Fathers also appear to hold different pain beliefs and perceptions, such as believing that pain following surgery is acceptable, boys should be able to tolerate pain better than girls, and children should be able to cope with their pain on their own (Kankkunen, Vehviläinen-Julkunen, Pietilä, & Halonen, 2003).

Sex differences (including differences in chromosomal and hormonal makeup) and gender differences (characterized as socially constructed roles and behaviors attributed to "masculine" and "feminine") can play a role in a youth's pain experience and expression. Girls are at an increased risk for chronic pain, especially after the onset of puberty, with a higher prevalence and greater frequency of pain being reported after adolescence (Moon & Unruh, 2013). Studies on sex differences in pain outcomes have been mixed; in experimental conditions, some studies have found that girls may have lower heat and cold pain thresholds than boys (Blankenburg et al., 2010), while others have found no differences (Goodman & McGrath, 2003). Furthermore, the majority of studies have found no differences in pain tolerance (the subjective intensity of pain that children are willing to accept in a given situation) or self-reported pain intensity between girls and boys across a variety of experimental conditions and assessments (Boerner, Birnie, Caes, Schinkel, & Chambers, 2014; Moon & Unruh, 2013). Sex differences may pose important implications for pain expression and response to treatment, with girls and boys displaying differential pre-treatment mood and anxiety (Boerner, Eccleston, Chambers, & Keogh, 2016). Finally, a youth's gender may also impact his/her pain experience. Differences have been found in how girls and boys cope with their pain, with girls being more likely to seek social support and boys being more likely to engage in behavioral distraction (Lynch, Kashikar-Zuck, Goldschneider, & Jones, 2007). Furthermore, parental responses to children's pain may differ by the child's gender, as described above.

Assessment: Pediatric Acute Pain

Pain Intensity

Pain intensity (how much something hurts) is an important aspect of the pain experience that is routinely sought by clinicians. Yet, pain is complex and a measure of intensity is an (necessary) oversimplification. Although the issues of reliability and validity are challenging when it comes to pain as a frequently changing and subjective experience, in the review of measures that follows, available reliability and validity data are discussed.

The Pieces of Hurt tool was designed by Hester (1979) and is also referred to as the Poker Chip Tool. It has been used with a wide age range (3–18 years) for pain from a variety of procedures (e.g., hospitalization, immunization, postoperative, venipuncture; Aradine, Beyer, & Tompkins, 1988; Beyer & Aradine, 1987, 1988; Gharaibeh & Abu-Saad, 2002; Goodenough et al., 1997; Hester, 1979; Suraseranivongse et al., 2005). Four plastic chips are used to represent "pieces of hurt"; the child is first asked whether something did/does hurt, and if the child says no, a score of zero is given. If the child indicates yes, the child is then asked to use the poker chips to indicate pain intensity ranging from one chip ("A Little Hurt") to four chips ("The Most Hurt"). The score is the number of chips selected. The measure has adequate content validity (Hester, 1979) and good construct validity in terms of both convergent and divergent validities (Beyer & Aradine, 1987, 1988; Gharaibeh & Abu-Saad, 2002; Goodenough et al., 1997; Hester, 1979; Suraseranivongse et al., 2005). Translations are available for use in Thailand (Suraseranivongse et al., 2005) and Jordan (Gharaibeh & Abu-Saad, 2002). The Pieces of Hurt tool was recommended in a systematic review of self-report measures of pain intensity, particularly for younger children (e.g., 3–7 years) due to the concreteness of the ordinal rating scale (Stinson et al., 2006). There are two notable challenges with the tool: (1) the chips need to be sterilized after each use, and (2) it does not use the more common 0–10 rating scale typically used in healthcare settings.

Designed for children between 3 and 12 years old, the Oucher uses two different scale formats depending on the child's age (Beyer, 1984; Beyer & Knott, 1998). Older children (5–12 years; Stinson et al., 2006; Tomlinson, von Baeyer, Stinson, & Sung, 2010) are asked to respond on a 0 to 100 numerical scale with higher scores indicating higher pain intensity. Younger children respond on a photographic faces scale ranging from 0 ("No Hurt") to 5 ("The Biggest Hurt You Could Ever Have"). "Faces scales" use a series of facial expressions depicting gradations in pain (or other state) intensity from none/absent to high/intense. The child is asked to match his/her internal experience with a face on the scale. In typically developing children, the ability to recognize facial expressions of emotion develops relatively early, which has been argued as an advantage of these scales (Bieri, Reeve, Champion, Addicoat, & Ziegler, 1990). There are different versions of the photographic scale of the Oucher depicting Caucasian, Hispanic, African American, and First Nations children (Shapiro, 1997; Villarruel & Denyes, 1991). Of note, all of these versions depict a male child. There is an Asian version of the Oucher which is scored 0–10 and shows a female child (Yeh, 2005). The Oucher has been successfully used to gather pain intensity from children following surgery (Beyer & Knott, 1998; Ramritu, 2000) and hospitalization (Beyer & Aradine, 1987, 1988). The creation of the scale was based on a conceptual framework which was detailed in the work of Beyer and colleagues (Beyer, Denyes, & Villaruel, 1992). Even young children (3–7 years) appear to agree with the ordering of the faces (Beyer & Aradine, 1986), and content validity is supported for the Asian, African American, and Hispanic versions (Villarruel & Denyes, 1991; Yeh, 2005). The original Oucher has demonstrated low to moderate levels of test-retest reliability (Belter, McIntosh, Finch, & Saylor, 1988), while the African American version has shown high test-retest reliability (Luffy & Grove, 2003). Convergent and divergent validity has been supported for the original, Asian, African American, and Hispanic versions (Beyer & Aradine, 1988; Beyer & Knott, 1998; Yeh, 2005).

The Faces Pain Scale-Revised (Hicks, von Baeyer, Spafford, van Korlaar, & Goodenough, 2001) is a commonly used single-item self-report measure of pain which was modified from the Faces Pain Scale (Bieri et al., 1990). Children are asked to look at the series of 6 faces which range from 0 to 10 with a neutral face on the far left to a face consistent with a facial expression demonstrating extreme pain on the far right, and then choose one that matches their experience. The FPS-R has been used with a number of different populations aged 4–19 years old, including both clinical and nonclinical samples, and youth undergoing a variety of medical procedures (e.g., Hicks et al., 2001; Lister et al., 2006; Miró & Huguet, 2004; Migdal, Chudzynska-Pomianowska, Vause, Henry, & Lazar, 2005; Newman et al., 2005; Taddio, Kaur

Soin, Schuh, Koren, & Scolnik, 2005; Wood et al., 2004). Strong psychometric support exists for the use of the FPS-R (Stinson et al., 2006; Tomlinson et al., 2010; von Baeyer, 2013) including content validity (Bieri et al., 1990; Hicks et al., 2001), convergent validity (Hicks et al., 2001; Miró & Huguet, 2004; Newman et al., 2005), and discriminant validity (Miró & Huguet, 2004; Stanford et al., 2006). There is evidence of interrater reliability with parents (e.g., Wood et al., 2004) and test-retest reliability (Miró & Huguet, 2004). The scale has been translated into over 30 languages. The acceptability of the FPS-R varies: when compared with cartoon-like faces (see Wong-Baker FACES scale below), the FPS-R is less preferred by nurses, children, and parents (Chambers, Hardial, Craig, Court, & Montgomery, 2005). However, children prefer the FPS-R better than a non-faces scale (Miró & Huguet, 2004).

Six cartoon-like faces ranging from a smiling "No Hurt" face to a crying face with tears for "Hurts Worst" make up the Wong-Baker FACES Pain Scale (Wong & Baker, 1988). This scale is widely used and has been described in numerous reviews as psychometrically sound (Stinson et al., 2006; Tomlinson et al., 2010; von Baeyer, 2013). There is evidence that the use of a smiling no pain face confounds pain intensity with affect and results in statistically significant differences in ratings (Chambers & Craig, 1998; Chambers, Giesbrecht, Craig, Bennett, & Huntsman, 1999). Importantly however, the clinical importance of these differences has not been established.

Visual Analogue scales (VAS) typically consist of a horizontal line with anchors placed on the far left ("No Pain") and far right ("Most Extreme Pain") of the line. The rater is asked to make a mark along the line to represent his/her pain intensity. For a line measuring 10 centimeters, the location of the mark is measured in millimeters, thus providing an interval score between 0 and 100. VAS have been used to measure various forms of acute pain including venipuncture, pain in the emergency department, and pain in hospitalized children (Beyer & Aradine, 1987, 1988; Migdal et al., 2005; Powell, Kelly, & Williams, 2001). There are a number of forms of VAS available which vary according to their orientation, anchors, whether other visual divisions are present, and length of the line (Stinson et al., 2006; von Baeyer, 2013). VAS show moderate to strong convergent validity (Beyer & Aradine, 1987, 1988; Migdal et al., 2005) and good discriminant validity (Beyer & Aradine, 1988). There is some evidence of test-retest reliability (Luffy & Grove, 2003) but more support is needed. VAS are affordable and easy to administer but do require careful photocopying to ensure there are no distortions to the line length. Preference data for the VAS compared to other self-report measures are inconclusive (Berntson & Svensson, 2001; Luffy & Grove, 2003). Appropriate use of the VAS requires ability to seriate and thus is most appropriate for children who are 8 years and older (Stinson et al., 2006).

The most commonly used measures of pain intensity are arguably numerical rating scales; these typically take the form of 0 ("No Pain At All") to 10 ("Most Pain Possible") (von Baeyer, 2013; von Baeyer et al., 2009). They may be administered in writing or verbally (VNS) and are recommended for use with children 8 years and older (von Baeyer et al., 2009). NRS has been used with a number of different populations aged 7–17 years old, including both clinical and nonclinical samples and youth undergoing a variety of medical procedures (e.g., Bailey, Daoust, Doyon-Trottier, Dauphin-Pierre, & Gravel, 2010; Miró, Castarlenas, & Huguet, 2009; von Baeyer et al., 2009). The psychometrics of NRS are well-established with demonstrated concurrent (von Baeyer et al., 2009) and discriminant validity (Miró et al., 2009), content validity (Bailey et al., 2010), and test-retest reliability (Bailey et al., 2010). Youth report preferring the VNS over a VAS and a verbal descriptor rating scale (Bailey et al., 2010).

Pain Location

Understanding the location of pain is important. Youth may be asked informally to either describe or point to the location(s) on their body where they feel pain. These methods presume that the child has the anatomical knowledge and ability to indicate the location and are willing to indicate it (Savedra, Tesler, Holzemer, Wilkie, & Ward, 1989). A more empirical, standardized approach which can be used to record pain localization over time is the use of body outline tools.

Originally used with 4–10-year-old children, the Eland Color Tool (Eland & Anderson, 1977) is designed to capture children's reports of pain intensity and location. Children are asked to choose four crayon colors to represent pain intensities ranging from "No Hurt" to "Worst Hurt." Children then choose the color matching their current pain intensity and color the body outline to indicate where they hurt. Although the appeal of this tool in using an interactive, familiar activity (coloring) is clear, the psychometrics are not. There is some limited evidence of construct validity but no information on reliability (Eland & Anderson, 1977; Guariso et al., 1999; Hamill, Lyndon, Liley, & Hill, 2014).

In a recent systematic review of pain location tools, the Adolescent Pediatric Pain Tool (APPT; Savedra, Holzemer, Tesler, & Wilkie, 1993) was the most widely used in the included literature (Hamill et al., 2014). Based on the adult McGill Pain Questionnaire (Melzack, 1983), the APPT was designed to be used with 8–17-year-old children; however, the tool has been actually used with a much broader age range (2–68 years; Fernandes, De Campos, Batalha, Perdigão, & Jacob, 2014). The APPT contains multiple assessment components including pain intensity (word-graphic rating scale), location (body outline), and quality (word list). In the body outline, the front and back of the body are depicted. The psychometrics of the APPT have been studied in both healthy and hospitalized youth in acute pain (Fernandes et al., 2014; Hamill et al., 2014). Adequate content validity, convergent validity, and test-retest reliability have been supported for all three components with the weakest evidence for the word list (Savedra et al., 1989; Tesler et al., 1991; Wilkie et al., 1990). It has recently been recommended for use with 8–17-year-old hospitalized children due to its strong psychometrics with this population (Fernandes et al., 2014). The APPT takes approximately 3–6 minutes to administer and scoring is relatively straightforward but may challenge feasibility in a busy clinical setting: a clear plastic overlay is placed over the body outline, the mark on the rating scale is measured, and the frequency and proportions of subgroups on the word list are calculated (e.g., sensory, affective). Younger children may also reverse the sides on the body outline and struggle with some of the words on the word list (Savedra et al., 1989; 1993; Wilkie et al., 1990).

Fear

In most cases, the experience of pain is at least somewhat threatening and urges us to "act" to reduce or eliminate it. Thus, fear, a proximal alarm reaction to a real or imagined threat, and anxiety as future-oriented apprehension are important constructs within the pain context (Asmundson et al., 2012; McMurtry et al., 2015; McMurtry et al., 2017). The general assessment of anxiety is covered elsewhere in this volume but a brief overview of measures assessing fear in pain contexts is warranted. Self-report measures of fear in the context of acute pain are much more limited than measures of pain intensity. A recent clinical practice guideline (Taddio et al., 2015) recommended the following measures of fear for the procedural pain context: the Children's Fear Scale (McMurtry, Noel, Chambers, & McGrath, 2011), a verbal rating scale, or a 0–10 numerical rating scale. The Children's Fear Scale shows a horizontal array of five gender-neutral faces ranging from a neutral facial expression on the left to a face showing extreme fear on the right-hand side (total score ranges from 0 to 4; McMurtry et al., 2011). Youth are asked to choose the face that shows their level of fear; the measure has also been used to gather parent-proxy report (McMurtry et al., 2011). The CFS has been used with 5–18-year-old children and adolescents undergoing venipuncture, experimental pain, surgery, vaccination, and treatment for ulcers. The CFS was developed from the Faces Anxiety Scale for adults (McKinley, Coote, & Stein-Parbury, 2003). The CFS has demonstrated evidence of construct (concurrent and discriminant validity), test-retest, and interrater reliability with children 5–10 years old undergoing venipuncture and is freely available online (McMurtry et al., 2011). Verbal descriptor scales analogous to those used for pain intensity can be used to assess for fear in this context, but their psychometrics are unclear. An example verbal descriptor scale could be: *how scared of [X] are/were you: not at all, a little bit, a medium amount, a lot, of very much/most possible?* (Taddio et al., 2015). For children 8 years and older, a 0 ("No Fear") to 10 ("Most Fear Possible") numerical rating scale could be used (Taddio et al., 2015). Understanding the focus of the fear is important for guiding treatment; of note, these various measures of fear could be targeted for fear of pain specifically or the situation more generally.

Assessment: Pediatric Chronic Pain

Pain Quality, Intensity, Frequency, and Duration

How youth describe their pain, or pain quality, can be helpful in determining the type of pain or etiology (Wilkie et al., 1990). A salient example is the "burning" quality often associated with neuropathic pain. There are few investigations in this area, and measures have not been developed which are designed to diagnose particular disorders/conditions. The APPT word list (Savedra et al., 1993) is the only tool assessing pain quality in youth with sufficient psychometric evidence.

Assessing pain intensity is an important part of case formulation and treatment planning. Some of the measures used in acute pain contexts to assess pediatric pain intensity have also demonstrated adequate psychometrics in discriminating pain intensity in chronic pain (e.g., Faces Pain Scale-Revised, Numerical Rating Scale, VAS; Beales, Keen, & Lennox-Holt, 1983; McGrath et al., 2008). For example, one study (Ruskin et al., 2014) of youth aged 8–17 years who presented in a pain clinic found that a verbally administered NRS was shown to have convergent validity and discriminant validity from a pain affect scale, which measures the emotional valence of pain. As can be seen by the question marks in Table 1, research on assessments of pain intensity in pediatric chronic pain populations is less developed than in acute contexts; some studies suggest that pain intensity should not even be the primary focus of chronic pain assessment (Ballantyne & Sullivan, 2015). For example, an interdisciplinary approach may emphasize a youth's level of functioning (including their physical, emotional, and role functioning), rather than their reported pain intensity (McGrath et al., 2008). Furthermore, youth-reported pain intensity should be interpreted in consideration of its associations with other domains of the youth's functioning and parent-proxy reports (von Baeyer, 2006).

Collecting multiple reports of pain may provide richer depictions of a child's pain over time. Pain diaries are a particularly helpful method of assessing pain intensity over time in combination with pain frequency and duration (Table 2).

Collecting data "in the moment" about a youth's pain may deliver more accurate reports of pain. Youth may overreport their pain when asked to rate it retrospectively, compared to when they use pain diaries (Andrasik, Burke, Attanasio, & Rosenblum, 2005; Stinson, 2009; van den Brink, Bandell-Hoekstra, & Abu-Saad, 2001). Pain diaries can also be administered electronically (e.g., through apps), and some research has shown that compliance is higher when using electronic pain diaries versus paper versions. One disadvantage of using an electronic pain diary is the possible financial burden of accessing the diary, as it is administered via an electronic device (e.g., smartphone; Stinson, 2009). Further, it may be a burden on the youth to complete the diary each day, and missing data can be ambiguous (e.g., does no pain report on that day necessarily indicate no pain or forgetting to complete it?). Parent-proxy pain diaries can also be administered, with youth and parent report generally showing interrater agreement (Andrasik et al., 2005; Vetter et al., 2014). However, parent-reported pain diaries may not always cor-

Table 2 Hypothetical pain diary of a youth with chronic pain suggesting that something related to school may be an exacerbating issue Some independent coping is implemented, but coping is limited in its diversity. A diary such as this could be used to identify patterns in pain (including triggers, exacerbating and protective factors) and functioning over time which could be used to guide treatment

Your name:					
Date (month, day, year) and time	Where in the body do you feel pain?	Intensity of pain (0 = no pain to 10 = severe pain)	What were you doing when you felt this pain?	How long did the pain last?	What did you do about the pain?
Jan 1, 2017, at 11:25 am	Stomach	7	At school	30 mins	Took two ibuprofen and went home
Jan 1, 2017, at 9:30 pm	Stomach and back	4	Doing homework	20 mins	Laid down with heat pack
Jan 3, 2017, at 8:30 am	Stomach and back	6	Getting ready for school	15 mins	Heat pack and rubbing

roborate youth pain diaries, especially for younger children (i.e., 8–12 years) or for mild pain that is not as observable (Vetter et al., 2014).

Physical Functioning

Youth with chronic pain may have difficulty being mobile and completing daily activities such as walking to and from school, completing household chores, and participating in valued extracurriculars (McGrath et al., 2008). Furthermore, sleep disruptions are common in this population and have been linked to worsened pain, greater functional disability, and decreased quality of life (Carter & Threlkeld, 2012; Long, Krishnamurthy, & Palermo, 2008), making sleep an important consideration for assessment.

Functional Disability The Functional Disability Inventory (FDI) is a 15-item measure that was originally developed for use with youth (8–17 years) with chronic abdominal pain. The measure has now been used in youth with multiple types of pain including headache, fibromyalgia, back pain, and musculoskeletal pain (Kashikar-Zuck et al., 2011). The FDI asks youth to rate their difficulty performing daily activities in home, school, recreational, and social domains on a scale ranging from 0 ("No Trouble") to 4 ("Impossible"). Examples of items include "Doing chores at home" and "Walking the length of a football field" (Kashikar-Zuck et al., 2011).

Total scores range from 0 to 60, with higher scores reflecting greater functional disability. Three levels of disability have been derived according to reported scores, ranging from no/minimal (0–12), moderate (13–29), and severe (≥ 30) (Kashikar-Zuck et al., 2011). Parent-proxy forms are also available, using the same items and scoring procedure. Correlations between youth and parent reports on the FDI range from moderate to strong (Reid, McGrath, & Lang, 2005; Walker & Greene, 1991). The FDI has also demonstrated adequate test-retest reliability (Claar & Walker, 2006; Walker & Greene, 1991), good to excellent internal consistency for both youth and parent versions (Walker & Greene, 1991), and moderate to strong concurrent and convergent validity with other measures of child health (Claar & Walker, 2006; Palermo et al., 2005; Walker & Greene, 1991). The FDI is quick and easy to administer and has been translated into many languages.

The Pediatric Quality of Life Inventory – Generic Core Scales (PedsQL) is a 23-item self-report tool designed to measure health-related quality of life in youth. Youth and parent forms are available for young children (5–7 years), children (8–12 years), and teenagers (13–18 years). A separate parent form is also available for use with toddlers (2–4 years). The PedsQL has been recommended for assessing physical functioning in children younger than 7 years (McGrath et al., 2008). The total scale contains four subscales assessing physical, emotional, social, and school functioning. Sample items on the physical functioning subscale include "It is hard for me to run" and "It is hard for me to do chores around the house." Items are rated on a 5-point scale ranging from 0 ("Never") to 4 ("Almost Always"). Higher scores indicate better health-related quality of life. Parent-proxy forms use the same items and scoring procedure. The PedsQL has demonstrated good construct validity and can distinguish between healthy youth and youth with chronic medical conditions (Varni, Seid, & Kurtin, 2001). Furthermore, youth and parent reports have shown moderate correlations (Powers, Patton, Hommel, & Hershey, 2004; Varni, Limbers, & Burwinkle, 2007). The PedsQL is quick and easy to administer and score, demonstrates strong psychometric properties, and has been translated into many languages.

Sleep Sleep disruptions play an important role in pediatric chronic pain. However, measurements of sleep have not widely been included in clinical trials (McGrath et al., 2008). In addition, there is currently no standardized measure of sleep specifically for use in pediatric chronic pain populations. A systematic review of sleep measures used in studies of pediatric chronic pain found two measures to be considered "well-established" according to evidence-based research: the Children's Sleep Habits Questionnaire (CSHQ) and the Adolescent Sleep-Wake Scale (ASWS) (de la Vega & Miró, 2013). Wrist actigraphy may be a nonintrusive, cost-effective, and user-friendly tool for assessing sleep in pediatric chronic pain patients. Actigraphy utilizes wrist movements via a small wristwatch-like device worn on the non-dominant hand and provides objective data on multiple sleep domains (e.g., sleep onset, number of nighttime awakenings, wake after sleep onset, etc.). Comparable validity with polysomnography has been demonstrated for use in adult populations (Lichstein et al., 2006). However, several issues with validity in pediatric populations have been raised, including inconsistencies across studies in the devices, software, and scoring algorithms that are used (Meltzer, Montgomery-Downs, Insana, & Walsh, 2012). To date, findings from actigraphy research in pediatric chronic pain populations have been mixed; some studies have found that youth with chronic pain experience more objective night awakenings and lower sleep efficiency compared to healthy youth, while larger studies have found no differences between youth with chronic pain and healthy youth on sleep outcomes via actigraphy (Valrie, Bromberg, Palermo, & Schanberg, 2013).

Sleep diaries, either on their own or incorporated within the pain diaries, or other standardized assessments of youth sleep could also be used, and parent-proxy reports of youth sleep may be helpful as well. For example, the Children's Sleep Habits Questionnaire (CSHQ) is a 33-item tool that asks parents to report and rate their young child's (4–10 years) sleep patterns (Owens, Spirito, & McGuinn, 2000). It yields a score on eight subscales including bedtime resistance, sleep-onset delay, sleep-duration, sleep anxiety, night wakings, parasomnias, sleep-disordered breathing, and daytime sleepiness. Across a clinical and community sample, the CSHQ demonstrated good internal consistency and discriminant validity (Owens et al., 2000).

The Children's Report of Sleep Patterns (CRSP) is a 62-item self-report assessment of school-aged children's sleep (8 to 12 years; Meltzer et al., 2013). It yields scores across three subscales: sleep patterns, sleep hygiene, and sleep disturbance. Similar to the CSHQ, the CRSP involves different forms of responses, including fill-in-the-blank questions (e.g., "What time did you go to bed last night?") and questions rated on a 5-point scale ranging from 0 ("Never") to 4 ("Always") (e.g., "How often do you have bad dreams?"). The CRSP has demonstrated good test-retest reliability, convergent and divergent reliability, and internal consistency (Meltzer et al., 2013).

Adolescent (12–18 years) sleep patterns may be assessed using the Adolescent Sleep-Wake Scale (ASWS) (LeBourgeois et al., 2005). The ASWS is a 28-item questionnaire that asks adolescents to report on the frequency of their sleep problem on a 6-point scale ranging from 6 ("Never") to 1 ("Always"). It yields scores on five subscales related to sleep quality: going to bed, sleep onset, sleep maintenance, wake after sleep onset, and wakefulness. A total sleep quality score can also be derived. Higher scores indicate better sleep quality. The ASWS has demonstrated good internal consistency on the total scale (α = 0.80–0.86) and poor to good internal consistency on the subscales (α = 0.60–0.82). A recent examination of the factor structure of the ASWS revealed a shorter, 10-item version loaded onto three subscales: Falling Asleep and Reinitiating Sleep, Returning to Wakefulness-Revised, and Going to Bed-Revised. Internal consistency for the subscales ranged from adequate to good (α = 0.84, α = 0.87, and α = 0.71, respectively) (Essner, Noel, Myrvik, & Palermo, 2016).

Psychosocial Factors Related to Chronic Pain

Psychological factors, such as anxiety and depression, can play important exacerbating or protective roles in a child's pain experience; the reader is directed to Chaps 10. https://doi.org/10.1007/978-3-319-93542-3_10 and 11 regarding their assessment. Pain catastrophizing, or an "exaggerated negative orientation" toward actual or anticipated pain (Sullivan, Bishop, & Pivik, 1995), has been associated with greater pain intensity and disability (Vervoort, Goubert, Eccleston, Bijttebier, & Crombez, 2005). Pain-related fear has been associated with high functional disability, depression, and school interference, as well as greater avoidance of and disengagement from daily activities (Simons, 2016). Furthermore, parental responses, as well as newly emerging factors including pain acceptance, pain self-efficacy, and optimism, have also been found to be associated with pediatric chronic pain outcomes.

Pain Catastrophizing The Pain Catastrophizing Scale for Children (PCS-C) is a 13-item self-report measure designed for youth aged 8–18 years. Responses to a variety of thoughts and feelings that youth might have when they are in pain are rated from 0 ("Not At All") to 4 ("Extremely") (Crombez et al., 2003). Examples of items include "When I am in pain, it's terrible and I think it's never going to get any better" and "When I am in pain, I can't keep it out of my mind." The PCS-C yields three subscales of rumination, magnification, and helplessness. Total scores on the PCS-C range from 0 to 52, with higher scores indicating greater pain catastrophizing. The PCS-C has demonstrated adequate internal consistency, criterion and construct validity, and test-retest reliability (Crombez et al., 2003; Pielech et al., 2014). Furthermore, a parent version of the PCS-C has demonstrated adequate internal consistency, construct validity, and criterion validity (Goubert, Eccleston, Vervoort, Jordan, & Crombez, 2006; Pielech et al., 2014). An advantage of utilizing the PCS-C in pediatric chronic pain populations is the recent determination of references points for catastrophizing for three levels: low (0–14), moderate (15–25), and high ($\geq$26) (Pielech et al., 2014).

Pain-Related Fear The Fear of Pain Questionnaire, Child Report (FOPQ-C) is a 24-item questionnaire used to assess pain-related fear in youth between 8 and 17 years (Simons, Sieberg, Carpino, Logan, & Berde, 2011). Youth are asked to rate the extent to which they agree with a list of items on a 5-point scale ranging from 0 ("Strongly Disagree") to 4 ("Strongly Agree"). Example items include "I walk around in constant fear of hurting" and "When I am in pain, I stay away from other people." The FOPQ-C yields scores on two subscales: fear of pain and avoidance of activities. Higher scores indicate higher pain-related fear and avoidance of activities. Furthermore, a 23-item parent version (FOPQ-P) has also been created for use in this population. In pilot testing, the FOPQ-C and FOPQ-P demonstrated high internal consistency, construct validity, criterion validity, and 1-month stability (Simons et al., 2011).

Parent Responses to Child's Pain The Adult Responses to Children's Symptoms (ARCS) is a 29-item tool designed for use with parents who have youth between 8 and 18 years of age (Van Slyke & Walker, 2006). Parents are asked how often they engage in a behavior on a 5-point scale ranging from 0 ("Never") to 4 ("Always"). Examples of items on the ARCS include "Let your child stay home from school" and "Tell your child and he/she needs to learn to be stronger." Recent factorial analyses found a four-factor structure of adult responses for youth with pain: protect, minimize, monitor, and distract (Noel et al., 2015). Confirmatory factor analyses have shown that the ARCS is a valid tool for use in pediatric chronic pain populations (Claar, Guite, Kaczynski, & Logan, 2010). Validity of the ARCS has been demonstrated differentially by subscale, with the protect subscale showing strong associations (Van Slyke & Walker, 2006), while the other subscales demonstrate poorer internal consistency. An examination of the sensitivity to change and responsiveness of the ARCS pre- and posttreatment for pediatric chronic pain revealed that the Protect and Monitor subscales demonstrated clinically meaningful reductions for youth (Noel et al., 2016).

Emerging Positive Psychological Factors There is an emerging trend to examine psychological factors that are in line with promoting well-being and optimal outcomes in youth with chronic pain. Some of these include pain acceptance, pain self-efficacy, and optimism, and each has been associated with better outcomes. Moreover, some of these factors plays a role in an individual's overall psychological flexibility (the ability to contact the present moment and to change or persist in behavior in order to achieve "valued goals"), which is the central component of Acceptance and Commitment Therapy (ACT). ACT has shown promising results in the treatment of pediatric chronic pain (Pielech, Vowles, & Wicksell, 2017). Therefore, assessing for these factors would be in line with a biopsychosocial approach and may also reveal important treatment targets for intervention.

Pain acceptance (living with pain without reaction, disapproval, or attempts to reduce/avoid it) has been associated with better school functioning, and improvements in depressive symptomatology, psychological distress, and functional impairment (Kalapurakkel, Carpino, Lebel, & Simons, 2015; McCracken, Gauntlett-Gilbert, & Eccleston, 2010). Currently, the most researched measure of pain acceptance in pediatric pain populations is the Chronic Pain Acceptance Questionnaire-Adolescent version (CPAQ-A; McCracken et al., 2010). The CPAQ-A is a 20-item self-report measure designed to assess pain acceptance in adolescents aged 10–18 years. Pain acceptance is measured by two factors: activity engagement and pain willingness. Items are rated on a scale ranging from 0 ("Never True") to 4 ("Always True"), with higher scores reflecting higher pain acceptance. Example items on the CPAQ-A include "My life is going well, even though I have chronic pain" and "I realize that I don't have to change my pain to get on with life." Initial investigations of the CPAQ-A have shown high internal consistency and good construct validity (McCracken et al., 2010; Wallace, Harbeck-Weber, Whiteside, & Harrison, 2011). A parent version of the CPAQ-A has also demonstrated good internal consistency and construct validity for use in parents with youth aged 8–17 years (Simons, Sieberg, & Kaczynski, 2011).

Pain self-efficacy (belief that one can function despite pain) has also been linked with better outcomes in youth with chronic pain (Tomlinson, Cousins, McMurtry, & Cohen, 2017), including increased functional ability (Carpino, Segal, Logan, Lebel, & Simons, 2014; Kalapurakkel et al., 2015), quality of life (Cramm, Strating, & Nieboer, 2013), and school functioning (Carpino et al., 2014). The Child Self-Efficacy Scale (CSE; Bursch et al., 2006) is a common 7-item self- and parent report measure for youth aged 8–18 years. Items are rated on a 5-point scale ranging from 1

("Very Sure") to 5 ("Very Unsure"). Examples of items include "How sure are you that you can take care of yourself when you have pain?" and "How sure are you that you can make it through a day of school when you have pain?" Lower scores indicate greater self-efficacy. High internal consistency and good construct validity have been demonstrated (Bursch et al., 2006).

Optimism (extent to which an individual holds favorable expectancies for the future) has been relatively understudied in chronic pain populations. However, findings from pediatric populations with cancer suggest that optimism is associated with lower reported pain intensity and better overall quality of life and emotional functioning (Mannix, Feldman, & Moody, 2009; Williams, Davis, Hancock, & Phipps, 2010). In one study of chronic pain in patients aged 8–17 years, optimism mediated the relation between pain catastrophizing and quality of life (Cousins, Cohen, & Venable, 2015). One measure of optimism that has been used in pediatric chronic pain studies is the Youth Life Orientation Test (YLOT). The YLOT is a 16-item measure of optimism developed for use with youth aged 8–12 years (Ey et al., 2005), but use has been expanded to 7–18-year-olds in some studies (Cousins et al., 2015; Williams et al., 2010). Items are rated on a 4-point scale ranging from 3 ("True For Me") to 0 ("Not True For Me"). Examples include "I'm always hopeful about my future" and "Usually, I don't expect things to go my way." The YLOT yields scores on a youth's optimism, pessimism, and global optimism. It has demonstrated good test-retest reliability, as well as convergent and discriminant validity (Ey et al., 2005).

Another psychosocial factor that has been associated with pediatric chronic pain outcomes, yet so far is relatively understudied, is the consideration of pain-related goals. In line with the pediatric fear-avoidance model, two distinct goal approaches have been identified: valued life goals and pain control goals (Fisher & Palermo, 2016). Valued life goals, such as those that are espoused by the psychological flexibility model, are associated with pain recovery. In contrast, a greater priority given to pain control goals is predicted to be related to greater fear, pain, and subsequent avoidance (Fisher & Palermo, 2016). Some evidence suggests that youth with chronic pain experience greater frustration with goals related to social and self-acceptance, health, and school compared to healthy youth (Massey, Garnefski, & Gebhardt, 2009; Stommen, Verbunt, & Goossens, 2016). In turn, higher goal frustration in these domains is associated with higher depression and lower quality of life (Fisher & Palermo, 2016).

The PROMIS Tools

A tool for comparing and evaluating chronic pain in children is the Patient-Reported Outcomes Measurement Information System (PROMIS®), developed by the US Department of Health and Human Services. The PROMIS® is a set of brief tools that assesses a youth's self-reported mental, physical, and social health, thus allowing for relative comparisons across these domains. Additionally, parent-proxy reports exist for most of the pediatric domains as well. The measures are publicly available without a license or fee. Standardized scoring allows for comparisons and interpretations to be made between measures and domains. For pain, the pediatric PROMIS® includes an 11-point NRS to assess pain intensity, a Pain Interference measure, and a Pain Behavior measure. The Pain Interference tool measures the social, cognitive, emotional, and physical consequences of pain on the child's life. During the development of the Pain Interference tool, evidence of reliability, construct validity, and discriminant validity were found (Amtmann et al., 2010). The Pain Behavior measure assesses for verbal, nonverbal, deliberate, and involuntary behaviors that typically indicate that a child is in pain to others. Psychometrically, scores from the Pain Behavior measure were found to be strongly correlated with pain intensity scores (Revicki et al., 2009). Given the advantages of the PROMIS® for use in clinical practice, further research on these measures in the assessment of pediatric pain is warranted.

Special Considerations: Pain in Children with Developmental Disabilities

In the following, the term developmental disabilities describe lifelong mental and/or physical disabilities that emerge in childhood. Developmental disabilities can impact functioning to differing degrees of severity across a number of adaptive domains (e.g., mobility, learning, communication; AAIDD, n.d.; Craig, 2006). Examples of developmental disabilities include autism spectrum disorder, Down syndrome, cerebral palsy, and intellectual disability.

Pain: Experience, Expression, Prevalence, and Impact

Inaccurate beliefs about pain in those with developmental disabilities developed within the unfortunate historical dehumanization and depersonalization directed toward these individuals (Sobsey, 2006). For many years, individuals held the belief that those with developmental disabilities were insensitive or indifferent to pain (Sobsey, 2006). Although research and understanding of pain in children with developmental disabilities remains limited in scope, to date there has been no evidence to support this belief; in fact, some findings suggest increased pain sensitivity compared to those without disabilities (e.g., intellectual disability or Down syndrome (Defrin, Pick, Peretz, & Carmeli, 2004); Autism: (Nader, Oberlander, Chambers, & Craig, 2004); Down syndrome (Valkenburg, Tibboel, & van Dijk, 2015)). Although literature regarding hyper- and hyposensitivity to pain in youth with developmental disabilities is mixed, it is clear that these youth can have limitations impacting their experience with, response to, and communication of pain (e.g., Dubois, Capdevila, Bringuier, & Pry, 2010; Valkenburg et al., 2015). Thus, rather than an inability to experience pain, pain expression of these individuals seems to differ (e.g., slower responses, differences in communication; Bottos & Chambers, 2006; Dubois et al., 2010; Valkenburg et al., 2015).

Compared to typically developing youth, those with developmental disabilities may be more likely to experience acute and chronic pain (Bottos & Chambers, 2006). For example, Stallard, Williams, Lenton, and Velleman (2001) found that 75% of a sample of youth with disabilities experienced pain within a 2-week period; 84% of those youth experienced pain on at least 5 days. High prevalence rates have also been found in a sample of youth with severe developmental disabilities: pain was experienced for multiple hours per week by more than one third of the sample (Breau, Camfield, McGrath, & Finley, 2003). These rates are much higher than in typically developing youth (e.g., Perquin et al., 2000). Parents of youth with disabilities have also reported beliefs that pain is something their children frequently experience and have learned to accept (Carter, McArthur, & Cunliffe, 2002). The sources of pain for these youth can vary greatly and may include comorbid and chronic conditions (e.g., gastrointestinal, congenital heart defects), medical procedures (e.g., needle procedures), unintentional injury (e.g., falling; Benini et al., 2004; Bottos & Chambers, 2006; Breau, Camfield et al., 2003), and others (e.g., earaches, stomachaches).

Beyond the short- and long-term consequences of unmanaged pain for typically developing youth, those with developmental disabilities are at an increased risk for negative consequences given their already limited cognitive and functional abilities (Breau, Camfield et al., 2007). Youth with developmental disabilities who are in pain may be less able to perform and practice necessary adaptive functioning skills including communication, daily living skills, motor skills, and socialization (Breau et al., 2007). There may also be a relation between experiencing pain and self-injury/aggression (Courtemanche, Black, & Reese, 2016; Courtemanche, Schroeder, Sheldon, Sherman, & Fowler, 2012). As unrecognized and untreated pain can negatively impact the quality of life of children with developmental disabilities, pain assessment is a critical task to ensure that children with developmental disabilities are living well. Given the unique challenges and needs of this population, special considerations are warranted.

Self-Report

In order to provide accurate self-reports of subjective painful experiences, a number of cognitive skills are necessary (e.g., understanding magnitude, seriation; von Baeyer et al., 2017). Unfortunately, these skills may be difficult for youth with developmental disabilities whose impairment is beyond the mild range. For example, when asked to provide self-report on a 0–5 numerical rating scale, only 21% of youth with intellectual disabilities were able to understand the necessary concepts (e.g., magnitude, ranking); all of these youth fell in the borderline or mild intellectual disability range (Fanurik, Koh, Harrison, Conrad, & Tomerun, 1998). Compounding the issue, the abilities these youth do possess may be negatively impacted when experiencing pain (Breau & Burkitt, 2009). As a result, their responses to measures using numerical or faces scales may be biased, inconsistent, or idiosyncratic. For example, similar to younger typically developing children (von Baeyer et al., 2017), those with developmental disabilities may show a bias toward choosing scale extremes (very low or very high pain; e.g., Ely, Chen-Lim, Carpenter II, Wallhauser, & Friedlaender, 2016).

Based on functional differences of youth with developmental disabilities, obtaining accurate self-report can be challenging but not impossible. Youth with mild to moderate levels of impairment are typically capable of providing some form of self-report (Benini et al., 2004; Fanurik, Koh, Schmitz, Harrison, & Conrad, 1999; Zabalia, Jacquet, & Breau, 2005). For example, Valkenburg et al. (2015) found that 80% of the youth with Down syndrome in their study could communicate that they were in pain, but the majority of these youth were unable to quantify or pinpoint where the pain was. Unfortunately, although a number of self-report tools have been utilized in research with youth who have disabilities (e.g., see Benini et al., 2004; Ely et al., 2016), these tools have not been validated for use with this population and may need to be adapted to match a youth's abilities (Benini et al., 2004; Ely et al., 2016). For example, in a sample of verbal youth with autism spectrum disorder, Ely et al. (2016) highlighted the need for individualized self-report accounting for factors such as language (e.g., use meaningful language that the child understands such as "hurt" or "cry") and method (e.g., opportunity to describe with words rather than numbers). Individual preferences regarding tools may also be important to consider (Ely et al., 2016). Finally, physical or motor limitations (e.g., use of hands) should not preclude a youth's ability to provide self-report and measures may also to be adapted accordingly (Crosta, Ward, Walker, & Peters, 2014).

Observational Reports

As in pain assessment with typically developing populations, a multimodal approach is recommended. It is common and recommended for the pain assessment process with youth with developmental disabilities to incorporate observational reports and judgments made by caregivers (Solodiuk et al., 2010; Taddio et al., 2015). Although observational assessment may be particularly useful when the youth is unable to provide any form of self-report (Quinn, Seibold, & Hayman, 2015), it also has a number of limitations and challenges. Most notably, youth with developmental disabilities often express their pain in different ways than typically developing youth and tend to engage in less help-seeking behaviors when in pain (Dubois et al., 2010; Gilbert-MacLeod, 2000). Accurate pain assessment may be even more difficult if pain is expressed in inconsistent ways within a given child (Bottos & Chambers, 2006; Fanurik et al., 1999). An individual's pain expression is also likely to be impacted by factors such as severity of pain, learned pain responses, level of intellectual impairment, and verbal ability (De Knegt et al., 2013; Defrin, Lotan, & Pick, 2006; Solodiuk, 2013).

Solodiuk (2013) asked parents to describe their children's pain responses and identified seven categories: vocalization (e.g., whimpering, crying), social behavior (e.g., withdrawal, hand-holding), facial expression (e.g., wincing, eye squinching), muscle tone (e.g., making fists, floppy arms), activity level (e.g., fatigued, increased activity), physiologic measures (e.g., heavy breathing, sweating), and self-injury (e.g., biting, head banging). Solodiuk's (2013) study and a recent systematic review (De Knegt et al., 2013) on pain behaviors of individuals with intellectual impairments were similar in that both studies identified vocalizations, social behavior, and facial expression as some of the most commonly reported pain behaviors; De Knegt et al.'s (2013) review also highlighted motor activity (e.g., activity level, body posture). Within each of these categories, pain responses can vary widely and be signaled through changes in either direction (e.g., increased or decreased vocalizations; withdrawal or comfort-seeking behavior; De Knegt et al., 2013; Solodiuk, 2013). A recent review by Crosta et al. (2014) explored the psychometric properties of four observational pain measures used in acute pain settings: (1) the Non-communicating Children's Pain Checklist-Postoperative Version (Breau, Finley, McGrath, & Camfield, 2002); (2) the revised Face, Leg, Activity, Cry, and Consolability scale (Malviya, Voepel-Lewis, Burke, Merkel, & Tait, 2006); (3) the Individualized Numeric Rating Scale (Solodiuk et al., 2010); and (4) the Pediatric Pain Profile (Hunt et al., 2004).

The Non-communicating Children's Pain Checklist-Postoperative Version (NCCPC-PV) is a 27-item measure designed to assist in observational pain assessment of young children and youth (3–18 years) with severe intellectual disabilities after surgery or painful medical procedures (Breau, Finley, et al., 2002). The NCCPC-PV asks caregivers to indicate how often a child showed a number of behaviors over a 10-min period ranging from 0 ("Not At All") to 3 ("Very Often"; Breau, Finley, et al., 2002; Breau, McGrath, Finley, & Camfield, 2009). The behaviors indicated on the NCCPC-PV are categorized into six subscales: vocal, social, facial, activity, body and limbs, and physiological (Breau et al., 2009). Examples of items include *crying (moderately loud), less interaction with others/withdrawn, furrowed brow,* and *not moving/less active/quiet* (Breau et al., 2009). Scores can be derived for each of the subscales, as well as combined to create a total score. To interpret, the total score can be compared to the cutoff scores, 6–10 = mild pain and > 11 = moderate to severe pain (Breau et al., 2009; Breau, Finley, et al., 2002). The NCCPC-PV demonstrates excellent internal consistency, interrater reliability, internal reliability (α = 0.91), and convergent validity (Breau, Finley, et al., 2002). A revised version (the Non-communicating Children's Pain Checklist-Revised [NCCPC-R]) has also been developed, and psychometric properties have been explored to help assist with pain assessment when the child is at home or in a residential setting (Breau, McGrath, et al., 2002).

The revised Face, Leg, Activity, Cry, and Consolability (r-FLACC) scale is a 5-item individualized measure designed for observational pain assessment of youth (4–21 years) with disabilities in hospital (Malviya et al., 2006). The r-FLACC asks the clinician to observe the youth and provide ratings from 0 to 2 across five subcategories, face, legs, activity, cry, and consolability, based on descriptions given within the measure (e.g., in the face subcategory, a score of 0 would be given if the youth had no particular expression or was smiling, while a score of 2 would be given if the youth had a consistent grimace or frown; Malviya et al., 2006). Caregivers who know the youth well may also add individualized behaviors (Malviya et al., 2006). The scores can be added together to create a total score from 0 to 10. A score from 0 to 3 is considered mild, 4–6 is moderate, and 7–10 is severe pain (Malviya et al., 2006). Psychometric evaluations of the r-FLACC have shown excellent interrater reliability as well as criterion and construct validity (Malviya et al., 2006). A Danish translation shows evidence of maintained psychometric properties (Pedersen, Rahbek, Nikolajsen, & Moller-Madsen, 2015).

The Individualized Numeric Rating Scale (INRS) is an adapted 0 ("No Pain") to 10 ("Worst Possible Pain") numeric rating scale on which caregivers provide descriptions of the youth's behavioral response to pain (Solodiuk et al., 2010). The INRS can be used for children older than 3 years (Solodiuk & Curley, 2003). It was initially designed to assist nurses in assessing and documenting pain in youth who are nonverbal following surgical procedures (Solodiuk et al., 2010). As such, nurses help parents to complete the INRS during a face-to-face interview; the youth's behavior on a usual day would be filled in under "0," and other pain behaviors would be placed accordingly on the scale (Solodiuk et al., 2010). The behavioral categories on the r-FLACC can be used to help guide parents in identifying pain behaviors (Solodiuk et al., 2010; Solodiuk & Curley, 2003). There is evidence of interrater reliability, convergent validity, and construct validity of the INRS (Solodiuk et al., 2010).

The Pediatric Pain Profile (PPP) is a 20-item observational measure developed for 1–18-year-old children with severe disabilities; the PPP can be used as a record across a number of settings including home, school, and respite (Hunt et al., 2004); part of this validation work appears to have been completed on a sample with recurrent, if not chronic, pain.[1] The PPP asks parents to rate how often a behavior occurs in a given time period ranging from 0 ("Never") to 3 ("A Great Deal"). Examples of items include *had disturbed sleep*, *resisted being moved*, *was hard to console or comfort*, and *appeared withdrawn/depressed*. The scores for each item are added together to create a total score ranging from 0 to 60, with higher scores indicating greater pain. A score of 0 should be given for missing items or items that the caregiver is unable to assess. Although each youth will have an individualized range of pain behaviors, the PPP includes general interpretation patterns based on research. The PPP demonstrates concurrent and face validity, interrater reliability, and construct validity (Hunt et al., 2004).

Each of the four measures reviewed in this section share some features including the assessment of children's facial expressions, physical activity, vocalization, and consolability. However, the format and methodology differ (Crosta et al., 2014). For example, the number of items on the checklists, level of parent involvement, and time to complete the measure (1–10 min) differ across measures (Crosta et al., 2014). At this time, the r-FLACC appears to have the most clinical utility for acute pain and has been recommended for this purpose (Chen-Lim et al., 2012; Crosta et al., 2014; Ely et al., 2016; Taddio et al., 2015). Importantly, however, a quality improvement study found that while nurses seemed to prefer the r-FLACC, parent preferences were split between the r-FLACC and the PPP (Chen-Lim et al., 2012). Still, another review focused on school settings suggested that the INRS may be the most useful (Quinn et al., 2015). Thus, the most useful or preferred observational assessment measure may vary depending on the setting, rater, and child.

Primary Caregivers, Attitudes, Beliefs, and Pain-Related Education

Given the complexity of pain assessment in youth with developmental disabilities, it is crucial for professionals and secondary caregivers to access information from those who know the youth well (Carter et al., 2002; Ely et al., 2016; Quinn et al., 2015). Parents typically know their children well, understand their capacity for self-report, and can serve as good proxy reporters of pain, particularly when using a structured pain assessment tool (Benini et al., 2004; Fanurik et al., 1999; Voepel-Lewis, Malviya, & Tait, 2005). They are able to describe their child's unique pain responses to others given their intimate knowledge of the youth's baseline behaviors, as well as pain history (Breau & Burkitt, 2009; Carter et al., 2002; Solodiuk, 2013). Furthermore, youth (e.g., verbal children with autism spectrum disorder) report seeking their parents for help communicating their pain or interpreting pain behaviors (Ely et al., 2016). Carter et al. (2002) found that parents see themselves as needing to take an active role in pain assessment and are happy to be consulted in this regard.

It is important for caregivers to conceptualize the pain assessment and communication process

---

[1] In the Hunt et al. (2004, p.278) validation study, one group of children was described as in pain "all of the time" or "some time each day".

as bidirectional between the youth and the caregiver. Although this is very important for typically developing youth as well as those with developmental disabilities, it may be particularly salient in the latter case given challenges in pain assessment and their vulnerability. Craig's (2009) social communication model of pain demonstrates the interplay between intra- and interpersonal characteristics that may impact pain-related decisions. For example, aside from the painful experience itself, a youth's pain may be impacted by the judgments/decisions made by those around them (e.g., caregivers) which, in turn, are related to how the youth expresses pain. These judgments and decisions may also be impacted by intrapersonal factors such as caregivers' experiences and pain−/disability-related beliefs (Craig, 2009). For example, caregivers may still hold beliefs that youth with developmental disabilities are less sensitive to pain (Breau, MacLaren, McGrath, Camfield, & Finley, 2003; Genik, McMurtry, & Breau, 2017). While it is unclear the extent to which these beliefs may impact care decisions, it is important that caregivers are aware of their beliefs and biases.

Although caregivers need to be knowledgeable about the "science" of pain (Hunt, Mastroyannopoulou, Goldman, & Seers, 2003), adequate pain-related education specific to children with developmental disabilities is lacking. Both healthcare and non-healthcare professionals lack confidence in these areas and believe that more education is needed (Carter, Simons, Bray, & Arnott, 2016; Genik, McMurtry, Breau, Lewis, & Freedman-Kalchman, 2017). Pilot work with children's respite workers demonstrated that targeted pain training can improve these caregivers' pain knowledge as well as their perceptions of the feasibility of and their own confidence and skill in pain assessment (Genik et al., 2017). Respite workers reported the pain training was highly valuable to their work (Genik et al., 2017). Further research in this area is necessary and ongoing.

Developmental Disabilities Case Study

Lyla Smith is a 10-year-old girl with Autism Spectrum Disorder and a moderate intellectual disability. She is typically a happy-go-lucky and healthy young girl but experiences significant gastrointestinal pain on occasion. Her family doctor believes that Lyla may have some food sensitivities but these have not been conclusively identified. Lyla can often verbally communicate her basic needs and desires; however, her understanding of spoken language is variable. She is able to communicate nonverbally through pointing if prompted. Conceptually, although Lyla has some understanding of differences in size, she cannot differentiate between more than two or three levels (e.g., small, medium, large). Lyla enjoys active play that involves gross motor skills such as climbing and running. She is easily irritated by certain fabrics and has difficulty in loud or crowded settings. She engages in a number of repetitive sensory-seeking behaviors such as rocking, spinning, and hand-flapping which appear to worsen when she is agitated.

Lyla receives weekly care by a respite provider and her grandparents. Each summer, Lyla attends an inclusive day camp with her sister. This summer, her regular respite provider was unavailable and a new worker, Petra, has been contracted out by the camp. When meeting Petra, Lyla's parents, Mr. and Mrs. Smith, completed an "all about me" booklet which described their daughter's typical demeanor and behavior, as well as her behavioral responses when she becomes upset. The Smiths completed the Pediatric Pain Profile (Hunt et al., 2004) which included Lyla's pain history and baseline information and provided it to Petra. The Smiths indicated that Lyla often becomes withdrawn when in pain and may appear oppositional (e.g., refusing to play games). They noted that while her repetitive and sensory-seeking behaviors may increase due to pain, there are also a number of other triggers. As such, increased sensory behaviors should not be exclusively used to determine whether pain is present.

On the first day of camp, Lyla began her day excited and engaged in the activities. She appeared happy during lunch and while on the jungle gym. After the transition from lunch to the swimming change room, Petra noticed Lyla sit in a corner and begin to rock. Despite showing Lyla her bathing suit, Lyla appeared disinterested in getting changed. Petra took a moment to consider her own beliefs and reaction to this situation (e.g., her past experience with other children and how they showed pain) and set those aside. She checked in with some of the other camp counselors to ask whether they had witnessed Lyla injure herself; no one had noticed this. She then took Lyla to a quiet place outside of the change room to determine whether her change in behavior was related to the crowded room and loud noises. When the behavior persisted, Petra referred to the documentation provided by Lyla's parents for history and baseline information. Based on the increased sensory-seeking behavior, her withdrawn and disinterested behavior, and the timing of onset (e.g., after lunch), the worker began to suspect that Lyla may be experiencing pain. She continued to observe Lyla for a few minutes, keeping an eye out for other pain behaviors identified by her parents in Lyla's PPP (e.g., holding her stomach). Lyla's worker then used language consistent with that used at home, to ask if she had any hurt. Lyla responded yes. Petra prompted Lyla to point to where her hurt was, and she was able to point to her stomach. She was unable to indicate the severity of her pain. After taking appropriate action (e.g., use of distraction and provision of a parent- and physician-approved pain medication[2]), Lyla's worker continued to informally observe Lyla throughout the day and reassess whether she was still experiencing pain.

Future Directions and Conclusions

Research on pediatric pain experience, expression, and treatment has progressed substantially in the past few decades. However, there are still substantive gaps in areas of the research literature. From a foundational knowledge perspective, given the importance of parental responses and the parent-child relationship on the child's pain experience, further investigations of fathers' roles on children's pain are warranted. Additionally, pain research has focused on more traditional psychopathological constructs and deficits; recent explorations into more positive psychological factors (e.g., pain acceptance, pain self-efficacy, optimism, etc.) have revealed an important avenue for future research to better understand the role of these factors in a youth's pain experience and outcomes and inform future treatment efforts.

Further work is also needed in validating *existing* pediatric pain measures for use across different populations, rather than the creation of new measures when current ones exist (cf. Tomlinson et al., 2010). For example, validation of existing pain intensity and location tools for use in youth with chronic pain is warranted. Studying the psychometrics of simplified pain intensity measures for preschool ages is needed (von Baeyer et al., 2017). There are also gaps at older ages, for example, in sleep assessment for youth with chronic pain, the CSHQ and ASWS have emerged as "well established" assessments (de la Vega & Miró, 2013), leaving a gap for appropriate assessment in youth aged 10–12 years old. Research into sleep assessments for younger children and sleep measures that can be administered in self-report format for younger

---

[2] Given that the purpose of this chapter is pain assessment, limited information regarding pain management has been provided throughout. Research regarding pain management in children with developmental disabilities is scarce. As such, the reader is referred to: (1) Belew et al. (2013) for pain in children with intellectual or developmental disabilities; (2) Taddio and Oberlander (2006) regarding pharmacological management of pain in children with developmental disabilities, and (3) to the general pediatric pain management literature for more information regarding other pain management strategies, including numerous chapters in the Oxford Textbook of Paediatric Pain (McGrath, Stevens, Walker, & Zempsky, 2013). There are also numerous systematic reviews, meta-analyses, and clinical practice guidelines on various treatments for acute and chronic pain (e.g., Eccleston et al., 2014; Fisher et al., 2014; Taddio et al., 2015).

ages are important (i.e., CRSP: Meltzer et al., 2013).

A multimodal approach to pediatric chronic pain assessment has necessitated the inclusion of various psychosocial measures that have yet to be validated for use in youth with chronic pain or have not been psychometrically examined beyond their initial validation (e.g., ASWS, LeBourgeois et al., 2005; CSE, Bursch et al., 2006). More work is also needed in terms of examining more recently established factor structures (e.g., ASWS, Essner et al., 2016; ARCS, Noel et al., 2015) in pediatric chronic pain populations, as well as exploring the validity of measures for wider age ranges (e.g., CPAQ-A, McCracken et al., 2010; YLOT, Ey et al., 2005). Tools that have been developed for use in patient registries, such as the PROMIS®, provide measurement of patient outcomes across health conditions and may show particular promise for future research driving the chronic pain field forward.

Considerable questions remain regarding pain (assessment) in youth with developmental disabilities. Novel work such as that conducted by Ely et al. (2016) can serve as a model – how can/do we gather self-report from youth with various developmental disabilities? What kind of modifications are most helpful? There has also been a lack of research examining the psychometric properties of pain measures designed to be used for non-procedure-related pain in youth with developmental disabilities; looking beyond the procedure-related pain context to include chronic or recurrent pain is critical.

Pediatric pain is a prevalent health concern for a significant number of youth that has drawn increased research attention in the past several decades. The biopsychosocial approach provides a framework to guide pediatric pain research, assessment, and management across a variety of contexts, presentations, and populations. Unsurprisingly then, there are many areas ripe for future work. Longitudinal work with collaboration across sites (e.g., through registries) may be particularly important to advance the field. It is clear that unmanaged acute pain is associated with significant short- and long-term deleterious consequences (McMurtry et al., 2015; Taddio et al., 2012). Chronic pain is associated with reduced physical, emotional, and social functioning, as well as increased healthcare costs (Groenewald et al., 2014). Comprehensive pediatric pain assessments can help identify the need for intervention and highlight relations between pain and other biological, psychological, and social variables that may be serving to exacerbate or perpetuate the pain in order to guide treatment. In acute pain, information regarding pain intensity, location, and pain-related fear are important for future pain management for a given youth (e.g., what strategies to use for the next needle) and for intervention research more generally. Chronic pain assessments require examination of other functional variables (e.g., sleep, mood, functional disability), as well as parental factors to guide treatment and assess treatment response. Special considerations for youth with developmental disabilities are critical in order to gain an accurate understanding of the youth's pain and maximize quality of life. This may involve a greater reliance on observational measures rather than self-reports, necessitating an understanding of various pain behaviors. In sum, evidence-based assessment guides treatment, and pain management is a human right (Brennan, Carr, & Cousins, 2007). Youth and their families deserve nothing less.

References

American Association on Intellectual and Developmental Disabilities (AAIDD). (n.d.). Is intellectual disability the same as developmental disabilities? In *Frequently asked questions on intellectual disability*. Retrieved from: https://aaidd.org/intellectual-disability/definition/faqs-on-intellectual-disability

Amtmann, D., Cook, K. F., Jensen, M. P., Chen, W., Choi, S., Revicki, D., ... Callahan, L. (2010). Development of a PROMIS item bank to measure pain interference. *Pain, 150*(1), 172–182.

Andrasik, F., Burke, E. J., Attanasio, V., & Rosenblum, E. L. (2005). Child, parent, and physician reports of a child's headache pain: Relationships prior to and following treatment. *Headache: The Journal of Head and Face Pain, 25*(8), 421–425. https://doi.org/10.1111/j.1526-4610.1985.hed2508421.x

Aradine, C., Beyer, J., & Tompkins, J. (1988). Children's pain perception before and after analgesia: A study of instrument construct validity and related issues. *Journal of Pediatric Nursing, 3*, 11–23.

Asmundson, G. J. G., Noel, M., Petter, M., & Parkerson, H. A. (2012). Pediatric fear-avoidance model of chronic pain: Foundation, application and future directions. *Pain Research and Management: The Journal of the Canadian Pain Society = Journal de La Société Canadienne Pour Le Traitement de La Douleur, 17*(6), 397–405.

Bailey, B., Daoust, R., Doyon-Trottier, E., Dauphin-Pierre, S., & Gravel, J. (2010). Validation and properties of the verbal numeric scale in children with acute pain. *Pain, 149*, 216–221.

Ballantyne, J. C., & Sullivan, M. D. (2015). Intensity of chronic pain — The wrong metric. *New England Journal of Medicine, 373*(22), 2098–2099. https://doi.org/10.1056/NEJMp1507136

Beales, J. G., Keen, J. H., & Lennox-Holt, P. J. (1983). The child's perception of the disease and the experience of pain in juvenile chronic arthritis. *Journal of Rheumatology, 10*, 61–65.

Belew, J. L., Barney, C. C., Schwantes, S. A., Tibboel, D., Valkenburg, A. J., & Symons, F. J. (2013). Pain in children with intellectual or developmental disabilities. In P. J. McGrath, B. J. Stevens, S. M. Walker, & W. T. Zempsky (Eds.), *Oxford textbook of paediatric pain* (pp. 147–156). Oxford: Oxford University Press. Location: New York, USA.

Belter, R. W., McIntosh, J. A., Finch, A. J., & Saylor, C. F. (1988). Preschoolers' ability to differentiate levels of pain: Relative efficacy of three self-report measures. *Journal of Clinical Child Psychology, 17*, 329–335.

Benini, F., Trapanotto, M., Gobber, D., Agosto, C., Carli, G., Drigo, P., … Zacchello, F. (2004). Evaluating pain induced by venipuncture in pediatric patients with developmental delay. *The Clinical Journal of Pain, 20*(3), 156–163. https://doi.org/10.1097/00002508-200405000-00005

Berntson, L., & Svensson, E. (2001). Pain assessment in children with juvenile chronic arthritis: A matter of scaling and rater. *Acta Pediatrica, 90*, 1131–1136.

Beyer, J. E. (1984). *The oucher: A user's manual and technical report.* Evanston, IL: Judson Press.

Beyer, J. E., & Aradine, C. R. (1986). Content validity of an instrument to measure young children's perceptions of the intensity of their pain. *Journal of Pediatric Nursing, 1*, 386–395.

Beyer, J. E., & Aradine, C. R. (1987). Patterns of pediatric pain intensity: A methodological investigation of a self-report scale. *The Clinical Journal of Pain, 3*, 130–141.

Beyer, J. E., & Aradine, C. R. (1988). Convergent and discriminant validity of a self-report measure of pain intensity for children. *Children's Health Care, 16*, 274–282.

Beyer, J. E., Denyes, M., & Villaruel, A. (1992). The creation, validation and continuing development of the oucher: A measure of pain intensity in children. *Journal of Pediatric Nursing, 7*, 335–346.

Beyer, J. E., & Knott, C. B. (1998). Construct validity estimation for the African-American and Hispanic versions of the Oucher scale. *Journal of Pediatric Nursing, 13*, 20–31.

Bieri, D., Reeve, R., Champion, G., Addicoat, L., & Ziegler, J. (1990). The faces pain scale for the self-assessment of the severity of pain experienced by children: Development, initial validation, and preliminary investigation for ratio scale properties. *Pain, 41*, 13–50.

Birnie, K.A., Boerner, K.E., & Chambers, C.T. (2013). Families and pain. In P.J. McGrath, B.J. Stevens, S.W. Walker and W.T. Zempsky (Eds.), *Oxford Textbook of Pediatric Pain* (pp. 111–118). New York, USA: Oxford University Press.

Blankenburg, M., Boeken, H., Hechler, T., Maier, C., Krumova, E., Scherens, A., … Zernikow, B. (2010). Reference values for quantitative sensory testing in children and adolescents: Developmental and gender differences of somatosensory perception. *Pain, 149*(1), 76–88.

Blount, R. L., & Loiselle, K. A. (2009). Behavioural assessment of pediatric pain. *Pain Research and Management, 14*(1), 47–52.

Boerner, K. E., Birnie, K. A., Caes, L., Schinkel, M., & Chambers, C. T. (2014). Sex differences in experimental pain among healthy children: A systematic review and meta-analysis. *Pain, 155*(5), 983–993.

Boerner, K. E., Eccleston, C., Chambers, C. T., & Keogh, E. (2016). Sex differences in the efficacy of psychological therapies for the management of chronic and recurrent pain in children and adolescents: A systematic review and meta-analysis. *Pain, 158*(4), 569–582.

Bottos, S., & Chambers, C. T. (2006). The epidemiology of pain in developmental disabilities. In T. F. Oberlander & F. J. Symons (Eds.), *Pain in children and adults with developmental disabilities.* Baltimore, MD: Paul H. Brookes Pub.

Breau, L. M., & Burkitt, C. (2009). Assessing pain in children with intellectual disabilities. *Pain Research and Management, 14*(2), 116–120.

Breau, L. M., Camfield, C. S., McGrath, P. J., & Finley, G. A. (2003). The incidence of pain in children with severe cognitive impairments. *Archives of Pediatrics and Adolescent Medicine, 157*(12), 1219–1226. https://doi.org/10.1001/archpedi.157.12.1219

Breau, L. M., Camfield, C. S., McGrath, P. J., & Finley, G. A. (2007). Pain's impact on adaptive functioning. *Journal of Intellectual Disability Research, 51*(2), 125–134. https://doi.org/10.1111/j.1365-2788.2006.00851.x

Breau, L. M., Finley, G. A., McGrath, P. J., & Camfield, C. S. (2002). Validation of the non-communicating Children's pain checklist-postoperative version. *Anesthesiology, 96*(3), 528–535 http://doi.org/00000542-200203000-00004

Breau, L. M., MacLaren, J., McGrath, P. J., Camfield, C. S., & Finley, G. A. (2003). Caregivers' beliefs regarding pain in children with cognitive impairment: Relation between pain sensation and reaction increases with severity of impairment. *The Clinical Journal of Pain, 19*(6), 335–344.

Breau, L. M., McGrath, P. J., Camfield, C. S., & Finley, G. A. (2002). Psychometric properties of the non-communicating Children's pain checklist - revised. *Pain, 99*, 349–357.

Breau, L. M., McGrath, P. J., Finley, G. A., & Camfield, C. S. (2009). Non-communicating children's pain checklist – postoperative version. Retrieved from http://pediatric-pain.ca/wp-content/uploads/2013/04/NCCPCPV_200901.pdf

Bursch, B., Tsao, J. C. I., Meldrum, M., & Zeltzer, L. K. (2006). Preliminary validation of a self-efficacy scale for child functioning despite chronic pain (child and parent versions). *Pain, 125*(1-2), 35–42. https://doi.org/10.1016/j.pain.2006.04.026

Brennan, F., Carr, D. B., Cousins, M. (2007). Pain management: a fundamental human right. *Anesthesia & Analgesia, 105*(1), 205–221.

Carpino, E., Segal, S., Logan, D., Lebel, A., & Simons, L. E. (2014). The interplay of pain-related self-efficacy and fear on functional outcomes among youth with headache. *The Journal of Pain: Official Journal of the American Pain Society, 15*(5), 527–534. https://doi.org/10.1016/j.jpain.2014.01.493

Carter, B., McArthur, E., & Cunliffe, M. (2002). Dealing with uncertainty: Parental assessment of pain in their children with profound special needs. *Journal of Advanced Nursing, 38*(5), 449–457. https://doi.org/10.1046/j.1365-2648.2002.02206.x

Carter, B., Simons, J., Bray, L., & Arnott, J. (2016). Navigating uncertainty: Health professionals' knowledge, skill, and confidence in assessing and managing pain in children with profound cognitive impairment. *Pain Research and Management, 2016*, 1–7. https://doi.org/10.1155/2016/8617182

Carter, B. D., & Threlkeld, B. M. (2012). Psychosocial perspectives in the treatment of pediatric chronic pain. *Pediatric Rheumatology, 10*(1), 15. https://doi.org/10.1186/1546-0096-10-15

Chambers, C. T., & Craig, K. D. (1998). An intrusive impact of anchors in children's faces pain scales. *Pain, 78*(1), 27–37.

Chambers, C. T., Giesbrecht, K., Craig, K. D., Bennett, S., & Huntsman, E. (1999). A comparison of faces scales for the measurement of pediatric pain: Children's and parents' ratings. *Pain, 83*, 25–35.

Chambers, C. T., Hardial, J., Craig, K. D., Court, C., & Montgomery, C. (2005). Faces scales for the measurement of postoperative pain intensity in children following minor surgery. *Clinical Journal of Pain, 21*, 277–285.

Chen-Lim, M. L., Zarnowsky, C., Green, R., Shaffer, S., Holtzer, B., & Ely, E. (2012). Optimizing the assessment of pain in children who are cognitively impaired through the quality improvement process. *Journal of Pediatric Nursing, 27*(6), 750–759. https://doi.org/10.1016/j.pedn.2012.03.023

Claar, R. L., Guite, J. W., Kaczynski, K. J., & Logan, D. E. (2010). Factor structure of the adult responses to Children's symptoms: Validation in children and adolescents with diverse chronic pain conditions. *Clinical Journal of Pain, 26*, 410–417.

Claar, R. L., & Walker, L. S. (2006). Functional assessment of pediatric pain patients: Psychometric properties of the functional disability inventory. *Pain, 121*(1-2), 77–84. https://doi.org/10.1016/j.pain.2005.12.002

Courtemanche, A., Schroeder, S., Sheldon, J., Sherman, J., & Fowler, A. (2012). Observing signs of pain in relation to self-injurious behaviour among individuals with intellectual and developmental disabilities. *Journal of Intellectual Disability Research, 56*(5), 501–515. https://doi.org/10.1111/j.1365-2788.2011.01492.x

Courtemanche, A. B., Black, W. R., & Reese, R. M. (2016). The relationship between pain, self-injury, and other problem behaviors in young children with autism and other developmental disabilities. *American Journal on Intellectual and Developmental Disabilities, 121*(3), 194–203. https://doi.org/10.1352/1944-7558-121.3.194

Cousins, L. A., Cohen, L. L., & Venable, C. (2015). Risk and resilience in pediatric chronic pain: Exploring the protective role of optimism. *The Journal of Pediatric Psychology, 40*(9), 934–942.

Craig, K. D. (2006). The construct and definition of pain in developmental disability. In T. F. Oberlander & F. J. Symons (Eds.), *Pain in children and adults with developmental disabilities*. Baltimore, MD: Paul H. Brookes Pub.

Craig, K. D. (2009). The social communication model of pain. *Canadian Psychology, 50*(1), 22–32. https://doi.org/10.1037/a0014772

Cramm, J. M., Strating, M. M. H., & Nieboer, A. P. (2013). The importance of general self-efficacy for the quality of life of adolescents with diabetes or juvenile rheumatoid arthritis over time: A longitudinal study among adolescents and parents. *Frontiers in Pediatrics, 1*, 40. https://doi.org/10.3389/fped.2013.00040

Crombez, G., Bijttebier, P., Eccleston, C., Mascagni, T., Mertens, G., Goubert, L., & Verstraeten, K. (2003). The child version of the pain catastrophizing scale (PCS-C): A preliminary validation. *Pain, 104*(3), 639–646.

Crosta, Q. R., Ward, T. M., Walker, A. J., & Peters, L. M. (2014). A review of pain measures for hospitalized children with cognitive impairment. *Journal for Specialists in Pediatric Nursing, 19*(2), 109–118. https://doi.org/10.1111/jspn.12069

De Knegt, N. C., Pieper, M. J. C., Lobbezoo, F., Schuengel, C., Evenhuis, H. M., Passchier, J., & Scherder, E. J. A. (2013). Behavioral pain indicators in people with intellectual disabilities: A systematic review. *Journal of Pain*. https://doi.org/10.1016/j.jpain.2013.04.016

de la Vega, R., & Miró, J. (2013). The assessment of sleep in pediatric chronic pain sufferers. *Sleep Medicine Reviews, 17*, 185–192.

Defrin, R., Lotan, M., & Pick, C. G. (2006). The evaluation of acute pain in individuals with cognitive impairment: A differential effect of the level of impairment. *Pain, 124*(3), 312–320. https://doi.org/10.1016/j.pain.2006.04.031

Defrin, R., Pick, C. G., Peretz, C., & Carmeli, E. (2004). A quantitative somatosensory testing of pain threshold in individuals with mental retardation. *Pain, 108*(1), 58–66. https://doi.org/10.1016/j.pain.2003.12.003

Dick, B. D., & Pillai Riddell, R. (2010). Cognitive and school functioning in children and adolescents with chronic pain: A critical review. *Pain Research and Management : The Journal of the Canadian Pain Society = Journal de La Société Canadienne Pour Le Traitement de La Douleur, 15*(4), 238–244.

Dubois, A., Capdevila, X., Bringuier, S., & Pry, R. (2010). Pain expression in children with an intellectual disability. *European Journal of Pain, 14*(6), 654–660. https://doi.org/10.1016/j.ejpain.2009.10.013

Eccleston, C., Palermo, T. M., Williams, A. C., Lewandowski Holley, A., Morley, S., Fisher, E., & Law, E. (2014). Psychological therapies for the management of chronic and recurrent pain in children and adolescents. *Cochrane Database of Systematic Reviews*. https://doi.org/10.1002/14651858.CD003968.pub4

Eland, J. M., & Anderson, J. E. (1977). The experience of pain in children. In A. Jacox (Ed.), *Pain: A sourcebook for nurses and other health care professionals*. Boston, MA: Little, Brown & Co.

Ely, E., Chen-Lim, M. L., Carpenter, K. M., II, Wallhauser, E., & Friedlaender, E. (2016). Pain assessment of children with autism Spectrum disorders. *Journal of Developmental and Behavioural Pediatrics, 37*(1), 53–61.

Essner, B., Noel, M., Myrvik, M., & Palermo, T. (2016). Examination of the factor structure of the adolescent sleep-wake scale (ASWS). *Behavioral Sleep Medicine, 13*(4), 296–307.

Ey, S., Hadley, W., Allen, D. N., Palmer, S., Klosky, J., Deptula, D., ... Cohen, R. (2005). A new measure of children's optimism and pessimism: The youth life orientation test. *Journal of Child Psychology and Psychiatry, and Allied Disciplines, 46*(5), 548–558. https://doi.org/10.1111/j.1469-7610.2004.00372.x

Fanurik, D., Koh, J. L., Harrison, R. D., Conrad, T. M., & Tomerun, C. (1998). Pain assessment in children with cognitive impairment: An exploration of self-report skills. *Clinical Nursing Research, 7*(2), 103–119. https://doi.org/10.1177/105477389800700202

Fanurik, D., Koh, J. L., Schmitz, M. L., Harrison, R. D., & Conrad, T. M. (1999). Children with cognitive impairment: Parent report of pain and coping. *Journal of Developmental and Behavioral Pediatrics*. https://doi.org/10.1097/00004703-199908000-00004

Fernandes, A. M., De Campos, C., Batalha, L., Perdigão, A., & Jacob, E. (2014). Pain assessment using the adolescent Pediatric pain tool: A systematic review. *Pain Research & Management, 19*, 212–218.

Fisher, E., Heathcote, L., Palermo, T. M., de C Williams, A. C., Lau, J., & Eccleston, C. (2014). Systematic review and meta-analysis of psychological therapies for children with chronic pain. *Journal of Pediatric Psychology, 39*, 763–782.

Fisher, E., & Palermo, T. M. (2016). Goal pursuit in youth with chronic pain. *Children, 3*, 36.

Forgeron, P. A., King, S., Stinson, J. N., McGrath, P. J., MacDonald, A. J., & Chambers, C. T. (2010). Social functioning and peer relationships in children and adolescents with chronic pain: A systematic review. *Pain Research and Management, 15*, 27–41.

Franck, L. S., Greenberg, C. S., & Stevens, B. (2000). Pain assessment in infants and children. *Pediatric Clinics of North America, 47*(3), 487–512. https://doi.org/10.1016/S0031-3955(05)70222-4

Gaskin, D. J., & Richard, P. (2012). The economic costs of pain in the United States. *The Journal of Pain, 13*(8), 715–724. https://doi.org/10.1016/j.jpain.2012.03.009

Gatchel, R. J., Peng, Y. B., Peters, M. L., Fuchs, P. N., & Turk, D. C. (2007). The biopsychosocial approach to chronic pain: Scientific advances and future directions. *Psychological Bulletin, 133*(4), 581–624.

Genik, L. M., McMurtry, C. M., & Breau, L. M. (2017). Caring for children with intellectual disabilities part 2: Detailed analyses of factors involved in respite workers' reported assessment and care decisions. *Research in Developmental Disabilities, 63*, 1–10. https://doi.org/10.1016/j.ridd.2017.01.021

Genik, L. M., McMurtry, C. M., Breau, L. M., Lewis, S. P., & Freedman-Kalchman, T. (2017). Pain in children with developmental disabilities: Development and preliminary effectiveness of a pain training workshop for respite workers. *The Clinical Journal of Pain, 34*(5), 428-437.

Gharaibeh, M., & Abu-Saad, H. (2002). Cultural validation of pediatric pain assessment tools: Jordanian perspective. *Journal of Transcultural Nursing, 13*, 12–18.

Gilbert-MacLeod, C. A. (2000). Everyday pain responses in children with and without developmental delays. *Journal of Pediatric Psychology, 25*(5), 301–308. https://doi.org/10.1093/jpepsy/25.5.301

Goodenough, B., Addicoat, L., Champion, G. D., McInerney, M., Young, B., Juniper, K., et al. (1997). Pain in 4- to 6-year-old children receiving intramuscular injections: A comparison of the faces pain scale with other self-report and behavioral measures. *The Clinical Journal of Pain, 13*, 60–73.

Goodman, J. E., & McGrath, P. J. (2003). Mothers' modeling influences children's pain ratings during a cold pressor task. *Pain, 104*, 559–565.

Goubert, L., Eccleston, C., Vervoort, T., Jordan, A., & Crombez, G. (2006). Parental catastrophizing about their child's pain. The parent version of the pain catastrophizing scale (PCS-P): A preliminary validation. *Pain, 123*, 254–263.

Groenewald, C. B., Essner, B. S., Wright, D., Fesinmeyer, M. D., & Palermo, T. M. (2014). The economic costs of chronic pain among a cohort of treatment-seeking adolescents in the United States. *Journal

of Pain, 15, 925–933. https://doi.org/10.1016/j.jpain.2014.06.002
Guariso, G., Mozrzymas, R., Gobber, D., Benini, F., Zancan, L., Zacchello, F. (1999). Self-report assessment of recurrent abdominal pain. Medical and Surgical Pediatrics, 21(6), 255–260.
Hamill, J. K., Lyndon, M., Liley, A., & Hill, A. G. (2014). Where it hurts: A systematic review of pain-location tools for children. Pain, 155, 851–858.
Hamilton, J. G. (1995). Needle phobia: A neglected diagnosis. The Journal of Family Practice, 41(2), 169–175.
Hester, N. O. (1979). The preoperational child's reaction to immunization. Nursing Research, 28, 250–255.
Hicks, C. L., von Baeyer, C. L., Spafford, P. A., van Korlaar, I., & Goodenough, B. (2001). The faces pain scale-revised: Toward a common metric in pediatric pain measurement. Pain, 93, 173–183.
Hockenberry, M., McCarthy, K., Taylor, O., Scarberry, M., Franklin, Q., Louis, C., & Torres, L. (2011). Managing painful procedures in children with cancer. Journal of Pediatric Hematology/Oncology, 33(2), 119–127.
Holley, A. L., Wilson, A. C., & Palermo, T. M. (2017). Predictors of the transition from acute to persistent musculoskeletal pain in children and adolescents: A prospective study. Pain e-pub ahead of print March 2017. https://doi.org/10.1097/j.pain.0000000000000817
Huguet, A., & Miró, J. (2008). The severity of chronic pediatric pain: An epidemiological study. The Journal of Pain : Official Journal of the American Pain Society, 9(3), 226–236. https://doi.org/10.1016/j.jpain.2007.10.015
Hunfeld, J. A., Perquin, C. W., Duivenvoorden, H. J., Hazebroek-Kampschreur, A. A., Passchier, J., van Suijlekom-Smit, L. W., & van der Wouden, J. C. (2001). Chronic pain and its impact on quality of life in adolescents and their families. Journal of Pediatric Psychology, 26(3), 145–153.
Hunt, A., Goldman, A., Seers, K., Mastroyannopoulou, K., Moffat, V., Oulten, K., & Brady, M. (2004). Clinical validation of the paediatric pain profile. Developmental Medicine and Child Neurology, 46(1), 9–18. https://doi.org/10.1017/S0012162204000039
Hunt, A., Mastroyannopoulou, K., Goldman, A., & Seers, K. (2003). Not knowing--the problem of pain in children with severe neurological impairment. International Journal of Nursing Studies, 40, 171–183. https://doi.org/10.1016/S0020-7489(02)00058-5
Jaaniste, T., Noel, M., & von Baeyer, C. L. (2016). Young children's ability to report on past, future, and hypothetical pain states. Pain, 157(11), 2399–2409. https://doi.org/10.1097/j.pain.0000000000000666
Kalapurakkel, S., Carpino, E. A., Lebel, A., & Simons, L. E. (2015). "Pain can't stop me": Examining pain self-efficacy and acceptance as resilience processes among youth with chronic headache. Journal of Pediatric Psychology, 40(9), 926–933. https://doi.org/10.1093/jpepsy/jsu091
Kankkunen, P. M., Vehviläinen-Julkunen, K. M., Pietilä, A.-M. K., & Halonen, P. M. (2003). Parents' perceptions of their 1-6-year-old children's pain. European Journal of Pain, 7(3), 203–211. https://doi.org/10.1016/S1090-3801(02)00100-3
Kashikar-Zuck, S., Flowers, S. R., Claar, R. L., Guite, J. W., Logan, D. E., Lynch-Jordan, A. M., … Wilson, A. C. (2011). Clinical utility and validity of the functional disability inventory among a multicenter sample of youth with chronic pain. Pain, 152(7), 1600–1607. https://doi.org/10.1016/j.pain.2011.02.050
King, S., Chambers, C. T., Huguet, A., MacNevin, R. C., McGrath, P. J., Parker, L., & MacDonald, A. J. (2011). The epidemiology of chronic pain in children and adolescents revisited: A systematic review. Pain, 152(12), 2729–2738. https://doi.org/10.1016/j.pain.2011.07.016
LeBourgeois, M. K., Giannotti, F., Cortesi, F., Wolfson, A. R., & Harsh, J. (2005). The relationship between reported sleep quality and sleep hygiene in Italian and American adolescents. Pediatrics, 115(1 Suppl), 257–265.
Lee, G. Y., & Stevens, B. J. (2013). Neonatal and infant pain assessment. In P. McGrath, B. Stevens, S. Walker, & W. Zempsky (Eds.), Oxford textbook of paediatric pain (pp. 353–369). Oxford: Oxford University Press.
Lewandowski, A. S., Palermo, T. M., Stinson, J., Handley, S., Chambers, C. T. (2010). Systematic review of family functioning in families of children and adolescents with chronic pain. The Journal of Pain, 11(11), 1027–1038.
Lichstein, K. L., Stone, K. C., Donaldson, J., Nau, S. D., Soeffing, J. P., Murray, D., … Aguillard, R. N. (2006). Actigraphy validation with insomnia. Sleep, 29(2), 232–239.
Liossi, C., & Howard, R. F. (2016). Pediatric chronic pain: Biopsychosocial assessment and formulation. Pediatrics, 138(5).
Lister, M. T., Cunningham, M. J., Benjamin, B., Williams, M., Tirrell, A., Schaumberg, D. A., et al. (2006). Microdebrider tonsillotomy vs electrosurgical tonsillectomy: A randomized, double-blind, paired control study of postoperative pain. Archives of Otolaryngology—Head and Neck Surgery, 132, 599–604.
Long, A. C., Krishnamurthy, V., & Palermo, T. M. (2008). Sleep disturbances in school-age children with chronic pain. Journal of Pediatric Psychology, 33(3), 258–268. https://doi.org/10.1093/jpepsy/jsm129
Luffy, R., & Grove, S. K. (2003). Examining the validity, reliability, and preference of three pediatric pain tools in African-American children. Pediatric Nursing, 29, 54–59.
Lynch, A. M., Kashikar-Zuck, S., Goldschneider, K. R., & Jones, B. A. (2007). Sex and age differences in coping styles among children with chronic pain. Journal of Pain and Symptom Management, 33(2), 208–216. https://doi.org/10.1016/j.jpainsymman.2006.07.014
Lynch, M. E. (2011). The need for a Canadian pain strategy. Pain Research and Management, 16(2), 77–80.
Malviya, S., Voepel-Lewis, T., Burke, C., Merkel, S., & Tait, A. R. (2006). The revised FLACC observational pain tool: Improved reliability and validity for pain assessment in children with cognitive

impairment. *Paediatric Anaesthesia.* https://doi.org/10.1111/j.1460-9592.2005.01773.x

Mannix, M. M., Feldman, J. M., & Moody, K. (2009). Optimism and health-related quality of life in adolescents with cancer. *Child: Care, Health and Development, 35*(4), 482–488. https://doi.org/10.1111/j.1365-2214.2008.00934.x

Massey, E. K., Garnefski, N., & Gebhardt, W. A. (2009). Goal frustration, coping and Well-being in the context of adolescent headache: A self-regulation approach. *European Journal of Pain, 13,* 977–984.

McCracken, L. M., Gauntlett-Gilbert, J., & Eccleston, C. (2010). Acceptance of pain in adolescents with chronic pain: Validation of an adapted assessment instrument and preliminary correlation analyses. *European Journal of Pain (London, England), 14*(3), 316–320. https://doi.org/10.1016/j.ejpain.2009.05.002

McGrath, P. J., Stevens, B. J., Walker, S. M., & Zempsky, W. T. (Eds.). (2013). *Oxford textbook of paediatric pain.* Oxford: Oxford University Press.

McGrath, P. J., Walco, G. A., Turk, D. C., Dworkin, R. H., Brown, M. T., Davidson, K., ... PedIMMPACT. (2008). Core outcome domains and measures for pediatric acute and chronic/recurrent pain clinical trials: PedIMMPACT recommendations. *The Journal of Pain, 9*(9), 771–783. https://doi.org/10.1016/j.jpain.2008.04.007

McKillop, H. N., & Banez, G. A. (2016). A broad consideration of risk factors in pediatric chronic pain: Where to go from here? *Children, 3,* 38.

McKinley, S., Coote, K., & Stein-Parbury, J. (2003). Development and testing of a faces scale for the assessment of anxiety in critically ill patients. *Methodological Issues in Nursing Research, 41,* 73–79.

McMurtry, C. M., Chambers, C. T., McGrath, P. J., & Asp, E. (2010). When "don't worry" communicates fear: Children's perceptions of parental reassurance and distraction during a painful pediatric medical procedure. *Pain, 150,* 52–58.

McMurtry, C. M., McGrath, P. J., & Chambers, C. T. (2006). Reassurance can hurt: Parental behavior and painful medical procedures. *The Journal of Pediatrics, 148,* 560–561.

McMurtry, C. M., Noel, M., Chambers, C. T., & McGrath, P. J. (2011). Children's fear during procedural pain: Preliminary investigation of the Children's fear scale. *Health Psychology, 30,* 780–788.

McMurtry, C. M., Pillai Riddell, R., Taddio, A., Racine, N., Asmundson, G. J. G., Noel, M., ... HELPinKidsandAdults Team. (2015). Far from "just a poke". *The Clinical Journal of Pain, 31*(10 Suppl), S3–S11. https://doi.org/10.1097/AJP.0000000000000272

McMurtry, C. M., Taddio, A., Noel, M., Antony, M. M., Chambers, C. T., Asmundson, G. J. G., ... Scott, J. (2016). Exposure-based interventions for the management of individuals with high levels of needle fear across the lifespan: A clinical practice guideline and call for further research. *Cognitive Behavior Therapy, 45*(3), 217–235.

McMurtry, C.M., Tomlinson, R.M., Genik, L.M. (2017). Cognitive behavioural therapy for anxiety and fear in pediatric pain contexts. *Journal of Cognitive Psychology, 31*(1), 41–56.

Meltzer, L. J., Avis, K. T., Biggs, S., Reynolds, A. C., Crabtree, V. M., & Bevans, K. B. (2013). The Children's report of sleep patterns (CRSP): A self-report measure of sleep for school-aged children. *Journal of Clinical Sleep Medicine, 9*(3), 235–245. https://doi.org/10.5664/jcsm.2486

Meltzer, L. J., Montgomery-Downs, H. E., Insana, S. P., & Walsh, C. M. (2012). Use of actigraphy for assessment in pediatric sleep research. *Sleep Medicine Reviews, 16*(5), 463–475.

Melzack, R. (1983). The McGill pain questionnaire. In R. Melzack (Ed.), *Pain measurement and assessment* (pp. 41–47). New York, NY: Raven Press.

Melzack, R., & Wall, P. D. (1965). Pain mechanisms: A new theory. *Science, 150*(3699), 971–979.

Merskey, H., & Bogduk, N. (1994). *Classification of chronic pain: Description of chronic pain syndromes and definitions of pain terms* (2nd ed.). Seattle, WA: IASP Press.

Migdal, M., Chudzynska-Pomianowska, E., Vause, E., Henry, E., & Lazar, J. (2005). Rapid, needle-free delivery of lidocaine for reducing the pain of venipuncture among pediatric subjects. *Pediatrics, 115,* 393–398.

Miró, J., & Huguet, A. (2004). Evaluation of reliability, validity, and preference for a pediatric pain intensity scale: The Catalan version of the faces pain scale—Revised. *Pain, 111,* 59–64.

Miró, J., Castarlenas, E., Huguet, A. (2009). Evidence for the use of a numerical rating scale to assess the intensity of pediatric pain. *European Journal of Pain, 13*(10), 1089–1095.

Moon, E. C., Chambers, C. T., Larochette, A.-C., Hayton, K., Craig, K. D., & McGrath, P. J. (2008). Sex differences in parent and child pain ratings during an experimental child pain task. *Pain Research and Management, 13*(3), 225–230.

Moon, E. C., & Unruh, A. M. (2013). The effects of sex and gender on child and adolescent pain. In P. J. McGrath, B. J. Stevens, S. W. Walker and W. T. Zempsky (Eds.), *Oxford Textbook of Pediatric Pain* (pp. 127–134). New York, United States of America: Oxford University Press.

Nader, R., Oberlander, T. F., Chambers, C. T., & Craig, K. D. (2004). Expression of pain in children with autism. *The Clinical Journal of Pain, 20*(2), 88–97. https://doi.org/10.1097/00002508-200403000-00005

Newman, C. J., Lolekha, R., Limkittikul, K., Luangxay, K., Chotpitayasunondh, T., & Chanthavanich, P. A. (2005). A comparison of pain scales in Thai children. *Archives of Disease in Childhood, 90,* 269–270.

Noel, M., Alberts, N., Langer, S. L., Levy, R. L., Walker, L. S., & Palermo, T. M. (2016). The sensitivity to change and responsiveness of the adult responses to Children's symptoms in children and adolescents with chronic pain. *Journal of Pediatric Psychology, 41,* 350–362.

Noel, M., Chambers, C. T., McGrath, P. J., Klein, R. M., & Stewart, S. H. (2012). The influence of children's pain memories on subsequent pain experience. *Pain, 153*(8), 1563.

Noel, M., Palermo, T. M., Essner, B., Zhou, C., Levy, R. L., Langer, S., et al. (2015). A developmental analysis of the factorial validity of the adult responses to Children's symptoms (ARCS) in children versus adolescents with chronic pain and pain-related chronic illness. *Journal of Pain, 16,* 31–41.

Owens, J. A., Spirito, A., & McGuinn, M. (2000). The Children's sleep habits questionnaire (CSHQ): Psychometric properties of a survey instrument for school-aged children. *Sleep, 23*(8), 1043–1051.

Palermo, T. M., & Chambers, C. T. (2006). Parent and family factors in pediatric chronic pain and disability: An integrative approach. *Pain, 119,* 1–4.

Palermo, T. M., & Eccleston, C. (2009). Parents of children and adolescents with chronic pain. *Pain, 146*(1-2), 15–17. https://doi.org/10.1016/j.pain.2009.05.009

Palermo, T. M., Kiska, R., Bloom, B. J., Owens, J. A., McGuinn, M., Nobile, C., ... Tarasiuk, A. (2005). Subjective sleep disturbances in adolescents with chronic pain: Relationship to daily functioning and quality of life. *The Journal of Pain : Official Journal of the American Pain Society, 6*(3), 201–207. https://doi.org/10.1016/j.jpain.2004.12.005

Palermo, T. M., Valrie, C. R., & Karlson, C. W. (2014). Family and parent influences on pediatric chronic pain: A developmental perspective. *The American Psychologist, 69*(2), 142–152. https://doi.org/10.1037/a0035216

Pedersen, L. K., Rahbek, O., Nikolajsen, L., & Moller-Madsen, B. (2015). The revised FLACC score: Reliability and validation for pain assessment in children with cerebral palsy. *Scandinavian Journal of Pain, 9,* 57–61. https://doi.org/10.1016/j.sjpain.2015.06.007

Perquin, C. W., Hazebroek-Kampschreur, A. A., Hunfeld, J. A., Bohnen, A. M., van Suijlekom-Smit, L. W., Passchier, J., & van der Wouden, J. C. (2000). Pain in children and adolescents: A common experience. *Pain, 87*(1), 51–58.

Pielech, M., Ryan, M., Logan, D., Kaczynski, K., White, M. T., & Simons, L. E. (2014). Pain catastrophizing in children with chronic pain and their parents: Proposed clinical reference points and reexamination of the pain catastrophizing scale measure. *Pain, 155*(11), 2360–2367. https://doi.org/10.1016/j.pain.2014.08.035

Pielech, M., Vowles, K., & Wicksell, R. (2017). Acceptance and commitment therapy for pediatric chronic pain: Theory and application. *Children, 4*(2), 10. https://doi.org/10.3390/children4020010

Powell, C. V., Kelly, A.-M., & Williams, A. (2001). Determining the minimum clinically significant difference in visual analogue pain score for children. *Annals of Emergency Medicine, 37,* 28–31.

Powers, S., Patton, S., Hommel, K., & Hershey, A. (2004). Quality of life in paediatric migraine: Characterization of age-related effects using PedsQL 4.0. *Cephalalgia, 24*(2), 120–127. https://doi.org/10.1111/j.1468-2982.2004.00652.x

Quinn, B. L., Seibold, E., & Hayman, L. (2015). Pain assessment in children with special needs: A review of the literature. *Exceptional Children, 82*(1), 44–57. https://doi.org/10.1177/0014402915585480

Ramritu, P. L. (2000). Use of the Oucher numeric and word graphic scale in children aged 9–14 years with post-operative pain. *Journal of Clinical Nursing, 9,* 763–773.

Reid, G. J., McGrath, P. J., & Lang, B. A. (2005). Parent-child interactions among children with juvenile fibromyalgia, arthritis, and healthy controls. *Pain, 113,* 201–210. https://doi.org/10.1016/j.pain.2004.10.018

Revicki, D. A., Chen, W.-H., Harnam, N., Cook, K. F., Amtmann, D., Callahan, L. F., ... Keefe, F. J. (2009). Development and psychometric analysis of the PROMIS pain behavior item bank. *Pain, 146*(1-2), 158–169. https://doi.org/10.1016/j.pain.2009.07.029

Ruskin, D., Lalloo, C., Amaria, K., Stinson, J. N., Kewley, E., Campbell, F., ... McGrath, P. A. (2014). Assessing pain intensity in children with chronic pain: Convergent and discriminant validity of the 0 to 10 numerical rating scale in clinical practice. *Pain Research and Management, 19*(3), 141–148.

Savedra, M., Holzemer, W., Tesler, M., & Wilkie, D. (1993). Assessment of postoperative pain in children and adolescents using the adolescent Pediatric pain tool. *Nursing Research, 42,* 5–9.

Savedra, M. C., Tesler, M. D., Holzemer, W. L., Wilkie, D. J., & Ward, J. A. (1989). Pain location: Validity and reliability of body outline markings by hospitalized children and adolescents. *Research in Nursing and Health, 12,* 307–314.

Schechter, N. L., Allen, D. A., & Hanson, K. (1986). Status of pediatric pain control: A comparison of hospital analgesic usage in children and adults. *Pediatrics, 77*(1), 11–15.

Schechter, N. L., Zempsky, W. T., Cohen, L. L., McGrath, P. J., McMurtry, C. M., & Bright, N. S. (2007). Pain reduction during pediatric immunizations: evidence-based review and recommendations. *Pediatrics, 119*(5), 1184–1198.

Shapiro, C. (1997). *Development of the Oucher pain assessment tool for Canadian aboriginal children.* Poster presentation at the conference of the Special Interest on Childhood Pain of the International Association for the Study of Pain, Helsinki, Finland.

Simons, L. E. (2016). Fear of pain in children and adolescents with neuropathic pain and complex regional pain syndrome. *Pain, 157*(1), S90–S97.

Simons, L. E., Sieberg, C. B., Carpino, E., Logan, D., & Berde, C. (2011). The fear of pain questionnaire (FOPQ): Assessment of pain-related fear among children and adolescents with chronic pain. *The Journal of Pain, 12*(6), 677–686.

Simons, L. E., Sieberg, C. B., & Kaczynski, K. J. (2011). Measuring parent beliefs about child acceptance of pain: A preliminary validation of the chronic pain acceptance questionnaire, parent report. *Pain,*

152(10), 2294–2300. https://doi.org/10.1016/j.pain.2011.06.018

Sobsey, D. (2006). Pain and disability in an ethical and social context. In T. F. Oberlander & F. J. Symons (Eds.), *Pain in children and adults with developmental disabilities*. Baltimore, MD: Paul H. Brookes Pub.

Solodiuk, J., & Curley, M. A. Q. (2003). Pain assessment in nonverbal children with severe cognitive impairments: The individualized numeric rating scale (INRS). *Journal of Pediatric Nursing, 18*(4), 295–299. https://doi.org/10.1016/S0882-5963(03)00090-3

Solodiuk, J. C. (2013). Parent described pain responses in nonverbal children with intellectual disability. *International Journal of Nursing Studies, 50*(8), 1033–1044. https://doi.org/10.1016/j.ijnurstu.2012.11.015

Solodiuk, J. C., Scott-Sutherland, J., Meyers, M., Myette, B., Shusterman, C., Karian, V. E., … Curley, M. A. Q. (2010). Validation of the individualized numeric rating scale (INRS): A pain assessment tool for nonverbal children with intellectual disability. *Pain, 150*(2), 231–236. https://doi.org/10.1016/j.pain.2010.03.016

Stallard, P., Williams, L., Lenton, S., & Velleman, R. (2001). Pain in cognitively impaired, non-communicating children. *Archives of Disease in Childhood, 85*(6), 460–462. https://doi.org/10.1136/adc.85.6.460

Stanford, E. A., Chambers, C. T., & Craig, K. D. (2006). The role of developmental factors in predicting young children's use of a self-report scale for pain. *Pain, 120*(1-2), 16–23. https://doi.org/10.1016/j.pain.2005.10.004

Stevens, B. J., Abbott, L. K., Yamada, J., Harrison, D., Stinson, J., Taddio, A., … Finley, G. A. (2011). Epidemiology and management of painful procedures in children in Canadian hospitals. *Canadian Medical Association Journal, 183*(7), 403–410.

Stinson, J. N. (2009). Improving the assessment of pediatric chronic pain: Harnessing the potential of electronic diaries. *Pain Research and Management, 14*(1), 59–64.

Stinson, J. N., Kavanagh, T., Yamada, J., Gill, N., & Stevens, B. (2006). Systematic review of the psychometric properties, interpretability, and feasibility of self-report pain intensity measures for use in clinical trials in children and adolescents. *Pain, 125*, 143–157.

Stommen, N. C., Verbunt, J. A., & Goossens, M. E. (2016). Future goals of adolescents and young adults with chronic musculoskeletal pain. *European Journal of Pain, 20*, 564–572.

Sullivan, M. J. L., Bishop, S., & Pivik, J. (1995). The pain catastrophizing scale: Development and validation. *Psychological Assessment, 7*(4), 524–532.

Suraseranivongse, S., Montapaneewat, T., Monon, J., Chainhop, P., Petcharatana, S., & Kraiprasit, K. (2005). Cross-validation of a self-report scale for postoperative pain in school-aged children. *Journal of the Medical Association of Thailand, 88*, 412–417.

Taddio, A., Ipp, M., Thivakaran, S., Jamal, A., Parikh, C., Smart, S., … Katz, J. (2012). Survey of the prevalence of immunization non-compliance due to needle fears in children and adults. *Vaccine, 30*(32), 4807–4812. https://doi.org/10.1016/j.vaccine.2012.05.011

Taddio, A., Katz, J., Illersich, A. L., & Koren, G. (1997). Effect of neonatal circumcision on pain response during subsequent routine vaccination. *The Lancet, 349*, 599–603.

Taddio, A., Kaur Soin, H., Schuh, S., Koren, G., & Scolnik, D. (2005). Liposomal lidocaine to improve procedural success rates and reduce procedural pain among children: A randomized controlled trial. *Canadian Medical Association Journal, 172*, 1691–1695.

Taddio, A., McMurtry, C. M., Shah, V., Riddell, R. P., Chambers, C. T., Noel, M., … HELPinKidsandAdults. (2015). Reducing pain during vaccine injections: Clinical practice guideline. *Canadian Medical Association Journal, 187*(13), 975–982. https://doi.org/10.1503/cmaj.150391

Taddio, A., & Oberlander, T. F. (2006). *Pharmacological management of pain in children and youth with significant neurological impairments. Pain in Children and Adults with Developmental Disabilities* (pp. 193–211). Baltimore, MD: Paul H. Brookes Publishing Co.

Tesler, M. D., Savedra, M. C., Holzemer, W. L., Wilkie, D. J., Ward, J. A., & Paul, S. M. (1991). The word-graphic rating scale as a measure of children's and adolescents' pain intensity. *Research in Nursing and Health, 14*, 361–371.

Tomlinson, D., von Baeyer, C. L., Stinson, J. N., & Sung, L. (2010). A systematic review of faces scales for the self-report of pain intensity in children. *Pediatrics, 126*, e1168–e1198.

Tomlinson, R. M., Cousins, L. A., McMurtry, C. M., & Cohen, L. L. (2017). The power of pain self-efficacy: Applying a positive psychology framework to pediatric pain. *Pediatric Pain Letter, 19*(1), 9.

Treede, R.-D., Rief, W., Barke, A., Aziz, Q., Bennett, M. I., Benoliel, R., … Wang, S.-J. (2015). A classification of chronic pain for ICD-11. *Pain, 156*(6), 1003–1007. https://doi.org/10.1097/j.pain.0000000000000160

Turk, D. C., & Monarch, E. S. (2002). Biopsychosocial perspective on chronic pain. In D. C. Turk & R. J. Gatchel (Eds.), *Psychological approaches to pain management: A practitioner's handbook* (2nd ed., pp. 3–30). New York, NY: Guilford Press.

Twycross, A., Voepel-Lewis, T., Vincent, C., Franck, L. S., & von Baeyer, C. L. (2015). A debate on the proposition that self-report is the gold standard in assessment of pediatric pain intensity. *The Clinical Journal of Pain, 31*(8), 707–712. https://doi.org/10.1097/AJP.0000000000000165

Unruh, A. M., & McGrath, P. J. (2013). History of pain in children. In P. J. McGrath, B. J. Stevens, S. W. Walker, & W. T. Zempsky (Eds.), *Oxford textbook of Pediatric pain* (pp. 3–12). New York, USA: Oxford University Press.

Valkenburg, A. J., Tibboel, D., & van Dijk, M. (2015). Pain sensitivity of children with down syndrome and their siblings: Quantitative sensory testing versus parental reports. *Developmental Medicine and Child Neurology, 57*(11), 1049–1055. https://doi.org/10.1111/dmcn.12823

Valrie, C. R., Bromberg, M. H., Palermo, T., & Schanberg, L. E. (2013). A systematic review of sleep in pediatric pain populations. *Journal of Developmental and Behavioral Pediatrics: JDBP, 34*(2), 120–128. https://doi.org/10.1097/DBP.0b013e31827d5848

van den Brink, M., Bandell-Hoekstra, E. N. G., & Abu-Saad, H. H. (2001). The occurrence of recall bias in pediatric headache: A comparison of questionnaire and diary data. *Headache: The Journal of Head and Face Pain, 41*(1), 11–20. https://doi.org/10.1046/j.1526-4610.2001.111006011.x

Van Slyke, D. A., & Walker, L. S. (2006). Mothers' responses to children's pain. *The Clinical Journal of Pain, 22*(4), 387–391.

Varni, J. W., Limbers, C. A., & Burwinkle, T. M. (2007). Parent proxy-report of their children's health-related quality of life: An analysis of 13,878 parents' reliability and validity across age subgroups using the PedsQL 4.0 generic Core scales. *Health and Quality of Life Outcomes, 5*, 2. https://doi.org/10.1186/1477-7525-5-2

Varni, J. W., Seid, M., & Kurtin, P. S. (2001). PedsQL 4.0: Reliability and validity of the Pediatric quality of life inventory version 4.0 generic core scales in healthy and patient populations. *Medical Care, 39*(8), 800–812.

Vervoort, T., Goubert, L., Eccleston, C., Bijttebier, P., & Crombez, G. (2005). Catastrophic thinking about pain is independently associated with pain severity, disability, and somatic complaints in school children and children with chronic pain. *Journal of Pediatric Psychology, 31*(7), 674–683. https://doi.org/10.1093/jpepsy/jsj059

Vetter, T. R., Bridgewater, C. L., Ascherman, L. I., Madan-Swain, A., & McGwin, G. L. (2014). Patient versus parental perceptions about pain and disability in children and adolescents with a variety of chronic pain conditions. *Pain Research and Management, 19*(1), 7–14.

Villarruel, A., & Denyes, M. (1991). Pain assessment in children: Theoretical and empirical validity. *Advances in Nursing Science, 14*, 32–41.

Voepel-Lewis, T., Malviya, S., & Tait, A. R. (2005). Validity of parent ratings as proxy measures of pain in children with cognitive impairment. *Pain Management Nursing, 6*(4), 168–174. https://doi.org/10.1016/j.pmn.2005.08.004

von Baeyer, C. L. (2006). Children's self-reports of pain intensity: Scale selection, limitations and interpretation. *Pain Research and Management, 11*(3), 157–162.

von Baeyer, C. L., Spagrud, L. J., McCormick, J. C., Choo, E., Neville, K., Connelly, M. A. (2009). Three new datasets supporting the use of the Numerical Rating Scale (NRS-11) for children's self-reports of pain intensity. *Pain, 143*(3), 223–227.

von Baeyer, C. L. (2013). Self-report: The primary source in assessment after infancy. In P. McGrath, B. Stevens, S. Walker, & W. Zempsky (Eds.), *Oxford textbook of paediatric pain* (pp. 370–378). Oxford: Oxford University Press.

von Baeyer, C. L., Jaaniste, T., Vo, H. L., Brunsdon, G., Lao, A. H. C., & Champion, G. D. (2017). Systematic review of self-report measures of pain intensity in 3-and 4-year-olds: Bridging a period of rapid cognitive development. *The Journal of Pain.* https://doi.org/10.1016/j.jpain.2017.03.005

Walker, L. S., Dengler-Crish, C. M., Rippel, S., & Bruehl, S. (2010). Functional abdominal pain in childhood and adolescence increases risk for chronic pain in adulthood. *Pain, 150*(3), 568–572. https://doi.org/10.1016/j.pain.2010.06.018

Walker, L. S., & Greene, J. W. (1991). The functional disability inventory: Measuring a neglected dimension of child health status. *Journal of Pediatric Psychology, 16*(1), 39–58.

Wallace, D. P., Harbeck-Weber, C., Whiteside, S. P. H., & Harrison, T. E. (2011). Adolescent acceptance of pain: Confirmatory factor analysis and further validation of the chronic pain acceptance questionnaire, adolescent version. *The Journal of Pain: Official Journal of the American Pain Society, 12*(5), 591–599. https://doi.org/10.1016/j.jpain.2010.11.004

Wilkie, D. J., Holzemer, W. L., Tesler, M. D., Ward, J. A., Paul, S. M., & Savedra, M. C. (1990). Measuring pain quality: Validity and reliability of children's and adolescents' pain language. *Pain, 41*, 151–159.

Williams, N. A., Davis, G., Hancock, M., & Phipps, S. (2010). Optimism and pessimism in children with cancer and healthy children: Confirmatory factor analysis of the youth life orientation test and relations with health-related quality of life. *Journal of Pediatric Psychology, 35*(6), 672–682. https://doi.org/10.1093/jpepsy/jsp084

Wong, D. L., & Baker, C. M. (1988). Pain in children: Comparison of assessment scales. *Pediatric Nursing, 14*, 9–17.

Wood, C., von Baeyer, C. L., Bourrillon, A., Dejos-Conant, V., Clyti, N., & Abitbol, V. (2004). Self-assessment of immediate post-vaccination pain after two different MMR vaccines administered as second dose in 3- to 6-year old children. *Vaccine, 23*, 127–131.

Yeh, C. H. (2005). Development and validation of the Asian version of the Oucher: A pain intensity scale for children. *Journal of Pain, 6*, 526–534.

Zabalia, M., Jacquet, D., & Breau, L. (2005). Role du niveau verbal sur l'expression et l'evaluation de la douleur chez des sujets deficients intellectuels. *Douleur et Analge, 2*, 67–72.

Eating Disorders

Pamela McPherson, Hannah K. Scott, Astik Joshi, and Raghu Gandhi

The Assessment of Eating Disorders in Children and Adolescents

The high mortality associated with eating disorders (ED) demands that all child and adolescent assessments include screening for ED. The core feature of ED is an unhealthy relationship with food which is driven by intense emotions that impair logical reasoning about eating behaviors and, in some ED, body image. ED typically begin in adolescence, often with dieting. The course of illness is typically chronic with a high rate of premature mortality, which is highest in anorexia nervosa (AN). In fact, AN has the highest mortality of all mental disorders (Campbell & Peebles, 2014; Stice, Marti, & Rohde, 2013) with the first 10 years of illness posing the greatest risk of death (Franko et al., 2013). Screening for ED during assessments is a necessity as early identification is critical to treatment success (Ackard, Richter, Egan, Engel, & Cronemeyer, 2014; Golden et al., 2015).

This chapter will focus on the major eating disorders – anorexia nervosa (AN), bulimia nervosa (BN), and binge eating disorder (BED). The other specified feeding and eating disorders (OSFED) including purging disorder (PD) and night eating syndrome (NES) will be briefly reviewed. An introduction to a range of proposed ED is included. Patients with disordered eating experience a very high rate of diagnostic crossover from one eating disorder to another; in fact, this is the rule, not the exception. Because the study of ED is best approached with this crossover in mind, this chapter integrates information regarding AN, BN, and BED.

Overview of Anorexia Nervosa, Bulimia Nervosa, and Binge Eating Disorder

In AN there is an obsessive control of food intake that is often coupled with excessive exercising and/or purging behaviors in a frantic effort to achieve an elusive body ideal. These behaviors lead to a dangerous loss of weight. Reports of the lifetime prevalence for adolescent females range from 0.3% to 1.7% (Smink, van Hoeken, Oldehinkel, & Hoek, 2014; Stice et al., 2013; Swanson, Crow, Le Grange, Swendsen, &

P. McPherson (✉)
Northwest Louisiana Human Services District, Shreveport, LA, USA
e-mail: Pamela.McPherson@LA.GOV

H. K. Scott · A. Joshi
Louisiana State University Health Sciences Center Shreveport, Shreveport, LA, USA

R. Gandhi
University of Minnesota, Minneapolis, MN, USA

Merikangas, 2011). Changes in diagnostic criteria, globalization of the western thinness ideal, increase in the recognition of mental illness, and variation in study methodology contribute to the range in prevalence data. Longitudinal studies have shown an increase in the incidence of new AN diagnoses since the 1970s (Steinhausen & Jensen, 2015). Epidemiological studies have consistently found increased incidence of AN in females with a 15:1 female to male ratio. The onset of AN is most often in late adolescence with a peak onset in males of ~13 years and ~15 years in females according to the Danish register study, which included nearly a million persons (Zerwas et al., 2015). AN typically begins in late adolescence. The onset is uncommon in middle age or before puberty. Approximately 85% of AN present before the age of 20 (Jagielska & Kacperska, 2017). Over time it is common for AN to progress to BED then BN (Nagl et al., 2016; Stice et al., 2013; Uher & Rutter, 2012). Male homosexuals have an increased risk for AN due to a body ideal in the gay community for slimness (Shearer et al., 2015). Historically female homosexuality was considered protective against eating disorders (Siever, 1994); current studies contradict this finding and propose a universal risk for all women, regardless of sexual preference (Bankoff, Marks, Swenson, & Pantalone, 2016).

In BN and BED, the rapid compulsive eating of large quantities of food is coupled with extreme distress and disgust which in BN leads to unhealthy compensatory behaviors to control weight gain. ED-related behaviors – including restrictive eating, excessive exercising, purging, and loss of control eating – ravage the body with acute physiological consequences that cause lasting damage or, worse, death. "Purging" is used in the broad sense of the word to signify any behavior intended to mitigate weight gain. Purging behaviors may include vomiting, chewing and spitting, using laxatives or enemas, and misusing medications. Reported lifetime prevalence for BN and BED in adolescents ranges from 0.9% to 2.6% and 1.6% to 3%, respectively (Smink et al., 2014; Stice et al., 2013; Swanson et al., 2011). BED is the most common ED (Hudson, Hiripi, Pope, & Kessler, 2007; Micali et al., 2017; Stice et al., 2013; Swanson et al., 2011). BN has a peak onset of 13 years in males and 18 years in females with a 60:1 female to male ratio (Zerwas et al., 2015). Rates of BN have been more stable than AN in recent decades (Steinhausen & Jensen, 2015).

Eating Disorders in Persons with Developmental Disabilities

Growing evidence supports an association between ED and autism spectrum disorders (ASD) (Zhou, McAdam, & Donnelly, 2017). In the early 1980s, a proposed link between AN and ASD was suggested (Gillberg, 1983) leading to the observation of similar difficulties in social, emotional, and cognitive functioning in the two disorders (Oldershaw, Treasure, Hambrook, Tchanturia, & Schmidt, 2011). There is an increased risk of AN/ASD comorbidity with studies reporting between 4% and 52.5% (Westwood & Tchanturia, 2017). While the association between AN and ASD requires additional research, it is clear that the presence of ASD symptoms in persons with AN is associated with poorer treatment outcomes and subsequent need for higher levels of care (Stewart, McEwen, Konstantellou, Eisler, & Simic, 2017; Westwood & Tchanturia, 2017). Patients with AN/ASD require intensive initial treatment, including more medication and, after stabilization, exhibit serious social deficits increasing risk of chronicity and future complications (Nazar et al., 2018).

Among other neurodevelopmental disorders, there is data connecting ADHD and ED. The association between ADHD and binging–/purging-type disorders, i.e., BN and AN binge/purge type, is significant (Nazar et al., 2016; Ptacek et al., 2016; Sala et al., 2017; Svedlund, Norring, Ginsberg, & von Hausswolff-Juhlin, 2017). In an analysis of National Longitudinal Study of Adolescent Health data, youth with ADHD were nearly three times more likely to have an ED (Bleck, DeBate, & Olivardia, 2014). For persons with BN and BED, more

ADHD symptoms predicted increased frequency of binge-eating episodes (Fernández-Aranda et al., 2013).

ED presenting in a patient with intellectual disability is the exception rather than the rule. There have been case reports of AN in person with ID (Clarke & Yapa, 1991; Counts, 2001; Räder, Specht, & Reister, 1989) but no significant established patterns. In fact, quite the opposite has been found – it has been postulated that higher-than-average intelligence may increase your risk for developing an ED (Schilder et al., 2017). Research of ED in young children and persons with developmental disabilities is limited. Young children and persons with cognitive delays may be partially protected from ED because they may lack the abstract thinking ability to fully consider their own body image and the cognitive capacity to sustain ED behaviors to the point of raising caregivers' concern. Some youth with neurodevelopmental delay may lack the ability to characterize their emotions or distress related to eating and may be less impacted by societal influences regarding weight and appearance (Small & Aplasca, 2016). Unhealthy eating by young children is most often characterized as a feeding disorder or sensory issue. This raises interesting questions regarding the relationship of FD to ED which, for now, go unanswered.

OSFED/UFED

Other specified feeding or eating disorder (OSFED) and unspecified feeding or eating disorder (UFED) are new categories in the DSM-5, replacing the eating disorder not otherwise specified (EDNOS) diagnosis of the DSM-IV (American Psychiatric Association, 1994, 2013). Both diagnoses apply to "presentations in which symptoms characteristic of a feeding or eating disorder cause clinically specific distress or impairment" (American Psychiatric Association, 2013), with OSFED allowing for explanation of the disorder and UFED used without explanation or when available details are limited or do not rise to the level of a specific ED/FD (American Psychiatric Association, 2013). The reorganization of the *Feeding and Eating Disorders* section of the DSM-5 aims to promote more effective clinical description, which in turn informs treatment options and the expected course of illness (Keel, Brown, Holland, & Bodell, 2012).

A point prevalence for OSFED of 5% was reported for adolescent females (Fairweather-Schmidt & Wade, 2014). In an 8-year prospective study, a lifetime prevalence of OSFED was reported as 11% in young women (Stice et al., 2013). UFED was studied in a group of 309 adolescents presenting for outpatient ED assessment; approximately two-thirds received an EDNOS diagnosis under DSM-IV criteria. When DSM-5 criteria were applied, only four received the UFED diagnosis (Fisher, Gonzalez, & Malizio, 2015). UFED has been identified in 1.41% to 4.7% in large prevalence studies (Hay, Girosi, & Mond, 2015; Wade & O'Shea, 2014). Compared to no ED, AN, and atypical AN, the UFED group was more likely to be overweight. Differences in severity, impairment, and distress among the ED and UFED groups were not significant (Wade & O'Shea, 2014).

The DSM-5 includes OSFED examples including *atypical AN* (AN in a normal or overweight individual who has experienced significant weight loss), *atypical BN* (BN with inappropriate compensatory behaviors not meeting frequency or duration criteria), *atypical BED* (binging not meeting frequency or duration criteria), *purging disorder* (PD), and *night eating syndrome* (NES) (American Psychiatric Association, 2013).

PD is characterized by purging behaviors without binging to effect weight or body contours (American Psychiatric Association, 2013). Keel notes that women with PD endorse less concern with body image and decreased severity of disordered eating compared to those with BN (Keel, 2017; Keel, Haedt, & Edler, 2005). The Missouri Adolescent Female Twin Study reported a 3.77% lifetime prevalence of PD and less heritability than other ED (Munn-Chernoff et al., 2015). Recently PD has been distinguished from BN by higher satiety peptide YY and lower ghrelin levels (Keel et al., 2018).

Clinically it must be remembered that "purging" is defined broadly to include any behavior intended to mitigate weight gain. Purging behaviors may include vomiting, using laxatives or enemas, chewing and spitting, and misusing medications (see diabulimia below).

Night eating syndrome (NES) was first described by Albert Stunkard in 1955. Stunkard described NES as a disorder characterized by morning anorexia to the point of not eating during morning hours and evening hyperphagia and/or insomnia (Stunkard, Grace, & Wolff, 1955). NES affects an estimated 1.5% of the population and is equally common in men and women (Vetrugno et al., 2006). NES is more common in persons with diabetes, major depression, and schizophrenia as well as those who are obese (de Zwaan, Müller, Allison, Brähler, & Hilbert, 2014; Hood, Reutrakul, & Crowley, 2014; Palmese et al., 2013). In a study of German 5- and 6-year-olds, night eating was reported in 1.1% (Lamerz et al., 2005).

DSM-5 criteria describe NES as recurrent episodes of night eating which cause distress or impairment (American Psychiatric Association, 2013). Proposed research diagnostic criteria are more stringent, specifying two or more episodes a week that include 25% of daily intake consumed after supper, memory for the eating, and at least three additional symptoms such as evening irritability or depression, insomnia, belief that eating is necessary in order to go back to sleep, lack of morning appetite or skipping breakfast more than four mornings a week, and a strong urge to eat after supper or during the night (Allison et al., 2010). The Night Eating Questionnaire (NEQ) for NES screening has been validated in children and adolescents and has been shown to supply important information beyond that typically reported by parents (Gallant et al., 2012).

Night eating syndrome can be distinguished from bulimia nervosa and binge eating disorder by the lack of associated compensatory behaviors, the timing of food intake, and the fact that the food intake is typically not considered excessive; however, persons with AN, BN, and BED may experience NES. NES also differs from sleep-related eating disorder (SRED). In NES there is full awareness of waking and eating. In SRED there is no memory of eating (O'Reardon, Peshek, & Allison, 2005). Clinically it is important to identify NES in children and adolescents because of the association with obesity and interference with sleep which has implications for school performance, growth, and behavior.

Numerous disordered eating patterns have been described in the literature, the most common of which are described below.

Orthorexia Nervosa

The term "orthorexia nervosa" (ON) was originally defined as "a fixation on eating proper food" by Bratman in 1997 (Bratman & Knight, 2004). In 2015, Moroze and colleagues proposed diagnostic criteria including an "obsessional preoccupation with eating 'healthy foods', focusing on concerns regarding quality and composition of meals" that causes severe impairment or distress (Moroze, Dunn, Craig Holland, Yager, & Weintraub, 2015). Koven and Senbonmatsu reported neuropsychological weaknesses in set shifting, emotional control, self-monitoring, and working memory in university students with ON (Koven & Senbonmatsu, 2013). ON shares features with AN and obsessive-compulsive disorder. Questions regarding prevalence, etiology, and treatment are *unanswered* (Koven & Abry, 2015).

Anorexia Athletica/Female Athlete Triad/Relative Energy Deficiency in Sport

Anorexia athletica (AA) refers to restricted calorie intake coupled with compulsive exercise in athletes. It has long been recognized that there is an increased risk for ED in certain sports, most notably wrestling, ballet, and gymnastics. More recently the increased risk of ED in college and high school athletes has become widely recognized. Due to the energy demands during teen years, adolescent athletes are at an increased risk for nutritional deficiencies and ED (Bingham, Borkan, & Quatromoni, 2015; Mehler & Andersen, 2017). The NEDA website (NationalEatingDisordersAssociation.org) has specific information for athletes, coaches, and trainers.

The International Olympic Committee (IOC) and the American College of Sports Medicine (ACSM) have issued position papers on female athlete triad (FAT) – inadequate caloric intake, amenorrhea, and reduced bone mineral density – directing coaches, trainers, and team physicians to monitor female athletes (Nattiv et al., 2007; Otis, Drinkwater, Johnson, Loucks, & Wilmore, 1997; Sherman & Thompson, 2006). Tools to screen female athletes for the FAT and ED have been developed (Wagner, Erickson, Tierney, Houston, & Bacon, 2016).

Recently the IOC proposed a new condition, relative energy deficiency in sport (RED-S), to expand and replace the FAT and recognize the risk to all athletes. The IOC Consensus Statement on RED-S states:

> The syndrome of RED-S refers to impaired physiological function including, but not limited to, metabolic rate, menstrual function, bone health, immunity, protein synthesis, cardiovascular health caused by relative energy deficiency. The cause of this syndrome is energy deficiency relative to the balance between dietary energy intake and energy expenditure required for health and activities of daily living, growth and sporting activities. (Mountjoy et al., 2014)

Twenty-seven North American scientists have challenged the scientific basis for RED-S and cautioned that it undermines decades of research and education around FAT (De Souza et al., 2014). The IOC subsequently issued additions to the 2014 Statement calling for support of RED-S and additional research (Mountjoy et al., 2015b). The RED-S Clinical Assessment Tool (RED-S CAT) has been developed to guide the assessment of athletes and monitor athlete's ability to compete safely (Mountjoy et al., 2015a). See Andersen's *Athletes and Eating Disorders* for a comprehensive, clinically oriented review of the special challenges faced by clinicians treating athletes (Mehler & Andersen, 2017, Chapter 12).

Loss of Control ED

Children and youth may experience binge eating, but not meet criteria for an ED leading Tanofsky-Kraff and colleagues to propose the diagnosis of loss of control eating disorder (LOC-ED) for children under 12 (Tanofsky-Kraff, Marcus, Yanovski, & Yanovski, 2008). Loss of control eating (LOC) has been strongly associated with ADHD (Reinblatt et al., 2015). LOC in childhood was a predictor of BED in a 5-year follow-up study (Hilbert & Brauhardt, 2014). The Research Domain Criteria domain of negative valence systems (acute threat, potential threat, sustained threat, loss, and frustrative nonreward) and neurobiological correlates of LOC-ED are under study (Tanofsky-Kraff, Engel, Yanovski, Pin, & Nelson, 2013; Vannucci, 2015). (See explanation of RDoC under Diagnostic Nosologies.) While LOC-ED requires additional study to establish diagnostic validity, the symptom of LOC, when present, should be assessed for age of onset, frequency, temporal patterns, preferred food, hoarding, hiding, amount eaten, emotion before, during and after eating, and hunger before and fullness after LOC (Matherne et al., 2015).

Diabulimia

Diabulimia is an "intentional insulin omission or manipulation to induce weight loss." Diabulimia is well recognized in the medical community. It is associated with poor control of diabetes and increased incidence of diabetes-related complications including visual impairment and renal dysfunction (Candler, Murphy, Pigott, & Gregory, 2017). There are modified versions of the SCOFF and EDI screening tools (see Table 2 for screening and assessment tools) for ED screening in youth with diabetes (Morgan, 2000; Zuijdwijk et al., 2014). Youth with diabetes are 2.4 times as likely to have an ED when compared to peers without diabetes. Youth with comorbid diabetes and an ED are more likely to misuse insulin than diabetic peers without ED, 42% and 11%, respectively (Jones, Lawson, Daneman, Olmsted, & Rodin, 2000). Mental health providers should monitor for signs of poorly controlled diabetes which may result in altered mental status including confusion, memory impairment, low energy level, and irritability. Mental health providers should screen youth with diabetes for ED and insulin misuse and coordinate care needs with a primary care provider. The Diabulimia Helpline (diabulimiahelpline.org) offers support, including a 24-h hotline, to both diabetics who have an ED and the professionals who treat them.

Muscle Dysmorphia/Bigorexia/Reverse Anorexia

Body builders first used the term "bigorexia" in the 1990s to describe the perception that one's body was too small (Sreshta, Pope, Hudson, & Kanayama, 2017). The DSM-5 has included muscle dysmorphia as a specifier under body dysmorphic disorder in the category of obsessive-compulsive and related disorders (American Psychiatric Association, 2013). Muscle dysmorphia has been associated with increased incidence of ED (Strother, Lemberg, Stanford, & Turberville, 2012).

Etiology of Eating Disorders

The assessment of ED is based on a foundation structure that is rapidly evolving as ED research advances. While no clear etiology has been identified for ED, new genetic and scanning technologies in the hands of skilled researchers pursuing multiple avenues of study require that the clinician review the ED literature frequently. The concepts of an "anorexigenic family" and ED as "a retreat from developing adult sexuality via a regression to the prepubertal relation to the parents" (Schmidt, 2003) have given way to a multifactorial causality with psychological, genetic, neurobiological, and sociocultural factors forming a complex web as important contributors (Becker, 2017; Meyre, Mayhew, Pigeyre, & Couturier, 2017). As each is examined below, the implications for the clinical assessment process will be highlighted.

Psychological Factors

Psychological factors include cognitive development and function, personality, and comorbid psychological disorders. Dissatisfaction with one's body requires the cognitive ability to formulate an accurate body image and compare this self-representation to a body ideal which entails a level of abstract thinking that begins to develop in the preteen years. In addition to cognitive factors, rapid growth during the preschool years complicates the young child's perception of their own body size while being able to accurately perceive another's body (Dunphy-Lelii, Hooley, McGivern, Guha, & Skouteris, 2014; León, González-Martí, Fernández-Bustos, & Contreras, 2017). The clinician must understand the child's developmental level and cognitive ability in order to assess concerns from children or parents regarding body perception and body dissatisfaction.

Adults with ED have shown neuropsychological impairment compared to controls, and in some parameters these deficits have persisted after weight restoration (Bosanac et al., 2007; Eneva, Murray, & Chen, 2017; Manasse et al., 2015; Weider, Indredavik, Lydersen, & Hestad, 2014). No association has been demonstrated between body size estimation and visual spatial memory or other select neuropsychological tasks (Øverås, Kapstad, Brunborg, Landrø, & Rø, 2017). Adults with BN but not AN have shown deficits in set shifting as measured by the Trail Making Test (Vall & Wade, 2015). In adults with BED, altered cortical function with increased impulsivity and compulsivity paired with executive function deficits has been implicated, as well as altered response to reward and food cues (Kessler et al., 2016). These findings have not been consistently replicated in youth, even in young teens with severe AN (Rose et al., 2017; van Noort, Pfeiffer, Ehrlich, Lehmkuhl, & Kappel, 2016). To address research and clinical consistency when using psychological tests, the "Ravello Profile" has been proposed as a standardized neuropsychological battery for the assessment of ED (Rose, Davis, Frampton, & Lask, 2011). A meta-analysis of fifteen studies using the Ravello Profile found visual memory and set shifting deficits in persons with AN (Stedal, Frampton, Landrø, & Lask, 2011). Neuropsychological research of youth with neurodevelopmental delays and ED is needed.

Personality development is a major task of adolescence that continues through young adulthood. Personality has genetic and environmental determinants with the balance favoring genetics early in life, tipping to the environment with age (Kandler, Bleidorn, Riemann, Angleitner, & Spinath, 2012). The contribution of personality factors to ED has been an area of study for over half a century with adolescent personality patterns aligning with research in adult populations. Research notes an increased incidence of high-functioning/perfectionistic, emotionally dysregulated, and avoidant/depressed personality types. Adolescents with the high-functioning/perfectionistic personality style have better treatment response and less comorbidity. The emotionally dysregulated group shows more difficulties with school and a greater history of adverse childhood events. Poor peer and maternal relationships are features of the avoidant/depressed group (Thompson-Brenner, Eddy, Satir, Boisseau, & Westen, 2008). Perfectionism is associated with disordered eating patterns, attempts at weight control, and predicts risk for bulimic behaviors (De Caro & Di Blas, 2016; García-Villamisar, Dattilo, & Del Pozo, 2012). Other personality characteristics with a reported association to ED include inflexibility and adherence to routine, restricted interest, rumination, social anhedonia, and alexithymia (Dell'Osso et al., 2016, 2017).

Youth with ED often have comorbid mental disorders. Anxiety disorders, oppositional defiant disorder, obsessive-compulsive disorder, ADHD, and ASD have all been reported as significant (Hudson et al., 2007; Rojo-Moreno et al., 2015; Swanson et al., 2011). The National Comorbidity Survey Replication Adolescent Supplement (NCS-A) reported lifetime ED with a comorbid disorder in ~55%, 88%, and ~84% of youth with AN, BN, BED, respectively, with 37% of the BED group reporting three or more comorbidities (Swanson et al., 2011). In a large prospective cross-sectional study, the risk for a comorbid anxiety disorder was ~7x, obsessive-compulsive disorder ~6x, and oppositional defiant disorder 11x when compared to youth without an ED (Rojo-Moreno et al., 2015). A systematic review and meta-analysis of ED and child abuse found child sexual abuse associated with BN and BED, while child physical abuse was associated with AN, BN, and BED (Caslini et al., 2016). Youth with ED and comorbid mental illness are at increased risk for poorer treatment outcomes including suicide (Cucchi et al., 2016).

Neurobiological Factors

The neuroscience of the complex gut-brain interactions controlling hunger and feeding behaviors has advanced remarkably with the advent of increasingly sophisticated neuroimaging technologies. The limbic system, parietal and frontal regions of the brain, plays roles in feeding behaviors with the amygdala-orbitofrontal circuit integrating mood and eating behaviors (Hill, Peck, Wierenga, & Kaye, 2016; Schwartz & Zeltser, 2013; Tanofsky-Kraff et al., 2013). Neurological correlates of altered responses to reward, punishment, and social distress in persons with ED have been identified (Frank, Shott, Hagman, & Mittal, 2013; Hill et al., 2016; Jarcho et al., 2015).

Neurotransmitters and hormones are messengers that regulate bodily functions. Dopamine, with genetically influenced signaling capacity, has been implicated in reward response to high calorie foods (Yokum, Marti, Smolen, & Stice, 2015). Endogenous opioids, stimulated by appetite dysfunction, binging, and excessive exercise, also impact reward response (Gorwood et al., 2016). Serotonin has been shown to regulate feeding decisions and satiety and may play a role in memory disturbances leading to impaired body image (Riva, 2016). The limbic-hypothalamic-pituitary-adrenal axis and the sympathetic-adrenal-medullary axis mediate stress responses which have been implicated in loss of control eating in BN and BED through the neurotransmitter adrenaline and noradrenaline and the hormone cortisol (Maniam & Morris, 2012; Tanofsky-Kraff et al., 2013). The hormones leptin and ghrelin, long studied for an association with obesity, are being investigated for their roles in ED (Knatz, Wierenga, Murray, Hill, & Kaye, 2015; Miller et al., 2014; Monteleone et al., 2018). Altered ghrelin has been associated with BED and BN with normalization after binge eating remits (Tanofsky-Kraff et al., 2013). Metabolic phenotypes have been identified for some neuromodulators (Duncan et al., 2017). (In contrast to the genotype determined by DNA, the phenotype describes how the genotype is expressed, including the influence of the external and internal environments.) In addition, hormonal changes associated with puberty in females have been associated with increased expression of ED-related behaviors (Bakalar, Shank, Vannucci, Radin, & Tanofsky-Kraff, 2015). Neurobiological factors inform the treatment of ED clinically and pharmacologically. Still, a medication has not been identified for the treatment of youth with ED. Recently a team from the University of California in San Diego has developed a neurobiologically based treatment protocol, the Neurobiologically Enhanced with Family Eating Disorder Trait Response Treatment (NEW FED TR) (Hill et al., 2016; Knatz et al., 2015).

Genetic Factors

Rapid genetic sequencing has allowed the expansion from behavioral genetic studies to the identification of candidate genes and most recently genome-wide association studies. To date, the latter has focused on AN. Behavioral genetic studies comparing monozygotic versus dizygotic twins have demonstrated increased concordance rates for AN which suggests that both the environment and genetics play a role in the development of the disease (Bulik et al., 2010). A recent genome-wide association study identified the first significant gene locus associated with AN, located on chromosome 12 (Duncan et al., 2017). This same gene locus is associated with type 1 diabetes and an array of autoimmune disorders. There are genetic correlations for AN and obesity, two extremes of weight regulation; shared genetic etiologies have been proposed (Baker, Schaumberg, & Munn-Chernoff, 2017; Hinney et al., 2017). Risk alleles have been identified linking AN with ASD and mood disorders (Bulik-Sullivan et al., 2015). Thaler and Steiger have hypothesized that epigenetic factors (factors which change gene expression without altering the DNA sequence) may contribute to ED presentation, mediated by perinatal complications, trauma, and malnutrition (Thaler & Steiger, 2017). Obtaining a detailed family history is critical as the risk of developing AN is up to 11 times greater for those with a first-degree relative with a history of the illness versus families with no history of AN (Yilmaz, Hardaway, & Bulik, 2015). Refer to Yilmaz et al. (2015) for a comprehensive review of the *Genetics and Epigenetics of Eating Disorders*.

Sociocultural and Environmental Factors

The relationship of ED to family, peers, media, culture, trauma, and race has been investigated with a focus on western societal values of thinness and weight bias (Becker, 2017, Chapter 20; Culbert, Racine, & Klump, 2015; Mitchison & Hay, 2014). Becker (2017) has categorized sociocultural influences into three domains: cultural values shaping core values of selfhood, local social structures, and global processes. Becker's classic study of the rise of ED in Fiji tracks the introduction of Western television programs in the 1990s to a shift in ideal body image and rise of ED in adolescent females (Becker et al., 2011). With industrialization and urbanization, Asian cultures have experienced shifts in local structures (eating habits and exercise) along with increased exposure to western media, foods, and body image which has led to a rise in ED (Pike, Dunne, & Grant, 2015).

Body dissatisfaction in children has been linked to poor self-esteem and the development of ED (Stice, Marti, & Durant, 2011). A comprehensive review of children's body image in girls found body dissatisfaction with a desire to be thinner increasing from the early school years through adolescence. For young boys, when dissatisfaction is reported, the desire for a thinner and larger body is approximately equal. Media exposure, perceived peer body dissatisfaction, and peer appearance conversations including teasing influenced dissatisfaction in girls (Paxton & Damiano, 2017). These factors continue to influence adolescents along with friends' dieting behaviors (Webb, Zimmer-Gembeck, & Donovan, 2014). Family is also a predictor of body dissatisfaction in children and adolescents with mothers' body dissatisfaction and comments showing an association with daughters' level of body dissatisfaction (Perez, Kroon Van Diest, Smith, & Sladek, 2016; Rohde, Stice, & Marti, 2015).

A review of weight bias found that children as young as 3 years old hold negative attitudes toward excess weight. A childhood bias against persons who are overweight or obese may be internalized as body dissatisfaction (Paxton & Damiano, 2017). For adolescent females but not males, binge eating by fathers/male friends was associated with girl's binge eating (Goldschmidt et al., 2014). The Eating Activity in Teens (EAT) study found significant differences in dissatisfaction across races, with females and males of Asian descent having the highest dissatisfaction and African American males having the lowest satisfaction (Bucchianeri et al., 2016). Activities that promote thinness such as wrestling, ballet, gymnastics, or modeling have been associated with an increased risk for ED.

There is a subculture that glorifies ED. Websites promoting anorexia (pro-an) and bulimia (pro-mia) abound with "how to" tips, advice, and images (The rise of pro-anorexia and pro-mia websites, n.d). Conversely, negative societal attitudes against persons with ED may contribute to failure to seek treatment and hide ED-related behaviors. A study using the Stigmatizing Attitudes and Beliefs About Bulimia Nervosa (SAB-BN) questionnaire revealed that stigma against ED was greater in males and people with a lower educational level (Griffiths et al., 2015; McLean et al., 2014). A systematic review of treatment barriers revealed stigma and shame as the most commonly reported reasons for not seeking ED therapy. Denial of the seriousness of ED was also common (Ali et al., 2017). Public health interventions to destigmatize ED provide education and tools to help individuals suffering from ED including motivational interviewing (Golden et al., 2016; McLean et al., 2014). The clinician should screen youth for idealized body and target weight, body dissatisfaction, perception of family and friend's weight-related attitudes, family and friend's dieting behavior, and media use.

Current Diagnostic Nosologies

The concepts underlying ED date back to the ancient Greeks with "anorexia" denoting "without hunger" and bulimia "ox hunger" (Fairburn & Brownell, 2002). Symptoms consistent with our modern diagnosis of AN have been described for centuries primarily as extreme forms of asceticism involving religious fasting. The first medical description consistent with AN appeared in 1694 followed by the designation of "anorexia nervosa" in the nineteenth century (Dell'Osso et al., 2016). BED and BN entered the medical literature much more recently. BED was described in 1959 as a behavior associated with obesity (Stunkard, 1959) and BN in 1979 was described as "an ominous variant of anorexia nervosa" (Russell, 1979) (Table 1).

ED are diagnosed according to the *Diagnostic and Statistical Manual* of the American Psychiatric Association (DSM) and/or the WHO International Classification of Diseases (ICD) (American Psychiatric Association, 2013; World Health Organization, 1992). In addition, research is guided by the National Institutes of Mental Health Research Domain Criteria (RDoC) (Cuthbert, 2014). The DSM and ICD nosologies base diagnoses on symptom constellations informed by research and clinical practice. Both have undergone multiple revisions and informed practice for over half a century. In the United States, the DSM-5 stipulates specific criteria for mental disorders for clinical practice and research, while the ICD 10 provides codes that are in use for billing purposes.

The RDoC was proposed in 2008 as a research framework for "classifying mental disorders

Table 1 Diagnostic Features of AN, BN, and BED

	Anorexia nervosa	Bulimia nervosa	Binge eating disorder

Core Features	Restricted energy intake leading to significantly low weight or failure to meet minimally expected weight in children and adolescents
	Intense fear of weight gain or getting fat or behaviors that interfere with weight gain
	Disturbance on how the body weight and shape are experienced, excessive self-evaluation of weight and shape, or denial of the seriousness of low body weight
		Recurrent episodes of binge eating including both:
		  Eating an excess of food in a short amount of time
		  A sense of lack of control over eating
		Compensatory behaviors after binging to prevent weight gain, i.e., self-induced vomiting, diuretics, laxative abuse, fasting, chewing and spitting, and medication manipulation
		Occurs ~ 1x/week for 3 months
		Body shape and weight have excess influence on self-evaluation
		BN does not occur at the same time as episodes of AN
			Recurrent episodes of binge eating which include both:
			  Eating an excess of food in a short amount of time
			  A sense of lack of control over eating
			The episodes have three or more of the following:
			  Eating more rapidly than normal
			  Eating until feeling uncomfortably full
			  Eating when not hungry
			  Eating alone due to embarrassment by amount of food consumed
			  Feelings of disgust with self, depression, or guilt after episode
			Distress during a binge episode
			No compensatory behavior is present as in BN or AN

Duration	No set duration to diagnose the disorder	Both binge eating and compensatory behavior occur on average 1x/week for 3 months	Binge eating occurs on average 1x/week for 3 months

Specifiers	Type: *restricting type* – dieting, fasting, and excessive exercise with no occurrence of binging or purging during a period of 3 months
	  Binge eating/purging type: self-induced vomiting and misuse of laxatives, diuretics, or enemas for 3 months
	Severity:
	  Mild: BMI ≥ 17 kg/m^2
	  Moderate: BMI 16–16.99 kg/m^2
	  Severe: BMI 15–15.99 kg/m^2
	  Extreme: BMI < 15 kg/m^2
		Severity
		  Mild: ~1–3 episodes/week
		  Moderate: ~4–7 episodes/ week
		  Severe: ~ 8–13 episodes per week
		  Extreme: ~ 14 or more episodes per week
			Mild: 1–3 binge-eating episodes per week
			Moderate: 4–7 binge-eating episodes per week
			Severe: 8–13 binge-eating episodes per week
			Extreme: 14 or more binge-eating episodes per week

Adpated from the DSM-5

based on dimensions of observable behavior and neurobiological measures," focusing on brain/behavior relationships to better inform DSM/ICD descriptive nosologies (National Institute of Mental Health, n.d). The RDoC framework is conceptualized as a matrix or table with rows detailing the five domains/constructs (negative valence systems, positive valence systems, cognitive systems, systems for social processes, and arousal/modulatory systems) and columns representing eight units of analysis (genes, molecules, cells, circuits, physiology, behavior, self-report, and paradigms) (Sanislow, 2016). The RDoC framework considers development and environmental influences across domains and is transdiagnostic, fostering research to compare domain characteristics within and between DSM/ICD categories (Cuthbert, 2014). In this framework the common features of ED with FD or other disorders can be explored methodically. The RDoC domains of negative valence systems (acute threat, potential threat, sustained threat, loss, and frustrative nonreward) are areas of early exploration (Tanofsky-Kraff et al., 2013; Vannucci et al., 2015). Wildes and Marcus (2015) provide a detailed review of utilization of RDoC in ED research.

AN was defined in the first edition of the DSM as a psychophysiological reaction. It was described as a "visceral expression of affect which may be thereby largely prevented from being conscious" in which "emotional factors play a causative role" (American Psychiatric Association, 1952). The DSM-II placed AN in Section VII – Special Symptoms "for the occasional patient whose psychopathology is manifest by a single symptom" in the subcategory of Feeding Disturbance (American Psychiatric Association, 1975). The DSM-III reclassified AN under the section Disorders Usually First Evident in Infancy, Childhood, or Adolescence (American Psychiatric Association, American Psychiatric Association. Task Force on Nomenclature and Statistics, 1980; American Psychiatric Association. Committee on Nomenclature and Statistics, & American Psychiatric Association. Work Group to Revise DSM-III, 1987). This classification may have contributed to the underdiagnosis of late-onset ED (American Psychiatric Association, American Psychiatric Association. Task Force on Nomenclature and Statistics, American Psychiatric Association. Committee on Nomenclature and Statistics, & American Psychiatric Association. Work Group to Revise DSM-III, 1980; Dell'Osso et al., 2016). The DSM-III introduced bulimia (American Psychiatric Association, American Psychiatric Association. Task Force on Nomenclature and Statistics, American Psychiatric Association. Committee on Nomenclature and Statistics, & American Psychiatric Association. Work Group to Revise DSM-III, 1980). The DSM-III-R renamed "bulimia" to "bulimia nervosa" (BN) and noted that AN and BN are "apparently related disorders, typically beginning in adolescence or early adult life"; this differentiated the ED and FD diagnoses and led to ED being placed in a separate category in the DSM-IV. When reviewing research using DSM-III and DSM-IV criteria, remember that these earlier editions include weight/body mass requirements to qualify for an AN diagnosis that are not DSM-5 requirements (American Psychiatric Association, 2013; American Psychiatric Association & American Psychiatric Association, 1994; American Psychiatric Association, American Psychiatric Association. Task Force on Nomenclature and Statistics, American Psychiatric Association. Committee on Nomenclature and Statistics, & American Psychiatric Association. Work Group to Revise DSM-III, 1980). The DSM-5 removed weight/BMI and changed duration requirements after clinical research noted that over 50% of clinical diagnoses did not meet strict AN criteria and were coded as ED not otherwise specified (EDNOS). This decision is supported by the findings of Mustelin et al. (2016) in their comparison of AN diagnoses under the DSM-IV and DSM-5 criteria in a Finnish female twin birth cohort study investigating those born between 1975 and 1979 ($n = 2825$). The prevalence of AN increased from 2.2% to 3.6% when DSM-5 criteria were introduced (Mustelin et al., 2016). In line with the growing recognition of a developmental progression of ED, the DSM-5 regrouped feeding and eating disorders together. The frequency criteria for BN were reduced from twice a week to once a week in DSM-5 (American Psychiatric Association, 2013).

Although Stunkard hypothesized that binge eating was a medical condition in 1959 (Stunkard, 1959), it was not until 1994 that BED was recognized as a provisional diagnosis in the DSM-IV (American Psychiatric Association & Apa, 1994). BED was included in the DSM-5 after the Eating Disorder Task Force found BED criteria to be reliable in differentiating individuals with BED from those with other eating disorders and obesity, and treatments for BED were distinct from other ED (Tanofsky-Kraff et al., 2013).

The ICD-10 code for AN specifies subtypes including restricting type, binge eating/purging, or unspecified. BN, also referred to as hyperorexia nervosa, and BED correspond to the DSM-IV criteria including the twice-per-week frequency (World Health Organization, 1992). Like DSM criteria, ICD-10 criteria have resulted in a higher prevalence rates of EDNOS in clinical practice (Uher & Rutter, 2012). The ICD-10 eating disorders revision committee has proposed changing the criteria for weight, amenorrhea, and duration to align with DSM-5 (Al-Adawi et al., 2013). The ICD-11, with revised ED codes, is scheduled for release in 2018 (WHO/ICD-11 Revision, 2017).

The Assessment of Eating Disorders

The goal of ED assessment is to reduce the risk of mortality and comorbid medical and psychological disability. Among adolescents with AN, the ratio of the number of deaths due to anorexia to the expected number of deaths (the standard mortality ratio, SMR) is the highest of all mental disorders highlighting the importance of screening and assessing for ED (Franko et al., 2013). Youth with eating disorders are at substantial risk of cardiac impairment, osteoporosis, esophageal rupture, dental disease, and neuropsychological impairment even when symptoms do not qualify the youth for the full diagnosis (Campbell & Peebles, 2014). Neuropsychological impairment includes a high incidence of comorbid psychiatric disorders as well as increased risk of impaired memory, learning, and executive function (Weider et al., 2014). The Institute for Health Metrics and Evaluation at the University of Washington reports on the global burden of disease (GBD) for 333 physical and mental disorders in 195 countries. Eating disorders (AN and BN combined) ranked 12th in causes of disability burden for 15–19-year-old females in high-income countries in the GBD 2013 study (Erskine, Whiteford, & Pike, 2016).

The assessment of ED involves the skilled application of a broad array of knowledge to the presenting complaint of the child and parent. This skill may be learned by reading and observation but can only be honed and perfected by practice. To assess ED, the clinician must first listen to the presenting concerns of the family and then follow the threads of the parents' observations and child's perceptions to assemble the diagnostic puzzle. This is especially challenging with the assessment of ED. Consider the assessment of Katelyn (not an actual patient) who was initially assessed to have ASD. She now presents years later for an assessment of externalizing behaviors.

> Katelyn is 15 years old receiving educational accommodations for ASD. She is of average height and slightly overweight, with a BMI of 27. She lives with her mother who reports that Katelyn has become more oppositional since entering high school. She doesn't want to get up in the morning or go to school and in the rush often misses breakfast. Her mother is worried that Katelyn is hanging with the wrong crowd because she has been skipping classes and her grades have dropped.

> You learn that Katelyn is struggling academically since being moved to regular classes with a 1-h academic support class each day. She doesn't like school and refuses to dress out for gym. On the bright side, although she has struggled to make friends in the past, she is pleased to have a new group of friends at school.

> Your initial treatment plan includes instruction on reconvening the individualized education plan (IEP) team at Katelyn's school and starting therapy to improve social skills and communication. You discuss Katelyn's need for increased supervision at school and at home including access to the internet and social media through electronic devices. Because it has been 5 years since Katelyn last received a comprehensive psychological testing, you schedule one for the following week.

If youth are referred from a medical primary care setting for ED treatment, the need for the assessment of eating-related behaviors is clear. Unhealthy eating or ED symptoms are far less likely to be the presenting complaint in a clinical psychology setting. Without direct inquiry into eating habits, dieting, and growth, an ED may be missed. ED in youth who are normal weight or overweight should not be overlooked for screening because youth with ED can be underweight, normal weight, or overweight. In children and adolescents, expected growth patterns for height and weight must be considered because failure to meet expected milestones may be a sign of ED. (See chapter 23 on obesity for specific instruments to monitor growth.) Additionally, the assessment can be challenging because youth may not have the skills to describe eating behaviors and related emotions or they may purposely hide disordered eating. Let's revisit Katelyn's story here:

> Prior to Katelyn's reevaluation, you note that during previous evaluation, she was fidgety yet cooperative and completed tasks in the expected time limits. Previous testing noted borderline intellectual functioning with memory and executive functioning consistent with IQ. Her history included social delays and strict adherence to preferred routines including starchy food preferences and challenging behaviors at meal time. You considered a diagnosis of avoidant restrictive feeding disorder.
>
> During the reevaluation you find Katelyn to be irritable and sluggish. Given past testing you are surprised at the decline in memory and her limited persistence. Katelyn and her mother report that she sleeps well. When discussing strengths, her mother reports that she is pleased that Katelyn has taken a new interest in her appearance and has recently talked about "slimming down." As you review eating habits and dieting attitude with Katelyn, you learn that she recently completed a unit on healthy eating at school and that she is dieting with her new friends. When you ask about the diet, she says her friends told her dieting was a secret. With coaxing, she explains that she and her friends chew food then spit it out. You administer the SCOFF Questionnaire (Hill, Reid, Morgan, & Hubert Lacey, 2009). The SCOFF reveals that Katelyn believes that she is fat and tries not to eat but ends up "thinking about food all the time." You explain to Katelyn and her mother that this raises concerns that Katelyn could have an eating disorder and that Katelyn's health and safety are the first priority. You write a safety plan (See Table 3) and refer Katelyn to her primary care provider for an evaluation.

Primary care providers track weight and growth patterns over time monitoring a youth's individual growth curve and pubertal development for deviations from expected trajectories. Professional organizations and practice guidelines call on primary care providers to screen all youth for eating disorders (Campbell & Peebles, 2014; Lock, La Via, & American Academy of Child and Adolescent Psychiatry (AACAP) Committee on Quality Issues (CQI), 2015; Nattiv et al., 2007). Screening includes direct inquiries about eating habits and may include screening instruments such as the SCOFF. (See Table 2 for additional assessment instruments.) Parents and children should be questioned about eating habits, especially feelings associated with loss of control when eating and dieting. Chewing and spitting out food rather than swallowing is associated with loss of control eating, greater comorbidity, and more severe ED (Makhzoumi et al., 2015). The evaluation of media access and use should include inquiry into the viewing of websites related to dieting or eating disorders. The genetics of eating disorders underscores the importance of asking about the history of eating disorders in family members. Youth should be queried privately to encourage the sharing of information that they might have difficulty expressing with parents present or that they may have withheld from parents.

A routine physical examination may note physical changes associated with ED. In addition to the physical changes of weight loss, cardiac changes (hypotension, bradycardia, heart murmur), poor healing of cuts and bruises, skin changes, hair loss, and lanugo (fine, downy hair) on the back, abdomen, and forearms can occur (Campbell & Peebles, 2014). With BN, dental issues and prominent cheeks may be physical signs which might also include Russell's sign, calluses formed on the knuckles with repeated self-induced vomiting (Daluiski, Rahbar, & Meals, 1997; Russell, 1979; Strumia, 2002).

It is equally important for the primary care provider to exclude medical conditions which may cause symptoms mimicking ED including thyroid abnormalities, diabetes, infectious diseases, gastrointestinal disorders, and pregnancy (Campbell & Peebles, 2014; DerMarderosian, Chapman, Tortolani, & Willis, 2018). This may necessitate EKG or blood tests to identify medical conditions and to further evaluate the effects of unhealthy eating. Blood tests can identify imbalances in electrolytes, such as the potassium, phosphorus, calcium, and sodium, which allow cells to function properly. The primary care provider may make referrals to specialists for further

Table 2 Selected eating disorder screening and assessment tools

Psychometric tool	Description
PhenX toolkit for ED (https://www.phenxtoolkit.org/index.php?pageLink=browse.conceptualgroups&id=3455&breadcrumbs=34493455)	The PhenX Toolkit of standard measures of phenotypes and environmental exposures in ED research. Twelve ED measures are available
Ravello Profile (Rose et al., 2011)	Standardized neuropsychological battery for the assessment of eating disorders highlighting visuospatial functioning, central coherence, and executive functioning
Eating Disorder Examination (EDE 17.0D) (Fairburn, Cooper, & O'Connor, 2018)	"Gold standard" assessment instrument for adults and youth older than 9 years of age. DSM-5 diagnosis, severity score, subscales, restraint, eating concern, weight concern, and shape concern. Available at no cost
Eating Disorder Examination 6.0 Questionnaire (EDE-Q) (Fairburn & Beglin, 2008)	A 28-item questionnaire adapted from the Eating Disorder Examination
Eating Disorder Examination-Questionnaire adapted for children (ChEDE-Q8) (Kliem et al., 2017)	An eight-item screen for AN, BN, and BED in children older than 7 years of age
Eating Disorder Assessment for DSM-5 (EDA-5) (Sysko et al., 2015)	Semi-structured interview for FD and ED. A child version is available. Both are available at no cost
Structured Interview For Anorexic And Bulimic Disorders for DSM-IV and ICD-10, 3rd revision (Fichter, Herpertz, Quadflieg, & Herpertz-Dahlmann, 1998)	Identifies lifetime and current ED. No DSM-5 version
Eating Pathology Symptoms Inventory (EPSI) (Forbush et al., 2013)	A 45-item self-report measure of body dissatisfaction, binge eating, cognitive restraint, purging, muscle building, restricting, excessive exercise, and negative attitudes toward obesity
SCOFF (Morgan, Reid, & Lacey, 1999)	A five-question quick screen for the core features of anorexia nervosa and bulimia nervosa. A modified version is available to screen persons with diabetes
Binge Eating Disorder Screener-7 (BEDS-7) (Herman et al., 2016)	A seven-item screening instrument for binge eating disorder
Eating Disorder Inventory-3 (Garner, 2004)	A 91-item scale identifying AN, BN, and BED. The EDI identifies ineffectiveness, interpersonal problems, affective problems, over control, and general psychological maladjustment. A child version is available
Kids Eating Disorder Survey (KEDS) (Childress, Jarrell, & Brewerton, 1993)	A 14-item self-report screening tool

assessment. An endocrinologist may be consulted for patients with diabetes who are at high risk for AN, BN, and BED (Raevuori et al., 2014). Youth with ASD are at increased risk of GI disorders including abdominal pain, constipation, diarrhea, gastroesophageal reflux, and food allergies which may require referral to a gastroenterologist. Although rare, a genetics consult may be obtained if binge eating raises concerns about Kleine-Levin, Prader-Willi, or fragile X-Prader-Willi subphenotype (see the chapter on Obesity) (Rosen & American Academy of Pediatrics Committee on Adolescence, 2010). The American Academy of Pediatrics and the American Academy of Child and Adolescent Psychiatry have published guidelines for the assessment of eating disorders which include grounds for hospitalization (Campbell & Peebles, 2014; Lock et al., 2015).

At her next visit, Katelyn's mother reports that she has monitored electronic use as you suggested and found that Katelyn had accessed an online Eating Disorder Screening Tool (Screening Tool, n.d) by following a link in a *Teen Vogue* article (Kronengold, 2017) sent to her by a friend. When talking with Katelyn privately, she shows you the pro-mia chat room she has joined with her friend. Further questions reveal that Katelyn believes that her mother and friends think she is fat. Katelyn has been thinking about purging. She does not understand the dangers of purging behaviors.

You discuss healthy behaviors and the risks of purging with Katelyn and her mother and provide the family with guidance for monitoring Katelyn. You reassure the family that Katelyn's prognosis is good because her ED was identified early and her symptoms are subthreshold (Stice et al., 2013). You collaborate care with her primary care provider.

Therapy begins with education about eating disorders and the recovery process. The National Eating Disorders Association website (NationalEatingDisordersAssociation.org) has numerous resources including a toolkit for parents. Parents may be shocked to learn their child has an eating disorder and may be hurt or angry upon learning their child has been secretive about ED behaviors. The initial phase of the outpatient treatment of ED requires a high level of family involvement. If constant supervision is required during initial outpatient treatment, parents may need assistance obtaining family medical leave (link to FMLA https://www.dol.gov/general/topic/benefits-leave/fmla) and homebound education or accommodations at school to monitor eating, limit exercise in physical education class, and monitor vital signs. The concept of an "anorexigenic family" (Schmidt, 2003) is outdated, but family therapy is indicated to improve communication and support recovery. Family-based treatment for eating disorders, the Maudsley approach, directs the clinician to provide specific instructions to parents for monitoring eating and exercise habits (Lock & Le Grange, 2015). The "Maudsley Parents" website (Maudsleyparents.org) offers extensive guidance for parents and professionals. When indicated, a weight restoration plan should be developed under medical guidance to avoid a potentially life-threatening condition called refeeding syndrome (DerMarderosian et al., 2018; Redgrave et al., 2015; Rosen & American Academy of Pediatrics Committee on Adolescence, 2010). "Refeeding syndrome" can occur as malnourished patients begin re-eating. It can occur at any BMI and requires prompt medical attention including blood work to identify the hypophosphatemia, hypokalemia, hypomagnesemia, and hypoglycemia characteristic of the syndrome. The junior MARISPAN (management of really sick patients with anorexia nervosa) guideline has been developed to manage refeeding safely (Marikar, Reynolds, & Moghraby, 2015; Redgrave et al., 2015). While any lifetime ED has been associated with increased suicidality (Chesney, Goodwin, & Fazel, 2014), death in ED is most likely to be due to the physiological abnormalities caused by restrictive eating and ED-related behaviors (Franko et al., 2013; Mehler & Brown, 2015). Cardiac arrhythmia is the most common medical complication leading to death (Becker, Grinspoon, Klibanski, & Herzog, 1999). A frank discussion of the medical risks of ED is critical and must include a safety plan because self-harming behaviors, suicidal ideation, and suicide are significantly increased in youth with ED (Cucchi et al., 2016; Lock et al., 2015; Rosen & American Academy of Pediatrics Committee on Adolescence, 2010; Zerwas et al., 2015). If there is a history of self-harming behaviors, the safety plan should include role playing with the child telling the parent about thoughts of self-harm as self-disclosure has been associated with decreased risk (Klomek et al., 2015). See Table 3 for suggestions on the initial treatment plan.

Table 3 Initial treatment planning suggestions

ED risk assessment	Detailed restoration plan	Safety plan
Weakness	Weight restoration	Ongoing screening for self-harming thoughts and behaviors
Dizziness	Refeeding	
Lethargy	Activity level	
Apathy	Nutritional requirements	
Irregular/rapid heartbeat	Parental responsibility for monitoring activity and refeeding	Identify stressors and triggers
Hypothermia		Written plan for coping with self-harming thoughts or behaviors
Lanugo		
Swollen checks		
Russell's sign	Electrolyte and protein monitoring	
Coordinate with primary care		

Summary

Youth with ED are among the most challenging patients to assess and treat. ED typically present during the teen years but often go untreated due to attempts to conceal the illness because of the stigmas of ED and mental health treatment. Mental health providers must be proactive in screening for ED. The high mortality and comorbidity of eating disorders coupled with diagnostic crossover require that mental health screening be based in a broad knowledge of ED and the common comorbidities – depression, anxiety, obsessive-compulsive disorder, and trauma. Coordination of care with medical providers, the school, and family is time-consuming but critical. Prevention efforts promoting healthy behaviors rather than body ideals and the early identification of youth with ED hold the best promise for treatment success. While ED research is expanding rapidly with neuropsychological, genetic, and neuroimaging informing the assessment and care of youth, additional research is needed to guide the assessment of youth with neurodevelopmental disorders.

References

Ackard, D. M., Richter, S., Egan, A., Engel, S., & Cronemeyer, C. L. (2014). The meaning of (quality of) life in patients with eating disorders: A comparison of generic and disease-specific measures across diagnosis and outcome. *The International Journal of Eating Disorders, 47*(3), 259–267.

Al-Adawi, S., Bax, B., Bryant-Waugh, R., Claudino, A. M., Hay, P., Monteleone, P., ... Uher, R. (2013). Revision of ICD – Status update on feeding and eating disorders. *Advances in Eating Disorders, 1*(1), 10–20.

Ali, K., Farrer, L., Fassnacht, D. B., Gulliver, A., Bauer, S., & Griffiths, K. M. (2017). Perceived barriers and facilitators towards help-seeking for eating disorders: A systematic review. *The International Journal of Eating Disorders, 50*(1), 9–21.

Allison, K. C., Lundgren, J. D., O'Reardon, J. P., Geliebter, A., Gluck, M. E., Vinai, P., ... Stunkard, A. J. (2010). Proposed diagnostic criteria for night eating syndrome. *The International Journal of Eating Disorders, 43*(3), 241–247.

American Psychiatric Association. (1952). *Diagnostic and statistical manual of mental disorders*. Amer Psychiatric Pub. Washington DC.

American Psychiatric Association. (2013). *Diagnostic and statistical manual of mental disorders (DSM-5®)*. American Psychiatric Pub Washington DC.

American Psychiatric Association, & Apa. (1994). *Dsm*. American Psychiatric Publishing Washington DC.

American Psychiatric Association, American Psychiatric Association. Task Force on Nomenclature and Statistics, American Psychiatric Association. Committee on Nomenclature and Statistics, & American Psychiatric Association. Work Group to Revise DSM-III. (1980). *Diagnostic and statistical manual of mental disorders*. Amer Psychiatric Pub Inc.

American Psychiatric Association. Committee on Nomenclature and Statistics. (1975). *DSM-II: Diagnostic and statistical manual of mental disorders*.

Bakalar, J. L., Shank, L. M., Vannucci, A., Radin, R. M., & Tanofsky-Kraff, M. (2015). Recent advances in developmental and risk factor research on eating disorders. *Current Psychiatry Reports, 17*(6), 42.

Baker, J. H., Schaumberg, K., & Munn-Chernoff, M. A. (2017). Genetics of anorexia nervosa. *Current Psychiatry Reports, 19*(11), 84.

Bankoff, S. M., Marks, A. K., Swenson, L. P., & Pantalone, D. W. (2016). Examining associations of sexual attraction and attitudes on Women's disordered eating behavior. *Journal of Clinical Psychology, 72*(4), 350–364.

Becker, A. E. (2017). Sociocultural influences on body image and eating disturbance. In B. Keely & W. Timothy (Eds.), *Eating disorders and obesity: A comprehensive handbook*. New York, NY: The Guilford Press.

Becker, A. E., Fay, K. E., Agnew-Blais, J., Khan, A. N., Striegel-Moore, R. H., & Gilman, S. E. (2011). Social network media exposure and adolescent eating pathology in Fiji. *The British Journal of Psychiatry: the Journal of Mental Science, 198*(1), 43–50.

Becker, A. E., Grinspoon, S. K., Klibanski, A., & Herzog, D. B. (1999). Eating disorders. *The New England Journal of Medicine, 340*(14), 1092–1098.

Bingham, M. E., Borkan, M. E., & Quatromoni, P. A. (2015). Sports Nutrition advice for adolescent athletes. *American Journal of Lifestyle Medicine, 9*(6), 398–402.

Bleck, J. R., DeBate, R. D., & Olivardia, R. (2014). The Comorbidity of ADHD and eating disorders in a nationally representative sample. *The Journal of Behavioral Health Services & Research, 42*(4), 437–451.

Bosanac, P., Kurlender, S., Stojanovska, L., Hallam, K., Norman, T., McGrath, C., ... Olver, J. (2007). Neuropsychological study of underweight and "weight-recovered" anorexia nervosa compared with bulimia nervosa and normal controls. *The International Journal of Eating Disorders, 40*(7), 613–621.

Bratman, S., & Knight, D. (2004). *Health food junkies: The rise of Orthorexia Nervosa - the health food eating disorder*. Broadway.

Bucchianeri, M. M., Fernandes, N., Loth, K., Hannan, P. J., Eisenberg, M. E., & Neumark-Sztainer, D. (2016). Body dissatisfaction: Do associations with disordered eating and psychological Well-being differ across race/ethnicity in adolescent girls and boys? *Cultural Diversity & Ethnic Minority Psychology, 22*(1), 137–146.

Bulik, C. M., Thornton, L., Root, T. L., Pisetsky, E. M., Lichtenstein, P., & Pedersen, N. L. (2010). Understanding the relation between anorexia nervosa and bulimia nervosa in a Swedish National Twin Sample. *Biological Psychiatry, 67*(1), 71–77.

Bulik-Sullivan, B., ReproGen Consortium, Finucane, H. K., Anttila, V., Gusev, A., Day, F. R., ... Genetic Consortium for Anorexia Nervosa of the Wellcome Trust Case Control Consortium. (2015). An atlas of genetic correlations across human diseases and traits. *Nature Genetics, 47*(11), 1236–1241.

Campbell, K., & Peebles, R. (2014). Eating disorders in children and adolescents: State of the art review. *Pediatrics, 134*(3), 582–592.

Candler, T., Murphy, R., Pigott, A., & Gregory, J. W. (2017). Fifteen-minute consultation: Diabulimia and disordered eating in childhood diabetes. *Archives of Disease in Childhood. Education and Practice Edition.* https://doi.org/10.1136/archdischild-2017-312689

Caslini, M., Bartoli, F., Crocamo, C., Dakanalis, A., Clerici, M., & Carrà, G. (2016). Disentangling the association between child abuse and eating disorders: A systematic review and meta-analysis. *Psychosomatic Medicine, 78*(1), 79–90.

Chesney, E., Goodwin, G. M., & Fazel, S. (2014). Risks of all-cause and suicide mortality in mental disorders: A meta-review. *World Psychiatry: Official Journal of the World Psychiatric Association, 13*(2), 153–160.

Childress, A. C., Jarrell, M. P., & Brewerton, T. D. (1993). The kids' eating disorders survey (KEDS): Internal consistency, component analysis, and reliability. *Eating Disorders, 1*(2), 123–133.

Clarke, D. J., & Yapa, P. (1991). Phenylketonuria and anorexia nervosa. *Journal of Mental Deficiency Research, 35*(Pt 2), 165–170.

Counts, D. (2001). An adult with Prader-Willi syndrome and anorexia nervosa: A case report. *The International Journal of Eating Disorders, 30*(2), 231–233.

Cucchi, A., Ryan, D., Konstantakopoulos, G., Stroumpa, S., Kaçar, A. Ş., Renshaw, S., ... Kravariti, E. (2016). Lifetime prevalence of non-suicidal self-injury in patients with eating disorders: A systematic review and meta-analysis. *Psychological Medicine, 46*(7), 1345–1358.

Culbert, K. M., Racine, S. E., & Klump, K. L. (2015). Research review: What we have learned about the causes of eating disorders - a synthesis of sociocultural, psychological, and biological research. *Journal of Child Psychology and Psychiatry, and Allied Disciplines, 56*(11), 1141–1164.

Cuthbert, B. N. (2014). The RDoC framework: Facilitating transition from ICD/DSM to dimensional approaches that integrate neuroscience and psychopathology. *World Psychiatry: Official Journal of the World Psychiatric Association, 13*(1), 28–35.

Daluiski, A., Rahbar, B., & Meals, R. A. (1997). Russell's sign. Subtle hand changes in patients with bulimia nervosa. *Clinical Orthopaedics and Related Research, 343*, 107–109.

De Caro, E. F., & Di Blas, L. (2016). A prospective study on the reciprocal influence between personality and attitudes, behaviors, and psychological characteristics salient in eating disorders in a sample of non-clinical adolescents. *Eating Disorders, 24*(5), 453–468.

De Souza, M. J., Williams, N. I., Nattiv, A., Joy, E., Misra, M., Loucks, A. B., ... McComb, J. (2014). Misunderstanding the female athlete triad: Refuting the IOC consensus statement on relative energy deficiency in sport (RED-S). *British Journal of Sports Medicine, 48*(20), 1461–1465.

de Zwaan, M., Müller, A., Allison, K. C., Brähler, E., & Hilbert, A. (2014). Prevalence and correlates of night eating in the German general population. *PLoS One, 9*(5), e97667.

Dell'Osso, L., Abelli, M., Carpita, B., Pini, S., Castellini, G., Carmassi, C., & Ricca, V. (2016). Historical evolution of the concept of anorexia nervosa and relationships with orthorexia nervosa, autism, and obsessive–compulsive spectrum. *Neuropsychiatric Disease and Treatment, 12*, 1651–1660.

Dell'Osso, L., Carpita, B., Gesi, C., Cremone, I. M., Corsi, M., Massimetti, E., ... Maj, M. (2017). Subthreshold autism spectrum disorder in patients with eating disorders. *Comprehensive Psychiatry, 81*, 66–72.

DerMarderosian, D., Chapman, H. A., Tortolani, C., & Willis, M. D. (2018). Medical considerations in children and adolescents with eating disorders. *Child and Adolescent Psychiatric Clinics of North America, 27*(1), 1–14.

Duncan, L., Yilmaz, Z., Gaspar, H., Walters, R., Goldstein, J., Anttila, V., ... Bulik, C. M. (2017). Significant locus and metabolic genetic correlations revealed in genome-wide association study of anorexia nervosa. *The American Journal of Psychiatry, 174*(9), 850–858.

Dunphy-Lelii, S., Hooley, M., McGivern, L., Guha, A., & Skouteris, H. (2014). Preschoolers' body-knowledge inaccuracy: Perceptual self-deficit and attitudinal bias. *Early Child Development and Care, 184*(11), 1757–1768.

Eneva, K. T., Murray, S. M., & Chen, E. Y. (2017). Binge-eating disorder may be distinguished by visuospatial memory deficits. *Eating Behaviors, 26*, 159–162.

Erskine, H. E., Whiteford, H. A., & Pike, K. M. (2016). The global burden of eating disorders. *Current Opinion in Psychiatry, 29*(6), 346–353.

Fairburn, C., Cooper, Z., & O'Connor M. (January 29, 2018). *Eating Disorder Examination* (17.0D. ed.). http://credo-oxford.com/pdfs/EDE_17.0D.pdf

Fairburn, C. G., & Beglin, S. (2008). Appendix II, eating disorder examination questionnaire (EDE-Q 6.0). In C. G. Fairburn (Ed.), *Cognitive behavior therapy and eating disorders*. New York, NY: Guilford Press.

Fairburn, C. G., & Brownell, K. D. (2002). *Eating disorders and obesity: A comprehensive handbook*. New York, NY: Guilford Press.

Fairweather-Schmidt, A. K., & Wade, T. D. (2014). DSM-5 eating disorders and other specified eating and feeding disorders: Is there a meaningful differentiation? *The International Journal of Eating Disorders, 47*(5), 524–533.

Fernández-Aranda, F., Agüera, Z., Castro, R., Jiménez-Murcia, S., Ramos-Quiroga, J. A., Bosch, R., ... Menchon, J. M. (2013). ADHD symptomatology in eating disorders: A secondary psychopathological measure of severity? *BMC Psychiatry, 13*, 166.

Fichter, M. M., Herpertz, S., Quadflieg, N., & Herpertz-Dahlmann, B. (1998). Structured interview for anorexic and bulimic disorders for DSM-IV and ICD-10: Updated (third) revision. *The International Journal of Eating Disorders, 24*(3), 227–249.

Fisher, M., Gonzalez, M., & Malizio, J. (2015). Eating disorders in adolescents: How does the DSM-5 change the diagnosis? *International Journal of Adolescent Medicine and Health, 27*(4), 437–441.

Forbush, K. T., Wildes, J. E., Pollack, L. O., Dunbar, D., Luo, J., Patterson, K., … Watson, D. (2013). Development and validation of the eating pathology symptoms inventory (EPSI). *Psychological Assessment, 25*(3), 859–878.

Frank, G. K., Shott, M. E., Hagman, J. O., & Mittal, V. A. (2013). Alterations in brain structures related to taste reward circuitry in ill and recovered anorexia nervosa and in bulimia nervosa. *The American Journal of Psychiatry, 170*(10), 1152–1160.

Franko, D. L., Keshaviah, A., Eddy, K. T., Krishna, M., Davis, M. C., Keel, P. K., & Herzog, D. B. (2013). A longitudinal investigation of mortality in anorexia nervosa and bulimia nervosa. *American Journal of Psychiatry, 170*(8), 917–925.

Gallant, A. R., Lundgren, J., Allison, K., Stunkard, A. J., Lambert, M., O'Loughlin, J., … Drapeau, V. (2012). Validity of the night eating questionnaire in children. *The International Journal of Eating Disorders, 45*(7), 861–865.

García-Villamisar, D., Dattilo, J., & Del Pozo, A. (2012). Depressive mood, eating disorder symptoms, and perfectionism in female college students: A mediation analysis. *Eating Disorders, 20*(1), 60–72.

Garner, D. M. 2004. EDI 3: Eating Disorder Inventory-3: Professional Manual, Psychological Assessment Resources.

Gillberg, C. (1983). Are autism and anorexia nervosa related? *The British Journal of Psychiatry: the Journal of Mental Science, 142*, 428.

Golden, N. H., Katzman, D. K., Sawyer, S. M., Ornstein, R. M., Rome, E. S., Garber, A. K., … Kreipe, R. E. (2015). Update on the medical management of eating disorders in adolescents. *The Journal of Adolescent Health: Official Publication of the Society for Adolescent Medicine, 56*(4), 370–375.

Golden, N. H., Schneider, M., Wood, C., & Committee on Nutrition, Committee on Adolescence, & Section On Obesity. (2016). Preventing obesity and eating disorders in adolescents. *Pediatrics, 138*(3). https://doi.org/10.1542/peds.2016-1649

Goldschmidt, A. B., Wall, M. M., Choo, T.-H. J., Bruening, M., Eisenberg, M. E., & Neumark-Sztainer, D. (2014). Examining associations between adolescent binge eating and binge eating in parents and friends. *The International Journal of Eating Disorders, 47*(3), 325–328.

Gorwood, P., Blanchet-Collet, C., Chartrel, N., Duclos, J., Dechelotte, P., Hanachi, M., … Epelbaum, J. (2016). New insights in anorexia nervosa. *Frontiers in Neuroscience, 10*, 256.

Griffiths, S., Mond, J. M., Li, Z., Gunatilake, S., Murray, S. B., Sheffield, J., & Touyz, S. (2015). Self-stigma of seeking treatment and being male predict an increased likelihood of having an undiagnosed eating disorder. *The International Journal of Eating Disorders, 48*(6), 775–778.

Hay, P., Girosi, F., & Mond, J. (2015). Prevalence and sociodemographic correlates of DSM-5 eating disorders in the Australian population. *Journal of Eating Disorders, 3*, 19.

Herman, B. K., Deal, L. S., DiBenedetti, D. B., Nelson, L., Fehnel, S. E., & Brown, T. M. (2016). Development of the 7-item binge-eating disorder screener (BEDS-7). *The Primary Care Companion to CNS Disorders, 18*(2). https://doi.org/10.4088/PCC.15m01896

Hilbert, A., & Brauhardt, A. (2014). Childhood loss of control eating over five-year follow-up. *The International Journal of Eating Disorders, 47*(7), 758–761.

Hill, L., Peck, S. K., Wierenga, C. E., & Kaye, W. H. (2016). Applying neurobiology to the treatment of adults with anorexia nervosa. *Journal of Eating Disorders, 4*, 31.

Hill, L. S., Reid, F., Morgan, J. F., & Hubert Lacey, J. (2009). SCOFF, the development of an eating disorder screening questionnaire. *The International Journal of Eating Disorders* NA–NA.

Hinney, A., Kesselmeier, M., Jall, S., Volckmar, A.-L., Föcker, M., Antel, J., … Hebebrand. (2017). Evidence for three genetic loci involved in both anorexia nervosa risk and variation of body mass index. *Molecular Psychiatry, 22*(2), 192–201.

Hood, M. M., Reutrakul, S., & Crowley, S. J. (2014). Night eating in patients with type 2 diabetes. Associations with glycemic control, eating patterns, sleep, and mood. *Appetite, 79*, 91–96.

Hudson, J. I., Hiripi, E., Pope, H. G., Jr., & Kessler, R. C. (2007). The prevalence and correlates of eating disorders in the National Comorbidity Survey Replication. *Biological Psychiatry, 61*(3), 348–358.

Jagielska, G., & Kacperska, I. (2017). Outcome, comorbidity and prognosis in anorexia nervosa. *Psychiatria Polska, 51*(2), 205–218.

Jarcho, J. M., Tanofsky-Kraff, M., Nelson, E. E., Engel, S. G., Vannucci, A., Field, S. E., … Yanovski, J. A. (2015). Neural activation during anticipated peer evaluation and laboratory meal intake in overweight girls with and without loss of control eating. *NeuroImage, 108*, 343–353.

Jones, J. M., Lawson, M. L., Daneman, D., Olmsted, M. P., & Rodin, G. (2000). Eating disorders in adolescent females with and without type 1 diabetes: Cross sectional study. *BMJ, 320*(7249), 1563–1566.

Kandler, C., Bleidorn, W., Riemann, R., Angleitner, A., & Spinath, F. M. (2012). Life events as environmental states and genetic traits and the role of personality: A longitudinal twin study. *Behavior Genetics, 42*(1), 57–72.

Kessler, R. M., Hutson, P. H., Herman, B. K., Potenza, M. N. (2016). The neurobiological basis of binge-eating disorder. *Neuroscience and Biobehavioral Reviews, 63*, 223–238.

Keel, P. K. (2017). Bulima Nervosa. In B. Kelly & W. Timothy (Eds.), *Eating disorders and obesity: A comprehensive handbook*. New York, NY: The Guilford Press.

Keel, P. K., Brown, T. A., Holland, L. A., & Bodell, L. P. (2012). Empirical classification of eating disorders. *Annual Review of Clinical Psychology, 8*, 381–404.

Keel, P. K., Eckel, L. A., Hildebrandt, B. A., Haedt-Matt, A. A., Appelbaum, J., & Jimerson, D. C. (2018). Disturbance of gut satiety peptide in purging disorder. *The International Journal of Eating Disorders, 51*(1), 53–61.

Keel, P. K., Haedt, A., & Edler, C. (2005). Purging disorder: An ominous variant of bulimia nervosa? *The International Journal of Eating Disorders, 38*(3), 191–199.

Kliem, S., Schmidt, R., Vogel, M., Hiemisch, A., Kiess, W., & Hilbert, A. (2017). An 8-item short form of the eating disorder examination-questionnaire adapted for children (ChEDE-Q8). *The International Journal of Eating Disorders, 50*(6), 679–686.

Klomek, A. B., Lev-Wiesel, R., Shellac, E., Hadas, A., Berger, U., Horwitz, M., & Fennig, S. (2015). The relationship between self-injurious behavior and self-disclosure in adolescents with eating disorders. *Eating and Weight Disorders: EWD, 20*(1), 43–48.

Knatz, S., Wierenga, C. E., Murray, S. B., Hill, L., & Kaye, W. H. (2015). Neurobiologically informed treatment for adults with anorexia nervosa: A novel approach to a chronic disorder. *Dialogues in Clinical Neuroscience, 17*(2), 229–236.

Koven, N., & Abry, A. (2015). The clinical basis of orthorexia nervosa: Emerging perspectives. *Neuropsychiatric Disease and Treatment, 11*, 385.

Koven, N. S., & Senbonmatsu, R. (2013). A neuropsychological evaluation of orthorexia nervosa. *Open Journal of Psychiatry, 03*(02), 214–222.

Kronengold, C. (2017, February 27). This 2-minute online test can tell you if you have an eating disorder. Retrieved January 30, 2018, from https://www.teenvogue.com/story/online-test-to-determine-eating-disorders

Lamerz, A., Kuepper-Nybelen, J., Bruning, N., Wehle, C., Trost-Brinkhues, G., Brenner, H., … Herpertz-Dahlmann, B. (2005). Prevalence of obesity, binge eating, and night eating in a cross-sectional field survey of 6-year-old children and their parents in a German urban population. *Journal of Child Psychology and Psychiatry, and Allied Disciplines, 46*(4), 385–393.

León, M.-P., González-Martí, I., Fernández-Bustos, J.-G., & Contreras, O. (2017). Percepción del Tamaño Corporal e Insatisfacción en Niños de 3 a 6 Años: Una Revisión Sistemática. *Anales de Psicología, 34*(1), 173.

Lock, J., La Via, M. C., & American Academy of Child and Adolescent Psychiatry (AACAP) Committee on Quality Issues (CQI). (2015). Practice parameter for the assessment and treatment of children and adolescents with eating disorders. *Journal of the American Academy of Child and Adolescent Psychiatry, 54*(5), 412–425.

Lock, J., & Le Grange, D. (2015). *Help your teenager beat an eating disorder* (2nd ed.). Guilford Publications. New York, New York

Makhzoumi, S. H., Guarda, A. S., Schreyer, C. C., Reinblatt, S. P., Redgrave, G. W., & Coughlin, J. W. (2015). Chewing and spitting: A marker of psychopathology and behavioral severity in inpatients with an eating disorder. *Eating Behaviors, 17*, 59–61.

Manasse, S. M., Forman, E. M., Ruocco, A. C., Butryn, M. L., Juarascio, A. S., & Fitzpatrick, K. K. (2015). Do executive functioning deficits underpin binge eating disorder? A comparison of overweight women with and without binge eating pathology. *The International Journal of Eating Disorders, 48*(6), 677–683.

Maniam, J., & Morris, M. J. (2012). The link between stress and feeding behaviour. *Neuropharmacology, 63*(1), 97–110.

Marikar, D., Reynolds, S., & Moghraby, O. S. (2015). Junior MARSIPAN (Management of Really Sick Patients with anorexia nervosa): Table 1. *Archives of Disease in Childhood - Education & Practice Edition, 101*(3), 140–143.

Matherne, C. E., Tanofsky-Kraff, M., Altschul, A. M., Shank, L. M., Schvey, N. A., Brady, S. M., … Yanovski, J. A. (2015). A preliminary examination of loss of control eating disorder (LOC-ED) in middle childhood. *Eating Behaviors, 18*, 57–61.

McLean, S. A., Paxton, S. J., Massey, R., Hay, P. J., Mond, J. M., & Rodgers, B. (2014). Stigmatizing attitudes and beliefs about bulimia nervosa: Gender, age, education and income variability in a community sample. *The International Journal of Eating Disorders, 47*(4), 353–361.

Mehler, P. S., & Andersen, A. E. (2017). *Eating disorders: A guide to medical care and complications*. Baltimore, MA: JHU Press.

Mehler, P. S., & Brown, C. (2015). Anorexia nervosa - medical complications. *Journal of Eating Disorders, 3*, 11.

Meyre, D., Mayhew, A., Pigeyre, M., & Couturier, J. (2017). An evolutionary genetic perspective of eating disorders. *Neuroendocrinology*. https://doi.org/10.1159/000484525

Micali, N., Martini, M. G., Thomas, J. J., Eddy, K. T., Kothari, R., Russell, E., … Treasure, J. (2017). Lifetime and 12-month prevalence of eating disorders amongst women in mid-life: A population-based study of diagnoses and risk factors. *BMC Medicine, 15*(1), 12.

Miller, R., Tanofsky-Kraff, M., Shomaker, L. B., Field, S. E., Hannallah, L., Reina, S. A., … Yanovski, J. A. (2014). Serum leptin and loss of control eating in children and adolescents. *International Journal of Obesity, 38*(3), 397–403.

Mitchison, D., & Hay, P. J. (2014). The epidemiology of eating disorders: Genetic, environmental, and societal factors. *Clinical Epidemiology, 6*, 89–97.

Monteleone, A. M., Castellini, G., Volpe, U., Ricca, V., Lelli, L., Monteleone, P., & Maj, M. (2018).

Neuroendocrinology and brain imaging of reward in eating disorders: A possible key to the treatment of anorexia nervosa and bulimia nervosa. *Progress in Neuro-Psychopharmacology & Biological Psychiatry, 80*(Pt B), 132–142.

Morgan, J. F. (2000). The SCOFF questionnaire: A new screening tool for eating disorders. *The Western Journal of Medicine, 172*(3), 164–165.

Morgan, J. F., Reid, F., & Lacey, J. H. (1999). The SCOFF questionnaire: Assessment of a new screening tool for eating disorders. *BMJ, 319*(7223), 1467–1468.

Moroze, R. M., Dunn, T. M., Craig Holland, J., Yager, J., & Weintraub, P. (2015). Microthinking about micronutrients: A case of transition from obsessions about healthy eating to near-fatal "orthorexia nervosa" and proposed diagnostic criteria. *Psychosomatics, 56*(4), 397–403.

Mountjoy, M., Sundgot-Borgen, J., Burke, L., Carter, S., Constantini, N., Lebrun, C., … Ljungqvist, A. (2014). The IOC consensus statement: Beyond the female athlete triad--relative energy deficiency in sport (RED-S). *British Journal of Sports Medicine, 48*(7), 491–497.

Mountjoy, M., Sundgot-Borgen, J., Burke, L., Carter, S., Constantini, N., Lebrun, C., … Ackerman, K. (2015a). RED-S CAT. Relative energy deficiency in sport (RED-S) clinical assessment tool (CAT). *British Journal of Sports Medicine, 49*(7), 421–423.

Mountjoy, M., Sundgot-Borgen, J., Burke, L., Carter, S., Constantini, N., Lebrun, C., … Ljungqvist, A. (2015b). Authors' 2015 additions to the IOC consensus statement: Relative energy deficiency in sport (RED-S). *British Journal of Sports Medicine, 49*(7), 417–420.

Munn-Chernoff, M. A., Keel, P. K., Klump, K. L., Grant, J. D., Bucholz, K. K., Madden, P. A. F., … Duncan, A. E. (2015). Prevalence of and familial influences on purging disorder in a community sample of female twins. *The International Journal of Eating Disorders, 48*(6), 601–606.

Mustelin, L., Silén, Y., Raevuori, A., Hoek, H. W., Kaprio, J., & Keski-Rahkonen, A. (2016). The DSM-5 diagnostic criteria for anorexia nervosa may change its population prevalence and prognostic value. *Journal of Psychiatric Research, 77*, 85–91.

Nagl, M., Jacobi, C., Paul, M., Beesdo-Baum, K., Höfler, M., Lieb, R., & Wittchen, H.-U. (2016). Prevalence, incidence, and natural course of anorexia and bulimia nervosa among adolescents and young adults. *European Child & Adolescent Psychiatry, 25*(8), 903–918.

National Institute of Mental Health. (n.d.). The National Institute of Mental Health Strategic Plan. Retrieved from https://web.archive.org/web/20081217154853/http://www.nimh.nih.gov/about/strategic-planning-reports/index.shtml

Nattiv, A., Loucks, A. B., Manore, M. M., Sanborn, C. F., Sundgot-Borgen, J., Warren, M. P., & American College of Sports Medicine. (2007). American College of Sports Medicine position stand. The female athlete triad. *Medicine and Science in Sports and Exercise, 39*(10), 1867–1882.

Nazar, B. P., Bernardes, C., Peachey, G., Sergeant, J., Mattos, P., & Treasure, J. (2016). The risk of eating disorders comorbid with attention-deficit/hyperactivity disorder: A systematic review and meta-analysis. *The International Journal of Eating Disorders, 49*(12), 1045–1057.

Nazar, B. P., Peynenburg, V., Rhind, C., Hibbs, R., Schmidt, U., Gowers, S., … Treasure, J. (2018). An examination of the clinical outcomes of adolescents and young adults with broad autism spectrum traits and autism spectrum disorder and anorexia nervosa: A multi Centre study. *The International Journal of Eating Disorders.* https://doi.org/10.1002/eat.22823

O'Reardon, J. P., Peshek, A., & Allison, K. C. (2005). Night eating syndrome: Diagnosis, epidemiology and management. *CNS Drugs, 19*(12), 997–1008.

Oldershaw, A., Treasure, J., Hambrook, D., Tchanturia, K., & Schmidt, U. (2011). Is anorexia nervosa a version of autism spectrum disorders? *European Eating Disorders Review: The Journal of the Eating Disorders Association, 19*(6), 462–474.

Otis, C. L., Drinkwater, B., Johnson, M., Loucks, A., & Wilmore, J. (1997). American College of Sports Medicine position stand. The female athlete triad. *Medicine and Science in Sports and Exercise, 29*(5), i–ix.

Øverås, M., Kapstad, H., Brunborg, C., Landrø, N. I., & Rø, Ø. (2017). Is overestimation of body size associated with neuropsychological weaknesses in anorexia nervosa? *European Eating Disorders Review: The Journal of the Eating Disorders Association, 25*(2), 129–134.

Palmese, L. B., Ratliff, J. C., Reutenauer, E. L., Tonizzo, K. M., Grilo, C. M., & Tek, C. (2013). Prevalence of night eating in obese individuals with schizophrenia and schizoaffective disorder. *Comprehensive Psychiatry, 54*(3), 276–281.

Paxton, S. J., & Damiano, S. R. (2017). The development of body image and weight Bias in childhood. *Advances in Child Development and Behavior, 52*, 269–298.

Perez, M., Kroon Van Diest, A. M., Smith, H., & Sladek, M. R. (2016). Body dissatisfaction and its correlates in 5- to 7-year-old girls: A social learning experiment. *Journal of Clinical Child and Adolescent Psychology: The Official Journal for the Society of Clinical Child and Adolescent Psychology, American Psychological Association, Division, 53*, 1–13.

Pike, K. M., Dunne, P. E., & Grant, A. (2015). Prevalence and incidence of eating disorders in Asian societies. In *The Wiley handbook of eating disorders* (pp. 64–78). Hoboken, NJ

Ptacek, R., Stefano, G. B., Weissenberger, S., Akotia, D., Raboch, J., Papezova, H., … Goetz, M. (2016). Attention deficit hyperactivity disorder and disordered eating behaviors: Links, risks, and challenges faced. *Neuropsychiatric Disease and Treatment, 12*, 571–579.

Räder, K., Specht, F., & Reister, M. (1989). Anorexia nervosa and down syndrome. *Praxis der Kinderpsychologie und Kinderpsychiatrie, 38*(9), 343–346.

Raevuori, A., Suokas, J., Haukka, J., Gissler, M., Linna, M., Grainger, M., & Suvisaari, J. (2014). Highly increased risk of type 2 diabetes in patients with binge eating disorder and bulimia nervosa. *The International Journal of Eating Disorders, 48*(6), 555–562.

Redgrave, G. W., Coughlin, J. W., Schreyer, C. C., Martin, L. M., Leonpacher, A. K., Seide, M., ... Guarda, A. S. (2015). Refeeding and weight restoration outcomes in anorexia nervosa: Challenging current guidelines. *The International Journal of Eating Disorders, 48*(7), 866–873.

Reinblatt, S. P., Mark Mahone, E., Tanofsky-Kraff, M., Lee-Winn, A. E., Yenokyan, G., Leoutsakos, J.-M. S., ... Riddle, M. A. (2015). Pediatric loss of control eating syndrome: Association with attention-deficit/hyperactivity disorder and impulsivity. *The International Journal of Eating Disorders, 48*(6), 580–588.

Riva, G. (2016). Neurobiology of anorexia nervosa: Serotonin dysfunctions link self-starvation with body image disturbances through an impaired body memory. *Frontiers in Human Neuroscience, 10*, 600.

Rohde, P., Stice, E., & Marti, C. N. (2015). Development and predictive effects of eating disorder risk factors during adolescence: Implications for prevention efforts. *The International Journal of Eating Disorders, 48*(2), 187–198.

Rojo-Moreno, L., Arribas, P., Plumed, J., Gimeno, N., García-Blanco, A., Vaz-Leal, F., ... Livianos, L. (2015). Prevalence and comorbidity of eating disorders among a community sample of adolescents: 2-year follow-up. *Psychiatry Research, 227*(1), 52–57.

Rose, M., Davis, J., Frampton, I., & Lask, B. (2011). The Ravello profile: Development of a global standard neuropsychological assessment for young people with anorexia nervosa. *Clinical Child Psychology and Psychiatry, 16*(2), 195–202.

Rose, M., Reville, M.-C., Iszatt, A., Levinson, S., Frampton, I., & Lask, B. (2017). Deconstructing planning ability in children and adolescents with anorexia nervosa. *Applied Neuropsychology. Child, 6*(4), 297–304.

Rosen, D. S., & American Academy of Pediatrics Committee on Adolescence. (2010). Identification and management of eating disorders in children and adolescents. *Pediatrics, 126*(6), 1240–1253.

Russell, G. (1979). Bulimia nervosa: an ominous variant of anorexia nervosa. *Psychological Medicine, 9*(3), 429–448.

Sala, L., Martinotti, G., Carenti, M. L., Romo, L., Oumaya, M., Pham-Scottez, A., ... Janiri, L. (2017). Attention-deficit/hyperactivity disorder symptoms and psychological comorbidity in eating disorder patients. *Eating and Weight Disorders: EWD*. https://doi.org/10.1007/s40519-017-0395-8

Sanislow, C. A. (2016). Updating the research domain criteria. *World Psychiatry: Official Journal of the World Psychiatric Association, 15*(3), 222–223.

Schilder, C. M. T., van Elburg, A. A., Snellen, W. M., Sternheim, L. C., Hoek, H. W., & Danner, U. N. (2017). Intellectual functioning of adolescent and adult patients with eating disorders. *The International Journal of Eating Disorders, 50*(5), 481–489.

Schmidt, U. (2003). Aetiology of eating disorders in the 21(st) century: New answers to old questions. *European Child & Adolescent Psychiatry, 12 Suppl, 1*, I30–I37.

Schwartz, G. J., & Zeltser, L. M. (2013). Functional organization of neuronal and humoral signals regulating feeding behavior. *Annual Review of Nutrition, 33*, 1–21.

Screening Tool. (n.d.). Retrieved January 30, 2018, from https://www.nationaleatingdisorders.org/screening-tool

Shearer, A., Russon, J., Herres, J., Atte, T., Kodish, T., & Diamond, G. (2015). The relationship between disordered eating and sexuality amongst adolescents and young adults. *Eating Behaviors, 19*, 115–119.

Sherman, R. T., & Thompson, R. A. (2006). Practical use of the International Olympic Committee medical commission position stand on the female athlete triad: A case example. *The International Journal of Eating Disorders, 39*(3), 193–201.

Siever, M. D. (1994). Sexual orientation and gender as factors in socioculturally acquired vulnerability to body dissatisfaction and eating disorders. *Journal of Consulting and Clinical Psychology, 62*(2), 252–260.

Small, L., & Aplasca, A. (2016). Child obesity and mental health. *Child and Adolescent Psychiatric Clinics of North America, 25*(2), 269–282.

Smink, F. R. E., van Hoeken, D., Oldehinkel, A. J., & Hoek, H. W. (2014). Prevalence and severity of DSM-5 eating disorders in a community cohort of adolescents. *The International Journal of Eating Disorders, 47*(6), 610–619.

Sreshta, N., Pope, H. G., Hudson, J. I., & Kanayama, G. (2017). *Muscle Dysmorphia*.

Stedal, K., Frampton, I., Landrø, N. I., & Lask, B. (2011). An examination of the Ravello profile - a neuropsychological test battery for anorexia nervosa. *European Eating Disorders Review: The Journal of the Eating Disorders Association, 20*(3), 175–181.

Steinhausen, H.-C., & Jensen, C. M. (2015). Time trends in lifetime incidence rates of first-time diagnosed anorexia nervosa and bulimia nervosa across 16 years in a Danish nationwide psychiatric registry study. *The International Journal of Eating Disorders, 48*(7), 845–850.

Stewart, C. S., McEwen, F. S., Konstantellou, A., Eisler, I., & Simic, M. (2017). Impact of ASD traits on treatment outcomes of eating disorders in girls. *European Eating Disorders Review: The Journal of the Eating Disorders Association, 25*(2), 123–128.

Stice, E., Marti, C. N., & Durant, S. (2011). Risk factors for onset of eating disorders: Evidence of multiple risk pathways from an 8-year prospective study. *Behaviour Research and Therapy, 49*(10), 622–627.

Stice, E., Marti, C. N., & Rohde, P. (2013). Prevalence, incidence, impairment, and course of the proposed DSM-5 eating disorder diagnoses in an 8-year prospective community study of young women. *Journal of Abnormal Psychology, 122*(2), 445–457.

Strother, E., Lemberg, R., Stanford, S. C., & Turberville, D. (2012). Eating disorders in men: Underdiagnosed, undertreated, and misunderstood. *Eating Disorders, 20*(5), 346–355.

Strumia, R. (2002). Bulimia and anorexia nervosa: cutaneous manifestations. *Journal of Cosmetic Dermatology, 1*(1), 30–34.

Stunkard, A. J. (1959). Eating patterns and obesity. *The Psychiatric Quarterly, 33*, 284–295.

Stunkard, A. J., Grace, W. J., & Wolff, H. G. (1955). The night-eating syndrome. *The American Journal of Medicine, 19*(1), 78–86.

Svedlund, N. E., Norring, C., Ginsberg, Y., & von Hausswolff-Juhlin, Y. (2017). Symptoms of attention deficit hyperactivity disorder (ADHD) among adult eating disorder patients. *BMC Psychiatry, 17*(1), 19.

Swanson, S. A., Crow, S. J., Le Grange, D., Swendsen, J., & Merikangas, K. R. (2011). Prevalence and correlates of eating disorders in adolescents. Results from the national comorbidity survey replication adolescent supplement. *Archives of General Psychiatry, 68*(7), 714–723.

Sysko, R., Glasofer, D. R., Hildebrandt, T., Klimek, P., Mitchell, J. E., Berg, K. C., … Walsh, B. T. (2015). The eating disorder assessment for DSM-5 (EDA-5): Development and validation of a structured interview for feeding and eating disorders. *The International Journal of Eating Disorders, 48*(5), 452–463.

Tanofsky-Kraff, M., Bulik, C. M., Marcus, M. D., Striegel, R. H., Wilfley, D. E., Wonderlich, S. A., & Hudson, J. I. (2013). Binge eating disorder: The next generation of research. *The International Journal of Eating Disorders, 46*(3), 193–207.

Tanofsky-Kraff, M., Engel, S., Yanovski, J. A., Pine, D. S., Nelson, E. E. (2013). Pediatric disinhibited eating: toward a research domain criteria framework. *The International Journal of Eating Disorders, 46*, 451–455.

Tanofsky-Kraff, M., Marcus, M. D., Yanovski, S. Z., & Yanovski, J. A. (2008). Loss of control eating disorder in children age 12 years and younger: Proposed research criteria. *Eating Behaviors, 9*(3), 360–365.

Thaler, L., & Steiger, H. (2017). Eating disorders and Epigenetics. *Advances in Experimental Medicine and Biology, 978*, 93–103.

The rise of pro-anorexia and pro-mia websites. (n.d.). Retrieved January 30, 2018, from http://www.sirc.org/articles/totally_in_control.shtml

Thompson-Brenner, H., Eddy, K. T., Satir, D. A., Boisseau, C. L., & Westen, D. (2008). Personality subtypes in adolescents with eating disorders: Validation of a classification approach. *Journal of Child Psychology and Psychiatry, and Allied Disciplines, 49*(2), 170–180.

Uher, R., & Rutter, M. (2012). Classification of feeding and eating disorders: Review of evidence and proposals for ICD-11. *World Psychiatry: Official Journal of the World Psychiatric Association, 11*(2), 80–92.

Vall, E., & Wade, T. D. (2015). Trail making task performance in inpatients with anorexia nervosa and bulimia nervosa. *European Eating Disorders Review: The Journal of the Eating Disorders Association, 23*(4), 304–311.

van Noort, B. M., Pfeiffer, E., Ehrlich, S., Lehmkuhl, U., & Kappel, V. (2016). Cognitive performance in children with acute early-onset anorexia nervosa. *European Child & Adolescent Psychiatry, 25*(11), 1233–1244.

Vannucci, A., Nelson, E. E., Bongiorno, D. M., Pine, D. S., Yanovski, J. A., & Tanofsky-Kraff, M. (2015). Behavioral and neurodevelopmental precursors to binge-type eating disorders: Support for the role of negative valence systems. *Psychological Medicine, 45*(14), 2921–2936.

Vetrugno, R., Manconi, M., Ferini-Strambi, L., Provini, F., Plazzi, G., & Montagna, P. (2006). Nocturnal eating: Sleep-related eating disorder or night eating syndrome? A videopolysomnographic study. *Sleep, 29*(7), 949–954.

Wade, T. D., & O'Shea, A. (2014). DSM-5 unspecified feeding and eating disorders in adolescents: What do they look like and are they clinically significant? *The International Journal of Eating Disorders, 48*(4), 367–374.

Wagner, A. J., Erickson, C. D., Tierney, D. K., Houston, M. N., & Bacon, C. E. W. (2016). The diagnostic accuracy of screening tools to detect eating disorders in female athletes. *Journal of Sport Rehabilitation, 25*(4), 395–398.

Webb, H. J., Zimmer-Gembeck, M. J., & Donovan, C. L. (2014). The appearance culture between friends and adolescent appearance-based rejection sensitivity. *Journal of Adolescence, 37*(4), 347–358.

Weider, S., Indredavik, M. S., Lydersen, S., & Hestad, K. (2014). Neuropsychological function in patients with anorexia nervosa or bulimia nervosa. *The International Journal of Eating Disorders, 48*(4), 397–405.

Westwood, H., & Tchanturia, K. (2017). Autism Spectrum disorder in anorexia nervosa: An updated literature review. *Current Psychiatry Reports, 19*(7), 41.

WHO| ICD-11 Revision . (2017). Retrieved from http://www.who.int/classifications/icd/revision/en/

Wildes, J. E., & Marcus, M. D. (2015). Application of the research domain criteria (RDoC) framework to eating disorders: Emerging concepts and research. *Current Psychiatry Reports, 17*(5), 30.

World Health Organization. (1992). *The ICD-10 classification of mental and Behavioural disorders: Clinical descriptions and diagnostic guidelines*. Geneva, Switzerland: World Health Organization.

Yilmaz, Z., Hardaway, J. A., & Bulik, C. M. (2015). Genetics and Epigenetics of eating disorders. *Advances in Genomics and Genetics, 5*, 131–150.

Yokum, S., Marti, C. N., Smolen, A., & Stice, E. (2015). Relation of the multilocus genetic composite reflecting high dopamine signaling capacity to future increases in BMI. *Appetite, 87*, 38–45.

Zerwas, S., Larsen, J. T., Petersen, L., Thornton, L. M., Mortensen, P. B., & Bulik, C. M. (2015). The incidence of eating disorders in a Danish register study: Associations with suicide risk and mortality. *Journal of Psychiatric Research, 65*, 16–22.

Zhou, Z. C., McAdam, D. B., & Donnelly, D. R. (2017). Endophenotypes: A conceptual link between anorexia nervosa and autism spectrum disorder. *Research in Developmental Disabilities.* https://doi.org/10.1016/j.ridd.2017.11.008

Zuijdwijk, C. S., Pardy, S. A., Dowden, J. J., Dominic, A. M., Bridger, T., & Newhook, L. A. (2014). The mSCOFF for screening disordered eating in pediatric type 1 diabetes. *Diabetes Care, 37*(2), e26–e27.

Assessment of Pediatric Feeding Disorders

Kathryn M. Peterson, Vivian F. Ibañez, Caitlin A. Kirkwood, Jaime G. Crowley, and Cathleen C. Piazza

Diagnosis and Prevalence

Most individuals eat multiple meals daily as part of their normal routine. Eating is an enjoyable activity for many, not just because food is an unconditioned primary reinforcer (Cooper, Heron, & Heward, 2007) and humans need it to survive, but also because eating often represents a meaningful social opportunity for friends and family to come together and interact (e.g., at restaurants or birthday parties, sitting around the dinner table). In fact, most typically eating individuals look forward to eating and demonstrate preferences for a large variety of foods. Given that food is often a potent reinforcer, many may assume that eating is a simple, instinctual process that would not be disrupted easily. In reality, feeding is a complex and dynamic operant behavior chain, consisting of many stages involving both nutritive and protective skills. Eating begins with accepting food or liquid into the mouth; forming that food or liquid into a bolus,; chewing (if necessary),; elevating the tongue and propelling food or liquid backward through the oral cavity; swallowing; and finally, retaining the food or liquid (Arvedson & Brodsky, 2002). A child's growth in height and weight is dependent on consistent daily intake of sufficient calories and nutrients (Kerwin, 1999). Thus, when there is a persistent disruption in the feeding process, caregivers should be concerned that the child might be at risk for the development of a feeding disorder.

Healthcare providers (e.g., pediatricians, licensed psychologists) diagnose a feeding disorder when a child is unable or unwilling to consume enough calories or a sufficient variety of solids and liquids to maintain adequate nutrition, hydration, and growth (Volkert & Piazza, 2012). Many children experience minor feeding difficulties during their toddler years, usually in the form of mild food selectivity (e.g., picky eating, refusing to eat presented foods). Often, these problems are typical and transient and will resolve over time in the absence of intervention. For some children, however, feeding problems are more severe and unlikely to resolve in the absence of intervention. For example, some children exhibit total food refusal and eat little to nothing by mouth, resulting in the need for support from tube feedings (e.g., nasogastric- or gastrostomy-tube feedings). Other children exhibit liquid dependency and rely exclusively on one calorically dense liquid (e.g., PediaSure) as the main source of daily nutrition. Some children exhibit more severe and persistent food selectivity and

K. M. Peterson · V. F. Ibañez · C. A. Kirkwood
J. G. Crowley · C. C. Piazza (✉)
University of Nebraska Medical Center's Munroe-Meyer Institute and Department of Pediatrics, Omaha, NE, USA
e-mail: cpiazza@unmc.edu

only eat certain foods of a specific type (e.g., starches), brand (e.g., McDonald's), color (e.g., white foods), texture (e.g., crunchy foods), temperature (e.g., warm milk), or presentation format (e.g., foods served on a specific plate). Estimates suggest that 25–45% of typically developing children and 80% of children with developmental disabilities have a feeding difficulty at some point in their lifetime (Manikam & Perman, 2000). In fact, certain subsets of the population are at greater risk for persistent feeding difficulties. These at-risk populations include children born prematurely (Arvedson & Brodsky, 2002) children with developmental disabilities (Babbitt, Hoch, & Coe, 1994); and children with certain genetic disorders such as autism spectrum disorder, Down syndrome, and cerebral palsy (Bandini et al., 2010). Children with complex medical conditions such as gastroesophageal reflux, bronchopulmonary dysplasia, short-gut syndrome, aspiration, and childhood cancer also may be at greater risk for developing a feeding disorder (Linscheid, Budd, & Rasnake, 1995).

Failing to eat or drink sufficient calories or nutrients to grow and maintain nutritional status can have devastating physical, psychological, and financial consequences for the child, the child's family, and society. Inadequate calories and nutrition are associated not only with poor growth but also long-term health, learning, and behavior problems (Freedman, Dietz, Srinivasan, & Berenson, 1999). For example, children who routinely refuse solids and liquids by mouth can experience poor weight gain; failure to thrive (i.e., deceleration of weight); malnutrition; dehydration; imbalances in electrolytes; impairments related to cognitive, emotional, or academic functioning; hospitalization; recurrent infections; a compromised immune system; dependency on tube feedings; and in severe cases if left untreated, death (Christophersen & Hall, 1978; Cohen, Piazza, & Navathe, 2006; Schwartz, 2000; Volkert & Piazza, 2012).

For these children, tube feedings can serve as a critical, life-saving solution. With recent advances in technology, surgeons can place the tube using minimally invasive procedures including laparoscopic techniques (Akay et al., 2010). However, there are several drawbacks to tube dependence. Even though tube placement is generally a relatively safe procedure, researchers have reported several major complications, including, but not limited to, skin infections, colonic fistulas, excessive bleeding, and esophageal tears (El-Matary, 2008). There also are minor complications associated with long-term dependency on tube feedings, such as superficial skin infections, vomiting, recurrent surgeries to resize the tube, and tube leakage or fallout, which occur in up to 50% of patients (El-Matary, 2008; Volkert, Patel, & Peterson, 2016). Another drawback includes the strain on caregivers given the response effort required to (a) maintain cleanliness of the tube and site, (b) conduct daily tube feedings, and (c) bring the child back to the hospital to address potential complications. Finally, another challenge is that tube feedings do not promote typical oral feeding or allow for feeding practice. As a result, the child may have even less motivation to eat or drink by mouth. In some cases, tube dependency might result in delayed oral-motor skills (e.g., chewing, tongue lateralization) due to inadequate opportunities to develop the skills needed for oral feeding (Piazza, 2008).

Liquid dependency on low-calorie liquids could place a child at risk for health problems if the caloric density is not sufficient to meet daily needs (Volkert, Patel, & Peterson, 2016). Alternatively, exclusive consumption of high-calorie liquids might result in deficiencies or excesses in vitamins and minerals if the liquid is not balanced in terms of macro- and micronutrients (Volkert, Patel, & Peterson, 2016). Children who consume nutrient-deficient diets consisting of foods that are high in fat (e.g., fast foods) or sugar (e.g., candy, soda) are likely at greater risk for acquiring severe health problems such as obesity, type 2 diabetes, chronic constipation, and hypertension (Freedman, Dietz, Srinivasan, & Berenson, 1999; Ludwig et al., 1999).

These types of feeding difficulties also may result in substantial distress for the family. Caregivers of children with feeding disorders have reported feelings of rejection, anger, anxiety, lack of self-confidence, stress, and depression

(Franklin & Rodger, 2003). Caregiver stress could likely be the result of a lifestyle that requires frequent contact with medical personnel (e.g., gastroenterologist) and unconventional feeding routines, as the caregivers are required to manage the child's medical and nutritional needs constantly (Franklin & Rodger, 2003; Winters, 2003). Most major social, cultural, and religious events (e.g., birthdays, holidays, weddings) involve consumption of food; therefore, this lifestyle often prevents families from engaging in typical activities due to the child's eating habits. For example, when a child only eats food from a specific restaurant, the family must alter vacation plans by only traveling to places near the specific restaurant. Children with total food and liquid refusal might not attend birthday parties because the child will not eat with the other children.

In addition to these physical and emotional health concerns, feeding disorders can be costly in terms of finances for the family and for society in general. Nicholls, Lynn, and Viner (2011) reported that feeding disorders are financially burdensome to healthcare systems, as 50% of the surveyed children from the study were hospitalized for their feeding disorder for a mean length of 32 days each. An independent analysis by the Nebraska Legislature's fiscal office showed that the state would save close to 1 million dollars over a 3-year period if 50 children received intervention to increase oral feeding and prevent gastrostomy-tube placement. In addition, the impact of feeding disorders on families who live in rural areas of the Midwest like Nebraska is magnified because the specialized services needed to treat pediatric feeding disorders are often nonexistent locally; thus, the emotional and financial costs of intervention are increased by the travel required to access intervention.

Etiology

Childhood feeding problems may occur in isolation or as the result of a complex interaction between physiological, medical, oral-motor, and environmental factors (Rommel, De Meyer, Feenstra, & Veereman-Wauters, 2003). Rommel et al. (2003) characterized the feeding disorders of 700 children referred for assessment and treatment of severe feeding difficulties as medical (86%), oral-motor (61%), behavioral (18%), or combined (e.g., medical, behavioral, and oral-motor; 60%). For example, a child who suffers from chronic gastroesophageal reflux disease may learn that eating and drinking often result in pain and discomfort. If the pain is significant enough, the child may begin refusing foods and liquids to avoid those feelings of discomfort in the future. In another situation, a child may develop feeding problems due to aversive experiences such as choking, gagging, or vomiting during or immediately after eating. The child may start avoiding the specific foods that were present during the aversive experience by engaging in excessive problem behavior whenever those or similar foods are presented. Over time, the parent attempts to avoid child problem behavior and begins only presenting the foods the child will eat willingly.

Many children with feeding disorders display oral-motor skill deficits, which could contribute to or serve as a causative factor for the feeding disorder. Children might display oral-motor skill deficits if they missed out on building critical prerequisite skills during early childhood, perhaps because they had not engaged in sufficient practice or gone through the appropriate milestones during development (e.g., due to medical conditions, tube dependence). In these situations, the child may refuse to eat because he or she does not possess the necessary skills or because he or she fatigues quickly when the eating response becomes too effortful. For example, children with oral-motor deficits may lack the necessary skills to efficiently chew or swallow solids and liquids safely. Anatomical abnormalities (e.g., cleft lip or palate) also can lead to feeding disorders in children (Palmer & Horn, 1978). If a child was not born with the necessary structures to eat, the child may not have the ability to consume solids or liquids orally without surgical intervention. Other children may develop "oral aversions" and refuse to let food or liquid near the mouth if they were exposed to invasive medical procedures involving tools in or near the mouth (e.g., laryngoscopy) or if they were exposed to noxious-tasting medications. Oral aversions may even affect other daily self-care routines, such as toothbrushing.

These conditions are often worsened by antecedent and consequent events in the natural environment. Children who experience chronic pain following oral feeds due to medical conditions or children who fatigue quickly during meals or do not have the necessary skills due to oral-motor delays often engage in problem behavior at mealtimes to escape or avoid the meal. If caregivers then provide escape from the meal or excessive attention following problem behavior in the form of coaxing (e.g., "please just take a little bite, you'll make mommy so happy") or reprimands (e.g., "You need to take your bites"), it is likely that child problem behavior will persist (Borrero, Woods, Borrero, Masler, & Lesser, 2010). Thus, it could be that problematic mealtime behavior occurs in isolation or as the result of an interaction of multiple factors (e.g., environmental events such as caregiver attention along with medical conditions). In our clinical practice, we have seen that even long after physicians treat symptoms of the medical condition (e.g., prescription medication for reflux), children with feeding disorders continue to engage in problem behavior at mealtimes. In these cases and others, persistence of problem behavior at mealtimes is likely due to the environmental events that now serve to strengthen and maintain the behavior over time (Piazza et al., 2003).

Assessment: Typical Versus Atypical Feeding

One approach to understanding the severity of a feeding problem is to compare the child's feeding behavior with typical developmental feeding patterns (Piazza, 2008). Because it is relatively common for children to demonstrate transient difficulties during feeding, professionals and caregivers might find it challenging to know when feeding problems warrant greater concern. Part of the challenge of answering this question is that feeding disorders are a heterogeneous group of problems (as described above). Many healthcare professionals will advise parents to wait before seeking treatment, given that the child will likely "grow out of" his or her feeding problem. This will be true for some children. That is, the feeding problems displayed by most children are often mild and many times resolve in the absence of intervention (Kerwin, 1999). By contrast, the feeding problems of children with atypical feeding patterns often persist and worsen over time (Lindberg, Bohlin, & Hagekull, 1991). In fact, Peterson, Piazza, and Ibañez (in press) recently compared an applied behavior-analysis intervention to a wait-list control with six participants diagnosed with autism spectrum disorder and food selectivity to determine whether waiting (up to 6 months) would result in the feeding problems resolving independent of treatment. After initial baseline assessments for both groups, children in the intervention group received applied behavior-analysis treatment for their food selectivity and children in the wait-list control group were asked to return home. Children in the intervention group demonstrated increases in independent acceptance across the 16 targeted novel or nonpreferred foods following applied behavior-analysis intervention. Children in the wait-list control group continued to refuse the 16 targeted novel or nonpreferred foods. Moreover, children in the wait-list control group did not demonstrate independent acceptance until they were exposed to the intervention. Overall, these results suggested that feeding problems might not resolve over time for children with atypical feeding patterns (e.g., food selectivity).

An objective way to compare typical to atypical feeding patterns often begins with an evaluation of the child's growth parameters. During wellness visits, a child's pediatrician will conduct physical exams that include taking the child's height and weight and plotting them on a growth chart to determine the child's growth curve (i.e., change in height and weight over time relative to other children of the same age and gender). The general expectation is that children consistently grow along their own curves. When the child's growth plateaus (i.e., weight or height stays the same across multiple months) or decelerates (i.e., the child fails to gain weight or grow taller, thereby failing to track continuously along his or her curve), there should be concern for a more serious feeding problem.

In addition to growth, practitioners must consider other factors relative to behavior and development and determine whether the child is engaging in feeding behavior that is generally age appropriate. For example, typically eating infants will accept breastmilk or formula readily after birth. Some infants have difficulty latching or may have problems initially coordinating the suck, swallow, breathe response. However, these difficulties typically resolve relatively quickly. Healthcare providers should become concerned about a possible feeding disorder when the infant consistently rejects or is unable to manage breast or bottle feedings, particularly if this lack of improvement is accompanied with slow or no weight gain (Piazza, 2008). According to typical developmental patterns, infants should begin to transition from breastmilk or formula to solid (pureed) baby foods around 4–6 months. It is typical for some tongue thrusting to occur, which might result in the infant temporarily pushing the food or liquid out of his or her mouth. However, for typically eating infants, replacing the food back into the infant's mouth provides sufficient practice to eliminate tongue thrusting over time. Healthcare providers might become concerned about a possible feeding disorder if they observe persistent tongue thrust that does not resolve with practice, as this behavior could result in low oral intake and lengthy meals (e.g., Gibbons, Williams, & Riegel, 2007). Most typically eating children transition to mashed table foods by 12 months of age and if they have teeth, demonstrate the ability to safely manage small bites of table-textured foods. By contrast, children with feeding disorders may display difficulties transitioning to baby, mashed, or table foods. These children might continue to depend on textures that are not age appropriate (e.g., purees) or show preference for one texture to the exclusion of others.

As children progress from a liquid to solid diet, most typically eating toddlers display preference for certain foods relative to others, with preferences sometimes rapidly shifting across foods. For this reason, picky eating might be tolerated for periods or go by unnoticed. Due to these circumstances, more chronic forms of picky eating are often misunderstood or underestimated and are associated with masked health risks given that most children who are selective eaters continue to grow well (Peterson, Piazza, &Ibañez, in press). Picky eating becomes a feeding disorder (i.e., food selectivity) when the child's selectivity results in severe nutrient deficiencies. For example, some children who consume a diet that is low in protein, fruit, and vegetables are likely deficient in iron, zinc, and vitamin C (Sullivan et al., 2002). Children with severe food selectivity often engage in more intense refusal (e.g., self-injury) with the introduction of novel or nonpreferred foods than do typically eating children. It also may be common for toddlers and preschoolers to vary their intake from day to day, consuming more calories on some days over others but generally obtaining enough calories to meet their needs, continue growing, and remain healthy. By contrast, children with feeding disorders often do not respond to hunger cues as typically eating children and can go multiple days without eating. This creates a potentially dangerous, life-threatening situation in which the child is likely failing to consume sufficient calories and nutrients to maintain adequate health and growth (Piazza, 2008).

Throughout childhood and even beyond the toddler years, caregivers should expect to see fairly consistent growth over time, in terms of weight and height. Thus, if the child experiences up to three consecutive months of weight loss, practitioners should be suspicious of a feeding disorder and recommend the child for services immediately.

Assessment: Interdisciplinary Team

The Pediatric Feeding Disorders Program in Omaha, Nebraska, provides a comprehensive, behavior-analytic approach to the treatment of pediatric feeding disorders through our assessment and intervention services. Children in our program range in age from birth to 18 years and often have comorbid medical conditions. Due to the complex etiology of pediatric feeding disorders, we use an interdisciplinary approach to assessment and intervention. An interdisciplinary team is often necessary to identify all possible contributing and maintaining factors before recommending treatment.

Our interdisciplinary team consists of a physician, speech-language pathologist, registered dietician, feeding therapists, behavior analysts, and licensed psychologists. We assemble members of this team to conduct initial intake evaluations before a child is admitted to our program and rely on input or recommendations from team members throughout the child's admission. For the intake evaluation specifically, we begin the process after we first receive a referral, usually from the child's pediatrician or medical specialist. At this point, we instruct caregivers to complete an intake packet and submit the necessary paperwork to schedule an evaluation in the clinic.

The *physician's* role on the interdisciplinary team is first to review the child's medical records for (a) significant and chronic medical conditions or illnesses (e.g., gastroesophageal reflux disease, intestinal failure), (b) history of frequent visits to the emergency room for dehydration or weight loss, (c) growth concerns (e.g., failure to thrive), or (d) dietary intolerances and severe food allergies. The physician also determines whether any additional medical workups or tests (e.g., endoscopy) are necessary. Overall, the physician must clear the child as medically fit to participate in feeding services before admission to our program. Following the intake evaluation, the physician continues to monitor the child's medical status throughout his or her admission by reviewing progress weekly. If the treatment team or physician identifies new concerns during the child's admission, the physician typically returns to the clinic to observe the child during mealtimes, schedules an examination relative to the child's medical needs, meets with the family to discuss the next course of action, and makes recommendations for treatment or additional testing as needed. The physician also manages acute or chronic medical problems and maintains contact with the child's physician or specialist as needed. Given that many children with feeding difficulties have medical comorbidities, this is a critical component of the child's assessment and admission.

During the intake evaluation, the *speech-language pathologist* assesses the child's oral-motor status and safety as an oral feeder and identifies delays or deficits. The speech-language pathologist first observes the child during an oral meal to assess the child's safety (e.g., chewing or swallowing concerns). The speech-language pathologist also schedules an interview with the child's caregivers to review the child's history relative to feeding in general (e.g., known history of choking or aspiration, child's ability to safely swallow, chew, and manage a variety of textures). If the speech-language pathologist identifies any potential risks (e.g., history of pneumonia, dysphagia, frequent coughing) during this assessment, he or she will likely refer the child for a modified-barium swallow study (Eicher et al., 2000). Based on the assessment and results of the swallow study (if necessary), the speech-language pathologist makes recommendations regarding solid and liquid textures (e.g., smooth, thickened), bolus (amount per bite or drink) sizes, and rates of presentation and provides recommendations regarding procedures to address any oral-motor deficits during the child's admission. Before admission, the speech-language pathologist must clear the child as a safe oral feeder who is not at risk for choking or aspiration. If the speech-language pathologist or the team identifies concerns along the way, the speech-language pathologist conducts observations of the child's meal and provides recommendations for safety precautions.

The *registered dietician* assesses the child's nutritional status and growth. Our registered dietician lives in another state but can attend intake evaluations virtually using a secure web-based platform. Before the intake evaluation, we ask caregivers to complete and submit a 3-day food log. The dietician analyzes the content of the food log to determine how many calories, on average, the child consumes daily and whether there are any nutrient deficiencies. During the intake evaluation, we measure the child's height and weight and plot the information on a growth chart. One of our feeding therapists takes a full-body picture of the child to send to the dietician, so she can assess the child's size and stature. The dietician then meets briefly with the caregivers to review the child's feeding and nutrition history. Throughout the child's admission, the dietician continues monitoring the child's growth, dietary intake, hydration, and elimination (e.g., urination, bowel movements, vomiting). The dietician also provides recommendations for formula and foods, based on the child's deficiencies and estimated caloric needs.

Feeding therapists are members of our program's staff who hold bachelor's or master's degrees in psychology, behavior analysis, education, or a related field (e.g., counseling). Given that we are a highly sought-after training site, feeding therapists also include trainees from across the country, including masters- or doctoral-level students, predoctoral interns, and postdoctoral fellows. Feeding therapists assist with the intake evaluation by preparing the foods and other session materials needed to conduct the meal observation. Feeding therapists also (a) observe and collect data on both child and caregiver behavior during the meal, (b) interview caregivers to complete any missing information from the intake packet, and (c) update the doctoral-level behavior analyst or licensed psychologist on the findings of the meal observation. Throughout the child's admission, feeding therapists implement the intervention, collect and graph data, and teach caregivers how to implement the procedures. Outside of the child's meals, feeding therapists prepare foods for the sessions and check in with supervisors for assessment or intervention decisions. At the beginning of the admission, we assign each child a team of feeding therapists who oversee the child's daily care.

Doctoral-level behavior analysts and *licensed psychologists* comprise two other critical members of the interdisciplinary team who use systematic assessment methods to identify the effects of environmental variables on feeding behavior (i.e., the conditions under which the child will and will not eat or drink). During the intake evaluation, the doctoral-level behavior analyst and licensed psychologist observe the caregiver conducting a meal as he or she typically would at home. These observations allow the behavior analyst and psychologist to identify some of the specific problems that may contribute to the child's feeding disorder. For example, caregivers might be more likely to terminate the meal early or provide attention in the form of reprimands and coaxing if the child is engaging in excessive problem behavior (e.g., head-turning, crying, pushing food away). At the end of the intake evaluation, the behavior analyst or psychologist meets with the family to provide diagnosis (discussed below) and treatment recommendations (i.e., outpatient versus intensive day treatment). Throughout the child's admission, the doctoral-level behavior analyst and licensed psychologist oversee the child's care, using empirically supported assessment tools (e.g., functional analysis) to guide intervention planning and decision-making. The doctoral-level behavior analyst and licensed psychologist oversee the therapeutic team who works directly with the child and oversee all aspects of intervention, including long-term maintenance and generalization of appropriate feeding behavior.

Assessment: Direct Observation

During the child's intake evaluation, we conduct direct observation assessments to gather information about the child's feeding difficulties. First, we conduct a *home baseline* assessment to observe the natural mealtime conditions (e.g., child and caregiver behavior) in the absence of treatment recommendations, structure, or intervention. The home baseline assessment provides an opportunity for direct observation of antecedent conditions, appropriate and inappropriate child behavior, and consequences provided by caregivers. For this assessment, we conduct one 5-min session with a few of the child's preferred foods (i.e., foods the child consistently eats) and one 5-min session with a few of the child's non-preferred foods (i.e., novel foods or foods the child refuses). We instruct caregivers to feed and interact with the child as they normally would at home.

After the home baseline assessment, we conduct a *standard outcome baseline* assessment to observe how the child responds when presented with solids and liquids with structure added to the meal. That is, we instruct caregivers to present a specific bolus (amount) of food or liquid during bite or drink presentations according to a fixed-time presentation schedule (e.g., fixed-time 30 s). We evaluate child responding during the standard outcome baseline assessment to gather initial data for which to compare later, after the child has been admitted to the program and is exposed to intervention. First, the therapist teaches the caregiver how to prepare an appropriate bolus on the utensil and models specific prompts he or she will use throughout the assessment (e.g., "Take a bite"). The therapist instructs the caregiver to present four different target foods (i.e., potato, green bean, pear, and chicken) prepared at pureed and table texture (e.g., small pieces at 1/4 in. by 1/4 in. by 1/4 in. in size) and a calorically dense, nutritionally complete liquid (e.g., milk mixed with Carnation Instant Breakfast). Depending on the child's age, we instruct caregivers to present the foods and liquids using both a self-feeder and nonself-feeder format in separate sessions, to assess the child's current skills and observe whether there are differences in caregiver-provided consequences. During each session of the standardized outcome baseline assessment, the therapist prompts the caregiver to present five bites or drinks approximately every 30 s and instructs the caregiver to otherwise respond as he or she would at home. If the parent misses a prompt or prepares an incorrect bolus, the therapist provides immediate corrective feedback.

Following the standard outcome baseline assessment, the therapist conducts a brief *interview* with the caregivers to fill any gaps that might be missing in the child's paperwork and review details or remaining questions regarding the child's feeding and medical history. The caregiver interview provides the therapist with an opportunity to gather additional information on the child's past and current medical diagnoses, prior services (e.g., occupational therapy, nutrition), typical meal format, and past and current food intake.

After members of the interdisciplinary team have completed their evaluations and met with other team members to review the child's history and current medical status, the licensed psychologist pulls together the relevant information to determine a diagnosis. The licensed psychologist gives a diagnosis of *avoidant/restrictive food intake disorder* when the presence of a feeding difficulty results in significant weight loss or nutritional deficiency, dependence on tube feedings or oral nutritional supplements, marked impairment with psychosocial functioning, or any combination of these conditions (American Psychiatric Association, 2013). The licensed psychologist provides a diagnosis of *feeding difficulties and mismanagement* when developmental delays in feeding, oral aversion, or feeding problems in infancy are present (World Health Organization, 1992). Based on the diagnosis and severity of the feeding disorder, the feeding team makes recommendations for the most appropriate level of service. The licensed psychologist or doctoral-level behavior analyst reviews the findings of the intake evaluation, diagnosis, and recommendations for treatment with the caregivers.

The feeding team recommends services at different levels based on clinical observations, past and current medical concerns, past and current food and liquid intake, current skill, and current growth. We typically recommend *intensive day-treatment* services when the child exhibits total food or liquid refusal; is liquid-, bottle-, or tube-dependent; has a diagnosis of failure to thrive or has recently lost a significant amount of weight; is currently eating fewer than 20 foods; engages in extreme problem behavior during the meal (e.g., self-injury, aggression, disruption, throwing food off the table); or a combination. We typically recommend weekly *outpatient* services, which we most often conduct via telehealth due to recent advances in technology, when the child exhibits food, texture, or brand selectivity, is not at risk for tube placement or a diagnosis of failure to thrive, has prerequisite feeding skills (e.g., eating pureed food but needs to advance to age-appropriate chewing), does not engage in high rates of problem behavior during the mealtime, or a combination. We recommend admission to the feeding and early intervention hybrid program called *SEEDS (Starting Early: Eating and Developmental Skills)* if the child is appropriate for outpatient services and has a diagnosis of autism spectrum disorder or developmental delays. The SEEDS program provides early intervention (e.g., skill acquisition, toilet training) and feeding services simultaneously. Currently, our program does not accept patients without insurance, but we work with other service providers, apply for grants or other coverage options, or refer to other providers as appropriate for patients without insurance.

Assessment: Initial Admission

Kerwin (1999) and Volkert and Piazza (2012) demonstrated in their reviews of the literature that interventions based on applied behavior analysis were the only ones with empirical support as treatment for pediatric feeding disorders. Given these findings, our pediatric feeding disorders program uses empirically supported assessment tools during the assessment of a child's feeding difficulties to indicate which empirically supported behavior-analytic interventions will be most effective.

At the beginning of every child's admission, regardless of the program (day treatment, outpatient, or SEEDS), we conduct additional assessments and evaluations. We always collect new growth information by obtaining a new height and weight for the child. After we take caregivers through basic paperwork and the consent process, we often initiate another series of more complex assessments. Given that several months may have elapsed between the intake evaluation and the first week of the child's admission, we first instruct caregivers to again implement the standard outcome baseline assessment, as outlined above. This time, we conduct multiple sessions of each condition (e.g., multiple sessions with purees, multiple sessions with table-textured bites) to obtain a more thorough assessment of how the child responds during structured, baseline contingencies. During the assessment, the feeding team (e.g., licensed psychologist or doctoral-level behavior analyst, feeding therapists) monitors the rate of inappropriate mealtime behavior and levels of acceptance, mouth clean (i.e., no food or liquid larger than a pea inside the mouth 30 s after acceptance; product measure for swallowing), and negative vocalizations to determine the next steps for assessment.

Preference Assessments

The purpose of a preference assessment is to identify stimuli that may serve as reinforcers for child behavior. Our program uses a variety of preference assessments, including the Reinforcer Assessment for Individuals with Severe Disabilities (RAISD; Fisher, Piazza, Bowman, & Amari, 1996), paired-choice preference assessment (Fisher et al., 1992), and a free-operant preference assessment (Roane, Vollmer, Ringdahl, & Marcus, 1998). In structured interviews, we ask caregivers to first identify stimuli (e.g., edibles, games, toys) their children are more likely to engage with or complete a task for using the RAISD. Based on the caregiver interview and the RAISD, we assess the child's preference for a few items using the paired-choice preference assessment to identify which items might function as reinforcers. During the assessment, the therapist presents each item in a pair with every other item across multiple trials. Observers collect data on how often the child *approaches* the items, defined as the child moving toward the object or event with his or her hand or body within 5 s of the presentation. Data collectors also measure *consumption*, defined as interaction with the item for longer than 5 s after the child approaches the item. If the child does not approach either item, data collectors score *no response*. After no response during a trial, the therapist removes both items, models interaction with the items, and presents the pair of items one additional time. If the child does not approach either item after the second presentation, the data collector once again scores no response, and the therapist removes the items from the child's reach and field of vision. Data collectors score *avoid* if the child pushes the item away. After the therapist has paired each item with every other item, the feeding team compares how often the child approached and consumed each item and ranks the items in terms of high, medium, or low preference. We use the top five highly preferred items during the functional analysis and intervention evaluations (see below).

We use the free-operant preference assessment arrangement to assess preference if the child engages in high rates of problem behavior in a chair, high rates of problem behavior whenever the therapist removes an item, is unable to indicate choice, or does not respond to any items during a paired-choice preference assessment. In a free-operant assessment, we present stimuli in a circle or semicircle around the child in an open space. We provide the child with noncontingent continuous access to the presented items. Observers record *item manipulation* during the 10-min assessment and use the total duration of time engaged with each item to rank preference.

Functional Analysis

After the standardd outcome baseline and preference assessments, the feeding therapists conduct a functional analysis of inappropriate mealtime behavior. Functional analyses (Iwata, Dorsey, Slifer, Bauman, & Richamn, 1994) involve the systematic manipulation of environmental events that may maintain problem behavior. In a functional analysis of inappropriate mealtime behavior, we arrange various antecedents (e.g., presenting a bite of nonpreferred food) and consequences (e.g., reprimands when the child does not take the bite) from the child's natural environment into different analogue conditions, so we can evaluate their separate effects on inappropriate mealtime behavior (Bachmeyer et al., 2009; Piazza et al., 2003). We evaluate child responding in the functional analysis using a pairwise design and use information from caregiver reports and direct observation of caregiver-fed meals to inform the conditions of each child's functional analysis. For example, we conduct escape, attention, and tangible conditions if we observed the caregiver delivering escape, attention, and access to tangible items following inappropriate mealtime behavior during the home baseline and standard outcome baseline assessments.

Before each five-bite session of the functional analysis, the feeder randomly selects one food from each of the food groups (i.e., fruit, protein, starch, and vegetable) from the child's list of target foods, resulting in the presentation of three foods once and one food twice. The feeder randomly selects the order to present the foods before each session and presents bites approximately every 30 s by touching the child's lips with the utensil and saying, "Take a bite." The feeder provides brief verbal praise for acceptance (e.g., "Good job taking your bite") and activates a timer for 30 s. The feeder conducts a mouth check when 30 s elapse (e.g., "Show me, ahh") while modeling an open mouth. The feeder provides brief verbal praise (e.g., "Good job swallowing your bite!") for mouth clean or delivers a verbal prompt to "Swallow your bite" and presents the next bite regardless of whether any food remains in the child's mouth at the check. If the child has food greater than the size of a pea inside the mouth after five bites, the feeder conducts a mouth check every 30 s until no food (larger than a pea) remains in the mouth or until 10 min elapse from the start of the session. The feeder provides no differential consequence for coughing, gagging, negative vocalizations, or vomiting. If the child does not accept the bite and does not engage in inappropriate mealtime behavior (e.g., head turns), the feeder holds the spoon stationary for 30 s across all conditions of the functional analysis. The feeder does not re-present expelled bites.

During the *control* condition, the feeder presents highly preferred stimuli, identified during the paired-choice preference assessment, on the tray at the beginning of the session and interacts with the child in the form of singing, playing, and telling stories throughout the session. The feeder provides no differential consequences if the child engages in inappropriate mealtime behavior. The purpose of this condition is to assess the frequency of inappropriate mealtime behavior when the child has free access to attention and preferred items. In the *escape* condition, the feeder removes the bite for 30 s immediately following the first instance of inappropriate mealtime behavior and presents the next bite at the end of the 30-s interval. The feeder does not provide attention or toys during this condition. The purpose of this condition is to assess the effects of negative reinforcement in the form of escape from bite presentations following inappropriate mealtime behavior. In the *attention* condition, the feeder delivers 30 s of continuous attention matched to the form that the caregiver delivered during the caregiver-fed meals described above (e.g., coaxing, reprimands, statements of concern) immediately following the first instance of inappropriate mealtime behavior and presents the next bite after the 30-s attention interval. No toys are available. The purpose of this condition is to assess the effects of social positive reinforcement in the form of caregiver attention. In the *tangible* condition, the feeder delivers a highly preferred item (identified in the preference assessment) for 30 s following the first instance of inappropriate mealtime behavior. After 30 s elapse, the feeder removes the item and presents the next bite. The purpose of this condition is to assess the effects of social positive reinforcement in the form of tangible items. We only conduct tangible conditions if we observe the caregiver deliver tangible items following inappropriate mealtime behavior during the home or standardized outcome baseline assessments.

Reinforcement Assessment

Often, we conduct a reinforcement assessment as the next step of the assessment process. Results of previous research have shown that positive-reinforcement-based interventions are ineffective for reducing inappropriate mealtime behavior for children with feeding disorders in the absence of escape extinction (Bachmeyer et al., 2009; Patel, Piazza, Martinez, Volkert, & Santana, 2002; Piazza, Patel, Gulotta, Sevin, & Layer, 2003; Reed et al., 2004). Even though functional analyses often reveal that inappropriate mealtime behavior is maintained by negative reinforcement in the form of escape from bites (Piazza et al., 2003), we conduct reinforcement assessments as a method to evaluate the least-restrictive procedures first. In addition, there may be some benefit to adding positive reinforcers to the meal for some children in that positive reinforcement may mitigate the undesirable side effects of escape extinction (e.g., crying, other forms of problem behavior). Therefore, we conduct an assessment to evaluate the effects of differential and noncontingent positive reinforcement in the absence of escape extinction for some children. We compare the effects of these positive-reinforcement based procedures using a multielement design, rapidly alternating between differential reinforcement, noncontingent reinforcement, and a control or no-reinforcement condition. We use the procedure described for the functional analysis (e.g., five-bite sessions, 30-s mouth checks, feeder rotates across target foods for each child). During the *differential reinforcement* condition, the feeder presents a preferred stimulus immediately following acceptance of the bite of target food. In the *noncontingent reinforcement* condition, the feeder provides continuous, noncontingent access to various preferred items (e.g., attention in the form of talking and singing, toys) regardless of acceptance or inappropriate mealtime behavior. In the *control* or no-reinforcement condition, the feeder presents the bite and provides no differential consequences following acceptance or inappropriate mealtime behavior. Escape from bites is available across all conditions. The feeder immediately removes the spoon if the child engages in inappropriate mealtime behavior.

The reinforcement assessment has yielded mixed results thus far. For most children, we have demonstrated that positive-reinforcement-based interventions alone are not sufficient to increase bite or drink acceptance and reduce inappropriate mealtime behavior to clinically acceptable levels. For some children, we have observed beneficial effects of positive reinforcement, such as lower levels of negative vocalizations or inappropriate mealtime behavior, but with no increases in levels of acceptance. Some caregivers, however, request the addition of positive reinforcement to the treatment package, reporting that the mealtime is more enjoyable. We will continue evaluating the effects of positive reinforcement for children with severe feeding disorders to determine whether there are any merits or challenges with adding positive reinforcers to the meal context. For example, even if including differential reinforcement with arbitrary tangible items (e.g., toys) results in slightly lower levels of negative vocalizations initially, it may make the meal appear less typical and require more effort on caregivers if they must include highly preferred items during every meal.

Baseline Evaluation

Consistent with the field of applied behavior analysis, we use single-case designs to evaluate interventions aimed at reducing inappropriate mealtime behavior and increasing alternative, appropriate feeding behavior (e.g., acceptance, swallowing). To do this, we begin by conducting baseline to determine patterns of responding before implementing the intervention. The baseline condition serves as a control for which to measure and compare the effects of intervention, and we use the results of the functional analysis to inform the baseline. For example, if the functional analysis reveals both social positive (e.g., attention) and negative reinforcement functions, we arrange the baseline condition so that the feeder delivers escape and attention immediately after instances of inappropriate mealtime behavior. Once we observe stable responding during baseline at a level or trend that would indicate the need for intervention, we proceed with our intervention evaluation, using any number of empirically supported design strategies (e.g., reversal, multielement, multiple baseline) and interventions.

Intervention Evaluation

Results of the functional analysis guide our intervention decisions because we use that information to design individualized, function-based treatments to achieve the most effective outcomes. Recall that most often, we observe that the child's inappropriate mealtime behavior is maintained by negative reinforcement in the form of escape from bites and drinks. When we identify escape as the function for inappropriate mealtime behavior, we most often select escape extinction as the first line of treatment. Research demonstrates that escape extinction is the most efficacious and well-supported intervention for pediatric feeding disorders (Kerwin, 1999; Volkert & Piazza, 2012) and that inappropriate mealtime behavior is likely to persist in the absence of escape extinction (Addison et al., 2003). In a feeding context, therapists implement escape extinction using non-removal of the spoon with or without physical guidance. That is, during structured sessions and across a time-based presentation schedule, the feeder presents the spoon to the child's lips and follows the child's lips until the child opens to accept the bite or drink, regardless of inappropriate mealtime behavior (e.g., head turns, batting at the spoon).

We typically evaluate the effectiveness of escape extinction using a reversal design. Once we observe high stable levels of acceptance and mouth clean and low, stable levels of inappropriate mealtime behavior during the intervention, we then remove the intervention to demonstrate functional control to determine whether escape extinction produced the change in responding. After a reduction in acceptance and mouth clean and an increase in inappropriate mealtime behavior during the return-to-baseline condition, we return to the intervention (i.e., escape extinction).

Occasionally, we include positive-reinforcement-based interventions in our treatment package, even if results of the reinforcement assessment demonstrate little to no effects with positive reinforcement alone. We include positive reinforcement if caregivers indicate a preference for the additional component. In addition, if escape extinction results in consistently high levels of negative vocalizations, inappropriate mealtime behavior, or other problem behavior, we may evaluate alternative strategies such as antecedent interventions instead of or in addition to the escape-extinction procedure (e.g., stimulus fading). If we observe an increase in corollary problem behavior (e.g., packing or pocketing food inside the mouth for extended periods of time, expulsion or spitting food or liquid) following acceptance during the intervention evaluation, we evaluate specific interventions to address these challenges. For example, research has demonstrated that a flipped-spoon procedure is effective at reducing packing for children with pediatric feeding disorders (Volkert, Vaz, Piazza, Frese, & Barnett, 2011).

Caregiver Training Evaluation

After we evaluate and determine which treatment is most effective, we teach caregivers to implement the treatment protocol using competency-based training as well as instructions, modeling, and feedback. We first train caregivers in the clinic where the child has demonstrated success with feeding. Before training, caregivers observe meals with the therapists feeding. We then collect data on the caregiver's integrity and provide in vivo feedback to praise correct implementation or give corrective guidance after implementation errors. We measure caregiver accuracy with the intervention protocols by assessing whether the caregiver holds the utensil in the correct location during a meal (i.e., ensuring that the utensil follows the child's lips during non-removal of the spoon) and whether the caregiver follows other critical components of the intervention (e.g., refraining from providing attention following inappropriate mealtime behavior during attention extinction). We systematically fade therapists from the meal as caregivers demonstrate high levels of treatment integrity and the child's behavior remains stable. After caregivers implement the procedures with high integrity in the clinic setting, we observe the caregivers conducting meals in the home and any other natural environments where the child eats (e.g., school, daycare) to ensure generalization. In addition, we observe all meals the caregivers conduct throughout the day as there are different variables at each meal that could interfere with correct protocol implementation.

Goal Evaluation

At the beginning of a child's admission, we set observable and measurable goals. We evaluate progress toward goal attainment at intermittent points throughout the child's admission. Often, our first goal is to increase the child's acceptance and mouth clean of a variety of solids, up to 16 target foods across all 4 major food groups and liquids (e.g., calorically dense and nutritionally complete formula) to 80% across all opportunities. That is, we expect that the child will begin (a) accepting the bite or drink within 5 s of the presentation and (b) swallowing the bite or drink within 30 s of the bite entering the mouth (i.e., mouth clean) during treatment. Another goal is to reduce inappropriate mealtime behavior to low levels (e.g., rate of <5 per min). After the child meets these initial goals, we teach caregivers (e.g., parents, grandparents, siblings) to implement the intervention procedures with high integrity (see above).

Throughout the child's admission, we also set goals to (a) increase variety of foods in the diet, (b) increase volume of oral intake while making simultaneous deductions to tube feedings, (c) increase meal efficiency by increasing the rate of bite and drink presentations and gradually increasing the bolus size (e.g., 2 cc, 4 cc, 6 cc, 10 cc), (d) maintain success as we work toward creating a more typical meal by removing structured components of the procedure (e.g., removal of prompts and mouth checks), and (e) teach other caregivers to implement the procedures with high integrity in other environments (i.e., generalization to daycare, school, home).

During follow-up outpatient services, we set other goals geared toward the child becoming an age-typical feeder. Before setting goals for building more advanced feeding skills, we conduct new assessments to determine the child's safety and readiness (e.g., whether the child chews and masticates the bites or attempts to swallow the bites whole). After we determine the child is ready, we set goals to (a) increase self-feeding and self-drinking, (b) increase chewing and other skills required to consume table-textured foods (e.g., lateralization), (c) increase consumption of age-appropriate portion-based meals involving both solids and liquids to ensure the child becomes more independent during meals, and (d) increase the child's acceptance and tolerance of foods presented in their natural forms (e.g., presenting a whole hot dog inside a hot dog bun).

During SEEDS (Starting Early: Eating and Developmental Skills) admissions, we set similar goals to increase appropriate feeding behavior (e.g., increase acceptance of a wider variety of nutritional foods) and reduce inappropriate mealtime behavior; however, we expand the service to include a variety of critical goals toward improving adaptive functioning for the child. We use the Verbal Behavior Milestones Assessment and Placement Program (VB-MAPP; Sundberg, 2008) or the Assessment of Basic Language and Learning Skills (Revised) (ABLLS-R; Partington, 2008) tools to determine each child's most critical areas of need. We then set individualized, observable, and measurable goals to target skill acquisition across a variety of domains, including self-help (e.g., appropriate toileting, handwashing, tooth brushing), social (e.g., greetings, sharing), academic (e.g., receptive and expressive identification of letters), and communication (e.g., mands and tacts). We also set behavior-reduction goals, when necessary, to decrease severe problem behavior (e.g., aggression, self-injury), noncompliance, resistance to change (e.g., difficulty with transitions), or elopement.

Conclusions

Pediatric feeding disorders are serious conditions that have a significant impact on the child's health, learning, and behavior. Failing to eat or drink sufficient calories or nutrients to grow and maintain nutritional status can have devastating physical, psychological, and financial consequences for the child, the child's family, and society. The difficulty lies in the many factors that contribute to these disorders. An interdisciplinary approach enables the feeding team to assess all relevant factors. Behavior analysts and behavioral psychologists play a critical role on this interdisciplinary team, given that they are uniquely equipped to assess and address specific environmental variables that likely affect feeding behavior. We use structured, systematic and empirically supported assessment tools to determine the environmental factors maintaining a child's inappropriate mealtime behavior and then use the results of these assessments to guide intervention decisions, set appropriate goals for the child, evaluate whether the intervention is effective, and teach caregivers to implement the effective interventions with high integrity across a variety of settings. These rigorous assessment strategies are part of the reason why researchers identified applied behavior analysis as the only empirically supported interventions for pediatric feeding disorders.

For many children, we have a good understanding of why feeding disorders develop (e.g., complex medical histories, environmental variables). For children with autism spectrum disorders, conclusions are less clear regarding the specific establishing operations or antecedent conditions that contribute to food selectivity and rigid eating patterns. Recent studies show that up to 80% of children with autism spectrum disorders display food selectivity. Researchers report that children with autism spectrum disorders often refuse healthy foods and replace them with a limited variety of calorie-dense, nutritionally deficient alternatives (e.g., cookies, chips) that are often high in fat, sugar, and sodium (Hubbard, Anderson, Curtin, Must, & Bandini, 2014; Schreck, Williams, & Smith, 2004). This type of food selectivity occurs in seemingly healthy children who may not have a significant medical history or obvious skill deficits to explain how the problem developed. Instead, children with autism spectrum disorder and food selectivity often insist upon sameness of mealtime routines (e.g., will only eat pizza from Pizza Hut if served from the box); display rigidity with the type, texture, or other stimulus properties of the foods (e.g., only eats white foods, only eats pureed foods); and engage in excessive problem behavior in the presence of novel foods. Given these behavior patterns, we often conceptualize food selectivity in this population as a manifestation of one of the characteristic symptoms of autism spectrum disorder (i.e., rigid or repetitive behavior patterns, behavior that is highly resistant to change; Turner, 1999). However, we still do not possess effective tools for which to fully assess this prevalent problem. Thus, future researchers should consider evaluating the conditions under which food selectivity emerges for children with autism spectrum disorder as well as the conditions under which the child is willing to eat. Hubbard, Anderson, Curtin, Must, and Bandini (2014) found that children with ASD refused more foods based on texture (77% versus 36%), taste or smell (49% versus 5%), and brand (15% versus 1%) than typically developing children. We could benefit from a more comprehensive assessment tool to identify the precise stimulus properties of foods most commonly consumed by children with autism spectrum disorder or other relevant antecedent conditions that result in food selectivity. An empirically supported assessment of this type could capture a comprehensive list of the stimulus conditions under which a child may or may not eat a variety of foods. This empirical assessment could then be used to guide strategies and prescribe intervention. For example, if an assessment indicates that a child will only consume foods that are white and crunchy (e.g., Club crackers), a clinician could arrange the stimulus conditions to match those that result in appropriate mealtime behavior (i.e., consumption) by first presenting a Club cracker to the child. After observing child acceptance and consumption of the Club cracker across sessions, the clinician could alter the stimulus properties of the Club cracker systematically to approximate a novel food (i.e., stimulus fading). This approach increases the likelihood that the child's behavior will either contact reinforcement following success after the initial demand or come under instructional control of the context and therapist. More refined and comprehensive assessment tools would allow us to systematically, rather than arbitrarily, select a "starting point" for the child. Smith, Iwata, Han-Leong, and Shore (1995) highlighted the importance of a more detailed analysis of establishing operations, and food selectivity appears to be a behavior that would greatly benefit from this approach.

References

Addison, L. R., Piazza, C. C., Patel, M. R., Bachmeyer, M. H., Rivas, K. M., Milnes, S. M., & Oddo, J. (2003). A comparison of sensory integrative and behavioral therapies as treatment for pediatric feeding disorders. *Journal of Applied Behavior Analysis, 45*, 455–471. https://doi.org/10.1901/jaba.2012.45-455

Akay, B., Capizzani, T. R., Lee, A. M., Drongowski, R. A., Geiger, J. D., Hirschl, R. B., & Mychaliska, G. B. (2010). Gastrostomy tube placement in infants and children: Is there a preferred technique? *Journal of Pediatric Surgery, 45*, 1147–1152. https://doi.org/10.1016/j.jpedsurg.2010.02.079

American Psychiatric Association. (2013). *Diagnostic and statistical manual of mental disorders* (4th ed., text rev.). Washington, DC: Author.

Arvedson, J. C., & Brodsky, L. (2002). *Pediatric swallowing and feeding: Assessment and management* (2nd ed.). San Diego, CA: Singular Publishing (2nd ed.). Albany, NY: Singular.

Babbitt, R. L., Hoch, T. A., & Coe, D. A. (1994). Behavioral feeding disorders. In D. Tuchman & R. Walters (Eds.), *Pediatric feeding and swallowing disorders: Pathology, diagnosis, and treatment*. San Diego, CA: Singular Publishing Group. https://doi.org/10.1097/00004703-199408000-00011

Bachmeyer, M. H., Piazza, C. C., Fredrick, L. D., Reed, G. K., Rivas, K. D., & Kadey, H. J. (2009). Functional analysis and treatment of multiply controlled inappropriate mealtime behavior. *Journal of Applied Behavior Analysis, 42*, 641–658. https://doi.org/10.1901/jaba.2009.42-641

Bandini, L. G., Anderson, S. E., Curtin, C., Cermak, S., Evans, E. W., Scampini, R., ... Must, A. (2010). Food selectivity in children with autism Spectrum disorders and typically developing children. *The Journal of Pediatrics, 157*, 259–264. https://doi.org/10.1016/j.jpeds.2010.02.013

Borrero, C. S., Woods, J. N., Borrero, J. C., Masler, E. A., & Lesser, A. D. (2010). Descriptive analyses of pediatric food refusal and acceptance. *Journal of Applied Behavior Analysis, 43*, 71–88. https://doi.org/10.1901/jaba.2010.43-71

Christophersen, E. R., & Hall, C. L. (1978). Eating patterns and associated problems encountered in normal children. *Issues in Comprehensive Pediatric Nursing, 3*, 1–16. https://doi.org/10.3109/01460867809087345

Cohen, S. A., Piazza, C. C., & Navathe, A. (2006). Feeding and nutrition. In I. L. Rubin & A. C. Crocker (Eds.), *Medical care for children and adults with developmental disabilities* (pp. 295–307). Baltimore: Paul H. Brooks Publishing Co.

Cooper, J. O., Heron, T. E., & Heward, W. L. (2007). *Applied behavior analysis* (2nd ed.). Upper Saddle River, N.J: Pearson Prentice Hall.

Eicher, P. S., Mcdonald-Mcginn, D. M., Fox, C. A., Driscoll, D. A., Emanuel, B. S., & Zackai, E. H. (2000). Dysphagia in children with a 22q11.2 deletion: Unusual pattern found on modified barium swallow. *The Journal of Pediatrics, 137*, 158–164. https://doi.org/10.1067/mpd.2000.105356

El-Matary, W. (2008). Percutaneous endoscopic gastrostomy in children. *Canadian Journal of Gastroenterology, 22*, 993–998. https://doi.org/10.1155/2008/583470

Fisher, W. W., Piazza, C. C., Bowman, L. G., & Amari, A. (1996). Integrating caregiver report with a systematic choice assessment. *American Journal on Mental Retardation, 101*, 15–25.

Fisher, W. F., Piazza, C. C., Bowman, L. G., Hagopian, L. P., Owens, J. C., & Slevin, I. (1992). A comparison of two approaches for identifying reinforcers for persons with severe and profound disabilities. *Journal of Applied Behavior Analysis, 25*, 491–498. https://doi.org/10.1901/jaba.1992.25-491

Franklin, L., & Rodger, S. (2003). Parents' perspectives on feeding medically compromised children: Implications for occupational therapy. *Australian Occupational Therapy Journal, 50*, 137–147. https://doi.org/10.1046/j.1440-1630.2003.00375.x

Freedman, D. S., Dietz, W. H., Srinivasan, S. R., & Berenson, G. S. (1999). The relation of overweight to cardiovascular risk factors among children and adolescents: The Bogalusa Heart Study. *Pediatrics, 103*, 1175–1182. https://doi.org/10.1542/peds.103.6.1175

Gibbons, B., Williams, K. E., & Riegel, K. (2007). Reducing tube feeds and tongue thrust: Combining an oral-motor and behavioral approach to feeding. *American Journal of Occupational Therapy, 61*, 394–401. https://doi.org/10.5014/ajot.61.4.384

Hubbard, K. L., Anderson, S. E., Curtin, C., Must, A., & Bandini, L. G. (2014). *Journal of the Academy of Nutrition and Dietetics, 114*, 1981–1987. https://doi.org/10.1016/j.jand.2014.04.017

Iwata, B. A., Dorsey, M. F., Slifer, K. J., Bauman, K. E., & Richamn, G. S. (1994). Toward a functional analysis of self-injury. *Journal of Applied Behavior Analysis, 27*, 197–209. https://doi.org/10.1901/jaba.1994.27-197

Kerwin, M. (1999). Empirically supported treatments in pediatric psychology: Severe feeding problems. *Journal of Pediatric Psychology, 24*, 193–214. https://doi.org/10.1093/jpepsy/24.3.193

Lindberg, L., Bohlin, G., & Hagekull, B. (1991). Early feeding problems in a normal population. *International Journal of Eating Disorders, 10*, 395–405. https://doi.org/10.1002/1098-108X(199107)10:4<395::AID-EAT2260100404>3.0.CO;2-A

Linscheid, T. R., Budd, K. S., & Rasnake, L. K. (1995). Pediatric feeding disorders. In M. C. Roberts (Ed.), *Handbook of pediatric psychology* (pp. 501–515). New York: Guilford.

Ludwig, D. S., Majzoub, J. A., Al-Zahrani, A., Dallal, G. E., Blanco, I., & Roberts, S. B. (1999). High glycemic index foods, overeating, and obesity. *Pediatrics, 103*, e26. https://doi.org/10.1542/peds.103.3.e26

Manikam, R., & Perman, J. A. (2000). Pediatric feeding disorders. *Journal of Clinical Gastroenterology, 30*, 34–46. https://doi.org/10.1097/00004836-200001000-00007

Milnes, S. M., & Piazza, C. C. (2013). Feeding disorders. In R. Hastings & J. Rojahn (Eds.), *International review of research in developmental disabilities: Challenging behavior* (Vol. 44, pp. 143–163). Waltham, MA: Academic Press.

Nicholls, D. E., Lynn, R., & Viner, R. M. (2011). Childhood eating disorders: British national surveillance study. *The British Journal of Psychiatry, 198*, 295–301. https://doi.org/10.1192/bjp.bp.110.081356

Palmer, S., & Horn, S. (1978). Feeding problems in children. In S. Palmer & S. Ekvall (Eds.), *Pediatric nutrition in developmental disorders* (pp. 107–129). Springfield, Ill: Charles C. Thomas.

Partington, J. W. (2008). *The assessment of basic language and learning skills – Revised (the ABLLS-R)*. Pleasant Hill, CA: Behavior Analysts.

Patel, M. R., Piazza, C. C., Martinez, C. J., Volkert, V. M., & Santana, C. M. (2002). An evaluation of two differential reinforcement procedures with escape extinction to treat food refusal. *Journal of Applied Behavior Analysis, 35*, 363–374. https://doi.org/10.1901/jaba.2002.35-363

Peterson, K. M., Piazza, C. C., & Ibañez, V. F., (under review) *Randomized controlled trial of applied behavior analysis versus wait-list control for food selectivity in participants with autism spectrum disorder*.

Piazza, C. C., Fisher, W. W., Brown, K. A., Shore, B. A., Patel, M. R., Katz, R. M., ... Blakely-Smith, A. (2003). Functional analysis of inappropriate mealtime behaviors. *Journal of Applied Behavior Analysis, 36*, 187–204. https://doi.org/10.1901/jaba.2003.36-187

Piazza, C. C., Patel, M. R., Gulotta, C. S., Sevin, B. S., & Layer, S. A. (2003). On the relative contribution of positive reinforcement and escape extinction in the treatment of food refusal. *Journal of Applied Behavior Analysis, 36*, 309–324. https://doi.org/10.1901/jaba.2003.36-309

Piazza, C. C. (2008). Feeding disorders and behavior: What have we learned? *Developmental Disabilities Research Reviews, 14*, 174–181. https://doi.org/10.1002/ddrr.22

Reed, G. K., Piazza, C. C., Patel, M. R., Layer, S. A., Bachmeyer, M. H., Bethke, S. D., & Gutshall, K. A. (2004). On the relative contributions of noncontingent reinforcement and escape extinction in the treatment of food refusal. *Journal of Applied Behavior Analysis, 37*, 24–42. https://doi.org/10.1901/jaba.2004.37-27

Roane, H. S., Vollmer, T. R., Ringdahl, J. E., & Marcus, B. A. (1998). Evalaution of a brief stimulus preference assessment. *Journal of Applied Behavior Analysis, 31*, 605–620. https://doi.org/10.1901/jaba.1998.31-605

Rommel, N., De Meyer, A. M., Feenstra, L., & Veereman-Wauters, G. (2003). The complexity of feeding problems in 700 infants and young children presenting to a tertiary care institution. *Journal of Pediatric Gastroenterology and Nutrition, 37,* 75–84. https://doi.org/10.1097/00005176-200307000-00014

Schreck, K. M., Williams, K. E., & Smith, A. F. (2004). A comparison of eating behaviors between children with and without autism. *Journal of Autism and Developmental Disorders, 34,* 433–438.

Schwartz, D. (2000). Failure to thrive: An old nemesis in the new millennium. *Pediatrics in Review, 21,* 257–264. https://doi.org/10.1542/pir.21-8-257

Smith, R. G., Iwata, B. A., Han-Leong, G., & Shore, B. A. (1995). Analysis of establishing operations for self-injury maintained by escape. *Journal of Applied Behavior Analysis, 28,* 515–535. https://doi.org/10.1901/jaba.1995.28-515

Sullivan, P. B., Juszczak, E., Lambert, B. R., Rose, M., Ford-Adams, M. E., & Johnson, A. (2002). Impact of feeding problems on nutritional intake and growth: Oxford feeding study II. *Developmental Medicine and Child Neurology, 44,* 461–467. https://doi.org/10.1111/j.1469-8749.2002.tb00307.x

Sundberg, M. L. (2008). *Verbal behavior milestones assessment and placement program: The VB-MAPP.* Concord, CA: AVB Press.

Turner, M. A. (1999). Annotation: Repetitive behavior in autism: A review of psychological research. *The Journal of Child Psychology and Psychiatry, 40,* 839–849.

The ICD-10 Classification of Mental and Behavioural Disorders. (1992). *Clinical descriptions and diagnostic guidelines.* Geneva: World Health Organization. https://doi.org/10.1177/146642409311300216

Volkert, V. M., Patel, M. R., & Peterson, K. M. (2016). Food refusal and selective eating. In J. K. Luiselli (Ed.), *Behavioral health promotion and intervention inintellectual disabilities* (pp. 137–161). Springer International Publishing. https://doi.org/10.1007/978-3-319-27297-9_7

Volkert, V. M., & Piazza, C. C. (2012). Empirically supported treatments for pediatric feeding disorders. In P. Sturmey & M. Herson (Eds.), *Handbook of evidence based practice in clinical psychology.* Hoboken, NJ: Wiley. https://doi.org/10.1002/9781118156391.ebcp001013

Volkert, V. M., Vaz, P. M., Piazza, C. C., Frese, J., & Barnett, L. (2011). Using a flipped spoon to decrease packing in children with feeding disorders. *Journal of Applied Behavior Analysis, 44,* 617–621. https://doi.org/10.1901/jaba.2011.44-617

Winters, N. C. (2003). Feeding problems in infancy and early childhood. *Primary Psychiatry, 10,* 30–34.

World Health Organization. (1992) . The ICD-10 classification of mental and behavioural disorders : clinical descriptions and diagnostic guidelines. Geneva : World Health Organization. http://www.who.int/iris/handle/10665/37958

Assessment of Obesity

Sarah Mallard Wakefield, Joshua Sanderson, and Pamela McPherson

The Assessment of Obesity in Children and Adolescents

Obesity is one of the most often discussed issues of our time and one with a lasting impact on the future health of the human race. The World Health Organization (WHO) considers it "one of the most serious public health challenges of the twenty-first century," (WHO Global Strategy on Diet, Physical Activity, and Health, 2018a), and the US Centers for Disease Control (CDC) has recognized obesity as a serious problem putting US children at risk for poor health (CDC Childhood Obesity Facts, 2017a). Obesity is not relegated to those places with an abundance of food but is growing at an alarming rate in low and middle income countries as well. For now, obesity remains highest in Western and industrialized countries. The Americas and Eastern Mediterranean regions have estimated rates of obesity up to 30–40%. Europe has somewhat lower rates from 20% to 30%, and the lowest documented rates by region are 10–20% in Southeast Asia, Western Pacific, and Africa (WHO, 2009).

In the United States, the CDC demonstrated a dramatic rise in obesity from the early 1970s until a leveling off in 2008. The National Center for Health Statistics at the CDC reported the prevalence of obesity in children 2–19 years of age to be approximately 17% overall between the years 2011 and 2014, up from around 5% in 1971 (Skinner, Perrin, & Skelton, 2016). Rates also increased with age from preschool (8.9%), to school age (17.5%), to adolescence (20.5%) (Ogden, Carroll, Fryar, & Flegal, 2015). The National Health and Nutrition Examination Survey (NHANES) indicated that another 14.9% of children 2–19 years of age are overweight (Skinner, Perrin, & Skelton, 2016) and thus at risk for obesity as adults (Guo, Wu, Chumlea, & Roche, 2002). Preschool- and elementary-aged children who are overweight are more than five times as likely to be overweight during adolescence, and up to 80% of overweight teens become obese adults (Nader, 2006).

The rising incidence of obesity is linked to significant health consequences and medical expenditures. Childhood overweight and obesity increase the risk for numerous disease conditions and a shortened life-span. Many of the health

S. M. Wakefield (✉)
Texas Tech University Health Sciences Center, Lubbock, TX, USA
e-mail: Sarah.Wakefield@ttuhsc.edu

J. Sanderson
Louisiana State University Health New Orleans, LA, USA

P. McPherson
Northwest Louisiana Human Services District, LA, USA

conditions associated with childhood obesity may not become apparent until adulthood. These include heart disease and stroke, osteoarthritis, and cancers of the breast, endometrium, and colon (WHO Global Strategy on Diet, Physical Activity, and Health: Why Does Childhood Overweight and Obesity Matter, 2018b). As the severity of obesity increases, abnormal cholesterol levels, blood pressure, and glucose metabolism become apparent at younger and younger ages. For yet unclear reasons, young males tend to show these signs earlier than young females despite similar severity of obesity (Skinner, Perrin, Moss, & Skelton, 2015).

Obesity is a costly condition for the United States. Trogdon et al. evaluated state- and payer-specific estimates of annual medical expenditures attributable to obesity. These annual expenses ranged from a low of $203 million for the state of Wyoming to $15,223 billion in California (2012). Children with obesity generally cost less than adults with obesity (Finkelstein & Trogdon, 2008), likely because they are not yet suffering many comorbid disease conditions. However, obese children do incur higher medical costs compared to normal-weight children. In analyzing the costs of medical care from infancy to early adulthood, Finkelstein estimated that greater than 19 thousand more dollars are spent on medical care for an obese child as compared to a normal-weight child (2014). When hospitalized for any reason, children with obesity incur higher costs per hospitalization and have longer stays (Trasande, Liu, Fryer, & Weitzman, 2009).

Diagnosis and Classification of Obesity

Definition of Obesity

Obesity is caused by consuming more calories than you expend, but it is more complex than simply counting calories in and calories out. Many additional factors affect and alter this calculation and require a more layered conceptualization of the individual with obesity. Appropriately and accurately categorizing obesity can assist with this more nuanced approach and therefore improve assessment and application of effective interventions.

Obesity is not a diagnosis listed in the fifth edition of the *Diagnostic and Statistical Manual* (DSM-5). It is, however, a diagnosable disease with an associated International Classification of Diseases (ICD-10) code. The WHO defines obesity as "abnormal or excessive fat accumulation that presents a risk to health" (WHO Health Topics, 2018c). Most clinical definitions designate obesity as a body mass index (BMI) above the 95th percentile on age- and gender-normed growth charts (Ogden et al., 2016; Ogden, Kuczmarski, Flegal, & Mei, 2002; Park, Woo, Jeong, & Yi, 2012), even for children younger than 2 years of age (Barlow, 2007). A diagnosis of overweight is designated at a BMI percentile greater than or equal to the 85th percentile but less than the 95th.

Classification of Obesity: Primary and Secondary

Obesity can be categorized as either primary or secondary. Primary obesity is caused directly by the imbalance of calories taken in compared to those expended. Primary obesity is further divided into exogenous or monogenic obesity. Exogenous obesity is the most common form of obesity in children and adolescents (Martos-Moreno et al., 2014). A child with exogenous obesity may appear to simply be taking in too many calories at a time or choosing unhealthy foods due to lack of self-control. However, exogenous obesity is believed to be caused by the interplay of genetic predisposition, nutrition, physical activity, and environmental risk factors. An example of exogenous obesity is a child who does not have access to high-fiber foods, and he snacks on candy bars brought home by his parent from work at a convenience station. His parent works overnights, and he is left for the evenings with his uncle who does not have transportation or live near public transportation. There are no public parks nearby, and he sits and watches the television for most of the evening. In exogenous obesity, there are multiple factors contributing to the energy imbalance. Monogenic obesity is a type of primary obesity seen in a minority of affected children in which a single gene mutation leads to early onset and severe obesity. In monogenic obesity, it is the gene mutation that contributes directly to overeating. Many of the causes of monogenic obesity include mutations in genes altering the function or utility of leptin, a hormone involved in regulating satiety. The deletion in chromosome 15 associated with Prader-Willi syndrome causes the most common type of severe, primary monogenic obesity (August et al., 2008).

Secondary obesity is due to weight gain that begins after the onset of a disease condition or the start date of a medication. In secondary obesity, weight gain is directly attributed to the illness or medication. A variety of illnesses and medications can contribute to weight gain and the development of obesity. The most common illnesses implicated in secondary obesity are hypothyroidism and Cushing syndrome (Martos-Moreno et al., 2014). Hypothyroidism is an illness in which the thyroid gland, which regulates metabolism, does not produce enough of the hormones needed to maintain adequate metabolism, and some of the body's processes begin to slow. Weight gain is an associated consequence of hypothyroidism. Many conditions can lead to a hypothyroid state. These include autoimmune disease, surgical removal of the thyroid, radiation, damage to the pituitary gland, and dysregulation of iodine (American Thyroid Association, n.d.). Cushing syndrome, also known as hypercortisolism, results from prolonged exposure to high cortisol levels and is associated with a fatty hump between the shoulder blades, a rounded face, and significant weight gain especially in the midsection. Cushing syndrome can be due to a pituitary gland tumor increasing adrenocorticotropic hormone (ACTH) which causes the adrenal glands to release more cortisol. It can also result from dysfunction in the adrenal glands or from an ACTH-secreting tumor elsewhere in the body. Glucocorticoid or steroid medications can also result in Cushing syndrome if used over a long period of time (Mayo Clinic, 2018). By this same mechanism, glucocorticoids alone can be a cause of secondary obesity. Many children taking chronic steroid medications for allergy conditions, some cancers, or autoimmune disorders are at increased risk for secondary obesity induced by medication. Antiepileptic medications can contribute to sedation and lethargy which could offset the body's energy balance and lead to weight gain. Antipsychotic medications are frequently implicated in the development of secondary obesity (Correll, 2008). Antipsychotics may increase sedation resulting in decreased physical activity and stimulate appetite by increasing the enzyme AMPK via interaction with histamine receptors (Kim, Huang, Snowman, & Snyder, 2007).

It is important to note that the etiology of obesity may not fall squarely into one category. The development of obesity may be due to both primary and secondary factors. Primary and secondary causes of obesity are summarized in Table 1.

Table 1 Primary and secondary causes of obesity

Primary obesity		Secondary obesity	
Exogenous	*Monogenic*	*Disease condition*	*Medication*
Genetic predisposition	Chromosome 15 (Prader-Willi)	Hypothyroidism	Antipsychotics
Excessive caloric intake	Leptin receptor	Cushing syndrome	Antiepileptics
Physical inactivity	MC4R	Polycystic ovarian syndrome	Glucocorticoids
Environmental factors	POMC	Growth hormone deficiency	
	PCSK1	Pseudohypoparathyroidism	
	SIM1	Resection of brain tumor	
	BDNF		
	NTRK2		

Risk Factors for Obesity

When evaluating risk and contributory factors for obesity, it is important to consider the etiology of the disease in order to implement an effective prevention or intervention strategy. For example, a child with primary, exogenous obesity may benefit from nutritional counseling for the individual and family regarding healthy food choices and/or enrollment in a program to increase physical activity. A child with primary, monogenic obesity would also benefit from these types of interventions but may also require restriction in access to certain foods or even medication to suppress hyperphagia. For a child with secondary obesity, treatment of the underlying condition or change in a contributory medication may be the only intervention necessary.

Regardless of the etiology, risk factors for obesity can be divided into biological, nutritional, and environmental. Furthermore, it is helpful to identify the ability to modify these factors. If a risk factor is modifiable or changeable, it is considered a *dynamic* risk factor. Those risk factors which cannot be changed with prevention or intervention strategies are considered *static* risk factors. Dynamic, or changeable, risk factors present the greatest opportunity for prevention and intervention strategies. Static risk factors, while unchangeable, aid in delineation of children who would benefit from earlier screening, prevention, and/or intervention strategies. Biological risk factors may be static or dynamic depending on their susceptibility to modification. Nutritional and environmental risk factors are usually dynamic in nature and present the most robust area for prevention and intervention strategies.

Dynamic Risk Factors

Biological risk factors for obesity that are dynamic and responsive to prevention or intervention span the developmental trajectory. Maternal history of obesity, before or during pregnancy, increases the risk of obesity for the child (Li, Law, Conte, & Power, 2009; Whitaker, Wright, Pepe, Seidel, & Dietz, 1997). Maternal smoking during pregnancy is another perinatal risk factor increasing the likelihood of obesity in later childhood (von Kries, Toschke, Koletzko, & Slikker, 2002). Early childhood risk factors include rapid infant weight gain due to overfeeding (Taveras et al., 2009), especially if the infant was not breastfed (Yan, Liu, Zhu, Huang, & Wang, 2014). Insufficient sleep throughout childhood is another biological risk factor associated with increased risk of obesity (Wu, Gong, Zou, Li, & Zhang, 2017).

Nutritional factors typically represent an area for successful prevention and intervention strategies independent of the etiology of obesity. Nutritional risk factors include the amount, type, and timing of food consumed. Without appropriate supervision, children may take in excessive amounts of food either in one sitting or by grazing throughout the day. Excessive intake of sugar-sweetened beverages and low intake of fruits and vegetables are especially associated with future obesity. Skipping breakfast and dining out at fast-food restaurants have been linked to increased caloric intake and future risk for obesity in children, as has eating while watching television (Spear et al., 2007).

Environmental factors present opportunities for prevention and intervention on both an individual and community level. Physical inactivity, excessive screen time, and exposure to teasing or bullying are significant risk factors for obesity so much that the American Academy of Pediatrics (AAP) provides directives to clinicians on appropriate screening and anticipatory guidance for well-child visits. Poor access to nutritious foods is another contributing factor.

The AAP has historically provided strong recommendations for promoting daily exercise and time limits on watching television, playing computers, or using other personal electronic devices (Children, Adolescents, and the Media, 2013; Council on Communications and Media & Brown, 2011). The AAP recently revised some of these time-based recommendations but continues to provide guidance on limiting the negative effects of media usage on the health of children (Shifrin, Brown, Hill, Jana, & Flinn, 2015). Exposure to teasing and bullying, especially in school-aged children, is both an environmental risk factor for obesity and a consequence of weight stigma. Overweight and obese children are at increased risk for being teased (Haines, Neumark-Sztainer, Eisenberg, & Hannan, 2006), and weight-teasing behavior can lead to an increased risk for further weight gain (Neumark-Sztainer et al., 2002). Limited access to public parks or other safe areas for play within a child's neighborhood is associated with more inside time, less physical activity, and a greater risk of obesity (Singh, Siahpush, & Kogan, 2010). Health food deserts, areas with restricted access to fresh fruits and vegetables, are associated with increased caloric intake and the development of obesity (Pérez-Escamilla et al., 2012). Children in lower socioeconomic groups are disproportionately exposed to these environmental risk factors and are thus at greater risk for obesity (Ogden, Carroll, Fryar, & Flegal, 2015).

Static Risk Factors

Static risk factors for obesity are typically biological in nature and include perinatal factors, age, sex, ethnicity, and genetic code or phenotype. Static risk factors can contribute to the development of both primary and secondary obesity. Early biological factors that increase later development of obesity include exposure to gestational diabetes in utero (Dabelea et al., 2000) and short sleep duration as an infant (Taveras, Rifas-Shiman, Oken, Gunderson, & Gillman, 2008).

The NHANES data indicated more than double the rate for obesity in adolescents (20.5%) compared to that of preschoolers. The prevalence of obesity in adults continues to climb even higher. In the United States, males appear to have a higher incidence of obesity in all age groups (Kuller, 2014), and ethnicity has also been correlated with obesity rates. The prevalence of obesity in non-Hispanic Asian youth is the lowest at 8.6% and Hispanic youth the highest at 21.9%. Non-Hispanic white and black youth have prevalence rates of 14.7% and 19.5%, respectively (Ogden, Carroll, Fryar, & Flegal, 2015).

Abnormalities in genes associated with hypothalamic development and leptin regulation have been associated with increased obesity rates (Martos-Moreno et al., 2014). The presence of any developmental disability has been independently correlated with an increased risk of obesity (Bandini, Curtin, Hamad, Tybor, & Must, 2005), and several genetic syndromes and neurodevelopmental disabilities have been specifically implicated and are discussed in more depth below.

Other Risk Factors

Endocrine disorders, mental health disorders, and the use of certain medications are risk factors that fall somewhere between dynamic and static as they are not always modifiable. Endocrine disorders such as hypothyroidism and Cushing syndrome discussed above may be a direct cause or significant risk factor for the development of obesity, but effective treatment can mitigate this risk.

Children with mental health disorders have increased risk for overweight or obesity (Patel et al., 2007). A diagnosis of depression has been positively correlated with increased risk, which may be more significant among females as compared to males (de Wit et al., 2010). In a systematic review of longitudinal studies, Luppino et al. indicated a reciprocal link between depression and obesity where each increased the risk of the other (2010). Subsequently, Amare et al. postulated that the genetic overlap between mood disorders and cardiometabolic diseases may be due to pleiotropic genes and shared biological pathways (Amare, Schubert, Klingler-Hoffmann, Cohen-Woods, & Baune, 2017). Further increasing risks of children with psychiatric symptoms are the medications used to target those symptoms. Prescriptions for antipsychotics rose dramatically from 1996 to 2001, primarily due to increased prescription to children (Findling & McNamara, 2004; Patel et al., 2005). In addition to stimulating appetite, the use of antipsychotic medications is associated with other adverse metabolic effects such as glucose and lipid abnormalities and sedation (Correll, 2008). These effects directly contribute to increased caloric intake, decreased physical activity, and increased morbidity.

Developmental and Mental Health Disorders Commonly Associated with Obesity

Obesity and Developmental Disorders

Children with developmental disabilities (DD) are at increased risk for obesity compared to peers with typical development (L. Bandini et al., 2015; Grondhuis & Aman, 2014; Neumeier, Grosso, & Rimmer, 2017). The National Health and Nutrition Examination Survey (NHANES), National Health Interview Survey (NHIS), and National Survey of Children's Health (NSCH) monitor the prevalence of obesity in youth with all reporting increased risk for youth with developmental disabilities. Risk increase from the most recent NHANES, NHIS, and NSCH data was 35%, 59%, and 27%, respectively (L. Bandini et al., 2015). Numerous authors have highlighted the need for additional research regarding developmental disorders and obesity including disorder-specific growth and body composition standard measurements (Grondhuis & Aman, 2014; Lobstein et al., 2015; Polfuss et al., 2016). This is critical as standard growth measures may not reflect the trajectory of youth with developmental disorders. Children with developmental disabilities are at increased risk for nutritional deficiencies as well as obesity. To aid in developing a balanced diet for all children, the American Academy of Pediatrics website healthychildren.org offers basic nutrition information ("Nutrition", n.d.).

Monogenic Syndromes Associated with Obesity

While risk factors for obesity have a strong genetic component in all populations, increased obesity in youth with genetic disorders may be a genetic phenotype or an associated risk. Obesity is an associated risk in Down syndrome, Williams syndrome, and fragile X (Raspa, Bailey, Bishop, Holiday, & Olmsted, 2010). Prader-Willi is the most commonly known genetic syndrome associated with obesity as part of the phenotype. Other syndromes with phenotypic obesity include congenital leptin deficiency, Bardet-Biedl, Cohen syndrome, Albright hereditary osteodystrophy, WAGR syndrome, and Alström syndrome (Grondhuis & Aman, 2014; Gunay-Aygun, Cassidy, & Nicholls, 1997; Gurnani, Birken, & Hamilton, 2015). For comprehensive information on genetic disorders, the reader is referred to the NIH Genetic and Rare Diseases Information Center (rarediseases.info.nih.gov).

Prader-Willi Syndrome

Prader-Willi syndrome (PWS) affects 1 in 15–25,000 infants, and although rare, it is the leading genetic cause of morbid obesity in children (Butler, 2011; "Health Supervision for Children With Prader-Willi Syndrome", 2011; Ho & Dimitropoulos, 2010). The AAP recommendations for the care of children with PWS include behavioral interventions to control hyperphagia. Children with PWS are at risk for pica, choking, and eating to the point of stomach rupture ("Health Supervision for Children With Prader-Willi Syndrome", 2011). Psychotic symptoms are more common in PWS than any other DD; therefore, treatment with antipsychotic medications is common and may exacerbate obesity (Ho & Dimitropoulos, 2010). Growth charts for youth with PWS are available at Prader-Willi Syndrome Association website (pwsa, 2017).

Down Syndrome

Down syndrome (DS) affects 1 in 800–1000 infants. Children with DS are at increased risk for obesity and associated medical complications including heart disease and sleep apnea (Basil et al., 2016; Hoffmire, Magyar, Connolly, Fernandez, & van Wijngaarden, 2014; Wee et al., 2014). In a 2011 systematic review and meta-analysis of obesity in youth with ID, children and adolescents with DS were at almost twice the risk of obesity compared to the ID group (Maiano, 2011). The American Academy of Pediatrics (AAP) healthcare guideline for DS advises parent education and regular screening for obesity (Bull & Committee on Genetics, 2011). The growth pattern of youth with DS does not follow the standard growth curve for body mass to height (Zemel et al., 2015). The Down Syndrome Growing Up Study (DSGS) growth and BMI charts can be used to monitor persons with Down syndrome. The DSGS growth charts are available on the Centers for Disease Control website (CDC, 2017a, 2017b). There is some question regarding the utility of DS-specific growth charts in identifying cardiometabolic risk (CMR). The relationship between BMI and CMR in children with DS continues to be an area needing investigation (Hatch-Stein et al., 2016).

Williams Syndrome

Williams syndrome (WS) affects 1 in 7500 to 10,000 infants. Children with Williams syndrome experience an increased incidence of cognitive challenges, ADHD, and anxiety disorders which often require intervention (Pober, 2010). Due to an increased incidence of cardiovascular disease in children with WS, the AAP recommends obesity monitoring and education for all children with this genetic syndrome (Cunniff, Frias, Kaye, & Moeschler, 2001). The Williams Syndrome Association provides syndrome-specific growth charts to aid clinicians in screening youth with this syndrome ("Growth Charts", 2010).

Fragile X Syndrome

The Fragile X Clinical and Research Consortium (FXCRC) data has identified an increased rate of obesity in male youth with fragile X syndrome (FXS) compared to typically developing peers, finding 31% and 18%, respectively. Interestingly, this has not held true for adults with FXS (Raspa, Bailey, Bishop, Holiday, & Olmsted, 2010). Youth with FXS often have comorbid ASD or ADHD (Bagni, Tassone, Neri, & Hagerman, 2012) which are independent risk factors for obesity. A Prader-Willi syndrome subphenotype of FXS has been identified in a small number of individuals who develop hyperphagia between 2 and 8 years of age. Youth with the PWS subphenotype are more likely to qualify for a diagnosis of autism than FXS youth without the subphenotype (Martínez-Cerdeño et al., 2017; Nowicki, Tassone, Ferranti, Ono, & Hagerman, 2006).

Obesity and Other Developmental Disabilities

Autism Spectrum Disorder

From preschool years, persons with autism spectrum disorder (ASD) are at increased risk for a lifelong struggle with weight and associated health risks (Hill, Zuckerman, & Fombonne, 2015; Matson, Matson, & Beighley, 2011; Phillips et al., 2014). In a large study (*n* = 5053) of youth with ASD ages 2–17, overweight and obesity were identified in 33.6% and 18%, respectively (Hill, Zuckerman, & Fombonne, 2015). The National Health Interview Survey (*n* = 9619) found 31% of youth with autism to be severely overweight (Phillips et al., 2014). A comprehensive review of overweight and obesity in ASD conducted by Matheson and Douglas (2017) highlights the need for additional research in this area.

Numerous risk factors for obesity have been identified in youth with ASD including genetics, medication (antipsychotics and antiepileptic medications), disordered sleep, energy balance, sensory issues, feeding issues, and family issues (Matheson & Douglas, 2017; Must et al., 2014; Segal et al., 2016). Autism Speaks has created a toolkit for parents to address feeding issues ("[No title]", n.d.)). The Healthy Weight Research Network has developed a research agenda to explore family-based behavioral treatment (FBT) and other issues related to maintaining a healthy weight in youth with ASD (Curtin, Must, Phillips, & Bandini, 2017).

Fetal Alcohol Spectrum Disorder

Although growth deficiency is a criteria for the diagnosis of fetal alcohol spectrum disorder (FASD), Fuglestad reported overweight/obesity in 40% of children and 42% of adolescents with partial FASD (Fuglestad et al., 2014). Youth with FASD report "never feeling full," snack more than typically developing peers, and experience more mealtime challenging behaviors (Amos-Kroohs et al., 2016; Werts, Van Calcar, Wargowski, & Smith, 2014). Additional information on addressing growth and other challenges experienced by youth with FASD can be found in the AAP FASD Toolkit (Academy of Pediatrics, n.d.).

Cerebral Palsy

Cerebral palsy (CP) is a disorder of poor muscle control due to an abnormality of brain development which occurs before, during, or after delivery. The CDC has reported that approximately 1 in 323 children is diagnosed with CP (Christensen et al., 2014). CP may present as spastic, dystonic, or mixed with the dystonic and mixed types being associated with a greater tendency to be overweight (Pinto, Alves, Mendes, & Ciamponi, 2016). A group in the Netherlands studied data sets from 2004 to 2014 of 7- to 18-year olds with spastic CP and found a trend toward substantial body mass and that BMI increases over the 10-year period. Body mass and BMI were 26% and 20% higher, respectively, in youth with CP compared to 6% and 7% increases in typically developing youth (Zwinkels et al., 2017). In a more recent study of Australian ambulatory youth with CP, 7.3% were overweight and 12.1% obese which were comparable to typically developing youth (Pascoe, Thomason, Graham, Reddihough, & Sabin, 2016). A wide range of physical impairments are associated with CP, and the relatively small sample sizes may account for variability in these studies.

Intellectual Disability

The increased risk for obesity among youth with an intellectual disability (ID) is well established (Maiano, 2011; Matson, Matson, & Beighley, 2011; Segal et al., 2016). The pooled prevalence estimates for overweight/obesity were 30% in children and 33% in adolescents in the Maiano et al. meta-analysis. North American youth held the greatest risk compared to youth in Europe, Southeast Asia, and the Western Pacific, and adolescents with ID were at 1.8 times the risk for obesity compared to typically developing teens (Maiano, 2011). Similarly, an analysis of 2011 NSCH data also found 10–17-year olds with ID to be at 1.89 times greater risk for obesity than typically developing youth (Segal et al., 2016). The National Health Interview Survey ($n = 9619$) found that in the United States, approximately 20% of youth with ID meet criteria for obesity compared with 13% of typically developing youth (Phillips et al., 2014). The etiology of increased rates of overweight and obesity in people with ID is multifactorial. Biological and genetic factors such as lower metabolic rate and an increased rate of hypothyroidism (Bhaumik, Watson, Thorp, & McGrother, 2008) contribute as does the increased rate of antipsychotic medication administration for treatment of comorbid mental illness (Newcomer, 2005). People with ID may also experience lack of access to leisure facilities, transport issues, and less income (Messent, Cooke, & Long, 2009), all contributing to decreased ability to engage in physical activity. Food choices may also be a risk factor. Biswas noted a likelihood of people with ID to engage in high consumption of sugary foods and low consumption of fruits and vegetables (2010).

Obesity and Mental Health Symptoms

The association between childhood obesity and mental health symptoms and vice versa has been recurrently emphasized; however, additional research is needed to understand these complex relationships (Avila et al., 2015; Rajan & Menon, 2017; Small & Aplasca, 2016). Internalizing and externalizing symptoms and psychosocial challenges have been linked with later obesity (Small & Aplasca, 2016). A German study of youth (47 females and males, aged 15–21) receiving inpatient treatment for extreme obesity found rates of mood (40%), anxiety (29.8%), somatoform (14.9%), and eating disorders (17%) greater than that of controls, with 70% of obese youth having a psychiatric diagnosis and most qualifying for multiple diagnoses. Psychiatric disorder onset was typically after the onset of obesity (Britz et al., 2000).

A meta-analysis of longitudinal studies of adolescents with obesity and depression found a 40% increased risk of depression in obese youth and a 70% increased risk of obesity in youth with depression. The association was found in females and males but was greater in females (Mannan, Mamun, Doi, & Clavarino, 2016). Two prospective longitudinal studies following teens to adulthood (combined n = 9963) found that obesity at 14 years of age was predictive of depression in adulthood for females (Herva et al., 2006; Marmorstein, Iacono, & Legrand, 2014). Anxiety and depression were found to be associated with adolescent obesity in females in a New York community cohort (n = 776) (Anderson, Cohen, Naumova, Jacques, & Must, 2007). An Australian study (n = 2243) found an association between childhood (age 7–15 years) overweight/obesity and later depression in females as well, but not an association with future anxiety disorders (Sanderson, Patton, McKercher, Dwyer, & Venn, 2011).

Eating disorders (ED) commonly present during adolescence with crossover from one disorder to another being the rule rather than the exception. The World Health Organization Mental Health Surveys and National Comorbidity Survey Replication found the correlation between binge eating disorder (BED) and obesity to be 36.2% and 42.4%, respectively (Hudson, Hiripi, Pope Jr, & Kessler, 2007; Kessler et al., 2013). An adolescent eating disorders program at the Mayo Clinic cautions that youth presenting for ED treatment often have a history of obesity, citing 45% of youth with a history of obesity and highlighting the importance of screening for ED symptoms in all youth (Lebow, Sim, & Kransdorf, 2015; Sim, Lebow, & Billings, 2013). While both underweight and overweight children have reported being teased, those considered very overweight based on BMI are the most likely to be teased by their peers. Project EAT (Eating Among Teens) demonstrated that teasing not only lowers an adolescent's self-esteem but that it also predicts disordered eating behaviors 5 years later (Haines, Neumark-Sztainer, Eisenberg, & Hannan, 2006). Weight-related bullying is the major source of teasing. In a recent multinational study, 69% of respondents classified weight-based teasing as serious (Puhl et al., 2016). Furthermore, weight-based stigma has been linked to increased somatization, depression, and stressful peer relationships beginning in the early school years (Harrist et al., 2016).

Sleep is an often under-characterized problem in children and adolescents with mental health symptoms. Only about 27% of high school and middle school students receive the recommended sleep according to the Youth Risk Behavior Surveys (YRBS) (Wheaton, Jones, Cooper, & Croft, 2018). The American Academy of Pediatrics has issued a technical report highlighting obesity among the consequences of sleep deficiency (Owens, 2014). Further evidence of the significant association between insufficient sleep and obesity has been provided by a meta-analysis which pooled data from over 35,000 adolescents (Wu, Gong, Zou, Li, & Zhang, 2017). Metabolic changes and poor eating habits induced by insufficient sleep have been implicated as factors increasing obesity in youth (Ogilvie et al., 2018; Sayin & Buyukinan, 2016). Sleep disorders including night eating syndrome, sleep apnea, and insomnia have been associated with obesity (Dikeos & Georgios, 2011).

Recommendations for Screening and Assessment

Screening for Obesity

Early problematic weight patterns are a predictor of increased morbidity later in life (Screening for Obesity in Children and Adolescents: US Preventive Services Task Force Recommendation Statement, 2010); therefore, early recognition of individuals at risk for obesity is key. The instrument should be easily accessible and simple to use and require minimal training in order to assure reliable use and consistency among clinical sites. Optimal characteristics of any screening instrument include ease of use combined with a high sensitivity. Having high sensitivity means that the screening instrument captures as close to 100% of the at-risk population as possible. The clinician can then further assess those individuals who screen positive for additional signs and symptoms of the condition.

Body mass index (BMI) is widely recognized as the primary screening instrument for obesity in adults. For children, the BMI percentile is used to compare BMI to population norms. BMI is a measure of weight in kilograms divided by height in meters squared (kg/m2), which suggests the proportionality of the individual (Skinner et al., 2014). BMI has been correlated with more invasive, time-consuming, and expensive measures of body fat such as skinfold thickness, bioelectrical impedance, and underwater weighting (Freedman, Horlick, & Berenson, 2013 Wohlfahrt-Veje et al., 2014). Body mass (also referred to as weight) and height measurements can be obtained during a clinical visit, and BMI is then calculated based on those values. The CDC provides recommendations for accurately measuring height and weight in a nonmedical setting (CDC, 2015b).

To measure height, the CDC recommends:

1. Remove the child or teen's shoes, bulky clothing, and hair ornaments, and unbraid the hair that interferes with the measurement.
2. Take the height measurement on flooring that is not carpeted and against a flat surface such as a wall with no molding.
3. Have the child or teen stand with the feet flat, together, and against the wall. Make sure the legs are straight, arms are at sides, and shoulders are level.
4. Make sure the child or teen is looking straight ahead and that the line of sight is parallel with the floor.
5. Take the measurement while the child or teen stands with the head, shoulders, buttocks, and heels touching the flat surface (wall). Depending on the overall body shape of the child or teen, all points may not touch the wall.
6. Use a flat headpiece to form a right angle with the wall, and lower the headpiece until it firmly touches the crown of the head.
7. Make sure the measurer's eyes are at the same level as the headpiece.
8. Lightly mark where the bottom of the headpiece meets the wall. Then, use a metal tape to measure from the base on the floor to the marked measurement on the wall to get the height measurement.
9. Accurately record the height to the nearest 1/8th inch or 0.1 centimeter.

The CDC recommends to measure weight using a digital scale on firm flooring after removal of shoes and any heavy clothing. The individual being measured should stand with both feet in the center of the scale. Weight is recorded to the nearest decimal fraction (i.e., 25.6 kilograms). The CDC also provides a BMI calculator for children and teens aged 2–19 (CDC, n.d.) to input these values. It is important to specify both age and gender of the individual in the calculation of BMI. After calculating the BMI, the clinician can use an age-, gender-, and often disability-normed growth chart to determine the BMI percentile and whether the patient is considered underweight, healthy weight, overweight, or obese for their age (Klein et al., 2010). The American Academy of Pediatrics (AAP) recommends annual screening for overweight and obesity beginning at the age of 2 (Barlow, 2007). It is essential to understand that while BMI can be helpful in recognizing those children at risk for or currently meeting criteria for obesity, an elevated BMI confers a need for further diagnostic assessment to determine the cause, whether primary or secondary, and to characterize the pertinent static and dynamic risk factors. Further assessment beyond the BMI calculation will provide pertinent details to support the development of an effective strategy for weight management and lowering the child's future risk of associated conditions.

Further Assessment of Contributory Factors for Obesity

When a child screens positive for overweight (85th percentile for BMI) or obesity (95th percentile for BMI), further assessment is required to identify the pertinent contributory factors. The goals of further assessment are to accurately diagnose the cause of obesity and to lay the groundwork for an effective intervention plan. Initial assessment should focus both on classifying the condition as primary or secondary and characterizing the biological, nutritional, and environmental factors in play. Over the course of the assessment, risk factors should be categorized as static or dynamic to further aid in the development of an appropriately targeted intervention. All children should be screened for age, biological sex, ethnicity, and socioeconomic status due to the increased rates of obesity dependent on these factors (Kuller, 2014; Ogden, Carroll, Fryar, & Flegal, 2015).

Assessment for Primary Exogenous Obesity

Most children presenting for further assessment after a positive obesity screen will meet criteria for primary exogenous obesity (Martos-Moreno et al., 2014). Because the factors contributing to primary exogenous obesity can exacerbate obesity independent of the cause, this is a good place to start in the assessment of all children with obesity. Primary exogenous obesity is due to a constellation of biological, nutritional, and environmental factors, and thus the assessment should begin with an investigation into each of these.

Biological Assessment

Biological assessment includes an investigation into family history of overweight or obesity including biological parents and siblings (Li, Law, Conte, & Power, 2009; Whitaker, Wright, Pepe, Seidel, & Dietz, 1997). The answers to these questions may signify a genetic predisposition to obesity. An assessment of developmental risk factors for primary exogenous obesity also includes questions about in utero exposure to gestational diabetes (Dabelea et al., 2000), maternal smoking during pregnancy (von Kries, Toschke, Koletzko, & Slikker, 2002), initial birth weight, whether the child received breast milk or formula (Yan, Liu, Zhu, Huang, & Wang, 2014), and weight gain during early childhood (Trasande, Liu, Fryer, & Weitzman, 2009).

Any mental health symptom may signify an increased risk for or consequence of obesity (Avila et al., 2015; Rajan & Menon, 2017; Small & Aplasca, 2016). This appears especially true for depressive symptoms (Mannan, Mamun, Doi, & Clavarino, 2016). Thus a thorough psychological evaluation of mood and other mental health symptoms, to include associated eating-disordered behaviors, is appropriate for all children presenting with overweight or obesity. It is also important to assess the child for his or her personal feelings about weight stigma.

A thorough assessment of sleep habits and quality is warranted, due to the effects of insufficient sleep on eating habits and metabolic changes (Sayin & Buyukinan, 2016). Sleep assessment should first determine if the child feels well rested during the day by inquiring about daytime fatigue and/or the need for daytime napping in a child older than preschool age. The clinician should assess for delayed sleep onset due to family engagements, lack of sleep hygiene and routine, and use of television or access to cellular phone while in bed. Parents or guardians are typically better suited to provide information regarding behaviors during sleep time such as snoring, apneic events, or abnormal leg movements (Moturi & Avis, 2010). The BEARS acronym can be helpful for initial assessment of sleep problems (Owens & Dalzell, 2005). The acronym stands for bedtime resistance/sleep onset delay; excessive daytime sleepiness; awakenings at night; regularity, patterns, and duration of sleep; and snoring and other symptoms.

Nutritional Assessment

A nutritional assessment should focus on both the type and amount of the food the child consumes on a regular basis and the social behaviors associated with mealtimes for the child and family. The clinician can begin by asking what the child's favorite meals are. In addition, it is helpful to assess what beverages are consumed for meals and snacks and the frequency, timing, length, and location of meals and snacks. Nutritional assessment should also include typical preparation methods used when cooking at home, cultural and ethnic family eating practices, and the current or past use of special diets (Hillou, 2017). Frequency of dining out and watching television during mealtimes are family mealtime practices that can greatly increase caloric intake (Colapinto, Fitzgerald, Taper, &

Veugelers, 2007Spear et al., 2007) and should be part of the nutritional assessment.

Environmental Assessment

Each child's environment is unique and thus requires an individualized assessment and some creativity on the part of the clinician. An environmental assessment will likely intertwine with both the biological and nutritional assessment. For example, taking a history of family obesity not only provides information about possible genetic predisposition to obesity, but it may also signify that the family regularly consumes high-fat/high-calorie foods. Furthermore, this may indicate that child is not exposed to healthy weight modeling (Faith, Scanlon, Birch, Francis, & Sherry, 2004) or that the family has limited access to healthy food choices.

As part of an environmental assessment for obesity, the clinician should investigate the child's daily physical activity and family exercise habits in addition to the amount of time spent using electronic devices during which the child is not significantly active. The clinician should also inquire regarding the child's relationship with parents and peers. Family psychological distress and negative interactions during mealtimes may contribute to utilizing food as a coping mechanism or other unhealthy attitudes toward food. Assessing peer relationships, including being bullied or bullying others, is part of all mental health assessments. The American Academy of Pediatrics has issued a policy statement calling upon healthcare providers to screen for testing in youth who are overweight and to be leaders in promoting healthy behaviors rather than stigmatizing obesity (Golden et al., 2016; Pont et al., 2017).

Assessment of the greater environment is also important so that the clinician will not recommend a strategy that is not achievable by the child and family. The clinician should ask where the family typically shops for food and what food choices are available within their weekly food budget. It is helpful to characterize the child's neighborhood as well regarding access to public parks and other safe areas for play.

Assessment of Primary Monogenic Obesity

Weight-related issues in addition to a developmental delay could be a sign of a genetic mutation as the cause of or contributing factor for obesity. Pertinent questions would target a history of delay in developmental milestones, difficulties in school, age of onset of weight gain, and any history of hyperphagia or lack of satiety. Assessment of the physical appearance of the child can point to a monogenic cause for obesity. Short stature or other phenotypic patterns such as elongated or elfin facies may suggest a genetic condition as a cause for weight abnormalities.

Assessment of Secondary Obesity

When evaluating the possibility of obesity as secondary to another illness or medication, the clinician should inquire about current medical illness requiring surveillance or treatment and current medication regimen. It is also useful to obtain a history of any illnesses or disease conditions for which the child has previously been treated and what medications they have been prescribed. The clinician is then able to formulate a timeline of medical symptoms and treatments to which the onset and/or exacerbation of weight gain can be temporally compared. Consideration of any history of illnesses that could result in obesity, like hypothyroidism or Cushing syndrome, in first- or second-degree relatives may suggest secondary obesity even if the child has yet to be diagnosed with any such illness.

Assessment Tools

Psychological assessment tools are important for clinical assessment and research. See Table 2. The clinician relies on tools to evaluate patients entering treatment and track response over time. Research informs clinical practice, demanding validated instruments that produce reliable results across time and populations. Many domains have been identified as relevant to obesity including body image perception, hunger, dietary intake, and activity level (Beechy, Galpern, Petrone, & Das, 2012). In addition, the stage of change or readiness for treatment is a critical part of the assessment

Table 2 Useful psychotropic measures

Instrument	Description
Readiness and Motivation Interview for Families (RMI-Family) (Ball et al., 2017)	Semistructured interview to determine readiness for treatment. Domains include treat foods, overeating, emotional eating, total physical activity, and screen time
Adolescent Sedentary Activity Questionnaire (ASAQ) (Hardy, Booth, & Okely, 2007)	Self-recorded activity log
3-Day Physical Activity Recall (Weston, Petosa, & Pate, 1997)	Youth code activity and intensity of activity on a log divided into 30-minute time intervals
The Child Eating Behavior Questionnaire (CEBQ) (Carnell & Wardle, 2007)	35-item parent report with 8 scales including emotional overeating
Questionnaire on Eating and Weight Patterns (QEWP) (Yanovski, Marcus, Wadden, & Timothy Walsh, 2014)	32-item self-report measure including loss of control eating and body silhouettes for self-identification, child and adolescent versions
Automated Self-Administered 24-Hour (ASA24®) Dietary Assessment Tool (Subar et al., 2012)	Standardized format for obtaining dietary intake. A version is available for children and adolescents
Body Figure Perception Scales (Collins & Elizabeth Collins, 1991)	Youth identify perceived or desired body using pictograms
SCOFF (Morgan, 2000)	Five-question quick screen for the core features of anorexia nervosa and bulimia nervosa. All weight-related assessments should screen for eating disorders

(Geller et al., 2015; Junne et al., 2016). Finally, all assessments should include screening for eating disorders. The five-question, SCOFF questionnaire has been designed for rapid screening for eating disorders (Morgan, 2000).

Medical Assessment

Regardless of the type of obesity identified during the assessment, it is appropriate to coordinate with the child's medical clinician for screening and monitoring of cholesterol, diabetes, and other medical sequelae of obesity. Medical clinicians could also assist with genetic testing if a monogenic cause is suspected but has not been affirmed or with screening and management in the case of secondary obesity.

Prevention and Intervention Strategies

Interventions are focused on modifying dynamic risk factors identified during the assessment and should proceed in a person- and culturally sensitive manner. Parents find the terms "fat" and "obese" objectionable and prefer "weight" or "unhealthy weight" when discussing their children (Puhl, Peterson, & Luedicke, 2011). Latino parents prefer "too much weight for his/her health or demasiado pesa para su salud" (Turer, Montaño, Lin, Hoang, & Flores, 2014). The use of motivational interviewing to determine parental and youth treatment goals and readiness for change is a patient-driven approach that respects individual preferences and reduces weight stigma (Daniels, Hassink, & Committee on Nutrition, 2015; Lock & Hillier, 2010; Perrin, Finkle, & Benjamin, 2007). Clinicians may provide education on healthy weight and assist the family in targeting lifestyle changes before considering more intensive therapies. Strategies for increased physical activity should be implemented. Exercise is necessary for a healthy lifestyle and has been associated with improved school performance and increased self-esteem (Martin et al., 2018). Parents may be referred to the USDA MyPlate website for family-friendly nutritional guidance ("MyPlate | Food and Nutrition Service", n.d.)). For more comprehensive dietary information, a dietitian should be consulted. For clinicians who wish to include evidence-based weight treatments, parent-only or family-based behavioral treatments addressing diet, activity level, and environmental factors with behavioral strategies have shown success (Altman & Wilfley, 2015). In very rare cases, weight loss surgery may be considered for more mature teens (Styne et al., 2017).

Acknowledgements Sarah Mallard Wakefield extends her special thanks to Ankit Chalia and Anu Vallabhaneni while Joshua Sanderson would like to thank Adina Suss for their contribution to the writing of this chapter.

Bibliography

[No title]. (n.d.). Retrieved January 19, 2018, from http://www.autismspeaks.org/sites/default/files/docs/sciencedocs/atn/feeding_guide.pdf

Altman, M., & Wilfley, D. E. (2015). Evidence update on the treatment of overweight and obesity in children and adolescents. *Journal of Clinical Child and Adolescent Psychology, 44*(4), 521–537.

Amare, A. T., Schubert, K. O., Klingler-Hoffmann, M., Cohen-Woods, S., & Baune, B. T. (2017). The genetic overlap between mood disorders and cardiometabolic diseases: A systematic review of genome wide and candidate gene studies. *Translational Psychiatry, 7*(1), e1007. https://search.proquest.com/docview/1862248629. https://doi.org/10.1038/tp.2016.261

American Academy of Pediatrics. (n.d.). FASD Expert Panel. *AAP FASD Toolkit. Aap. Org/fasd. Accessed.*

American Thyroid Association. (n.d.). Hypothyroid (Underactive). Retrieved February 3, 2018, from www.thyroid.org/hypothyroidism/

Amos-Kroohs, R. M., Fink, B. A., Smith, C. J., Chin, L., Van Calcar, S. C., Wozniak, J. R., & Smith, S. M. (2016). Abnormal eating behaviors are common in children with fetal alcohol Spectrum disorder. *The Journal of Pediatrics, 169*, 194–200.e1.

Anderson, S. E., Cohen, P., Naumova, E. N., Jacques, P. F., & Must, A. (2007). Adolescent obesity and risk for subsequent major depressive disorder and anxiety disorder: Prospective evidence. *Psychosomatic Medicine, 69*(8), 740–747.

August, G. P., Caprio, S., Fennoy, I., Freemark, M., Kaufman, F. R., Lustig, R. H., ... Endocrine Society. (2008). Prevention and treatment of pediatric obesity: An endocrine society clinical practice guideline based on expert opinion. *The Journal of Clinical Endocrinology and Metabolism, 93*(12), 4576–4599. https://doi.org/10.1210/jc.2007-2458

Avila, C., Holloway, A. C., Hahn, M. K., Morrison, K. M., Restivo, M., Anglin, R., & Taylor, V. H. (2015). An overview of links between obesity and mental health. *Current Obesity Reports, 4*(3), 303–310.

Ayaso-Maneiro, J., Domínguez-Prado, D. M., & García-Soidan, J. L. (2014). Influence of weight loss therapy programs in body image self-perception in adults with intellectual disabilities. *International Journal of Clinical and Health Psychology, 14*(3), 178–185.

Bagni, C., Tassone, F., Neri, G., & Hagerman, R. (2012). Fragile X syndrome: Causes, diagnosis, mechanisms, and therapeutics. *The Journal of Clinical Investigation, 122*(12), 4314–4322.

Ball, G. D. C., Spence, N. D., Browne, N. E., O'Connor, K., Srikameswaran, S., Zelichowska, J., ... Geller, J. (2017). The readiness and motivation interview for families (RMI-family) managing pediatric obesity: Study protocol. *BMC Health Services Research, 17*(1), 261.

Bandini, L., Danielson, M., Esposito, L. E., Foley, J. T., Fox, M. H., Frey, G. C., ... Humphries, K. (2015). Obesity in children with developmental and/or physical disabilities. *Disability and Health Journal, 8*(3), 309–316.

Bandini, L. G., Curtin, C., Hamad, C., Tybor, D. J., & Must, A. (2005). Prevalence of overweight in children with developmental disorders in the continuous National Health and nutrition examination survey (NHANES) 1999–2002. *The Journal of Pediatrics, 146*(6), 738–743. https://doi.org/10.1016/j.jpeds.2005.01.049

Bandini, L. G., Fleming, R. K., Scampini, R., Gleason, J., & Must, A. (2013). Is body mass index a useful measure of excess body fatness in adolescents and young adults with down syndrome? *Journal of Intellectual Disability Research, 57*(11), 1050–1057.

Barlow, S. E. (2007). Expert committee recommendations regarding the prevention, assessment, and treatment of child and adolescent overweight and obesity: Summary report. *Pediatrics, 120*(6), S164. https://doi.org/10.1542/peds.2007-2329c

Biswas, A.B., Vahabzadeh, A., Hobbs, T., Healy, J.M. (2010). Obesity in people with learning disabilities: possible causes and reduction interventions. *Nurs Times. 106*:16–8.

Basil, J. S., Santoro, S. L., Martin, L. J., Healy, K. W., Chini, B. A., & Saal, H. M. (2016). Retrospective study of obesity in children with down syndrome. *The Journal of Pediatrics, 173*, 143–148.

Beechy, L., Galpern, J., Petrone, A., & Das, S. K. (2012). Assessment tools in obesity — Psychological measures, diet, activity, and body composition. *Physiology & Behavior, 107*(1), 154–171.

Bioulac, S., Lode-Kolz, K., Micoulaud-Franchi, J.-A., Chalumeau, F., Monteyrol, P.-J., & Philip, P. (2017). Is it attention deficit hyperactivity disorder, sleep disorder breathing... or both? *Sleep Medicine, 40*, e37.

Bhaumik, S., Watson, J. M., Thorp, C. F., Tyrer, F. and McGrother, C. W. (2008). Body mass index in adults with intellectual disability: distribution, associations and service implications: a population-based prevalence study. *Journal of Intellectual Disability Research*, 52:287–298. doi:10.1111/j.1365-2788.2007.01018.x

Britz, B., Siegfried, W., Ziegler, A., Lamertz, C., Herpertz-Dahlmann, B. M., Remschmidt, H., ... Hebebrand, J. (2000). Rates of psychiatric disorders in a clinical study group of adolescents with extreme obesity and in obese adolescents ascertained via a population based study. *International Journal of Obesity and Related Metabolic Disorders, 24*(12), 1707–1714.

Bull, M. J., & Committee on Genetics. (2011). Health supervision for children with down syndrome. *Pediatrics, 128*(2), 393–406.

Butler, M. G. (2011). Prader-Willi syndrome: Obesity due to genomic imprinting. *Current Genomics, 12*(3), 204–215.

Carnell, S., & Wardle, J. (2007). Measuring behavioural susceptibility to obesity: Validation of the child eating behaviour questionnaire. *Appetite, 48*(1), 104–113.

CDC. (2015a). *About child & teen BMI*. Retrieved February 4, 2018, from https://www.cdc.gov/healthyweight/assessing/bmi/childrens_bmi/about_childrens_bmi.html

CDC. (2015b). *Measuring children's height and weight accurately at home*. Retrieved February 3, 2018, from https://www.cdc.gov/healthyweight/assessing/bmi/childrens_bmi/measuring_children.html

CDC. (2017a). *Childhood obesity facts: Prevalence of childhood obesity in the United States, 2011–2014*. Retrieved January 26, 2018, from https://www.cdc.gov/obesity/data/childhood.html

CDC. (2017b, Sept 7). Growth Charts | Down Syndrome | Birth Defects | NCBDDD | CDC. Retrieved January 9, 2018, from https://www.cdc.gov/ncbddd/birthdefects/downsyndrome/growth-charts.html

CDC. (n.d.). *BMI percentile calculator for child and teen*. Retrieved February 3, 2018, from https://nccd.cdc.gov/dnpabmi/Calculator.aspx

Children, Adolescents, and the Media. (2013). Council on communications and media. *Pediatrics, 132*(5), 958–961. https://doi.org/10.1542/peds.2013-2656

Christensen, D., Van Naarden Braun, K., Doernberg, N. S., Maenner, M. J., Arneson, C. L., Durkin, M. S., … Yeargin-Allsopp, M. (2014). Prevalence of cerebral palsy, co-occurring autism spectrum disorders, and motor functioning – Autism and developmental disabilities monitoring network, USA, 2008. *Developmental Medicine and Child Neurology, 56*(1), 59–65.

Colapinto, C. K., Fitzgerald, A., Taper, L. J., & Veugelers, P. J. (2007). Children's preference for large portions: Prevalence, determinants, and consequences. *Journal of the Academy of Nutrition Dietitics, 107*(7), 1183–1190.

Collins, M. E., & Elizabeth Collins, M. (1991). Body figure perception scale. *PsycTESTS Dataset*. https://doi.org/10.1037/t31645-000

Correll, C. U. (2008). Antipsychotic use in children and adolescents: Minimizing adverse effects to maximize outcomes. *FOCUS The Journal of Lifelong Learning in Psychiatry, 6*, 368–378.

Council on Communications and Media, & Brown, A. (2011). Media use by children younger than 2 years. *Pediatrics, 128*(5), 1040–1045. https://doi.org/10.1542/peds.2011-1753

Cunniff, C., Frias, J. L., Kaye, C. I., & Moeschler, J. (2001). *Health care supervision for children with Williams syndrome*. Retrieved from https://arizona.pure.elsevier.com/en/publications/health-care-supervision-for-children-with-williams-syndrome

Curtin, C., Must, A., Phillips, S., & Bandini, L. (2017). The healthy weight research network: A research agenda to promote healthy weight among youth with autism spectrum disorder and other developmental disabilities. *Pediatric Obesity, 12*(1), e6–e9.

Dabelea, D., Hanson, R. L., Lindsay, R. S., Pettitt, D. J., Imperatore, G., Gabir, M. M., … Knowler, W. C. (2000). Intrauterine exposure to diabetes conveys risks for type 2 diabetes and obesity: A study of discordant sibships. *Diabetes, 49*(12), 2208–2211. https://doi.org/10.2337/diabetes.49.12.2208

Daniels, S. R., Arnett, D. K., Eckel, R. H., Gidding, S. S., Hayman, L. L., Kumanyika, S., … Williams, C. L. (2005). Overweight in children and adolescents: Pathophysiology, consequences, prevention, and treatment. *Circulation, 111*(15), 1999–2012. https://doi.org/10.1161/01.CIR.0000161369.71722.10

Daniels, S. R., Hassink, S. G., & Committee On Nutrition. (2015). The role of the pediatrician in primary prevention of obesity. *Pediatrics, 136*(1), e275–e292.

De Hert, M., & D, V. (2011). Guidelines for screening and monitoring of cardiometabolic risk in schizophrenia: Systematic evaluation. *British Journal of Psychiatry, 199*, 99–105.

De Wit, L., Luppino, F., van Straten, A., Penninx, B., Zitman, F., & Cuijpers, P. (2010). Depression and obesity: A meta-analysis of community-based studies. *Psychiatry Research, 178*(2), 230–235. https://www.sciencedirect.com/science/article/pii/S016517810900170X. https://doi.org/10.1016/j.psychres.2009.04.015

de Wit, L., Luppino, F., van Straten, A., Penninx, B., Zitman, F., & Cuijpers, P. (2010). Depression and obesity: A meta-analysis of community-based studies. *Psychiatry Research, 178*(2), 230–235. https://doi.org/10.1016/j.psychres.2009.04.015

Demattia, L., Lemont, L., & Meurer, L. (2007). Do interventions to limit sedentary Behaviours change behaviour and reduce childhood obesity. *Obesity Reviews, 8*(1), 69–81.

Dikeos, D., & Georgios, G. (2011). Medical comorbidity of sleep disorders. *Current Opinion in Psychiatry, 24*(4), 346–354.

Eden, K., & Randle-Phillips, C. (2017). Exploration of body perception and body dissatisfaction in young adults with intellectual disability. *Research in Developmental Disabilities, 71*, 88–97.

Faith, M. S., Scanlon, K. S., Birch, L. L., Francis, L. A., & Sherry, B. (2004). Parent-child feeding strategies and their relationships to child eating and weight status. *Obesity Research, 12*(11), 1711–1722. https://doi.org/10.1038/oby.2004.212

Findling, R. L., & McNamara, N. K. (2004). Atypical antipsychotics in the treatment of children and adolescents: Clinical applications. *The Journal of Clinical Psychiatry, 65*(Suppl 6), 30–44.

Finkelstein, E. A., Graham, W. C., & Malhotra, R. (2014). Lifetime direct medical costs of childhood obesity. *Pediatrics, 133*(5), 854–862.

Finkelstein, E. A., & Trogdon, J. G. (2008). Public health interventions for addressing childhood overweight: Analysis of a business. *American Journal of Public Health, 98*(3), 411–415.

Fitch, A., Fox, C., Gross, A., Heim, C., Judge-Dietz, J., Kauffman, T., ... Webb, B. (2013). *Institute for clinical systems improvement: Prevention and management of obesity for children and adolescents*. Retrieved February 2, 2018 from https://www.icsi.org/_asset/tn5cd5/ObesityChildhood.pdf

Freedman, D. S., Horlick, M., & Berenson, G. S. (2013). A comparison of the slaughter skinfold-thickness equations and BMI in predicting body fatness and cardiovascular disease risk factor levels in children. *The American Journal of Clinical Nutrition, 98*(6), 1417–1424.

Fuglestad, A. J., Boys, C. J., Chang, P.-N., Miller, B. S., Eckerle, J. K., Deling, L., ... Wozniak, J. R. (2014). Overweight and obesity among children and adolescents with fetal alcohol spectrum disorders. *Alcoholism, Clinical and Experimental Research, 38*(9), 2502–2508.

Geller, J., Avis, J., Srikameswaran, S., Zelichowska, J., Dartnell, K., Scheuerman, B., ... Ball, G. (2015). Developing and pilot testing the readiness and motivation interview for families in pediatric weight management. *Canadian Journal of Dietetic Practice and Research: A Publication of Dietitians of Canada, 76*(4), 190–193.

Golden, N. H., Schneider, M., Wood, C., Committee On Nutrition, Committee On Adolescence, & Section On Obesity. (2016). Preventing obesity and eating disorders in adolescents. *Pediatrics, 138*(3), e20161649–e20161649.

Goodman, E., & Whitaker, R. (2002). A prospective study of the role of depression in the development and persistence of adolescent obesity. *Pediatrics, 110*(3). https://doi.org/10.1542/peds.110.3.497

Grondhuis, S. N., & Aman, M. G. (2014). Overweight and obesity in youth with developmental disabilities: A call to action. *Journal of Intellectual Disability Research, 58*(9), 787–799.

Growth Charts. (2010, January 26). Retrieved January 10, 2018, from http://williams-syndrome.org/growth-charts/growth-charts

Gunay-Aygun, M., Cassidy, S. B., & Nicholls, R. D. (1997). Prader-Willi and other syndromes associated with obesity and mental retardation. *Behavior Genetics, 27*(4), 307–324.

Guo, S. S., Wu, W., Chumlea, W. C., & Roche, A. F. (2002). Predicting overweight and obesity in adulthood from body mass index values in childhood and adolescence. *The American Journal of Clinical Nutrition, 76*(3), 653–658. https://doi.org/10.1093/ajcn/76.3.653

Gurnani, M., Birken, C., & Hamilton, J. (2015). Childhood obesity: Causes, consequences, and management. *Pediatric Clinics of North America, 62*(4), 821–840.

Haines, J., Neumark-Sztainer, D., Eisenberg, M. E., & Hannan, P. J. (2006). Weight teasing and disordered eating behaviors in adolescents: Longitudinal findings from project EAT (eating among teens). *Pediatrics, 117*(2), 209–215.

Hardy, L. L., Booth, M. L., & Okely, A. D. (2007). The reliability of the adolescent sedentary activity questionnaire (ASAQ). *Preventive Medicine, 45*(1), 71–74.

Harrist, A. W., Swindle, T. M., Hubbs-Tait, L., Topham, G. L., Shriver, L. H., & Page, M. C. (2016). The social and emotional lives of overweight, obese, and severely obese children. *Child Development, 87*(5), 1564–1580.

Hatch-Stein, J. A., Zemel, B. S., Prasad, D., Kalkwarf, H. J., Pipan, M., Magge, S. N., & Kelly, A. (2016). Body composition and BMI growth charts in children with down syndrome. *Pediatrics, 138*(4). https://doi.org/10.1542/peds.2016-0541

Herva, A., Laitinen, J., Miettunen, J., Veijola, J., Karvonen, J. T., Läksy, K., & Joukamaa, M. (2006). Obesity and depression: Results from the longitudinal northern Finland 1966 birth cohort study. *International Journal of Obesity, 30*(3), 520–527.

Hill, A. P., Zuckerman, K. E., & Fombonne, E. (2015). Obesity and autism. *Pediatrics, 136*(6), 1051–1061.

Hillou, F. (2017). Pediatric nutrition assessment. International Pediatric Summit, Dubai. Retrieved February 3, 2018 from http://www.ipsummit.me/ips-pdf/Pediatric-Nutrition-Assessment-Final-Farah.pdf

Ho, A. Y., & Dimitropoulos, A. (2010). Clinical management of behavioral characteristics of Prader-Willi syndrome. *Neuropsychiatric Disease and Treatment, 6*, 107–118.

Hoffmire, C. A., Magyar, C. I., Connolly, H. V., Fernandez, I. D., & van Wijngaarden, E. (2014). High prevalence of sleep disorders and associated comorbidities in a community sample of children with down syndrome. *Journal of Clinical Sleep Medicine, 10*(4), 411–419.

Hudson, J. I., Hiripi, E., Pope, H. G., Jr., & Kessler, R. C. (2007). The prevalence and correlates of eating disorders in the National Comorbidity Survey Replication. *Biological Psychiatry, 61*(3), 348–358.

Junne, F., Ziser, K., Mander, J., Martus, P., Denzer, C., Reinehr, T., ... Ehehalt, S. (2016). Development and psychometric validation of the "parent perspective University of Rhode Island Change Assessment-short" (PURICA-S) questionnaire for the application in parents of children with overweight and obesity. *BMJ Open, 6*(11), e012711.

Kelly, A. S., Barlow, S. E., Rao, G., Inge, T. H., Hayman, L. L., Steinberger, J., ... Council on Clinical Cardiology. (2013). Severe obesity in children and adolescents: Identification, associated health risks, and treatment approaches: A scientific statement from the American Heart Association. *Circulation, 128*, 1689–1712.

Kessler, R. C., Berglund, P. A., Chiu, W. T., Deitz, A. C., Hudson, J. I., Shahly, V., ... Xavier, M. (2013). The prevalence and correlates of binge eating disorder in the World Health Organization world mental health surveys. *Biological Psychiatry, 73*(9), 904–914.

Kim, S., Huang, A., Snowman, A., & Snyder, S. (2007). Antipsychotic drug-induced weight gain mediated by histamine H1 receptor-linked activation. *Proceedings of the National Academy of Sciences*.

Klein, J. D., Sesselberg, T. S., Johnson, M. S., O'Connor, K. G., Cook, S., Coon, M., ... Washington, R. (2010). Adoption of body mass index guidelines for screening and counseling in pediatric practice. *Pediatrics, 125*(2), 265–272. https://doi.org/10.1542/peds.2010-1130

Krebs, N. F., Himes, J. H., Jacobson, D., Nicklas, T. A., Guilday, P., & Styne, D. (2007). Assessment of child and adolescent overweight and obesity. *Pediatrics, 120*(Supplement), S228. https://doi.org/10.1542/peds.2007-2329D

Kuller, L. H. (2014). Incidence of childhood obesity in the United States. *The New England Journal of Medicine, 370*(17), 1659 Retrieved from http://www.ncbi.nlm.nih.gov/pubmed/24758624

Lebow, J., Sim, L. A., & Kransdorf, L. N. (2015). Prevalence of a history of overweight and obesity in adolescents with restrictive eating disorders. *Journal of Adolescent Health Care: Official Publication of the Society for Adolescent Medicine, 56*(1), 19–24.

Li, L., Law, C., Conte, R. L., & Power, C. (2009). Intergenerational influences on childhood body mass index: The effect of parental body mass index trajectories. *The American Journal of Clinical Nutrition, 89*(2), 551–557. https://doi.org/10.3945/ajcn.2008.26759

Lobstein, T., Jackson-Leach, R., Moodie, M. L., Hall, K. D., Gortmaker, S. L., Swinburn, B. A., ... McPherson, K. (2015). Child and adolescent obesity: Part of a bigger picture. *The Lancet, 385*(9986), 2510–2520.

Lock, K., & Hillier, R. (2010). The prevention of childhood obesity in primary care settings: Evidence and practice. In E. Walters, B. Swinburn, J. Seidell, & R. Uauy (Eds.), *Preventing childhood obesity* (pp. 94–104). West Sussex: Blackwell pub.

Luppino, F. S., de Wit, L. M., Bouvy, P. F., Stijnen, T., Cuijpers, P., Penninx, B. W. J. H., & Zitman, F. G. (2010). Overweight, obesity, and depression: A systematic review and meta-analysis of longitudinal studies. *Archives of General Psychiatry, 67*(3), 220–229. https://doi.org/10.1001/archgenpsychiatry.2010.2

Lurie, A., & Lurie, R. H. (2018). *Health promotion and public education*. Retrieved from www.clocc.net/.

Maiano, C. (2011). Prevalence and risk factors of overweight and obesity among children and adolescents with intellectual disabilities. *Obesity Reviews: An Official Journal of the International Association for the Study of Obesity*. Retrieved from http://onlinelibrary.wiley.com/doi/10.1111/j.1467-789X.2010.00744.x/full

Mannan, M., Mamun, A., Doi, S., & Clavarino, A. (2016). Prospective associations between depression and obesity for adolescent males and females- a systematic review and meta-analysis of longitudinal studies. *PLoS One, 11*(6), e0157240.

Marmorstein, N. R., Iacono, W. G., & Legrand, L. (2014). Obesity and depression in adolescence and beyond: Reciprocal risks. *International Journal of Obesity, 38*(7), 906–911.

Martin, A., Booth, J. N., Laird, Y., Sproule, J., Reilly, J. J., & Saunders, D. H. (2018). Physical activity, diet and other behavioural interventions for improving cognition and school achievement in children and adolescents with obesity or overweight. *Cochrane Database of Systematic Reviews., 1*, CD009728. https://doi.org/10.1002/14651858.cd009728.pub3

Martínez-Cerdeño, V., Lechpammer, M., Noctor, S., Ariza, J., Hagerman, P., & Hagerman, R. (2017). FMR1 premutation with Prader-Willi phenotype and fragile X-associated tremor/ataxia syndrome. *Clinical Case Reports, 5*(5), 625–629.

Martos-Moreno, et al. (2014). Principles and pitfalls in the differential diagnosis and management of childhood. *Advances in Nutrition, 5*(3), 299S–305S. https://doi.org/10.3945/an.113.004853 PMID- 24829481 http://www.ncbi.nlm.nih.gov/pubmed/26633046

Matheson, B. E., & Douglas, J. M. (2017). Overweight and Obesity in Children with Autism Spectrum Disorder (ASD): a Critical Review Investigating the Etiology, Development, and Maintenance of this .... *Journal of Autism and Developmental Disorders*. Retrieved from http://link.springer.com/article/10.1007/s40489-017-0103-7

Matson, M. L., Matson, J. L., & Beighley, J. S. (2011). Comorbidity of physical and motor problems in children with autism. *Research in Developmental Disabilities, 32*(6), 2304–2308.

Mayo Clinic. (2018). *Cushing syndrome*. www.mayoclinic.org/diseases-conditions/cushing-syndrome/symptoms-causes/syc-20351310. Retrieved February 3, 2018.

Messent, P. R., Cooke, C. B., Long, J. (2009). Primary and secondary barriers to physically active healthy lifestyles for adults with learning disabilities. *Disability and Rehabilitation, 21*:9, 409–419, DOI:10.1080/096382899297396

Morgan, J. F. (2000). The SCOFF questionnaire: A new screening tool for eating disorders. *The Western Journal of Medicine, 172*(3), 164–165.

Moturi, S., & Avis, K. (2010). Assessment and treatment of common pediatric sleep disorders. *Psychiatry (Edgmont), 7*(6), 24–37.

Must, A., Curtin, C., Hubbard, K., Sikich, L., Bedford, J., & Bandini, L. (2014). Obesity prevention for children with developmental disabilities. *Current Obesity Reports, 3*(2), 156–170.

MyPlate | Food and Nutrition Service. (n.d.). Retrieved February 5, 2018, from https://www.fns.usda.gov/tn/myplate

Nader, P. R. (2006). Identifying risk for obesity in early childhood. *Pediatrics, 118*(3), 594–601.

Neumark-Sztainer, D., Falkner, N., Story, M., Perry, C., Hannan, P. J., & Mulert, S. (2002). Weight-teasing among adolescents: Correlations with weight status and disordered eating behaviors. *International Journal of Obesity and Related Metabolic Disorders, 26*(1), 123–131.

Neumeier, W. H., Grosso, C., & Rimmer, J. H. (2017). Obesity and Individuals with Intellectual and Developmental Disabilities. Retrieved from http://rrtcadd.org/wp-content/uploads/2017/09/2017_0923_obesity_brief.pdf

Newcomer, J.W. (2005). CNS Drugs 19(Suppl 1): 1. https://doi.org/10.2165/00023210-200519001-00001

Nowicki, S. T., Tassone, F., Ferranti, J., Ono, M. Y., & Hagerman, R. J. (2006). 69 the Prader-Willi clinical Subphenotype of fragile x syndrome. *Journal of Investigative Medicine, 54*(1), S91.4–S9S91.

Nutrition. (n.d.). Retrieved January 19, 2018, from http://www.healthychildren.org/english/healthy-living/nutrition/pages/default.aspx

Ogden, C. L., Carroll, M. D., Fryar, C. D., & Flegal, K. M. (2015). Prevalence of obesity among adults and youth: United States, 2011–2014. *NCHS Data Brief,* (219), 1. Retrieved from http://www.ncbi.nlm.nih.gov/pubmed/26633046

Ogden, C. L., Carroll, M. D., Lawman, H. G., Fryar, C. D., Kruszon-Moran, D., Kit, B. K., & Flegal, K. M. (2016). Trends in obesity prevalence among children and adolescents in the United States, 1988–1994 through 2013–2014. *Journal of the American Medical Association, 315*(21), 2292–2299. https://doi.org/10.1001/jama.2016.6361. http://www.ncbi.nlm.nih.gov/pubmed/11773541. https://doi.org/10.1542/peds.109.1.45

Ogden, C. L., Kuczmarski, R. J., Flegal, K. M., & Mei, Z. (2002). Centers for disease control and prevention 2000 growth charts for the United States: Improvements to the 1977 National Center for Health Statistics Version. *Pediatrics, 109*(1), 45–60. https://doi.org/10.1542/peds.109.1.45

Ogilvie, R. P., Lutsey, P. L., Widome, R., Laska, M. N., Larson, N., & Neumark-Sztainer, D. (2018). Sleep indices and eating behaviours in young adults: Findings from project EAT. *Public Health Nutrition, 21*(4), 689–701.

Olvera, R. L., Williamson, D. E., Fisher-Hoch, S. P., Vatcheva, K. P., & McCormick, J. B. (2015). Depression, obesity, and metabolic syndrome: Prevalence and risks of comorbidity in a population-based representative sample of Mexican Americans. *The Journal of Clinical Psychiatry, 76*(10), e1300 Retrieved from http://www.ncbi.nlm.nih.gov/pubmed/26528653

Owens, J. (2014). Adolescent Sleep Working Group, And Committee On Adolescence. Insufficient sleep in adolescents and young adults: An update on causes and consequences. *Pediatrics, 134*(3), e921–e932.

Owens, J. A., & Dalzell, V. (2005). Use of the "BEARS" sleep screening tool in a pediatric residents' continuity clinic: A pilot study. *Sleep Medicine, 6*(1), 63–69.

Park, K.-J., Woo, J. S., Jeong, S. S., & Yi, J. H. (2012). Continuous. *The Korean Journal of Thoracic and Cardiovascular Surgery, 45*(1), 19–23. http://synapse.koreamed.org/search.php?where=aview&id=10.5090%2Fkjtcs.2012.45.1.19&code=1051KJTCS&vmode=FULL. https://doi.org/10.5090/kjtcs.2012.45.1.19

Pascoe, J., Thomason, P., Graham, H. K., Reddihough, D., & Sabin, M. A. (2016). Body mass index in ambulatory children with cerebral palsy: A cohort study. *Journal of Paediatrics and Child Health, 52*(4), 417–421.

Patel, N., Hariparsad, M., Matias-Akthar, M., Sorter, M. T., Barzman, D. H., Morrison, J. A., ... MP, D. B. (2007). Body mass indexes and lipid profiles in hospitalized children and adolescents exposed to atypical antipsychotics. *Journal of Child and Adolescent Psychopharmacology, 17*(3), 303–311.

Patel, N. C., Crismon, M. L., Hoagwood, K., Johnsrud, M. T., Rascati, K. L., Wilson, J. P., & Jensen, P. S. (2005). Trends in the use of typical and atypical antipsychotics in children and adolescents. *Journal of the American Academy of Child and Adolescent Psychiatry, 44*, 548–556.

Pérez-Escamilla, R., Obbagy, J. E., Altman, J. M., Essery, E. V., McGrane, M. M., Wong, Y. P., ... Williams, C. L. (2012). Dietary energy density and body weight in adults and children: A systematic review. *Journal of the Academy of Nutrition and Dietetics, 112*(5), 671–684 https://doi.org/10.1016/j.jand.2012.01.020

Perrin, E. M., Finkle, J. P., & Benjamin, J. T. (2007). Obesity prevention and the primary care pediatrician's office. *Current Opinion in Pediatrics, 19*(3), 354–361.

Phillips, K. L., Schieve, L. A., Visser, S., Boulet, S., Sharma, A. J., Kogan, M. D., ... Yeargin-Allsopp, M. (2014). Prevalence and impact of unhealthy weight in a national sample of US adolescents with autism and other learning and behavioral disabilities. *Maternal and Child Health Journal, 18*(8), 1964–1975.

Pinto, V. V., Alves, L. A. C., Mendes, F. M., & Ciamponi, A. L. (2016). The nutritional state of children and adolescents with cerebral palsy is associated with oral motor dysfunction and social conditions: A cross sectional study. *BMC Neurology, 16*, 55.

Pober, B. R. (2010). Williams-Beuren syndrome. *The New England Journal of Medicine, 362*(3), 239–252.

Polfuss, M., Papanek, P., Meyer-Wentland, F., Moosreiner, A., Wilkas, L. R., & Sawin, K. J. (2016). Body composition measurement in children with cerebral palsy, Spina bifida and spinal cord injury: A systematic review of the literature. *Comprehensive Child and Adolescent Nursing, 39*(3), 166–191.

Pont, S. J., Puhl, R., Cook, S. R., Slusser, W., Section On Obesity, & Obesity Society. (2017). Stigma experienced by children and adolescents with obesity. *Pediatrics, 140*(6). https://doi.org/10.1542/peds.2017-3034

Puhl, R. M., & Heuer, C. A. (2009). The stigma of obesity: A review and update. *Obesity, 17*, 941–964. https://doi.org/10.1038/oby.2008.636

Puhl, R. M., Latner, J. D., O'Brien, K., Luedicke, J., Forhan, M., & Danielsdottir, S. (2016). Cross-national perspectives about weight-based bullying in youth: Nature, extent and remedies. *Pediatric Obesity, 11*(4), 241–250.

Puhl, R. M., Peterson, J. L., & Luedicke, J. (2011). Parental perceptions of weight terminology that providers use with youth. *Pediatrics, 128*(4), e786–e793.

pwsa. (2017, January 6). Important Medical Growth Charts – Prader-Willi Syndrome Association (USA). Retrieved January 10, 2018, from http://www.pwsausa.org/important-medical-growth-charts/

Rajan, T. M., & Menon, V. (2017). Psychiatric disorders and obesity: A review of association studies. *Journal of Postgraduate Medicine, 63*(3), 182–190.

Raspa, M., Bailey, D. B., Bishop, E., Holiday, D., & Olmsted, M. (2010). Obesity, food selectivity, and physical activity in individuals with fragile X syndrome. *American Journal on Intellectual and Developmental Disabilities, 115*(6), 482–495.

Riggs, N. R., Sakuma, K. L., & Pentz, M. A. (2007). Preventing risk for obesity by promoting self-regulation and decision-making skills: Pilot results from the PATHWAYS to health program (PATHWAYS). *Evaluation Review, 31*(3), 287–310.

Sanderson, K., Patton, G. C., McKercher, C., Dwyer, T., & Venn, A. J. (2011). Overweight and obesity in childhood and risk of mental disorder: A 20-year cohort study. *The Australian and New Zealand Journal of Psychiatry, 45*(5), 384–392.

Sayin, F. K., & Buyukinan, M. (2016). Sleep duration and media time have a major impact on insulin resistance and metabolic risk factors in obese children and adolescents. *Childhood Obesity, 12*(4), 272–278.

Screening for Obesity in Children and Adolescents: US Preventive Services Task Force Recommendation Statement. (2010). US preventive services task force. *Pediatrics, 25*(2), 361–367. https://doi.org/10.1542/peds.2009-2037

SE, M. C., & Committee on Genetics. (2011). Clinical report—Health supervision for children with Prader-Willi syndrome. *Pediatrics, 127*(1), 195–204.

Sedky, K., Bennett, D. S., & Carvalho, K. S. (2014). Attention deficit hyperactivity disorder and sleep disordered breathing in pediatric populations: A meta-analysis. *Sleep Medicine Reviews, 18*(4), 349–356.

Segal, M., Eliasziw, M., Phillips, S., Bandini, L., Curtin, C., Kral, T. V. E., … Must, A. (2016). Intellectual disability is associated with increased risk for obesity in a nationally representative sample of US. children. *Disability and Health Journal, 9*(3), 392–398.

Shifrin, D., Brown, A., Hill, D., Jana, L., & Flinn, S. K. (2015). Growing up digital: Media research symposium. *American Academy of Pediatrics*. Retrieved from: https://www.aap.org/en-us/Documents/digital_media_symposium_proceedings.pdf

Sim, L. A., Lebow, J., & Billings, M. (2013). Eating disorders in adolescents with a history of obesity. *Pediatrics, 132*(4), e1026–e1030.

Singh, G. K., Siahpush, M., & Kogan, M. D. (2010). Neighborhood socioeconomic conditions, built environments, and childhood obesity. *Health Affairs, 29*(3), 503–512. https://doi.org/10.1377/hlthaff.2009.0730

Skinner AC, Skelton JA. Prevalence and trends in obesity and severe obesity among children in the United States, 1999–2012. JAMA Pediatr. 2014;168(6):561–566. doi:10.1001/jamapediatrics.2014.21

Skinner, A. C., Perrin, E. M., Moss, L. A., & Skelton, J. A. (2015). Cardiometabolic risks and severity of obesity in children and young adults. *New England Journal of Medicine, 373*(14), 1307–1317. https://doi.org/10.1056/NEJMoa1502821

Skinner, A. C., Perrin, E. M., & Skelton, J. A. (2016). Prevalence of obesity and severe obesity in US children, 1999–2014. *Obesity (Silver Spring, Md.), 24*(5), 1116–1123. http://www.ncbi.nlm.nih.gov/pubmed/27112068. https://doi.org/10.1002/oby.21497

Small, L., & Aplasca, A. (2016). Child obesity and mental health. *Child and Adolescent Psychiatric Clinics of North America, 25*(2), 269–282.

Sondike, S. B., Copperman, N., & Jacobson, M. S. (2003). Effects of a low-carbohydrate diet on weight loss and cardiovascular risk factor in overweight adolescents. *Journal of Pediatrics, 142*(3), 253–258.

Spear, B. A., Barlow, S. E., Ervin, C., Ludwig, D. S., Saelens, B. E., Schetzina, K. E., & Taveras, E. M. (2007). Recommendations for treatment of child and adolescent overweight and obesity. *Pediatrics, 120*(Supplement), S288. http://pediatrics.aappublications.org/cgi/content/abstract/120/Supplement_4/S254. https://doi.org/10.1542/peds.2007-2329F

Stunkard, A. (2000). Old and new scales for the assessment of body image. *Perceptual and Motor Skills, 90*(3 Pt 1), 930.

Styne, D. M., Arslanian, S. A., Connor, E. L., Farooqi, I. S., Murad, M. H., Silverstein, J. H., & Yanovski, J. A. (2017). Pediatric obesity-assessment, treatment, and prevention: An Endocrine Society clinical practice guideline. *The Journal of Clinical Endocrinology and Metabolism, 102*(3), 709–757.

Subar, A. F., Kirkpatrick, S. I., Mittl, B., Zimmerman, T. P., Thompson, F. E., Bingley, C., … Potischman, N. (2012). The automated self-administered 24-hour dietary recall (ASA24): A resource for researchers, clinicians, and educators from the National Cancer Institute. *Journal of the Academy of Nutrition and Dietetics, 112*(8), 1134–1137.

Taveras, E. M., Rifas-Shiman, S. L., Belfort, M. B., Kleinman, K. P., Oken, E., & Gillman, M. W. (2009). Weight status in the first 6 months of life and obesity at 3 years of age. *Pediatrics, 123*(4), 1177–1183. http://pediatrics.aappublications.org/cgi/content/abstract/123/4/1177. https://doi.org/10.1542/peds.2008-1149

Taveras, E. M., Rifas-Shiman, S. L., Oken, E., Gunderson, E. P., & Gillman, M. W. (2008). Short sleep duration in infancy and risk of childhood overweight. *Archives of Pediatrics & Adolescent Medicine, 162*(4), 305–311. https://doi.org/10.1001/archpedi.162.4.305

Trasande, L., Liu, Y., Fryer, G., & Weitzman, M. (2009). Effects of childhood obesity on hospital care and costs, 1999–2005. *Health Aff (Millwood), 28*(4), W751–W760.

Trogdon, J. G., Finkelstein, E. A., Feagan, C. W., & Cohen, J. W. (2012). State- and payer-specific estimates of annual medical expenditures attributable to obesity. *Obesity (Silver Spring), 20*(1), 214–220. https://doi.org/10.1038/oby.2011.169 Epub 2011 June 16.

Turer, C. B., Montaño, S., Lin, H., Hoang, K., & Flores, G. (2014). Pediatricians' communication about weight with overweight Latino children and their parents. *Pediatrics, 134*(5), 892–899.

Utzinger, L. M., Gowey, M. A., Zeller, M., Jenkins, T. M., Engel, S. G., Rofey, D. L., ... Teen Longitudinal Assessment of Bariatric Surgery (Teen-LABS) Consortium. (2016). Loss of control eating and eating disorders in adolescents before bariatric surgery. *The International Journal of Eating Disorders, 49*(10), 947–952.

von Kries, R., Toschke, A. M., Koletzko, B., & Slikker, W. (2002). Maternal smoking during pregnancy and childhood obesity. *American Journal of Epidemiology, 156*(10), 954–961. http://www.ncbi.nlm.nih.gov/pubmed/12419768. https://doi.org/10.1093/aje/kwf128

Wang, Y., & Lim, H. (2012). The global childhood obesity epidemic and the association between socio-economic status and childhood obesity. *International Review of Psychiatry, 24*(3), 176–188. http://www.ncbi.nlm.nih.gov/pubmed/22724639. https://doi.org/10.3109/09540261.2012.688195

Washington, R. (2012). New National Heart, Lung, and Blood Institute integrated cardiovascular guidelines: Management of Pediatric Obesity. *Pediatric Annals, 41*, e127–e133. https://doi.org/10.3928/00904481-20120625-07

Wee, S. O., Pitetti, K. H., Goulopoulou, S., Collier, S. R., Guerra, M., & Baynard, T. (2014). Impact of obesity and down syndrome on peak heart rate and aerobic capacity in youth and adults. *Research in Developmental Disabilities, 36C*, 198–206.

Werts, R. L., Van Calcar, S. C., Wargowski, D. S., & Smith, S. M. (2014). Inappropriate feeding behaviors and dietary intakes in children with fetal alcohol spectrum disorder or probable prenatal alcohol exposure. *Alcoholism, Clinical and Experimental Research, 38*(3), 871–878.

Weston, A. T., Petosa, R., & Pate, R. R. (1997). Validation of an instrument for measurement of physical activity in youth. *Medicine and Science in Sports and Exercise, 29*(1), 138–143.

Wheaton, A. G., Jones, S. E., Cooper, A. C., & Croft, J. B. (2018). Short sleep duration among middle school and high school students — United States, 2015. *MMWR. Morbidity and Mortality Weekly Report, 67*(3), 85–90.

Whitaker, R. C., Wright, J. A., Pepe, M. S., Seidel, K. D., & Dietz, W. H. (1997). Predicting obesity in young adulthood from childhood and parental obesity. *The New England Journal of Medicine, 337*(13), 869–873. https://doi.org/10.1056/NEJM199709253371301

WHO. (2009). *Obesity and overweight.* http://www.who.int/mediacentre/factsheets/fs311/en/

WHO. (2018a). *Global strategy on diet, physical activity, and health: Childhood overweight and obesity.* Retrieved January 30, 2018, from http://www.who.int/dietphysicalactivity/childhood/en/

WHO. (2018b). *Global strategy on diet, physical activity, and health: Why does childhood overweight and obesity matter?* Retrieved January 30, 2018, from http://www.who.int/dietphysicalactivity/childhood_consequences/en/

WHO. (2018c). *Health topics: Obesity.* Retrieved January 30, 2018, from http://www.who.int/topics/obesity/en/

Wohlfahrt-Veje, C., Tinggaard, J., Winther, K., Mouritsen, A., Hagen, C. P., Mieritz, M. G., ... Main, K. M. (2014). Body fat throughout childhood in 2647 healthy Danish children: Agreement of BMI, waist circumference, skinfolds with dual X-ray absorptiometry. *European Journal of Clinical Nutrition, 68*(6), 664–670.

Wu, Y., Gong, Q., Zou, Z., Li, H., & Zhang, X. (2017). Short sleep duration and obesity among children: A systematic review and meta-analysis of prospective studies. *Obesity Research & Clinical Practice, 11*(2), 140–150.

Yan, J., Liu, L., Zhu, Y., Huang, G., & Wang, P. P. (2014). The association between breastfeeding and childhood obesity: A meta-analysis. *BMC Public Health, 14*(1), 1267. http://www.ncbi.nlm.nih.gov/pubmed/25495402. https://doi.org/10.1186/1471-2458-14-1267

Yanovski, S. Z., Marcus, M. D., Wadden, T. A., & Timothy Walsh, B. (2014). The questionnaire on eating and weight Patterns-5: An updated screening instrument for binge eating disorder. *The International Journal of Eating Disorders, 48*(3), 259–261.

Zemel, B. S., Pipan, M., Stallings, V. A., Hall, W., Schadt, K., Freedman, D. S., & Thorpe, P. (2015). Growth charts for children with down syndrome in the United States. *Pediatrics, 136*(5), e1204–e1211.

Zwinkels, M., Takken, T., Ruyten, T., Visser-Meily, A., Verschuren, O., & Sport-2-Stay-Fit study group. (2017). Body mass index and fitness in high-functioning children and adolescents with cerebral palsy: What happened over a decade? *Research in Developmental Disabilities, 71*, 70–76.

Assessment of Toileting Problems

Esther Hong and Johnny L. Matson

Introduction

Individuals with intellectual and developmental disabilities experience impairments in a wide range of skill areas including adaptive, motor, cognitive, social, and motor skills. Adaptive behavior includes a wide range of abilities such as self-care, daily living, occupational, and safety skills. Deficits in adaptive skills can significantly limit socialization, independent living, and overall quality of life (Kroeger & Sorensen-Burnworth, 2009; Matson & LoVullo, 2009). Toilet training is a crucial developmental milestone for learning adaptive and prosocial skills and achieving independence. Despite its significance, toilet training has been somewhat neglected in the adaptive behavior research (Matson, Horovitz, & Sipes, 2011).

Assessment of a child's level of adaptive functioning should be conducted prior to the initiation of toilet training to ensure that the child possesses the prerequisite skills to successfully master toileting skills. The assessment may consist of a review of the child's developmental and medical history, structured and semi-structured interviews with the primary caregiver(s), rating scales, checklists, and/or standardized measures. A comprehensive evaluation of the information collected during the assessment process should be used to guide training procedure decisions and to set realistic training goals. This chapter will review the methods and measures available to assess for toileting and other related skills. Additional considerations for the evaluation of toilet training readiness will be discussed.

Enuresis and Encopresis

There is a dearth of research addressing the assessment and evaluation of toileting problems (Matson, Neal, Hess, & Kozlowski, 2011). To further complicate this issue, definitions used to describe incontinent behavior vary considerably across the existing literature. For example, Matson and LoVullo (2009) found that the terms "encopresis," "soiling," and "constipation" were used interchangeably, with no clear distinctions in definition in regard to treatment implications.

The *Diagnostic and Statistical Manual of Mental Disorders*, Fifth Edition (DSM-5; American Psychiatric Association [APA], 2013), provides specific diagnostic criteria for two types of elimination disorders: enuresis and encopresis. Individuals meet criteria for enuresis if they exhibit the following diagnostic features: (a) repeated voiding of urine into bed or clothes,

E. Hong (✉) · J. L. Matson
Department of Psychology, Louisiana State University, Baton Rouge, LA, USA
e-mail: ehong1@lsu.edu

whether involuntary or intentional; (b) voiding of urine must occur at least twice a week for at least 3 consecutive months or must cause clinically significant distress or impairment in social, academic, or other important areas of functioning; (c) chronological age is at least 5 years (or a mental age of 5 years for children with developmental delays); and (d) urinary incontinence is not attributable to the physiological effects of a substance or another medical condition. Individuals who meet the diagnostic criteria for enuresis are given a subtype of "nocturnal only" (i.e., passage of urine only during nighttime sleep), "diurnal only" (i.e., passage of urine during waking hours), or "nocturnal and diurnal" (i.e., a combination of the nocturnal and diurnal subtypes).

Individuals meet criteria for encopresis if they exhibit the following diagnostic features: (a) repeated passage of feces into inappropriate places (e.g., clothing, floor), whether involuntary or intentional; (b) at least one such event occurs each month for at least 3 months; (c) chronological age is at 4 years old (or a mental age of 4 years for children with developmental delays); and (d) the fecal incontinence is not attributable to the psychological effects of a substance or another medical condition except through a mechanism involving constipation. Individuals who meet the diagnostic criteria of encopresis are given a subtype of "with constipation and overflow incontinence" (i.e., there is evidence of constipation on physical examination or by history) or "without constipation and overflow incontinence" (i.e., there is no evidence of constipation on physical examination or by history).

Assessment of Toileting Problems

While cultural factors influence age norms for toilet training, toilet training is usually initiated when the child is around 2–3 years of age (Schum et al., 2002), with some children showing readiness to train as early as 18 months (Brazelton, 1962). By 3–4 years of age, most typically developing children achieve daytime and nighttime continence (Brazelton, 1962; Cocchiola Jr., Martino, Dwyer, & Demezzo, 2012; Heron, Joinson, Croudace, & von Gontard, 2008). By definition, children with intellectual or developmental disabilities lag behind their typically developing peers (Matson & LoVullo, 2009) and exhibit impairments across a range of skill domains; toileting problems are common in this population. As a result, individuals with intellectual and developmental disabilities face more obstacles to toilet training and may begin toilet training at a later age than their typically developing peers.

To assess for adaptive functioning and other factors contributing to toileting problems, a comprehensive assessment, including a medical examination, clinical interview, and collection of baseline behavioral data (Dalrymple & Ruble, 1992), may be warranted. The medical assessment can rule out potential physiological causes of incontinence and is especially important for individuals with certain developmental disabilities or genetic conditions. For example, some individuals with cerebral palsy have unique urinary problems due to hypotonia in the muscles that control the bladder (Cocchiola Jr. & Redpath, 2017), which would warrant a medical or pharmacological intervention rather than a behavioral one.

A clinical interview with the primary caregiver can provide valuable information regarding the child's toileting behavior and potential functions of these behaviors. The structure of the clinical interviews can vary across individual cases, as they should be customized to address the parent or primary caregivers' concerns and the skills and deficits of each child. Using rating scales, checklist, semi-structured interviews, and/or standardized measures, the clinician can assess for the child's functioning across multiple skill domains (e.g., language, adaptive, motor, cognition) as well as for challenging behaviors that may be interfering with toilet training procedures. This is particularly important when assessing for prerequisite skills to toilet training, which will be discussed in detail later in this chapter.

During the interview, the clinician should also assess for several primary caregiver factors that contribute to successful toilet training. Some caregiver factors related to successful toilet training include level of motivation, the ability to notice the subtle cues and behaviors of their child, and consistent and reliable implementation of the behavioral methods of toilet training (Kroeger & Sorensen, 2010). Primary caregivers are a crucial part of the toilet training process because they are the ones who are responsible for the implementation and monitoring of toilet training procedures (Kroeger, Weber, & Smith, 2017). Further, caregivers of children with intellectual and developmental disabilities may need additional training on behavioral principles and contingencies, so their ability to receive training and feedback should be considered. In addition, caregivers of children with autism spectrum disorder (ASD) face more challenges during toilet training because they must identify and respond to the nuanced needs of their children by, for example, reading their child's nonverbal cues indicating toileting behavior (Kasari, Sigman, Mundy, & Yirmiya, 1988). As such, the strengths and weaknesses of primary caregivers should be considered when determining toilet training procedures.

Lastly, the assessment should incorporate baseline data of the child's toileting behaviors. Baseline data are needed to get a sense of the child's toileting problems prior to the training but are also necessary to monitor the child's progress and training effectiveness. The caregiver may be asked by the clinician to take data on the frequency of incontinence occurrences, latency between occurrences, setting of successful and unsuccessful voids, and ratings of stool consistencies (Chase, Homsy, Siggaard, Sit, & Bower, 2004). Primary caregivers may also be asked to report on the types of challenging behaviors observed during toilet training attempts. Taken together, these data provide a good picture of the child's toileting problems and can be used to select the appropriate toilet training protocol. Specific measurement methods will be discussed later in the chapter.

It is important to note that when assessing for toileting problems in children with intellectual and developmental disabilities, the diagnosis should be guided by developmental age, not by chronological age. A variety of other factors should also be considered during the assessment, as the initiation of toilet training and types of procedures used are influenced by cultural, familial, historical (Warzak, Kennedy, & Bond, 2017), and many other variables.

Early assessment and intervention of toileting problems are crucial in achieving long-term success in toileting training. That is, the earlier toileting problems are identified and treated, the better the outcome for successful continence. Singh, Masey, and Morton (2006) found that children who were not toilet-trained by age 8 were not likely to retain continence later in life. Further, unsuccessful toilet training has been associated with decreased learning in adaptive and prosocial domains. A comprehensive assessment of developmental, behavioral, and physical readiness should be conducted in a timely manner to determine the appropriate time to initiate toilet training (Warzak, Kennedy, & Bond, 2017).

Prerequisite Skills

During the assessment, the clinician should also assess for certain prerequisite skills that are necessary for successful toilet training. The American Academy of Pediatrics (AAP, 1998) recommended that parents should not push their child into toilet training unless the child is developmentally ready or shows signs of readiness. Child readiness was described using the three-force model: (1) physiologic maturation (e.g., able to sit, walk, dress, undress), (2) external feedback (i.e., understands and responds to instruction), and (3) internal feedback (e.g., motivation, desire to imitate). That is, the child should have prerequisite adaptive, motor, language, social, and cognition skills prior to the initiation of toilet training.

Other researchers evaluating the prerequisite skills for toilet training individuals with intellectual and developmental disabilities also recommended assessing for similar prerequisite skills (Baker & Brightman, 1997; Kroeger &

Sorensen-Burnworth, 2009). In their review of the existing literature, Kroeger and Sorensen (2010) found that the following prerequisite skills were stated as "necessary" skills to initiate toilet training: (1) regular urinary and bowel voiding, with infrequent dribbling, (2) child is able to void urine in large amount, (3) child demonstrated ability to sit on the toilet, and (4) absence of counter-indicated medical conditions. Warzak, Kennedy, and Bond (2017) also reported on the commonly suggested prerequisite skills (from Harris, 2004; Foxx & Azrin, 1973; Frauman & Brandon, 1996). These skills included the following: (a) physiological readiness (e.g., normal bladder capacity, sits independently, perceives full bladder), (b) one to two bowel movements per day, (c) periods of time between voids, (d) recognizes being wet or soiled, (e) motor abilities (e.g., dexterity, walking), (f) pulls pants up and down, (g) imitates behavior, (h) follows directions, (i) unafraid of toilet or flush, (j) understands words for elimination, and (k) understands the social expectations that bladder emptying takes place in toilet.

Many children with intellectual and developmental disabilities may not have many of these prerequisite skills due to impairments in the adaptive, motor, language, social, and cognition skill domains. Of these prerequisite skills, the ability to follow and comply with instructions may be one of the most crucial skills for successful toilet training. In particular, children with ASD may experience more difficulties in regard to compliance with the toileting procedures if other core features of ASD (i.e., repetitive, restricted, repetitive patterns of behavior or interests; deficits in social communication; APA, 2013) have not been addressed. If restricted, repetitive behaviors and/or interests are not addressed prior to toilet training, certain toileting interventions, such as reinforcement-based interventions, may not be effective. That is, the reinforcement the child receives from repetitive behavior itself may be more reinforcing than the reinforcement received from appropriate toileting behavior (Cocchiola Jr. & Redpath, 2017).

In addition, many individuals with ASD, as well as individuals with intellectual and developmental disabilities, exhibit challenging behaviors (e.g., noncompliance, aggression, self-injurious behavior, tantrum; Jang, Dixon, Tarbox, & Granpeesheh, 2011), which may interfere with toilet training. If a child is exhibiting high rates of noncompliance and challenging behaviors during toilet training, the clinician may consider putting the training procedure on hold, in order to conduct an assessment of the topography and function of the challenging behaviors. Toilet training should resume only after the challenging behaviors have been managed and/or decreased.

Assessment Measures

At the time this chapter was written, there were no diagnostic measures designed to assess enuresis or encopresis. Toileting problems are usually assessed using informal methods under the umbrella of adaptive or daily living skills (Matson & LoVullo, 2009). One exception is the Profile of Toileting Issues (POTI), which was designed to screen for toileting problems in individuals with intellectual disabilities.

Profile of Toileting Issues (POTI)

The *Profile of Toileting Issues* (*POTI*; Matson, Dempsey, & Fodstad, 2010) was designed to screen for toileting problems in individuals with intellectual disabilities between the ages of 4 years through adulthood who are suspected of having a diagnosis of enuresis or encopresis. The POTI is a 56-item checklist scale that is completed by a clinician, with the individual's primary caregiver serving as the respondent. Respondents are asked to rate items regarding toileting, accidents, social/emotional problems, and physical problem. Based on the caregiver's report, items are scored as "X," does not apply; "0," no problem present; or "1," problem present. A total POTI score is calculated by summing the responses (i.e., 0 or 1). Higher total scores indicate more significant toileting issues. The POTI can also assess for potential functions of toileting issues, such as pain, social difficulties, motor issues, noncompliance, and medical conditions (Matson et al., 2011). The POTI was found to have strong internal consistency and good interrater reliability (Matson et al., 2011).

Matson and colleagues (2011) found that the most commonly endorsed items among 108 adults with intellectual and developmental disabilities included items regarding supplements and medication (i.e., requires the use of fiber supplements/laxatives to defecate [68.6%], on a medication with a known side effect of constipation [66%]) and incontinence (i.e., has toileting accidents during the day [60.1%], has had wet underwear in the past month [57.5%], has toileting accidents during the night [54.9%], has had soiled underwear in the past month [49.7%]).

The authors also evaluated the relationship between the frequency of endorsed items and participant characteristics. Specifically, level of intellectual impairment (i.e., profound, severe, moderate, or mild), ambulatory ability, fiber or laxative use, and verbal ability were evaluated. A significantly higher total POTI score was found among participants who had more severe levels of intellectual disability than those who were non-ambulatory, using fiber or laxatives, and nonverbal. These findings suggest that individual characteristics can inform treatment and the level of support needed throughout the course of toilet training.

Adaptive Behavior Measures

Vineland Adaptive Behavior Scales, Third Edition (Vineland-3)

The Vineland Adaptive Behavior Scales, Third Edition (Vineland-3; Sparrow, Cicchetti, & Saulnier, 2016), is a widely used measure that was designed to assess adaptive behavior in individuals from birth to 90 years old. The Vineland-3 is most commonly used to assess for adaptive skills and deficits in individuals with intellectual disabilities, developmental delays, ASD, and other impairments (Cicchetti, Carter, & Gray, 2013). The Vineland-3 can aid in the diagnosis of intellectual and developmental disabilities and provide detailed information regarding specific developmental domains.

The Vineland-3 has two versions: the comprehensive, full-length version and the domain-level, abbreviated version. In addition, there are several forms available for each version: the interview form, parent/caregiver form, and teacher form. Items related to toileting skills are included in both versions of the Vineland-3. Items are rated on a 3-point Likert scale; a score of "0" indicates that the individual does not perform the behavior or never performs it unless helped/prompted, "1" indicates that the individual sometimes performs the behavior without being helped/prompting, and "2" indicates that the individual performs the behavior most of the time without being helped/prompted.

The comprehensive interview form has toileting items under daily living skill domain, personal subdomain. Related items include the following: "defecates in a toilet or potty chair; parent or caregiver may initiate," "is toilet-trained during the day; may require help with undressing, flushing, wiping, or washing hands, but must initiate using the toilet," "is toilet-trained during the night; may require help with undressing, flushing, wiping, or washing hands, but must initiate using the toilet," and "uses the toilet during the day and at night without help; must wipe, flush, and wash hands by himself/herself."

The domain-level interview form provides domain scores and an adaptive behavior composite score. Domains include communication, daily living skills, and socialization as well as optional motor skills and maladaptive behavior. The daily living skill domain has three subdomains: personal, domestic, and community. Toilet training is assessed using three items: "urinates in a toilet or potty chair; parent or caregiver may initiate," "defecates in a toilet or potty chair; parent or caregiver may initiate," and "uses the toilet during the day and at night without help; must wipe, flush, and wash hands by himself/herself." Follow-up questions regarding how the child uses the toilet or potty chair and how much assistance is needed during toileting are asked. Item scores are summed with the other daily living skills item scores to produce an overall daily living skills score.

Given that toileting items are grouped under a total daily living skills score, toileting problems may not be detected or addressed unless the clinician or primary caregiver is specifically assessing for toileting behavior. Thus, when conducting broad adaptive assessments of individuals suspected to have intellectual and developmental disabilities, it is incumbent on the clinician to be aware of specific adaptive deficits, such as toileting problems, and gather additional information.

Adaptive Behavior Assessment System, Third Edition (ABAS-3)

The Adaptive Behavior Assessment System, Third Edition (ABAS-3; Harrison & Oakland, 2015), is an adaptive behavior rating scale that is used to evaluate adaptive behavior across the life span, from 0 to 89 years of age. The five forms of the ABAS-3, which include the parent/primary caregiver form (ages 0–5), teacher/daycare provider form (ages 2–5), parent form (ages 5–21), teacher form (ages 5–21), and adult form (ages 16–89), allow for information to be gathered across various informants and settings. All five forms take approximately 20 min to complete.

Respondents report on the following 11 skill areas: (1) communication, (2) functional preacademics, (3) self-direction, (4) leisure, (5) social, (6) community use, (7) home or school living, (8) health and safety, (9) self-care, (10) motor, and (11) work. Some skill areas are not evaluated across all age categories (e.g., work). Raters provide an ability rating and a frequency rating (i.e., "1," never/almost never; "2," sometimes; or "3," always/almost always). Following completion of the measure, an adaptive composite score on the individual's overall level of adaptive functioning is computed. This measure also provides scores at the domain level (i.e., conceptual, social, practical). Within the conceptual domain, the following skill areas are assessed: communication, functional preacademics, and self-direction. Within the social domain, the following skill areas are assessed: leisure and social. Within the practical domain, the following skill areas are assessed: community use, home living, health and safety, and self-care. Scores can also be reported on the individual skill areas. Items related to toileting skills are assessed within the "self-care" skill area, under the practical domain.

Adaptive Behavior Scales (ABS)

The Adaptive Behavior Scales was developed by the American Association on Mental Deficiency (AAMD) to assess for adaptive functioning in individuals with intellectual and developmental disabilities. There are two versions of the ABS: the Adaptive Behavior Scales-Residential and Community, Second Edition (ABS-RC:2), and the Adaptive Behavior Scales-School, Second Edition (ABS-S:2). The measure is completed by the examiner, based on the report of a parent/caregiver or another individual who has knowledge of the individual's adaptive abilities.

The ABS-RC:2 was developed for individuals living in residential and community settings and can be used for individuals through 79 years of age. The ABS-RC:2 is divided into two parts. Part one assesses for areas of personal independence and responsibility in daily living, while Part two assesses for social behaviors. Part one is comprised of ten subdomains: (1) independent functioning, (2) physical development, (3) economic activity, (4) language development, (5) numbers and time, (6) domestic activity, (7) prevocational/vocational activity, (8) self-direction, (9) responsibility, and (10) socialization. Each subdomain contains specific skills. For example, specific skills, such as toilet use, eating, cleanliness, care of clothing, etc., are included within the independent functioning domain. Respondents rate each item according to the level of difficulty (i.e., 0, 1, 2, or 3) the individual experiences with the task, with "0" being the least difficult and "3" being the most difficult. Other items are answered as "yes" or "no," dependent on the individual ability to complete the item task. Part two is comprised of eight subdomains: (1) social behavior, (2) conformity, (3) trustworthiness, (4) stereotyped and hyperactive behavior, (5) sexual behavior, (6) self-abusive behavior, (7) social engagement, and (8) disturbing interpersonal behavior.

Respondents rate the frequency of the item occurrence: "0" if the individual never engages in the behavior, "1" if the individual occasionally engages in the behavior, and "2" if the individual frequently engages in the behavior.

The ABS-S:2 is very similar to the ABS-RC:2 and is used to assess the adaptive functioning of school-aged children (through 21 years of age), in the school setting, and can help identify if the child is falling behind compared to their peers. The measure is completed by the examiner (i.e., the trained professional), based on the informant's report. Like the ABS-RC:2, the ABS-S:2 is divided into two parts. Part one contains nine subdomains: (1) independent functioning, (2) physical development, (3) economic activity, (4) language development, (5) numbers and time, (6) prevocational/vocational activity, (7) self-direction, (8) responsibility, and (9) socialization. Part two contains seven subdomains that assess for behaviors related to personality and behavioral disorders, which include (1) social behavior, (2) conformity, (3) trustworthiness, (4) stereotyped and hyperactive behavior, (5) self-abusive behavior, (6) social engagement, and (7) disturbing interpersonal behavior.

A strength of the ABS is that it assesses for adaptive functioning as well as for social and challenging behaviors. This measure may be a good screening tool for identifying toileting issues in individuals with known disruptive and/or challenging behaviors that may interfere with toilet training procedures.

Adaptive Behavior Evaluation Scale, Third Edition

The Adaptive Behavior Evaluation Scale, Third Edition (ABES-3; McCarney & House, 2017), is a rating form that takes approximately 15–20 min to complete. The ABES-3 was designed to guide educators in the evaluation of adaptive behavior in students who are experiencing behavior and learning problems in the classroom. As such, this measure can be completed by teachers and educators who have concerns regarding their students' adaptive functioning, to screen for intellectual disorders, learning disorders, and/or physical impairments.

The ABES-3 assesses for adaptive functioning across three domains, conceptual, social, and practical, as defined by the AAMD. The conceptual domain includes the communication and functional academics subdomains; the social domain includes the social, leisure, and self-direction subdomains; the practical domain includes the self-care, home living, community use, health and safety, and work subdomains. There are two versions of the ABES-3: the home version (ABES-3: 4–12 Home Version Rating Form) and the school version (ABES-3: 4–12 School Version Rating Form). In addition, there are home and school versions of the measure for individuals aged 13–18 years.

Items are rated on a Likert scale, to the extent to which the individual engages in the behavior: "0," not developmentally appropriate for age; "1," does not display the behavior/skill; "2," is developing the behavior/skill; "3," displays the behavior/skill inconsistently; "4," displays the behavior/skill most of the time; or "5," displays the behavior/skill consistently. While there is only one item that screens for toileting problems (i.e., "takes care of toileting needs"), a rating of a 3 or below on this item may prompt the clinician to probe further regarding the toileting behavior.

Developmental Measures

After toileting problems are identified, the clinician may consider assessing the child's developmental readiness for toilet training by using structured and/or indirect measures of developmental readiness. For children with intellectual and developmental disabilities, the developmental age of the child, not the chronological age, should guide treatment decisions regarding toilet training.

Battelle Developmental Inventory, Second Edition (BDI-2)

A developmental measure that can assess for toileting problems and prerequisite skills for successful toilet training is the *Battelle Developmental Inventory, Second Edition* (BDI-2; Newborg, 2005). The BDI-2 is an early childhood measure that measures a child's developmental progress across several domains including personal/social, adaptive, motor, communication, and cognition. The BDI-2 was designed to assess children from birth to age 7 years and 11 months. Items are scored on a scale of 0 to 2 through direct observation and interaction with the child. A score of "0" indicates no ability, "1" indicates emerging ability, and "2" indicates ability present. Domain raw scores are converted to age equivalents, percentile ranks, and developmental quotients, with the developmental quotient representing the child's general level of functioning.

The toileting subdomain is included under the adaptive domain. There are six items related to toileting, including the following: "expresses need to go to bathroom," "controls bowel movements regularly," "washes and dries hands without assistance," "sleeps through night without wetting bed," "takes care of own toileting needs," and "takes bath or shower without assistance." As with the Vineland-3, toileting problems can be overlooked if the clinician or caregiver is not concerned with toileting behavior. Nevertheless, the BDI-2 may aid in screening for toileting problems while evaluating the level of functioning across several developmental domains.

Bayley Scales of Infant and Toddler Development, Third Edition

The Bayley Scales of Infant and Toddler Development, Third Edition (Bayley-III; Bayley, 2006), is another developmental measure than can assess for toileting problems and developmental level of prerequisite skills but in a younger population. The Bayley-III was designed to assess the developmental functioning of infants and toddlers, aged 1–42 months, across five developmental domains. These domains include cognitive, language (receptive and expressive), motor (fine and gross), social-emotional, and adaptive (conceptual, social, and practical) behavior. This instrument is a structure instrument that incorporates a combination of testing methods. As such, the Bayley-III can take approximately 50–90 min to administer. To assess for cognitive, language, and motor skills, the trained clinician presents several structured tasks to the child. The social-emotional and adaptive domains are evaluated using a questionnaire, which is completed by the primary caregiver. The questionnaire used in this portion of the Bayley-III is the Adaptive Behavior Assessment System, Second Edition (ABAS-II; Harrison & Oakland, 2003), the former version of the ABAS-III, which was discussed in the adaptive measures section of this chapter. The primary caregiver reports the child's level of functioning in specific skill areas, which include communication, community use, health and safety, leisure, self-care, self-direction, functional pre-academics, home living, social, and motor. The respondent rates each item regarding the child's ability level, "0," not able; "1," never when needed; "2," sometimes when needed; or "3," always when needed. Self-care (i.e., toileting) skills are included within the adaptive-practical domain.

The Bayley-III provides composite scores and percentile ranks for all five developmental domains. With these data, the clinician can determine if the toddler is at the developmental age that is appropriate for the initiation of toilet training or if the toddler is exhibiting developmental delays compared to toddlers of the same age. If the toddler has low scores on the receptive and expressive language subtests, this may indicate that the toddler does not yet possess the skills to follow the toilet training instructions or vocally initiate toileting attempts. Information gathered from the Bayley-III should guide the clinician's decision regarding the initiation of toilet training, and the types of accommodations, if any, should be made to the toilet training procedures.

Ages and Stages Questionnaire

Another developmental screening measure designed to identify developmental delays in infants and young children (i.e., 1–60 months old) is the Ages and Stages Questionnaires: A Parent-Completed Child Monitoring System, Third Edition (ASQ-3; Squires et al., 2009). The ASQ-3 is a questionnaire that is completed by primary caregiver and only takes about 10–15 min to complete. The ASQ-3 includes 21 questionnaires, as the questionnaires are separated by age intervals (i.e., 2, 4, 6, 8, 9, 10, 12, 14, 16, 18, 20, 22, 24, 27, 30, 33, 36,42, 48, 54, and 60 months). Each questionnaire includes 30 items across 5 developmental domains: communication, gross motor, fine motor, problem-solving, and personal-social. In addition, primary caregivers are encouraged to complete the ASQ: Social-Emotional, Second Edition (ASQ: SE-2), which assess for social-emotional development in young children. It is recommended that the ASQ:SE-2 is used in conjunction with the ASQ-3, to obtain a broader understanding of the child's development and to determine if the child is developmentally ready for toilet training.

While developmental screening measures, such as the ASQ-3, can be used to assess for a child's level of functioning, they can and should be used to monitor treatment progress, treatment efficacy, and development of the child across age intervals.

Assessment of Challenging Behaviors

As previously discussed, the ability to follow and comply with instructions is an essential prerequisite skill for successful toilet training. While some adaptive measures screen for challenging behaviors (e.g., ABS), the presence of challenging behaviors may be overlooked and underreported when caregivers present their toileting concerns to a doctor or clinician. While the current chapter will not go into much detail regarding the assessment of challenging behaviors, it is important to note some measures that can provide valuable information regarding the challenging behaviors that are present during toileting attempts. Some examples include the Child Behavior Checklist (CBCL) and the Behavior Problem Inventory (BPI).

The CBCL (Achenbach, 1991) is an informant-based rating tool that assesses for challenging behaviors in children and adolescents aged 2–18 years. The 100-item checklist provides information regarding the individual's behaviors across various behavior scales (e.g., withdrawn, anxious/depressed, sleep problems, somatic problems, aggressive, destructive, attention problems, hyperactive, etc.). The BPI (Rojahn, Matson, Lott, Esbensen, & Smalls, 2001) is 52-item, informant-based rating tool that assesses for challenging behaviors in individuals with intellectual and developmental disabilities. The BPI provides information regarding the frequency and severity of three categories of challenging behaviors: self-injurious behavior, stereotyped behavior, and aggressive/destructive behavior.

Informant-based measures of challenging behaviors are quick to administer and provide valuable, supplemental information when assessing for toileting problems, particularly in individuals with intellectual and developmental disabilities, including ASD.

Behavioral Interventions

The proper assessment of toileting problems and prerequisite skills is essential when determining which training protocol will be most appropriate and effective for the individual. A wide range of behavioral methods and interventions have been found to be effective in toilet training individuals with intellectual and developmental disabilities. Some methods include graduated guidance, reinforcement-based training (i.e., positive reinforcement, negative reinforcement), scheduled sittings, elimination schedules, punishment procedures, hydration, manipulation of stimulus control, priming, and video modeling (Bainbridge & Smith Myles, 1999; Kroeger & Sorensen-Burnworth, 2009). More specifically, behavioral procedures based on the principles of applied behavior analysis (ABA) have been found to be effective in teaching toileting skills to children with intellectual and developmental disorders (Wingate, Falcomata, & Ferguson, 2017). According to Azrin and Foxx (1971), toilet training is a social process that relies on operant-based behavioral principles. As such, procedures including reinforcement, punishment, and stimulus control have been found to be effective methods of toilet training.

In fact, reinforcement is a key feature of ABA because the delivery of a reinforcer presents an immediate consequence following the behavior and increases the likelihood that the appropriate behavior will increase in the future (Cooper, Heron, & Heward, 2007). Positive reinforcement, which involves the delivery of a preferred item or activity, has been found to be effective in increasing toileting skills in children (Azrin & Foxx, 1971) and in adults (Halligan & Luyben, 2009). Prior to implementing positive reinforcement procedures, the clinician and/or caregiver should conduct a preference assessment to identify which items (e.g., toy, food) or activity (e.g., no longer sitting on the potty chair) is most reinforcing for the child. The delivery of the child's most preferred item and/or activity will increase the likelihood of successful toileting occurring in the future. However, if a preference assessment is not conducted prior to implementing the toileting procedures, the behavioral contingencies will not be established, and the child may not respond well to treatment.

If the child is not motivated to earn positive reinforcement, negative reinforcement procedures may be used. In negative reinforcement, the removal of a non-preferred item and/or activity increases the likelihood of successful toileting. Similar to positive reinforcement procedures, the caregiver and/or clinician should identify the non-preferred item or activity prior to or early in the toilet training procedures to ensure that the appropriate behavioral contingencies are being established. Rolider and Van Houten (1985) found that negative reinforcement procedures were effective in reducing soiling and increasing successful voiding in a typically developing 12-year-old girl. For this participant, not sitting on the potty chair for an extended period of time (i.e., negative reinforcement) was reinforcing, which resulted in toilet training success.

In addition to these reinforcement procedures, prompting procedures are usually incorporated into toilet training procedures. There are a variety of prompting procedures that can be used (e.g., model, gesture, verbal, physical, etc.) depending on the specific skills and deficits of the child. Given that children with intellectual and developmental disabilities have impairments across various skill domains, the primary caregiver and/or clinician should identify certain areas or skills that the child may need assistance with. Using the data collected from the clinical interview, adaptive, or developmental measures, the clinician can make adjustments to established toilet training procedures, to increase more opportunities for success. For example, if a child has low fine motor skills, the caregiver may provide a physical prompt and help the child pull down his or her underwear. If a child has limited verbal skills, the caregiver may provide a verbal prompt (e.g., "Do you need to go potty?") to assist the child with initiation. Providing a variety of prompts during the initial stages of toilet training will allow the child to receive direct reinforcement for all successful attempts at appropriate toileting behavior (Wingate, Falcomata, & Ferguson, 2017).

Monitoring Progress

Following the primary caregiver's initial report of toileting problems, the clinician may instruct the caregiver to take data on the child's current adaptive and/or toileting behaviors, to get a baseline level of functioning and/or to evaluate if a formal toilet training procedure is warranted. If the toileting problems appear to be due to deficits in a specific prerequisite skill, a focused intervention, rather than a formal toileting procedure, may be recommended.

An essential component of ABA-based toileting procedures is the measurement of the child's progress. For children who do require a formal toilet training procedure, caregivers may be instructed to take data on toileting behavior throughout the course of training. This allows both the caregiver and clinician to monitor the child's progress and ensure that the treatment is effective in reducing toileting problems and increasing appropriate toileting skills (Warzak, Kennedy, & Bond, 2017). With high rates of regression of toilet training (up to 30%; Ohta, Nagai, Hara, & Saski, 1987), monitoring treatment progress is especially important among individuals with intellectual and developmental disabilities so that procedures can be adjusted, as needed. Ongoing assessment and data collection ensures that toileting skills will be maintained over time and generalized across people and settings. When determining what type of data tracking method to assign to the caregiver, the clinician should consider certain variables, such as caregiver factors, the child's developmental level, and the level of support the caregiver will need to provide during the toilet training procedure. The measurement method should be relatively easy and feasible for caregivers to collect. If measurement methods are complex and intensive, it is not likely that the caregiver will take reliable data, if at all (Friman & Poling, 1995).

There are several measurement procedures that have been used to monitor behavior during toilet training procedures. Given that toileting attempts, successes, and problems occur throughout the day, it is not feasible to expect caregivers to take data on all occurrences of toileting behavior. One solution to this issue is the time sampling method. Time sampling involves dividing longer amounts of time into smaller intervals and taking data during that specified interval of time. There are several types of time sampling: whole-interval, partial-interval, and momentary time sampling (Warzak, Kennedy, & Bond, 2017). During whole-interval time sampling, the caregiver will take data on the target behavior throughout the entire designated time interval. During partial-interval time sampling, the caregiver will record if the target behavior did or did not occur during the designed time interval. Momentary time sampling involves recording if the target behavior did or did not occur at the end of a designated time interval. For example, a 10-minute observation period may be separated into ten 1-minute intervals. At the end of the 1-minute interval, the caregiver will record if the behavior did or did not occur during that designated time interval. The optimal method of time sampling procedures may vary across individuals, based on training goals and caregiver and child factors.

Time sampling provides valuable data on the frequency and duration of behavior. For this measurement procedure, it is important to provide clear, concise definitions of target behavior, to ensure that the caregiver takes reliable data. In addition, the clinician should assess if the caregiver is able to accurately identify what the target behavior looks like. However, if the caregiver is unable to observe or reliably identify the target behavior, other methods of measurement may be used.

One such method is permanent product recording, which involves taking data after the target behavior has occurred. Rather than taking data on the behavior itself, the effect of the behavior on the environment is measured (Cooper, Heron, & Heward, 2007). For example, a caregiver may detect and record when a void has occurred, by feeling the wetness of the child's diaper (Simon & Thompson, 2006). A limitation of permanent product recording is that it does not provide much information regarding the frequency, duration, or setting in which the voiding is occurring. As such, permanent product recording is usually used in conjunction with other measurement methods.

If the child exhibits challenging behaviors during toileting attempts, the caregiver may take data on the frequency, duration, and/or rate of the challenging behaviors exhibited during the toilet training procedures. Taking descriptive data on the events that happened before the challenging behavior (i.e., antecedent data) as well as on the events that happened after the occurrence of the challenging behavior (i.e., consequence data) provides the clinician with valuable information regarding which contingencies should or should not be implemented into the toilet training procedures.

Regardless of which measurement method is being used, the key to monitoring toilet training progress is to obtain reliable data that is representative of the child's behaviors. If the caregiver is not implementing the toileting training procedures and behavioral contingencies accurately, the data provided by the caregiver will not be an accurate representation of the child's progress. In order to ensure that the caregiver is taking accurate data, the clinician may consider incorporating a procedural integrity component into the measurement procedures.

An easy method of measuring procedural integrity is to create a checklist of steps of the procedure for the caregiver to follow along with. A clear and concise layout of the procedures will guide the caregiver during the implementation of the procedures and help the caregivers adhere to the treatment protocol.

Another way to verify if data is being accurately recorded is to take interobserver agreement (IOA) data. The IOA procedure requires that two (or more) individuals independently take data during the same observation period. Then, the data from the two observers are compared to evaluate if there is agreement between their data. If there is a high percentage of overlap in their data, this indicates that the data were reliably and consistently recorded. While IOA procedures are common in behavioral research, it is not commonly incorporated into toilet training research (Warzak, Kennedy, & Bond, 2017). This may simply be due to the fact that there is usually not a second caregiver who is available to take data during toilet training procedures.

Several measurement methods can be used to gather baseline behavioral data (i.e., behavior prior to the initiation of training procedures) and monitor progress throughout the training procedure. Collecting data during the training procedures is crucial in evaluating treatment effectiveness and troubleshooting any issues that may arise during treatment. To obtain reliable and accurate data, the most feasible measurement method should be selected, according to caregiver factors, the child's skills and deficits, and type of challenging behavior.

Conclusion

Individuals with intellectual and developmental disabilities have impairments across a range of skill domains, including adaptive, language, cognition, social, and motor skills. Consequently, they face greater obstacles during toilet training than their typically developing peers. A comprehensive assessment of the child's developmental and medical history, prerequisite skills, caregiver factors, and current toileting behavior is essential in guiding decisions regarding toilet training initiation and procedures. A combination of screening tools for toileting problems (i.e., POTI), adaptive behavior, development across domains, and challenging behaviors should be used to assess for the presence of toileting problems and to identify the child's level of functioning across various skill areas. Once toilet training procedures have been implemented, clinicians and caregivers should monitor toileting behaviors throughout the training process in order to assess for treatment efficacy and behavioral changes, if any.

However, given that toileting skills are usually assessed within the broad daily living skills or self-care subdomains of adaptive behavior assessments, toileting problems may easily get overlooked and go undetected. More research on the evaluation of measures designed to detect toileting problems, enuresis, and encopresis are warranted. Further, more research on group differences (e.g., age, diagnosis, level of functioning, motor skills) would be beneficial in improving assessment methods and treatment efficacy for toileting problems.

References

Achenbach, T. M. (1991). *Manual for the child behavior checklist and revised child behavior profile*. Burlington: University of Vermont Department of Psychiatry.

American Academy of Pediatrics. (1998). *Toilet training: Guidelines for parents*. Elk Grove Village, IL: AAP.

American Psychiatric Association. (2013). *Diagnostic and statistical manual of mental disorders* (5th ed.). Washington, DC: American Psychiatric Association.

Azrin, N. H., & Foxx, R. M. (1971). A rapid method of toilet training the institutionalized retarded. *Journal of Applied Behavior Analysis, 4*, 89–99.

Bainbridge, N., & Smith Myles, B. (1999). The use of priming to introduce toilet training to a child with autism. *Focus on Autism and Other Developmental Disabilities, 14*(2), 106–109.

Baker, B. L., & Brightman, A. J. (1997). *Steps to independence: Teaching everyday skills to children with special needs*. Baltimore, MD: Paul H. Brookes.

Bayley, N. (2006). *Bayley scales of infant and toddler development, third edition: Administration manual*. San Antonio, TX: Harcourt Assessment.

Brazelton, T. B. (1962). A child-oriented approach to toilet training. *Pediatrics, 29*, 121–128.

Chase, J. W., Homsy, Y., Siggaard, C., Sit, F., & Bower, W. F. (2004). Functional constipation in children. *The Journal of Urology, 171*, 2641–2643.

Cicchetti, D. V., Carter, A. S., & Gray, S. A. O. (2013). Vineland adaptive behavior scales. In F. R. Volkmar (Ed.), *Encyclopedia of autism spectrum disorders*. New York: Springer.

Cocchiola, M. A., Jr., Martino, G. M., Dwyer, L. J., & Demezzo, K. (2012). Toilet training children with autism and developmental delays: An effective program for school settings. *Behavior Analysis in Practice, 5*(2), 60–64.

Cocchiola, M. A., Jr., & Redpath, C. C. (2017). Special populations: Toilet training children with disabilities. In J. L. Matson (Ed.), *Clinical guide to toilet training children* (pp. 227–250). Cham: Springer Nature.

Cooper, J. O., Heron, T. E., & Heward, W. L. (2007). *Applied behavior analysis* (2nd ed.). Upper Saddle River, NJ: Pearson Prentice Hall.

Dalrymple, N. J., & Ruble, L. A. (1992). Toilet training and behaviors of people with autism: Parent views. *Journal of Autism and Developmental Disorders, 22*(2), 265–275.

Foxx, R. M., & Azrin, N. H. (1973). *Toilet training persons with developmental disabilities: A rapid program for day and nighttime independent toileting*. Harrisburg, PA: Help Services Press.

Frauman, A. C., & Brandon, D. H. (1996). Toilet training for the child with chronic illness. *Pediatric Nursing, 22*(6), 469–493.

Friman, P., & Poling, A. (1995). Making life easier with effort: Basic findings and applied research on response effort. *Journal of Applied Behavior Analysis, 28*, 583–590.

Halligan, S. M., & Luyben, P. D. (2009). Prompts, feedback, positive reinforcement, and potty training. *Journal of Prevention & Intervention in the Community, 37*, 177–186.

Harris, A. (2004). Toilet training children with learning difficulties: What the literature tells us. *British Journal of Nursing, 13*(13), 773–777.

Harrison, P. L., & Oakland, T. (2003). *Adaptive behavior assessment system–second edition*. San Antonio, TX: The Psychological Corporation.

Harrison, P., & Oakland, T. (2015). *Adaptive behavior assessment system* (3rd ed.). San Antonio, TX: Harcourt Assessment.

Heron, J., Joinson, C., Croudace, T., & von Gontard, A. (2008). Trajectories of daytime wetting and soiling in a United Kingdom 4 to 9-year old population birth cohort study. *The Journal of Urology, 179*(5), 1970–1975.

Jang, J., Dixon, D. R., Tarbox, J., & Granpeesheh, D. (2011). Symptom severity and challenging behavior in children with ASD. *Research in Autism Spectrum Disorders, 5*(3), 1028–1032.

Kasari, C., Sigman, M., Mundy, P., & Yirmiya, N. (1988). Caregiver interactions with autistic children. *Journal of Abnormal Child Psychology, 16*, 45–56.

Kroeger, K. A., & Sorensen-Burnworth, R. (2009). Toilet training individuals with autism and other developmental disabilities: A critical review. *Research in Autism Spectrum Disorders, 3*, 607–618.

Kroeger, K., & Sorensen, R. (2010). A parent training model for toilet training children with autism. *Journal of Intellectual Disability Research, 54*(6), 556–567.

Kroeger, K. A., Weber, S., & Smith, J. (2017). Risk factors. In J. L. Matson (Ed.), *Clinical guide to toilet training children* (pp. 33–62). Cham: Springer Nature.

Matson, J. L., Dempsey, T., & Fodstad, J. C. (2010). *The profile of toileting issues (POTI)*. Baton Rouge, LA: Disability Consultants, LLC.

Matson, J. L., Horovitz, M., & Sipes, M. (2011). Characteristics of individuals with toileting problems and intellectual disability using the profile of toileting issues (POTI). *Journal of Mental Health Research in Intellectual Disabilities, 4*, 53–63.

Matson, J. L., Neal, D., Hess, J. A., & Kozlowski, A. M. (2011). Assessment of toileting difficulties in adults with intellectual disabilities: An examination using the profile of toileting issues (POTI). *Research in Developmental Disabilities, 32*, 176–179.

Matson, J. L., & LoVullo, S. V. (2009). Encopresis, soiling and constipation in children and adults with developmental disability. *Research in Developmental Disabilities, 30*(4), 799–807.

Matson, J. L., Neal, D., Hess, J. A., & Kozlowski, A. M. (2011). Assessment of toileting difficulties in adults with intellectual disabilities: An examination using the profile of toileting issues (POTI). *Research in Developmental Disabilities, 32*, 176–179.

McCarney, S. B., & House, S. N. (2017). *Adaptive behavior evaluation scale- third edition (ABES-3)*. Columbia, MO: Hawthorne.

Newborg, J. (2005). *Batelle developmental inventory* (2nd ed.). Itasca, IL: Riverside Publishing.

Ohta, M., Nagai, Y., Hara, H., & Saski, M. (1987). Parental perception of behavioral symptoms in Japanese autistic children. *Journal of Autism and Developmental Disorders, 17*, 549–563.

Rolider, A., & Van Houten, R. (1985). Treatment of constipation-caused encopresis by a negative reinforcementprocedure. *Journal of Behavior Therapy and Experimental Psychiatry, 16*(1), 67–70.

Rojahn, J., Matson, J. L., Lott, D., Esbensen, A. J., & Smalls, Y. (2001). The behavior problems inventory: An instrument for the assessment of self-injury, stereotyped behavior and aggression/destruction in individuals with developmental disabilities. *Journal of Autism and Developmental Disorders, 31*, 577–588.

Simon, J. L., & Thompson, R. H. (2006). The effects of undergarment type on the urinary continence of toddlers. *Journal of Applied Behavior Analysis, 30*(3), 363–368.

Schum, T. R., Kolb, T. M., McAuliffe, T. L., Simms, M. D., Underhill, R. L., & Lewis, M. (2002). Sequential acquisition of toilet-training skills: A descriptive study of gender and age differences in normal children. *Pediatrics, 109*(3), 1–7.

Singh, B., Masey, H., & Morton, R. (2006). Levels of continence in children with cerebral palsy. *Pediatric Nursing, 18*(4), 23–26.

Sparrow, S. S., Cicchetti, D. V., & Saulnier, C. A. (2016). *Vineland adaptive behavior scales, third edition (Vineland-3)*. Bloomington, MN: Pearson.

Squires, J., Bricker, D., Twombly, E., Nickel, R., Clifford, J., Murphy, K., … Farrell, J. (2009). *Ages & stages questionnaires, 3rd edition (ASQ-3)*. Baltimore: Paul H. Brookes.

Warzak, W. J., Kennedy, A. E., & Bond, K. (2017). Monitoring progress in toilet training. In J. L. Matson (Ed.), *Clinical guide to toilet training children* (pp. 105–117). Cham: Springer Nature.

Wingate, H. V., Falcomata, T. S., & Ferguson, R. (2017). In J. L. Matson (Ed.), *Clinical guide to toilet training children* (pp. 119–167). Cham: Springer Nature.

Assessment of Fine and Gross Motor Skills in Children

Maya Matheis and Jasper A. Estabillo

Assessment of Fine and Gross Motor Skills in Children

Motor skills refer to the movement and coordination of one's muscles and body (Haibach-Beach, Reid, & Collier, 2011). Motor skills are typically divided into gross and fine motor abilities. Gross motor skills require coordination of an individual's arms, legs, and other large body parts for actions such as running, jumping, and throwing (Haibach-Beach, Reid, & Collier, 2011). Because these skills incorporate larger body parts and movements, the development of gross motor skills is necessary for proprioception, core stabilization, and body control (Piek, Dawson, Smith, & Gasson, 2008). Fine motor skills require coordination of smaller movements between the fingers, hands, and feet for actions such as picking up and grasping small objects (e.g., pincer grasp; Piek, Dawson, Smith, & Gasson, 2008). These actions involve dexterity in order to manipulate smaller movements and objects. Development of various gross and fine motor skills begins in infancy, and throughout childhood, individuals experience tremendous physical and developmental growth that typically progresses in a predictable sequence (Gerber, Wilks, & Erdie-Lalena, 2010); as such, tracking of developmental milestones allows for assessment of a child's developmental functioning, and monitoring of motor skills development in children is important for identifying children who may be at risk for various developmental delays (Gerber, Wilks, & Erdie-Lalena, 2010; Ghassabian et al., 2016).

The achievement of motor milestones is critical to overall development in children because as the child ages and progresses in motor development (e.g., crawling to walking), they are increasingly able to explore and interact with their environment (Gibson, 1988; Oudgenoeg-Paz, Mulder, Jongmans, van der Ham, & Van der Stigchel, 2017). This exploration of the environment provides the child with learning opportunities to develop cognitive, language, and social skills (Alcock & Krawczyk, 2010; Ghassabian et al., 2016; Gibson, 1988; Hitzert, Roze, Van Braeckel, & Bos, 2014; Houwen, van der Putten, & Vlaskamp, 2014; Piek, Dawson, Smith, & Gasson, 2008). As the child encounters novel stimuli in the environment, they are able to develop language (e.g., learning new words to label items in the setting), communicate with others, and develop social skills, as well as cognitive skills such as problem solving (Alcock & Krawczyk, 2010; Clearfield, 2011; Leonard & Hill, 2014; Walle & Campos, 2014).

Because motor skills emerge earlier in development, they are typically most noticeable by

---

M. Matheis (✉) · J. A. Estabillo
Department of Psychology, Louisiana State University, Baton Rouge, LA, USA

parents and caregivers (Piek, Dawson, Smith, & Gasson, 2008). Due to their early nature and influence on subsequent development of other skills, motor skills should be monitored in case of developmental concerns (Gerber, Wilks, & Erdie-Lalena, 2010). This chapter will provide an overview of assessment of fine and gross motor skills as they relate to childhood disorders.

Typical Motor Development

Throughout childhood, individuals are interacting with their environments through direct and indirect actions which foster their development. Theoretically, individuals' learning and acquisition of knowledge has been tied to their development of various motor behaviors (Piaget, 1953). From very early ages, children are learning through exploration via motor development.

Therefore, understanding of normal developmental milestones is necessary for assessment and identification of developmental delays (Gerber, Wilks, & Erdie-Lalena, 2010). Although the rate of acquisition varies greatly across individuals, motor skills typically progress in a sequential order within a certain timeframe. Given the variation in skills achievement, skills are not considered delayed unless the individual has not met the milestone past the recommended age. Table 1 includes various early motor milestones and the typical age of achievement.

Motor Skill Deficits

Comorbidity with Other Childhood Disorders

Motor deficits are common in various childhood disorders. This section will review a number of childhood disorders and the gross motor deficits associated with them.

Global Developmental Delay and Intellectual Disability Symptoms of global developmental delay (GDD) and intellectual disability (ID) include deficits in both intellectual and adaptive

Table 1 Typical motor milestones

Age in months	Milestone
2	Holds head up, pushes up when lying on stomach
4	Holds head steady (neck control), starts to roll over, brings hands to mouth
6	Rolls over both directions, starts to sit unsupported
9	Stands with support, sits unsupported, crawls
12	Walks supported, stands independently
18	Walks independently, drinks from cup, eats with spoon
24	Runs, climbs on furniture unassisted
36	Climbs independently, runs smoothly, walks up and down steps
48	Hops, catches bounced ball, cuts with scissors (supervised)
60	Uses utensils, swings, stands on one foot for at least 10 s

Adapted from the World Health Organization (2006) and Centers for Disease Control and Prevention (2017)

functions which affect one's skills in conceptual, social, and practical domains (American Psychiatric Association, 2013). Whereas individuals with ID have impairments in both cognitive functioning and adaptive behaviors, a diagnosis of GDD is reserved for children under the age of 5 who display significant delays in multiple developmental domains (American Psychiatric Association, 2013). Onset of GDD and ID is in the developmental period, with delayed developmental skills often apparent by age 2 (Institute of Medicine (U.S.), Boat, Wu, & National Academies of Sciences, Engineering, and Medicine, 2015). The motor deficits observed in individuals with GDD and ID range from mild to severe and across fine and gross motor skills. For individuals with mild ID, they may achieve motor milestones within normal limits but later exhibit difficulties with gross and fine motor skills (Vuijk, Hartman, Scherder, & Visscher, 2010). Often individuals with mild ID may not be identified until school age, when their academic and learning difficulties become more apparent (Institute of Medicine (U.S.) et al., 2015). Severe and profound ID are more commonly associated with an underlying genetic or neurological cause such as Down syndrome, Prader-Willi syndrome, fragile X syndrome, and Angelman syndrome (Flint, 2001; Karam et al., 2015). Researchers have indicated that there is a relationship between cognitive and motor functioning such that more severe ID is associated with greater motor impairment (Vuijk, Hartman, Scherder, & Visscher, 2010). Given that GDD and ID are characterized by impaired adaptive behaviors, which are related to motor skills, assessment of the individual's fine and gross motor difficulties is an essential component of evaluation.

Autism Spectrum Disorder Autism spectrum disorder (ASD) is a neurodevelopmental disorder characterized by marked deficits in social communication behaviors and the presence of restricted and repetitive behaviors and interests (American Psychiatric Association, 2013). Although not characteristic of ASD, motor deficits are also often observed in individuals with the disorder (Colombo-Dougovito & Reeve, 2017; Liu, 2013). Delayed achievement of motor milestones (e.g., crawling, walking) is often the first developmental concern reported by parents and caregivers of children who are later diagnosed with ASD (Chawarska et al., 2007; Lloyd, MacDonald, & Lord, 2013). An estimated 80% of children with ASD have motor difficulties, with the delays exhibited becoming more significant with age (Landa & Garrett-Mayer, 2006; Lloyd, MacDonald, & Lord, 2013). Common deficits include gross motor impairments such as difficulties in coordinating upper and lower limbs during balance, agility, and speed tasks (Bhat, Landa, & Galloway, 2011; Ghaziuddin & Butler, 1998; Miyahara et al., 1997). A number of researchers have also found that individuals with ASD display abnormal or ataxic gait (Calhoun, Longworth, & Chester, 2011; Kindregan, Gallagher, & Gormley, 2015; MacDonald, Lord, & Ulrich, 2014). Various motor deficits are common in individuals with ASD; however, the impairments observed have not been found to differ from the motor deficits observed in individuals with other developmental delays (Ozonoff et al., 2008). The presence of comorbid ID, though, has been found to be associated with more severe motor deficits in individuals with ASD (Smith, Maenner, & Seltzer, 2012).

For individuals with ASD, motor deficits are common, and when assessing the difficulties experienced by those with the disorder, considerations such as functioning level and the presence of ID should be made.

Language Disorders Language disorders include impairments in the acquisition and use of speech and language, in which both expressive and receptive language skills may be affected (American Psychiatric Association, 2013). A number of children with various speech delays and disorders also display motor deficits (Missiuna, Gaines, & Pollock, 2002), with some researchers finding that between 40 and 90% of children with speech problems also have motor impairments (Hill, 2001). The types of motor impairments observed in children with speech and language disorders are non-specific, such that they may exhibit gross and/or fine motor difficulties (Gaines & Missiuna, 2007; Missiuna, Gaines, & Pollock, 2002). These deficits may include difficulty with visuomotor skills, coordination, and timing (Sanjeevan et al., 2015; Zelaznik & Goffman, 2010). The significant overlap between speech deficits and motor impairments may not only suggest a relationship between the two skills but also a common underlying etiology in these difficulties.

Cerebral Palsy Cerebral palsy (CP) is a neurological disorder that affects an individual's movement and muscle coordination, including muscle control, tone, posture, and fine and gross motor skills (Parsons, 2011). It is the most common cause of motor disability in children (Kirby et al., 2011). CP is caused by brain injury or abnormal brain development affecting motor skills (Bax, 2008). The motor impairments and severity of deficits exhibited by individuals with CP vary across those with the disorder, such that some individuals may have complete paralysis while others may display milder difficulties such as tremors (Parsons, 2011).

Given the range and severity of motor deficits due to CP, considerations must be made when assessing motor function in children with the disorder.

There are several classification systems to describe the individual's type and severity of CP, with the Gross Motor Function Classification System (GMFS) created to address the goals set by the World Health Organization and Surveillance of Cerebral Palsy (R. Palisano, Rosenbaum, Bartlett, & Livingston, 2007). The GMFS is a multi-level system that describes the individual's level of abilities and impairments and is often used with other classification systems to provide additional information regarding the location and severity of impairments (Palisano, Rosenbaum, Bartlett, & Livingston, 2007). The GMFCS has five levels across four age bands that focus on voluntary movements with particular emphasis on sitting and ambulation, with level I indicating functional limitations less than what is often associated with CP and level V indicating severe functional limitations. The system was designed for professionals familiar with a child's current motor abilities to quickly classify the appropriate functioning level. Initial development of the GMFCS involved nominal group process and Delphi survey methods to determine content validity (Palisano et al., 2008; Palisano, Rosenbaum, Bartlett, & Livingston, 2008). Interrater reliability has been demonstrated to be excellent ($G = 0.93$), while test-retest reliability was found to be adequate ($G = 0.79$; Wood & Rosenbaum, 2000).

Dysgraphia Dysgraphia is a learning disability characterized by fine motor difficulties that may result in poor or illegible handwriting below what would be expected based on the child's age and education level (Berninger, Richards, & Abbott, 2015; Döhla & Heim, 2016). In the *Diagnostic and Statistical Manual of Mental Disorders*, Fifth Edition (DSM-5; American Psychiatric Association, 2013), there is no specific diagnosis of "dysgraphia." Individuals with these difficulties may meet criteria for a specific learning disorder with impairments in written expression (e.g., spelling accuracy, grammar and punctuation accuracy, clarity or organization of written expression); however, this may not fully capture the individual's deficits in handwriting. The problems the individual may have with writing may include poor and inconsistent letter formation and spacing, difficulty with spatial planning, and impairments with composition (Chung & Patel, 2016). It has been suggested that these deficits may be due to difficulties with visual processing (Döhla & Heim, 2016), visual memory (Vlachos & Karapetsas, 2003), or other visuomotor skills (Mäki, Voeten, Vauras, & Poskiparta, 2001). Because difficulties with handwriting may affect a child's academic skills, it is necessary to assess motor skills to determine fine motor function.

Genetic Disorders Individuals with various genetic disorders, including Down syndrome, Williams syndrome, fragile X syndrome, and Prader-Willi syndrome, have also been found to exhibit motor deficits. Though the genetic causes and phenotypes of each disorder vary, researchers have found a number of motor deficits to also be present (Chapman & Hesketh, 2000; Loveland & Kelley, 1991; Mervis & Klein-Tasman, 2000; Summers & Feldman, 1999). The types of impairments as well as severity range across each disorder and individual. As such, clinicians should consider the possible influence of the symptoms of the individual's genetic disorder when assessing motor skills.

Relationship Between Motor Skills and Adaptive Behaviors

Adaptive behaviors are independent daily living skills, as expected by the individual's age and cultural standards of the community (American Psychiatric Association, 2013; Bullington, 2011). The domains of adaptive behaviors include conceptual, social, and practical adaptive behavior and are skills related to self-care, community living, communication, and socialization (Bullington, 2011). Adaptive behaviors are central to the assessment of developmental disabilities in individuals because they often predict severity and prognosis, as well as assist with determining eligibility for services (Tassé et al., 2012). Across developmental disabilities, both fine and gross motor skills deficits have been found to be associated with difficulties with adaptive behaviors and daily living skills (Di Nuovo & Buono, 2011; Fu, Lincoln, Bellugi, & Searcy, 2015; MacDonald, Lord, & Ulrich, 2014; Tremblay, Richer, Lachance, & Côté, 2010; Vos et al., 2013). This may be due to the involvement of many fine and gross motor skills for successful independent living skills (e.g., pincer grasp for buttoning clothing). Coordination of both fine and gross motor skills is necessary for the development of various self-care and community living skills. Therefore, motor skills are a significant component of adaptive behaviors.

DSM-5 Motor Disorders

Developmental Coordination Disorder
Developmental coordination disorder (DCD) is a neurodevelopmental disorder characterized by significantly impaired coordination of motor skills, which may manifest as clumsiness and delayed or inaccurate motor performance (American Psychiatric Association, 2013). Skill level is significantly below what would be expected for the child's age and learning opportunities, and these impairments interfere with the child's ability to perform adaptive and occupational behaviors (American Psychiatric Association, 2013). As these deficits may also be observed in other disorders, DCD is not diagnosed if these impairments may be better explained by ID, CP, or other disorders which may affect one's movement (Wilmut, Du, & Barnett, 2016). Although these symptoms begin to manifest during an individual's developmental period, due to the variation in attainment of developmental milestones, this disorder is not typically diagnosed until after age 5 to provide adequate learning opportunities (American Psychiatric Association, 2013). As such, DCD intends to describe children who are "clumsy" and have significant motor incoordination in the absence of any underlying neurological pathology (Cairney & King-Dowling, 2015). Therefore, when assessing for DCD, it is necessary to rule out other possible disorders which may be affecting the individual's motor coordination.

The impairments observed in children with DCD vary across individuals and with the individual's age. Across individuals with DCD, deficits may include skills related to motor planning, visual-spatial reasoning, and other gross and fine motor skills (P. H. Wilson, Ruddock, Smits-Engelsman, Polatajko, & Blank, 2013). As the core feature of DCD is motor abilities that are significantly below what would be expected of same-aged peers, the deficits observed differ across ages (Cairney & King-Dowling, 2015). At younger ages, these skills may include walking, while at older ages, these deficits may refer to running and coordination with throwing and catching (Cairney & King-Dowling, 2015; Wilson, Ruddock, Smits-Engelsman, Polatajko, & Blank, 2013).

Assessment of Motor Skills

The assessment of motor skills involves the examination of motor functioning and motor development. Developmental screening is frequently used to identify children who have delays in motor development, with primary care providers often performing screening with preschool-aged children as part of routine medical care (Tieman, Palisano, & Sutlive, 2005). After screening, children who appear to have a delay in motor development may be referred for more comprehensive neurodevelopmental or physical assessment.

A comprehensive assessment of motor functioning with children should include an interview with a parent/caregiver, during which information pertaining to pre- and perinatal health, developmental milestones, adaptive skills, motor functioning, and family history should be collected. A structured interview or parent/caregiver questionnaire may be helpful in obtaining such information (see Review of Assessment Measures for more information). Table 2 also outlines a series of questions that can easily be integrated into clinical interviews that are likely to reveal relevant information. Assessment of developmental functioning, cognitive functioning, academic achievement, and neuromotor status should be integrated with the assessment as necessary to provide

Table 2 Recommended questions for parents/caregivers related to motor functioning and development

Parent/caregiver interview
Was your child born prematurely? If so, at how many weeks gestation?
Where there any complications during the pregnancy?
How much did your child weigh at birth?
At what age did your child first:
Sit up independently?
Crawl?
Walk independently?
Do you have any concerns about your child's motor skills?
Does your child have difficulty with daily tasks, such as dressing, fastening buttons, tying shoes, using utensils, or brushing teeth?
Does your child seem overly clumsy?
Does your child have difficulty with handwriting or using scissors?
Does your child have difficulty throwing or kicking a ball?
How does your child's motor coordination compare to other children his/her age?
Has anyone in your family been diagnosed with a developmental, neurological, or psychiatric disorder?

information needed to understand contributing factors and to rule out possible causes.

There are a number of standardized measures available to measure motor functioning in children. Norm-referenced measures allow for the comparison of an individual's score to the average performance of the normative sample and are helpful for identifying developmental delays and areas of impairment. Criterion-referenced measures assess an individual's performance related to a specific skill or area of functioning. For example, a norm-referenced measure would compare a child's ability to stand to typically developing children of the same age, while a criterion-referenced measure would assess the child's progress toward standing. Tieman, Palisano, and Sutlive (2005) outline five important factors to consider when selecting an appropriate measure for the assessment of motor functioning in children: the purpose of the evaluation (e.g., diagnostic, service eligibility, progress monitoring), characteristics of the child (e.g., age, functional abilities, language abilities), the developmental or functional areas requiring examination (e.g., gross/fine motor skills, self-care, mobility), the setting (e.g., home environment, clinic setting), and any external constraints (e.g., time, equipment, cost). The psychometrics properties of a measure should also be considered.

Standardized measures should be administered by a professional with a knowledge base in child development, experience testing children with disabilities, and knowledge related to test and score interpretation. Administration and scoring should be practiced several times with different children before clinically administering the measure, with particular attention paid to reviewing the test manual. During administration of a standardized measure, the examiner should simultaneously observe how the child performs tasks in order to gain information about the quality of movement in addition to evaluating the skill based on the measure's scoring criteria. Particular attention should be paid to oral motor skills (e.g., closing mouth, shaping lips), eye movements (e.g., eye tracking, pupil dilation), facial expressions, muscle bulk and texture, joint flexibility, grip strength, hand dominance, gross motor skills (e.g., running, hopping, balancing), fine motor skills (e.g., coloring, stacking blocks, using scissors), and motor planning.

Review of Assessment Measures

Fifteen measures of motor development and function for children have been selected for review in this chapter (see Table 3). These measures were selected as they are commonly used and have evidence of reliability and validity. For ease of reference, they are divided into three categories: those that assess motor skills through assessment of performance, those designed to assess developmental functioning overall, and those that are based on informant report.

Performance-Based Assessment of Motor Skills

Performance-based measures of motor skills require the examiner to observe and evaluate the performance of discrete skills based on predetermined criteria. Required tasks vary across measures and age bands, although

Assessment of Fine and Gross Motor Skills

Table 3 Summary of motor skill assessment measures

Measure	Target population	Age	Type	Assessment time
AIMS	Infants with motor difficulties	0–18 months	Test of motor skills	20–30 min
BDI-2	Children at risk for developmental difficulties	0–7.11 years	Test of developmental functioning	60–90 min
Bayley-III	Young children at risk for developmental difficulties	1–42 months	Test of developmental functioning	30–90 min
Beery VMI	Individuals with visual-motor integration difficulties	2–99 years	Test of motor skills	10–20 min
BOT-2	Children and youth with typical development or moderate motor deficits	4–21 years	Test of motor skills	Full form, 45–60 min Short form, 15–20 min
DCDQ'07	Children with coordination disorders	5–15 years	Parent/caregiver questionnaire	10–15 min
DIAL-4	Young children at risk for developmental difficulties	2.6–5.11 years	Test of developmental functioning	30–45 min
ESI-R	Young children at risk for developmental difficulties	3–5.11 years	Test of developmental functioning	10–15 min
GMFM	Children with CP	2–12 years	Test of motor skills	45–60 min
MAP	Preschool-aged children at risk for developmental difficulties	2.9–5.8 years	Test of developmental functioning	30–40 min
Movement ABC-2 performance test	Children and adolescents with motor impairments	3–16 years	Test of motor skills	20–40 min
Movement ABC-2 checklist	Children with motor impairments	5–12 years	Checklist	10 min
MSEL-AGS	Young children	0–68 months	Test of developmental functioning	15–60 min
PDMS-2	Young children with motor impairments	0–5 years	Test of motor skills	45–60 min
Vineland-3 interview form	Individuals with disabilities	0–90+ years	Interview for parent/caregiver	20–40 min
Vineland-3 parent/caregiver form	Individuals with disabilities	0–90+ years	Parent/caregiver questionnaire	10–20 min
Vineland-3 teacher form	Individuals with disabilities	3–21 years	Teacher questionnaire	10–15 min

common gross motor tasks include those such as sitting, walking, running, balancing, throwing/catching large balls, and climbing stairs. Common fine motor tasks include grasping, manipulation of small objects, writing, and using scissors. These tests require that examiners be trained in test administration, scoring, and interpretation to ensure reliable results.

Alberta Infant Motor Scales (AIMS) The AIMS is an assessment scale designed to assess motor development in infants from birth until the attainment of independent walking (Piper, Pinnell, Darrah, Maguire, & Byrne, 1992). It is comprised of 58 items that assess infant movement in 4 positions (i.e., prone, supine, sitting, and standing) that typically can be scored within 20–30 min. Each item is scored by an administrator with knowledge of normal infant motor development as "observed" or "not observed" to generate subscale scores for each position as well as a total score, with higher scores indicating more mature motor development. Percentile ranks, standardized scores, and age-equivalent scores are based on a standardization sample of 2220 infants between the ages of 1 week and 18 months living in the providence of Alberta between 1990 and 1992. Concurrent validity has been established with the Peabody Developmental Motor Scales (PDMS), $r = 0.97$, and the Bayley Scales of Infant Development (BSID-II), $r = 0.98$ (Piper, Darrah, Maguire, & Redfern, 1994; Piper, Pinnell, Darrah, Maguire, & Byrne, 1992). The predictive validity of the AIMS in classifying children with abnormal motor development was found to be good, with cutoff scores at the tenth percentile at 4 months (sensitivity of 77.3%; specificity of 81.7%) and the fifth percentile at 8 months (sensitivity of 86.4%; specificity of 93.0%) providing maximized specificity and sensitivity rates (Darrah, Piper, & Watt, 1998). Interrater and test-retest reliability have also been established (Piper, Darrah, Maguire, & Redfern, 1994; Piper, Pinnell, Darrah, Maguire, & Byrne, 1992). Despite these solid psychometric properties, concern has been raised regarding its outdated normative data (Fleuren, Smit, Stijnen, & Hartman, 2007).

The Beery-Buktenica Developmental Test of Visual-Motor Integration (Beery VMI) The Beery VMI is a measure designed to assess the integration of visual and motor abilities in individuals across the lifespan that can be administered in individual or group format (Beery & Beery, 2010). It is available as a full form and short form, with the full form being appropriate for all ages and the short form designed for children aged 2–7. The full form consists of 25 geometric forms that are copied by the examinee in a test booklet, the first 15 of which comprise the short form. Both versions of the Beery VMI can be administered in about 10–15 min. The Beery VMI is supplemented by two additional standardized tests, Visual Perception and Motor Coordination, which allow for the assessment of visual and motor contributions to performance on the Beery VMI. As these are timed tests, the Visual Perception test is administered in exactly 3 min and the Motor Coordination test in 5 min. The Visual Perception test consists of 30 items in which the examinee is asked to visually identify figures that are progressively smaller and more intricate. The Motor Coordination test consists of 30 increasingly complex shapes in which the examinee is asked to draw within a targeted area.

Raw scores from the Beery VMI and its two supplemental tests are converted into standard scores, scaled scores, percentile ranks, and age and grade equivalents. The Beery VMI has been normed 6 times with a total of 12,500 individuals over a span of 40 years, most recently in 2010. Internal consistency coefficients of the Beery VMI, Visual Perception, and Motor Coordination tests have been estimated to range from 0.83 to 0.96 across age ranges (Beery & Beery, 2010). Overall test-retest reliability coefficients were reported by the manual as 0.88 for the Beery VMI, 0.84 for Visual Perception, and 0.85 for Motor Coordination. Interrater reliability coefficients were reported as 0.93 for the Beery VMI, 0.98 for Visual Perception, and 0.94 for Motor Coordination. Construct validity of the Beery VMI has been examined, with Rasch analysis indicating that it is unidimensional (Brown, Unsworth, & Lyons, 2009; Mao, Li, & Lo, 1999). Predictive validity has also been established, with performance on the Beery VMI predicting performance in elementary school (Paro & Pianta, 2000; Pianta & McCoy, 1997).

Bruininks-Oseretsky Test of Motor Proficiency, Second Edition (BOT-2) The BOT-2 is a standardized measure of fine and gross motor skills in children and youth aged 4–21 years (Bruininks & Bruinicks, 2005). The assessment is designed for individuals with functioning ranging from typical development to moderate fine and/or gross motor difficulties. The BOT-2 consists of eight subtests (i.e., fine motor precision, fine motor integration, manual dexterity, bilateral coordination, balance, running speed and agility, upper limb coordination, strength) consisting of tasks that are scored by the examiner. Composite scores are generated in four motor areas (i.e., fine manual control, manual coordination, body coordination, strength and agility) as well as a total motor composite. The full form consists of 53 items and is typically completed in 45–60 min. A short form is available for screening purposes which includes 14 total items from across the 8 subtests generating a single score of motor proficiency and which can be administered in 15–20 min. Scores from both the full and short forms can be converted into standard scores, while those from the full form can also be converted into age-equivalent scores. The normative sample for the BOT-2 included 1520 children and youth between the ages of 4 and 21 from across the United States (Deitz, Kartin, & Kopp, 2007). Both the short form and full form of the BOT-2 have been demonstrated to have good to excellent test-retest and interrater reliability in healthy children (Bruininks & Bruinicks, 2005). The full form has also been demonstrated to have excellent test-retest reliability in children with ID (Wuang & Su, 2009). Validity has been established through studies examining internal structure, differentiation of clinical and nonclinical groups, and correlation with the PDMS-2 (Bruininks & Bruinicks, 2005).

Gross Motor Function Measure (GMFM) The GMFM is a measure developed to assess the motor functioning of children with CP (Russell, Rosenbaum, Wright, & Avery, 2013). It is designed as an evaluative measure to assess change over time or response to intervention. The original 88-item measure (GMFM-88) has been updated to a 66-item measure (GMFM-66), which requires less administration time. According to the manual, the GMFM-88 is the preferred choice for children who are very young, those who have severe motor limitations, and children who may have motor difficulties unrelated to CP (Russell, Rosenbaum, Wright, & Avery, 2013). Due to differences in item weights between populations, the GMFM-66 is recommended for use only with children with CP. Items from both versions of the GMFM are grouped into five dimensions (i.e., lying and rolling; sitting; crawling and kneeling; standing; walking, running, and jumping). Based on observation, the examiner scores a child's performance on each item on a 4-point scale (i.e., 1, 2, 3, or 4). Scores for each dimension are calculated as a percentage of the maximum score, with a total score then calculated by averaging percentage scores across the five dimensions. The GMFM is criterion-referenced, and thus normative data is not available. Both the GMFM-66 and GMFM-88 have been demonstrated to have excellent test-retest reliability (intraclass correlation coefficient [ICC] = 0.99) and face validity (Russell et al., 2000).

Movement Assessment Battery for Children (Movement ABC-2) The Movement ABC-2 is a measure designed to assess motor performance in children and adolescents aged from 3 to 16 years, developed from the Test of Motor Impairment (TOMI; Henderson, Sugden, & Barnett, 2007; Stott, Moyes, & Henderson, 1972). The Movement ABC-2 Performance Test is complementary to the Movement ABC-2 Checklist, which is described below (see the "Informant-based Measures" section). The Movement ABC-2 Performance Test consists of eight items involving fine and gross motor tasks grouped into three subscales (i.e., manual dexterity, aiming and catching, static and dynamic balance) and takes approximately 20–40 min to administer. Norms have been established based on a standardization sample of 395 children across three age bands (i.e., 3–6, 7–10, 11–16 years). Estimates of test-retest reliability across the subscales range from adequate to good among typically developing children (Henderson, Sugden, & Barnett, 2007). Internal consistency, $\alpha = 0.90$, and test-retest reliability, ICC = 0.97, have been demonstrated to be excellent among children with DCD (Wuang, Su, & Su, 2012). Research related to the validity of the Movement ABC-2 Performance Test is limited, although extensive evidence is available for previous versions of the measure (Brown & Lalor, 2009).

Peabody Developmental Motor Scales, Second Edition (PDMS-2) The PDMS-2 is a standardized test of motor functioning designed for children aged 5 and under (Folio & Fewell, 2000). The test includes 249 items across 6 subtests, which are subdivided into fine motor

(FM) and gross motor (GM) composites and that combine to create a total motor (TM) composite. The FM composite consists of 98 items from 2 subtests (i.e., grasping, visual-motor integration), while the GM composite consists of 151 items from 4 subtests (i.e., reflexes, stationary, locomotion, object manipulation). A child's performance on each item is scored by the examiner on a 3-point scale (i.e., 0, 1, or 2) based on specified item criteria. Standard scores, percentiles, and age-equivalent scores are available for each subtest. Scores from the FM, GM, and TM composites are converted into developmental quotient (DQ) scores. Research has demonstrated the PDMS-2 composite scores to have good to excellent test-retest reliability (ICC = 0.88–1.00) and acceptable sensitivity to change among children with CP (Wang, Liao, & Hsieh, 2006). Among a group of children with and without fine motor problems, the FM composite of the PDMS-2 was found to have excellent test-retest and interrater reliability (r = 0.84–0.99; van Hartingsveldt, Cup, & Oostendorp, 2005). Convergent validity has been established between the TM composite and the Bayley Scales of Infant and Toddler Development (Connolly, McClune, & Gatlin, 2012; Provost et al., 2004).

Measures of Developmental Functioning

Measures of developmental functioning aim to provide a comprehensive assessment of global development and are used frequently in the assessment and screening of developmental disorders. These measures are particularly helpful when assessing children who may be experiencing delays in multiple areas of development. Results from these measures yield valuable information regarding an individual's overall level of functioning as well as areas of strength and weakness, which can be used to inform diagnostic evaluations, determination of service eligibility, treatment planning, and the need for continued evaluation. Motor functioning is a common domain within measures that assess general developmental functioning. Some of the measures have scales addressing motor skills that can be administered independently, while others are designed to be administered within the full test battery. The assessment of motor skills within developmental measures involves the observation and assessment of skills, requiring that examiners be well trained in administration and scoring.

Battelle Developmental Inventory, Second Edition (BDI-2) The BDI-2 is a standardized assessment of developmental skills for children aged birth through 7 years and 11 months (Newborg, 2005). It is comprised of 450 items grouped into 5 domains (i.e., adaptive, personal/social, communication, motor, and cognitive), which can be administered independently of one another. When all five domains are administered, total assessment time is estimated to range from 60 to 90 min. The standardization data was collected in 2002–2003 based on a sample of 2500 children from across the United States; this original standardization data was reweighted in 2016 with the BDI-2 Normative Update. In regard to psychometric properties, the BDI-2 manual indicates internal consistency coefficients ranging from 0.98 to 0.99 for the total score, with averages across domains ranging from 0.85 to 0.95 (Newborg, 2005). Test-retest reliability coefficients for total BDI-2 score ranged from 0.93 to 0.94 across age groups and from 0.77 to 0.90 across domains and age ranges. Interrater reliability coefficients ranged from 0.97 to 0.99. The BDI-2 was found to correlate with the Bayley Scales of Infant and Toddler Development, the Wechsler Preschool and Primary Scale of Intelligence (WPPSI), and the Vineland Adaptive Behavior Scales (Newborg, 2005).

Bayley Scales of Infant and Toddler Development, Third Edition (Bayley-III) The Bayley-III is an individually administered assessment of developmental functioning for young children aged 1 month to 42 months (Bayley, 2006). It is comprised of two scales based on parent/caregiver questionnaires (i.e., social-emotional, adaptive behavior) and three scales scored by the examiner (i.e., cognitive, language, motor) based on observation of skills. Scoring for the testing components of the Bayley-III is either 1 (credit) or 0 (no credit). The Adaptive Behavior Assessment System, Second Edition (ABAS-II), serves as the adaptive behavior scale of the Bayley-III. The motor scale consists of fine motor and gross motor subtest. Total administration time ranges from 30 to 90 min, depending on the age of the child. Scaled scores, percentile ranks, and developmental age scores are available for scales and subtests. The total raw score of the Bayley-III can be converted into a standard score. Normative data for the cognitive, language, and motor scales is based on a standardization sample of 1700 children across 17 age groups; the normative sample for the social-emotional scale is based on a sample of 465 children, while that of the adaptive behavior scale is based on a sample of 1350 children. According to the manual, the Bayley-III has been demonstrated to have internal consistency coefficients ranging from 0.76 to 0.98 across scales (Bayley, 2006). The majority of test-retest reliability coefficients across scales and age ranges were in the .70s and .80s, with correlation increasing as age increased. Interrater reliability coefficients of the adaptive behavior scale were estimated to range between 0.59 and 0.86. Validity has been established through confirmatory factor analysis and correlation with the PDMS-2 and the WPPSI-III (Bayley, 2006; Connolly, McClune, & Gatlin, 2012).

Developmental Indicators for the Assessment of Learning, Fourth Edition (DIAL-4) The DIAL-4 is an individually administered screening of developmental function for children aged 2 years and 6 months to 5 years and 11 months (Mardell & Goldenberg, 2011). The test is designed to be used to screen large groups of children efficiently through the use of multiple testing stations for each of the three domains scored based on performance (i.e., motor, language, concepts), making it particularly useful for school settings. Items on these scales are scored on a scale of 0–4 based on task and skill demonstration. Two additional domains (i.e., self-help development, social-emotional development) are scored based on ratings on a 3-point Likert scale from a parent/caregiver or teacher. The full measure can be administered in approximately 30–45 min. The motor domain assesses both gross and fine motor functioning; it is not designed to be administered independent of the other domains. Standard scores and percentile ranks are available for a total score and each of the domains following completion of the fully assessment. The normative sample included 1400 children, 700 parents, and 700 teachers from across the United States. The DIAL-4 manual reports internal reliability coefficients across ages to range from the .80s to .90s (Mardell & Goldenberg, 2011). Test-retest reliability coefficients ranged from 0.64 to 0.95 between the English and Spanish versions, and interrater reliability ranged from 0.89 to 0.98. Moderate correlation was found between the concepts and language domains and the ESP cognitive/language domain (0.51 and 0.61), although correlation was low (0.21) between the DIAL-4 motor and ESP motor domain (Mardell & Goldenberg, 2011). The DIAL-4 and the ESP examine different motor tasks, which may account for the low correlation between the two motor scales. The DIAL-4 total score was found to correlate highly with the Differential Ability Scales, Second Edition (DAS-II) General Conceptual Ability score (0.73), supporting its use as a screener for possible cognitive delays (Mardell & Goldenberg, 2011).

Early Screening Inventory-Revised (ESI-R) The ESI-R is an individually administered test designed to screen young children for special education services (Meisels et al., 2008). Two forms of the ESI are available based on age group: the ESI Preschool (ESI-P) is appropriate for children aged 3 years to 4 years and 5 months, and the ESI Kindergarten (ESI-K) is appropriate for those aged 4 years and 6 months to 5 years and 11 months. It is comprised of three scales (i.e., visual-motor/adaptive, language and cognition, gross motor skills). The visual-motor/adaptive scale includes items targeting fine motor skills and visuomotor integration, while the gross motor scale includes those targeting gross motor coordination.

The ESI-R is typically administered in 15–20 min. Cutoffs are available for total scores on the ESI-P and ESI-K across age bands indicating into which of three classifications (i.e., "OK," "Rescreen," "Refer") the examinee scored. The ESI-R was originally standardized using a sample of 6031 children from across the United States and updated in 2006 with an additional 1200 cases. The ESI-R manual reports that both the ESI-P and ESI-K have sensitivity of at least 0.92 and specificity of 0.80 (Meisels et al., 2008). In regard to the ESI-K, interrater reliability was reported to be 0.97, and test-retest reliability coefficients ranged from 0.79 to 0.84. Reliability was not examined in the ESI-P. A strong correlation (0.73) was found between both the ESI-K and ESI-P, respectively, with the McCarthy Scales of Children's Abilities establishing convergent validity.

Miller Assessment of Preschoolers (MAP) The MAP is an individually administered test designed to assess the developmental functioning of children aged 2 years and 9 months up to 5 years and 8 months (Miller, 1988). As a broad developmental measure, the MAP provides a developmental overview and is designed to identify young children who may be at risk for developmental difficulties. It is comprised of five performance indices (i.e., foundations, coordination, verbal, nonverbal, complex tasks), two of which target motor skills: the foundation index assesses basic fine and gross motor skills and the coordination index assesses complex gross, fine, and oral motor skills. The MAP can typically be completed in 30–40 min. The total raw score of the MAP as well as the raw score of each of the indices can be transformed into percentile scores. The normative sample for the MAP was comprised of 1200 preschoolers from across the United States (Miller, 1988). The test manual reports good to excellent interrater and test-retest reliability across performance indices (Miller, 1988). More recently, construct validity has been demonstrated via strong correlation with the Pediatric Examination of Educational Readiness (PEER), another developmental measure (Parush, Yochman, Jessel, Shapiro, & Mazor-Karsenty, 2002). Additionally, the MAP has been demonstrated to differentiate between 5-year-olds with extremely low birth weight and those born full term (Leosdottir, Egilson, & Georgsdottir, 2006), as well as between preschool-aged children with and without prenatal drug exposure (Fulks & Harris, 2005). While the psychometrics appear to be sound, updated normative data and research pertaining to reliability are needed.

Mullen Scales of Early Learning: American Guidance Service Edition (MSEL:AGS) The MSEL:AGS is a widely used multidomain test designed to assess the development of young children (Mullen, 1995). It consists of 5 individual scales, 4 that cover children aged 0–68 months (i.e., visual reception, fine motor, receptive language, expressive language) and 1 for children aged 0–33 months (i.e., gross motor), which can be administered independently of one another. The fine motor scale consists of 30 items, requires minimal language skills, and measures visual-motor planning and control, motor imitation, and manipulation of objects. The gross motor scale consists of 35 items that measure motor control and mobility. The time required for administration for the full test varies by age, with the manual estimating 15 min for 1-year-olds, 30 min for 4-year-olds, and 60 min for 5-year-olds. Raw scores for each scale can be converted into standardized T scores, percentile ranks, and age equivalents. Administration of the full test generates an Early Learning Composite (ELC) standard score. Standardization is based on a normative sample of 1849 children aged 2 days–69 months from across the United States between 1981 and 1989 who did not have physical or mental disabilities. The manual reports psychometric properties of the original MSEL. Convergent validity was established through moderate correlation with the BSID and Peabody Developmental Motor Scales (Mullen, 1995). Test-retest reliability was high for the gross motor scale (0.96) and ranged from 0.82 to 0.85 for the other scales, while interrater reliability was reported to be high (0.91–0.99; Mullen, 1995). Concerns related to this measure include outdated norms and the exclusion of children with disabilities from the standardization sample (Lee, 2013).

Informant-Based Measures

Informant-based measures of motor functioning are based on report of skills from adults familiar with the child's functioning, such as a parent/caregiver or teacher. They are particularly useful for screening purposes, as they take less time to complete, require less training for administration and scoring, and are typically less expensive than performance-based measures. They are also frequently administered within testing batteries to allow for data collection from multiple sources.

Developmental Coordination Disorder Questionnaire 2007 (DCDQ'07) The DCDQ'07 is a brief parent questionnaire designed to assist in the identification of DCD in children aged 5–15 years (B. N. Wilson, Kaplan, Crawford, & Roberts, 2007). It consists of 15 items that ask parents to compare their child's motor performance to that of typically developing peers on a 5-point Likert scale. As the measure is brief, it can typically be completed by parents in about 10–15 min. The measure consists of three factors (i.e., control during movement, fine motor and handwriting, and general coordination). Scores from each of the three factors are computed along with a total score. Scores are interpreted across three age bands and two score ranges: "Indication of, or Suspect for, DCD" and "Probably not DCD." Overall sensitivity of the DCDQ'07 is reported to be 84.7% and the specificity to be 70.8% (Wilson, Kaplan, Crawford, & Roberts, 2007). Construct validity has been demonstrated through moderate correlation ($r = 0.55$) with the Movement ABC (Wilson et al., 2009) in addition to exploratory and confirmatory factor analysis (Hua et al., 2015). Internal consistency and test-retest reliability were found to be excellent (Hua et al., 2015).

Movement Assessment Battery for Children Checklist (Movement ABC-2 Checklist) The Movement ABC-2 Checklist is an informant-based checklist that is complementary to the Movement ABC-2 Performance Test (Henderson, Sugden, & Barnett, 2007). It is comprised of 30 items and takes approximately 10 min to complete. The checklist is designed to be completed by an adult familiar with the child, such as a parent/caregiver, teacher, or service provider. It has been found to discriminate between children with and without motor impairment when completed by teachers (Schoemaker, Niemeijer, Flapper, & Smits-Engelsman, 2012). Internal consistency was found to be excellent, $\alpha = 0.94$, and moderate correlation with the Performance Test and DCDQ'07 has been established (Schoemaker, Niemeijer, Flapper, & Smits-Engelsman, 2012). However, evidence is needed regarding test-retest and interrater reliability.

Vineland Adaptive Behavior Scales, Third Edition (Vineland-3) The Vineland-3 is a group of measures of adaptive behavior that are widely used in the assessment of individuals with disabilities (Sparrow, Cicchetti, & Saulnier, 2016). It is available in three formats: (1) the Interview Form, which is administered by a professional to a respondent who can reliably report on the adaptive behavior on the individual; (2) the Parent/Caregiver Form, which is completed by a parent or caregiver using a rating scale format; and (3) the Teacher Form, which is completed by a teacher using a questionnaire format. The Interview Form and Parent/Caregiver Form provide normative scores for individuals of all ages, from birth to over 90 years of age, whereas the Teacher Form provides normative scores for individuals aged 3–21. All three formats follow the same domain/subdomain format, which includes three domains that comprise the Adaptive Behavior Composite (i.e., communication, daily living skills, socialization) and two optional domains (i.e., motor skills, maladaptive behavior). For each of the domains and for the Adaptive Behavior Composite, standard scores, percentile ranks, and age equivalents are available.

The normative sample for Vineland-3 was recently updated. The Interview and Parent/Caregiver Forms included 2560 aged 0–80+ years from across the United States; the sample for the Teacher Form included 1415 students aged 3–18 years from across the United States. Both samples included individuals with a range of disabilities, including ID, developmental delay, autism, and speech/language impairments. The motor skills domain is comprised of two subdomains (i.e., gross motor, fine motor) and is normed for individuals aged 0–9 years. While optional for the Adaptive Behavior Composite, the motor skills domain is not designed for administration independent of the other domains. According to the Vineland-3 manual, all forms of the Vineland-3 demonstrate strong psychometric properties. ICCs ranged from 0.83 to 0.9 across domains and forms (Sparrow, Cicchetti, & Saulnier, 2016). Test-retest reliability coefficients ranged from 0.71 to 0.94 across domains and forms, and interrater reliability coefficients ranged from 0.61 to 0.87. Validity has been established through correlation with the Bayley-III and Adaptive Behavior Assessment System (ABAS-3) as well as through differential scoring of clinical subsamples.

Conclusion

Motor development is directly tied to the development of cognitive, language, and social skills. The assessment of motor skills and functioning in children provides valuable information toward the screening of developmental delays, the identification of neurodevelopmental disorders, intervention planning, and progress monitoring. There are a number of standardized measures that assess motor functioning in children, including those specifically examining fine and/or gross motor skills, measures of developmental functioning, and informant-report-based interviews and questionnaires. When selecting an appropriate measure, attention should be paid to child characteristics and the purpose of the evaluation. As part of a comprehensive assessment, standardized measures should be paired with parent/caregiver interview and clinical examination of cognitive, adaptive, and physical functioning.

References

Alcock, K. J., & Krawczyk, K. (2010). Individual differences in language development: Relationship with motor skill at 21 months. *Developmental Science*, *13*(5), 677–691. https://doi.org/10.1111/j.1467-7687.2009.00924.x

American Psychiatric Association. (2013). *Diagnostic and statistical manual of mental disorders* (5th ed.). Washington, DC: American Psychiatric Association.

Bax, M. C. O. (2008). Terminology and classification of cerebral palsy. *Developmental Medicine & Child Neurology*, *6*(3), 295–297. https://doi.org/10.1111/j.1469-8749.1964.tb10791.x

Bayley, N. (2006). *Bayley scales of infant and toddler development, third edition: Technical manual*. San Antonio, TX: Harcourt.

Beery, K. E., & Beery, N. A. (2010). *The Beery-Buktenica developmental test of visual-motor integration (Beery VMI)*. Bloomington, MN: Pearson.

Berninger, V. W., Richards, T. L., & Abbott, R. D. (2015). Differential diagnosis of dysgraphia, dyslexia, and OWL LD: Behavioral and neuroimaging evidence. *Reading and Writing*, *28*(8), 1119–1153. https://doi.org/10.1007/s11145-015-9565-0

Bhat, A. N., Landa, R. J., & Galloway, J. C. (2011). Current perspectives on motor functioning in infants, children, and adults with autism spectrum disorders. *Physical Therapy*, *91*(7), 1116–1129.

Brown, T., & Lalor, A. (2009). The movement assessment battery for children—Second edition (MABC-2): A review and critique. *Physical & Occupational Therapy in Pediatrics*, *29*(1), 86–103. https://doi.org/10.1080/01942630802574908

Brown, T., Unsworth, C., & Lyons, C. (2009). An evaluation of the construct validity of the developmental test of visual-motor integration using the Rasch measurement model. *Australian Occupational Therapy Journal*, *56*(6), 393–402. https://doi.org/10.1111/j.1440-1630.2009.00811.x

Bruininks, R. H., & Bruinicks, B. D. (2005). *Bruininks-Oseretsky test of motor proficiency, second edition (BOT-2)*. Minneapolis, MN: Pearson.

Bullington, E. A. (2011). Adaptive behavior. In S. Goldstein & J. A. Naglieri (Eds.), *Encyclopedia of child behavior and development*. New York: Springer.

Cairney, J., & King-Dowling, S. (2015). Developmental coordination disorder. In J. L. Matson (Ed.), *Comorbid conditions among children with autism spectrum disorders* (pp. 303–322). New York: Springer.

Calhoun, M., Longworth, M., & Chester, V. L. (2011). Gait patterns in children with autism. *Clinical biomechanics*, *26*(2), 200–206. https://doi.org/10.1016/j.clinbiomech.2010.09.013

Chapman, R. S., & Hesketh, L. J. (2000). Behavioral phenotype of individuals with down syndrome. *Mental Retardation and Developmental Disabilities Research Reviews*, *6*(2), 84–95. https://doi.org/10.1002/1098-2779

Chawarska, K., Paul, R., Klin, A., Hannigen, S., Dichtel, L. E., & Volkmar, F. (2007). Parental recognition of developmental problems in toddlers with autism spectrum disorders. *Journal of Autism and Developmental Disorders*, *37*(1), 62–72.

Chung, P., & Patel, D. R. (2016). Dysgraphia. In J. Merrick & J. Merrick (Eds.), *Child and adolescent health yearbook 2015* (pp. 27–38). Hauppauge, NY: Nova Science Publishers.

Clearfield, M. W. (2011). Learning to walk changes infants' social interactions. *Infant Behavior and Development, 34*(1), 15–25. https://doi.org/10.1016/j.infbeh.2010.04.008

Colombo-Dougovito, A. M., & Reeve, R. E. (2017). Exploring the interaction of motor and social skills with autism severity using the SFARI dataset. *Perceptual and Motor Skills, 124*(2), 413–424. https://doi.org/10.1177/0031512516689198

Connolly, B. H., McClune, N. O., & Gatlin, R. (2012). Concurrent validity of the Bayley-III and the Peabody developmental motor scale–2. *Pediatric Physical Therapy, 24*(4), 345. https://doi.org/10.1097/PEP.0b013e318267c5cf

Centers for Disease Control and Prevention. (2017, October 16). *Developmental Milestones*. Retrieved from https://www.cdc.gov/ncbddd/actearly/milestones/index.html

Darrah, J., Piper, M., & Watt, M.-J. (1998). Assessment of gross motor skills of at-risk infants: Predictive validity of the Alberta infant motor scale. *Developmental Medicine & Child Neurology, 40*(7), 485–491. https://doi.org/10.1111/j.1469-8749.1998.tb15399.x

Deitz, J. C., Kartin, D., & Kopp, K. (2007). Review of the Bruininks-Oseretsky test of motor proficiency, second edition (BOT-2). *Physical & Occupational Therapy in Pediatrics, 27*(4), 87–102. https://doi.org/10.1080/J006v27n04_06

Di Nuovo, S., & Buono, S. (2011). Behavioral phenotypes of genetic syndromes with intellectual disability: Comparison of adaptive profiles. *Psychiatry Research, 189*(3), 440–445. https://doi.org/10.1016/j.psychres.2011.03.015

Döhla, D., & Heim, S. (2016). Developmental dyslexia and dysgraphia: What can we learn from the one about the other? *Frontiers in Psychology, 6*. https://doi.org/10.3389/fpsyg.2015.02045

Fleuren, K. M. W., Smit, L. S., Stijnen, T., & Hartman, A. (2007). New reference values for the Alberta infant motor scale need to be established. *Acta Paediatrica, 96*(3), 424–427. https://doi.org/10.1111/j.1651-2227.2007.00111.x

Flint, J. (2001). Genetic basis of cognitive disability. *Dialogues in Clinical Neuroscience, 3*(1), 37.

Folio, M. K., & Fewell, R. F. (2000). *Peabody developmental motor scales: Examiner's manual* (2nd ed.). Austin, TX: PRO-ED.

Fu, T. J., Lincoln, A. J., Bellugi, U., & Searcy, Y. M. (2015). The association of intelligence, visual-motor functioning, and personality characteristics with adaptive behavior in individuals with Williams syndrome. *American Journal on Intellectual and Developmental Disabilities, 120*(4), 273–288. https://doi.org/10.1352/1944-7558-120.4.273

Fulks, M.-A. L., & Harris, S. R. (2005). Predictive accuracy of the miller assessment for preschoolers in children with prenatal drug exposure. *Physical & Occupational Therapy in Pediatrics, 25*(1–2), 17–37. https://doi.org/10.1080/J006v25n01_03

Gaines, R., & Missiuna, C. (2007). Early identification: Are speech/language-impaired toddlers at increased risk for developmental coordination disorder? *Child: Care, Health and Development, 33*(3), 325–332. https://doi.org/10.1111/j.1365-2214.2006.00677.x

Gerber, R. J., Wilks, T., & Erdie-Lalena, C. (2010). Developmental milestones: Motor development. *Pediatrics in Review, 31*(7), 267. https://doi.org/10.1542/pir.31-7-267

Ghassabian, A., Sundaram, R., Bell, E., Bello, S. C., Kus, C., & Yeung, E. (2016). Gross motor milestones and subsequent development. *Pediatrics, 138*(1), e20154372–e20154372. https://doi.org/10.1542/peds.2015-4372

Ghaziuddin, M., & Butler, E. (1998). Clumsiness in autism and Asperger syndrome: A further report. *Journal of Intellectual Disability Research: JIDR, 42*(Pt 1), 43–48.

Gibson, E. (1988). Exploratory behavior in the development of perceiving, acting, and the acquiring of knowledge. *Annual Review of Psychology, 39*, 1–42.

Haibach-Beach, P., Reid, G., & Collier, D. (2011). *Motor learning and development* (1st ed.). Champaign, IL: Human Kinetics.

Henderson, S. E., Sugden, D. A., & Barnett, A. L. (2007). *Movement assessment battery for children* (2nd ed.). London: Pearson.

Hill, E. L. (2001). Non-specific nature of specific language impairment: A review of the literature with regard to concomitant motor impairments. *International Journal of Language & Communication Disorders, 36*(2), 149–171. https://doi.org/10.1080/13682820010019874

Hitzert, M. M., Roze, E., Van Braeckel, K. N. J. A., & Bos, A. F. (2014). Motor development in 3-month-old healthy term-born infants is associated with cognitive and behavioural outcomes at early school age. *Developmental Medicine & Child Neurology, 56*(9), 869–876. https://doi.org/10.1111/dmcn.12468

Houwen, S., van der Putten, A., & Vlaskamp, C. (2014). A systematic review of the effects of motor interventions to improve motor, cognitive, and/or social functioning in people with severe or profound intellectual disabilities. *Research in Developmental Disabilities, 35*(9), 2093–2116. https://doi.org/10.1016/j.ridd.2014.05.006

Hua, J., Gu, G., Zhu, Q., Wo, D., Liu, M., Liu, J.-Q., ... Duan, T. (2015). The reliability and validity of the developmental coordination disorder Questionnaire'07 for children aged 4-6 years in mainland China. *Research in Developmental Disabilities, 47*, 405–415. https://doi.org/10.1016/j.ridd.2015.10.006

Institute of Medicine (U.S.). (2015). In T. F. Boat, J. T. Wu, & National Academies of Sciences, Engineering, and Medicine (Eds.), *Mental disorders and disabilities among low-income children*. Washington, DC: National Academies Press.

Karam, S. M., Riegel, M., Segal, S. L., Félix, T. M., Barros, A. J. D., Santos, I. S., ... Black, M. (2015). Genetic causes of intellectual disability in a birth cohort: A population-based study. *American Journal of Medical Genetics Part A, 167*(6), 1204–1214. https://doi.org/10.1002/ajmg.a.37011

Kindregan, D., Gallagher, L., & Gormley, J. (2015). Gait deviations in children with autism spectrum disorders: A review. *Autism Research and Treatment, 2015*, 1–8. https://doi.org/10.1155/2015/741480

Kirby, R. S., Wingate, M. S., Van Naarden Braun, K., Doernberg, N. S., Arneson, C. L., Benedict, R. E., ... Yeargin-Allsopp, M. (2011). Prevalence and functioning of children with cerebral palsy in four areas of the United States in 2006: A report from the Autism and Developmental Disabilities Monitoring Network. *Research in Developmental Disabilities, 32*(2), 462–469. https://doi.org/10.1016/j.ridd.2010.12.042

Landa, R., & Garrett-Mayer, E. (2006). Development in infants with autism spectrum disorders: A prospective study. *Journal of Child Psychology and Psychiatry, 47*(6), 629–638. https://doi.org/10.1111/j.1469-7610.2006.01531.x

Lee, E. B. (2013). Mullen scales of early learning. In *Encyclopedia of autism spectrum disorders* (pp. 1941–1946). New York, NY: Springer. https://doi.org/10.1007/978-1-4419-1698-3_596

Leonard, H. C., & Hill, E. L. (2014). Review: The impact of motor development on typical and atypical social cognition and language: A systematic review. *Child and Adolescent Mental Health, 19*(3), 163–170. https://doi.org/10.1111/camh.12055

Leosdottir, T., Egilson, S. T., & Georgsdottir, I. (2006). Performance of extremely low birthweight children at 5 years of age on the Miller assessment for preschoolers. *Physical & Occupational Therapy in Pediatrics, 25*(4), 59–72. https://doi.org/10.1080/J006v25n04_05

Liu, T. (2013). Sensory processing and motor skill performance in elementary school children with autism spectrum disorder. *Perceptual and Motor Skills, 116*(1), 197–209. https://doi.org/10.2466/10.25.PMS.116.1.197-209

Lloyd, M., MacDonald, M., & Lord, C. (2013). Motor skills of toddlers with autism spectrum disorders. *Autism, 17*(2), 133–146. https://doi.org/10.1177/1362361311402230

Loveland, K. A., & Kelley, M. L. (1991). Development of adaptive behavior in preschoolers with autism or down syndrome. *American Journal on Mental Retardation, 96*(1), 13–20.

MacDonald, M., Lord, C., & Ulrich, D. A. (2014). Motor skills and calibrated autism severity in young children with autism spectrum disorder. *Adapted Physical Activity Quarterly, 31*(2), 95–105.

Mäki, H. S., Voeten, M. J. M., Vauras, M. M. S., & Poskiparta, E. H. (2001). Predicting writing skill development with word recognition and preschool readiness skills. *Reading and Writing, 14*(7), 643–672. https://doi.org/10.1023/A:1012071514719

Mao, H.-F., Li, W., & Lo, J.-L. (1999). Construct validity of Beery's developmental test of visual-motor integration for Taiwanese children. *The Occupational Therapy Journal of Research, 19*(4), 241–257. https://doi.org/10.1177/153944929901900402

Mardell, C., & Goldenberg, D. (2011). *DIAL 4: Developmental indicators for the assessment of learning*. Bloomington, MN: Pearson.

Meisels, S. J., Marsden, D. B., Wiske, M. S., Henderson, L. W., Pearson (Firm), & PsychCorp (Firm). (2008). *Early screening inventory revised: ESI-R*. New York: Pearson.

Mervis, C. B., & Klein-Tasman, B. P. (2000). Williams syndrome: Cognition, personality, and adaptive behavior. *Mental Retardation and Developmental Disabilities Research Reviews, 6*(2), 148–158. https://doi.org/10.1002/1098-2779

Miller, L. J. (1988). *The Miller assessment for preschoolers*. San Antonio, TX: Pearson.

Missiuna, C., Gaines, B. R., & Pollock, N. (2002). Recognizing and referring children at risk for developmental coordination disorder: Role of the speech-language pathologist. *Journal of Speech-Language Pathology and Audiology, 25*(4), 172–179.

Miyahara, M., Tsujii, M., Hori, M., Nakanishi, K., Kageyama, H., & Sugiyama, T. (1997). Brief report: Motor incoordination in children with Asperger syndrome and learning disabilities. *Journal of Autism and Developmental Disorders, 27*(5), 595–603.

Mullen, E. M. (1995). *Mullen scales of early learning: AGS edition*. Circle Pines, MN: American Guidance Service.

Newborg, J. (2005). *Battelle developmental inventory* (2nd ed.). Itasca, IL: Riverside.

Oudgenoeg-Paz, O., Mulder, H., Jongmans, M. J., van der Ham, I. J. M., & Van der Stigchel, S. (2017). The link between motor and cognitive development in children born preterm and/or with low birth weight: A review of current evidence. *Neuroscience & Biobehavioral Reviews, 80*, 382–393. https://doi.org/10.1016/j.neubiorev.2017.06.009

Ozonoff, S., Young, G. S., Goldring, S., Greiss-Hess, L., Herrera, A. M., Steele, J., ... Rogers, S. J. (2008). Gross motor development, movement abnormalities, and early identification of autism. *Journal of Autism and Developmental Disorders, 38*(4), 644–656. https://doi.org/10.1007/s10803-007-0430-0

Palisano, R. J., Rosenbaum, P., Bartlett, D., & Livingston, M. H. (2008). Content validity of the expanded and revised Gross Motor Function Classification System. *Developmental Medicine & Child Neurology, 50*(10), 744–750. https://doi.org/10.1111/j.1469-8749.2008.03089.x

Palisano, R., Rosenbaum, P., Bartlett, D., & Livingston, M. (2007). *Gross motor function classification system - expanded and revised*. CanChild Centre for Childhood Disability Research: McMaster University.

Palisano, R., Rosenbaum, P., Walter, S., Russell, D., Wood, E., & Galuppi, B. (2008). Development and reliability of a system to classify gross motor function in children with cerebral palsy. *Developmental Medicine & Child Neurology, 39*(4), 214–223. https://doi.org/10.1111/j.1469-8749.1997.tb07414.x

Paro, K. M. L., & Pianta, R. C. (2000). Predicting children's competence in the early school years: A meta-analytic review. *Review of Educational Research, 70*(4), 443–484. https://doi.org/10.3102/00346543070004443

Parsons, J. P. (2011). Cerebral palsy. In S. Goldstein & J. A. Naglieri (Eds.), *Encyclopedia of child behavior and development* (pp. 327–328). Boston, MA: Springer US.

Parush, S., Yochman, A., Jessel, A. S., Shapiro, M., & Mazor-Karsenty, T. (2002). Construct validity of the miller assessment for preschoolers and the pediatric examination of educational readiness for children. *Physical & Occupational Therapy in Pediatrics, 22*(2), 7–27. https://doi.org/10.1080/J006v22n02_02

Piaget, J. (1953). *The origin of the intelligence in the child*. London: Routledge.

Pianta, R. C., & McCoy, S. J. (1997). The first day of school: The predictive validity of early school screening. *Journal of Applied Developmental Psychology, 18*(1), 1–22. https://doi.org/10.1016/S0193-3973(97)90011-3

Piek, J. P., Dawson, L., Smith, L. M., & Gasson, N. (2008). The role of early fine and gross motor development on later motor and cognitive ability. *Human Movement Science, 27*(5), 668–681. https://doi.org/10.1016/j.humov.2007.11.002

Piper, M. C., Darrah, J., Maguire, T. O., & Redfern, L. (1994). *Motor assessment of the developing infant*. Philadelphia: Saunders.

Piper, M. C., Pinnell, L. E., Darrah, J., Maguire, T., & Byrne, P. J. (1992). Construction and validation of the Alberta Infant Motor Scale (AIMS). *Canadian Journal of Public Health/Revue Canadienne de Sante Publique, 83*(Suppl 2), S46–S50.

Provost, B., Heimerl, S., McClain, C., Kim, N.-H., Lopez, B. R., & Kodituwakku, P. (2004). Concurrent validity of the Bayley scales of infant development II motor scale and the Peabody developmental motor scales-2 in children with developmental delays. *Pediatric Physical Therapy, 16*(3), 149–156. https://doi.org/10.1097/01.PEP.0000136005.41585.FE

Russell, D. J., Avery, L. M., Rosenbaum, P. L., Raina, P. S., Walter, S. D., & Palisano, R. J. (2000). Improved scaling of the gross motor function measure for children with cerebral palsy: Evidence of reliability and validity. *Physical Therapy, 80*(9), 873–885. https://doi.org/10.1093/ptj/80.9.873

Russell, D. J., Rosenbaum, P., Wright, M., & Avery, L. M. (2013). *Gross motor function measure (GMFM-66 & GMFM-88): Users manual* (2nd ed.). Hoboken, NJ: Wiley.

Sanjeevan, T., Rosenbaum, D. A., Miller, C., van Hell, J. G., Weiss, D. J., & Mainela-Arnold, E. (2015). Motor issues in specific language impairment: A window into the underlying impairment. *Current Developmental Disorders Reports, 2*(3), 228–236. https://doi.org/10.1007/s40474-015-0051-9

Schoemaker, M. M., Niemeijer, A. S., Flapper, B. C. T., & Smits-Engelsman, B. C. M. (2012). Validity and reliability of the movement assessment battery for Children-2 checklist for children with and without motor impairments. *Developmental Medicine & Child Neurology, 54*(4), 368–375. https://doi.org/10.1111/j.1469-8749.2012.04226.x

Smith, L. E., Maenner, M. J., & Seltzer, M. M. (2012). Developmental trajectories in adolescents and adults with autism: The case of daily living skills. *Journal of the American Academy of Child & Adolescent Psychiatry, 51*(6), 622–631. https://doi.org/10.1016/j.jaac.2012.03.001

Sparrow, S. S., Cicchetti, D. V., & Saulnier, C. A. (2016). *Vineland adaptive behavior scales, third edition*. Minneapolis, MN: Pearson Assessments.

Stott, D. H., Moyes, F. A., & Henderson, S. E. (1972). *Test of motor impairment*. Guelph, Ontario: Department of Psychology, University of Guelph, Ontario.

Summers, J. A., & Feldman, M. A. (1999). Distinctive pattern of behavioral functioning in Angelman syndrome. *American Journal on Mental Retardation, 104*(4), 376–384. https://doi.org/10.1352/0895-8017

Tassé, M. J., Schalock, R. L., Balboni, G., Bersani, H., Borthwick-Duffy, S. A., Spreat, S., ... Zhang, D. (2012). The construct of adaptive behavior: Its conceptualization, measurement, and use in the field of intellectual disability. *American Journal on Intellectual and Developmental Disabilities, 117*(4), 291–303. https://doi.org/10.1352/1944-7558-117.4.291

Tieman, B. L., Palisano, R. J., & Sutlive, A. C. (2005). Assessment of motor development and function in preschool children. *Mental Retardation and Developmental Disabilities Research Reviews, 11*(3), 189–196. https://doi.org/10.1002/mrdd.20074

Tremblay, K. N., Richer, L., Lachance, L., & Côté, A. (2010). Psychopathological manifestations of children with intellectual disabilities according to their cognitive and adaptive behavior profile. *Research in Developmental Disabilities, 31*(1), 57–69. https://doi.org/10.1016/j.ridd.2009.07.016

van Hartingsveldt, M. J., Cup, E. H., & Oostendorp, R. A. (2005). Reliability and validity of the fine motor scale of the Peabody developmental motor scales-2. *Occupational Therapy International, 12*(1), 1–13. https://doi.org/10.1002/oti.11

Vlachos, F., & Karapetsas, A. (2003). Visual memory deficit in children with dysgraphia. *Perceptual and Motor Skills, 97*(3_suppl), 1281–1288.

Vos, R. C., Becher, J. G., Ketelaar, M., Smits, D.-W., Voorman, J. M., Tan, S. S., ... Dallmeijer, A. J. (2013). Developmental trajectories of daily activities in children and adolescents with cerebral palsy. *Pediatrics, 132*(4), e915–e923. https://doi.org/10.1542/peds.2013-0499

Vuijk, P. J., Hartman, E., Scherder, E., & Visscher, C. (2010). Motor performance of children with mild intellectual disability and borderline intellectual functioning. *Journal of Intellectual Disability Research, 54*(11), 955–965. https://doi.org/10.1111/j.1365-2788.2010.01318.x

Walle, E. A., & Campos, J. J. (2014). Infant language development is related to the acquisition of walking.

Developmental Psychology, 50(2), 336–348. https://doi.org/10.1037/a0033238

Wang, H.-H., Liao, H.-F., & Hsieh, C.-L. (2006). Reliability, sensitivity to change, and responsiveness of the Peabody developmental motor scales–second edition for children with cerebral palsy. *Physical Therapy, 86*(10), 1351–1359. https://doi.org/10.2522/ptj.20050259

Wilmut, K., Du, W., & Barnett, A. L. (2016). Gait patterns in children with developmental coordination disorder. *Experimental Brain Research, 234*(6), 1747–1755. https://doi.org/10.1007/s00221-016-4592-x

Wilson, B. N., Crawford, S. G., Green, D., Roberts, G., Aylott, A., & Kaplan, B. J. (2009). Psychometric properties of the revised developmental coordination disorder questionnaire. *Physical & Occupational Therapy in Pediatrics, 29*(2), 182–202. https://doi.org/10.1080/01942630902784761

Wilson, B. N., Kaplan, B. J., Crawford, S. G., & Roberts, G. (2007). *Developmental coordination disorder questionnaire-2007 (DCDQ'07)*. Alberta, Canada: Children's Hospital Research Center.

Wilson, P. H., Ruddock, S., Smits-Engelsman, B., Polatajko, H., & Blank, R. (2013). Understanding performance deficits in developmental coordination disorder: A meta-analysis of recent research: Review. *Developmental Medicine & Child Neurology, 55*(3), 217–228. https://doi.org/10.1111/j.1469-8749.2012.04436.x

Wood, E., & Rosenbaum, P. (2000). The gross motor function classification system for cerebral palsy: A study of reliability and stability over time. *Developmental Medicine and Child Neurology, 42*(5), 292–296.

Wuang, Y.-P., & Su, C.-Y. (2009). Reliability and responsiveness of the Bruininks–Oseretsky test of motor proficiency-second edition in children with intellectual disability. *Research in Developmental Disabilities, 30*(5), 847–855. https://doi.org/10.1016/j.ridd.2008.12.002

Wuang, Y.-P., Su, J.-H., & Su, C.-Y. (2012). Reliability and responsiveness of the movement assessment battery for children–second edition test in children with developmental coordination disorder. *Developmental Medicine & Child Neurology, 54*(2), 160–165. https://doi.org/10.1111/j.1469-8749.2011.04177.x

WHO Multicentre Growth Reference Study Group. (2006). WHO motor development study: Windows of achievement for six gross motor development milestones. *Acta Paediatrica, 450*, 86–95.

Zelaznik, H. N., & Goffman, L. (2010). Generalized motor abilities and timing behavior in children with specific language impairment. *Journal of Speech Language and Hearing Research, 53*(2), 383. https://doi.org/10.1044/1092-4388(2009/08-0204)

Index

A
AAMD adaptive behavior scales, 74
ABDS, *see* Adaptive Behavior Diagnostic Scale (ABDS)
Aberrant Behavior Checklist (ABC), 137
ABI, *see* Adaptive Behavior Inventory (ABI)
Abnormal cholesterol levels, 434
Academic achievement assessments
    academic skill, 106
    basic reading, 107
    clinical judgment, 106
    DSM-5, 106
    greatest diagnostic certainty, 106
    identify and classify learning disabilities, 106
    low academic achievement, 106
    mathematics
        career and job opportunities, 110
        child's ability, 110
        WIAT-III, 110–111
        WJ-IV ACH, 110–111
        youth's ability, 110
    psychometric evidence, 106
    reading
        central academic skill, 107
        child's reading abilities, 107
        components, 107
        WIAT-III, 107–108
        WJ-IV ACH, 108
    SLD, 106
    total reading, 107
    WIAT-III, 106
    WJ-IV ACH, 107
    writing
        components, 109
        WIAT-III, 109
        WJ-IV ACH, 109–110
Academic intervention
    design, 96
    educational treatment programs, 95
    environmental supports, learning gains, 96, 97
    monitor progress, 98
    support implementation, 97
    task completion, 96

Academic skills
    ADHD, 83
    causality, 83
    direct academic assessment, 91
        CATs, 91
        CBM (*see* Curriculum-based measurement (CBM))
        RtI/MTSS models, 90
        universal screening data, 94, 95
    DSM-5 (*see* Diagnostic and statistical manual of mental disorders (DSM-5))
    IDEA (*see* Individuals with Disabilities Education Improvement Act (IDEA))
    intelligence tests, 88
    interventions (*see* Academic intervention)
    measures
        achievement, 89
        adaptive behavior, 89
    molar assessments, 98
    poor academic achievement, 83
    psychopathology assessments, 83, 84
    rating scales, 89
    RtI/MTSS approaches, 98
    specific treatment planning, 98
    standardized norm-referenced tests, 90
Achenbach system, 197
Achenbach System of Empirically Based Assessment (ASEBA), 25, 26, 250
Achenbach System of Empirically Based Assessment (ASEBA) Teacher Report Form, 193
Acid test, 268
Acquisition deficits, 302
Actigraphy
    advantages, 346
    computer analysis, 345
    disadvantages, 346
    practice parameters, 346
    recording device and sleep measure, 346
    sensitivity, 346
    sleep diaries, 346
    specificity, 346
    visual analysis, activity levels, 345

Acute pain
  assessment (*see* Assessment, pediatric acute pain)
  and fear, 362
  fear and anxiety, 363
  pediatric fear-avoidance model, 362
  vaccinations, 362
Adaptive behavior
  ABAS-3, 458
  ABS, 458, 459
  assessment, 44
  deficits, 453
  definition, 44
  screening tools, for toileting problems, 464
  Vineland-3, 457, 458
Adaptive Behavior Assessment System, Second Edition (ABAS-II), 460
Adaptive Behavior Assessment System, Third Edition (ABAS-3), 45, 46, 73–74, 458
Adaptive Behavior Diagnostic Scale (ABDS), 75
The Adaptive Behavior Evaluation Scale, Third Edition (ABES-3), 459
Adaptive Behavior Inventory (ABI), 74–75
Adaptive behavior scales (ABS), 458, 459
  AAMD, 74
  ABAS-3, 73–74
  ABDS, 75
  ABI, 74–75
  activities of daily living, 71
  assessment, 72
  DABS, 76
  defined, AAIDD, 72
  individuals with developmental disabilities, 72
  intellectual and developmental disabilities, 72
  SIB-R, 75
  Vineland-III, 72–73
Adaptive behaviors
  and motor skills, 470–471
The Adaptive Behavior Evaluation Scale, Third Edition (ABES-3), 459
The Adaptive Behavior Scales-Residential and Community, Second Edition (ABS-RC2), 458
The Adaptive Behavior Scales-School, Second Edition (ABS-S2), 459
Adolescents
  assessment scales, 6
  CAPA, 2
  CBCL, 5
  checklists, 4
  DICA, 2
  differential diagnosis, 8
  DISC, 3
  ISCA, 2
  Kiddie-SADS/K-SADS, 2
  mental health-based assessments, 1
  observations, 3, 4
  psychopathology, 6
  RCADS, 7
  SCARED, 6
The Adolescent Pediatric Pain Tool (APPT), 368
The Adolescent Sleep-Wake Scale (ASWS), 371, 372, 380

Adrenocorticotropic hormone (ACTH), 435
The Adult Responses to Children's Symptoms (ARCS), 373
Ages and Stages Questionnaires, Third Edition (ASQ-3), 78–79, 460, 461
Aggression
  anger, 254
  and antisocial, 254
  and CD (*see* Conduct disorder (CD))
  CU traits, 249
  instrumental, 254
  physical, 246
  symptoms, 245
Alberta Infant Motor Scales (AIMS), 473, 474
Alphabet Writing Fluency, 109
American Academy of Child and Adolescent Psychiatry (AACAP), 403
American Academy of Pediatrics (AAP), 438
American Association on Intellectual and Developmental Disabilities (AAIDD), 71
American College of Sports Medicine (ACSM), 395
Anorexia athletica (AA), 394, 395
Anorexia nervosa (AN)
  and ASD, 392
  case reports, 393
  Danish register study, 392
  diagnostic criteria, 392
  diagnostic features, 399–402
  epidemiological studies, 392
  female homosexuality, 392
  food intake, 391
  mental disorders, 391
  middle age/before puberty, 392
Anorexigenic family, 396, 405
Antecedent-behavior-consequence (A-B-C) recording, 268, 271–274
Antiepileptic medications, 435
Antipsychotic medications, 435
Anxiety, 207
Anxiety Disorder Interview Schedule: Child and Parent versions (ADIS: C/P), 192
Anxiety disorders
  assessment
    behavioral observation, 199–201
    behavioral responses, 193–195
    cognitive responses, 195
    community health clinics/busy hospitals, 195
    cost- and time-efficient approach, 195
    physiological responses, 193
    structured and semi-structured interviews, 193, 194
  behaviors, 189
  characteristic symptoms, 190
  children and adults, 189
  comorbidity, 191
  confirmation bias, 191, 192
  diagnostic labeling, 191
  etiology and maintenance, 190–191
  evidence-based assessments, 191
  mental health, 189
  multiple informants, 192–193

Index

negative thoughts, 189
physiological responses, 189
prevalence rate, 189
psychopathology, 191
selected disorder-specific assessments, 198–199
self-, informant- and clinician reports
    Achenbach system, 197
    CASI, 198
    CATS, 198
    MASC-2, 197
    PARS, 198
    RCMAS-2, 197
    SCARED, 197
    STAI, 197, 198
semi-structured interview, 192
semi-structured/structured interviews
    ADIS:C/P, 195, 196
    DICA, 196
    DISC-IV, 196
    K-SADS, 196
social problems, 189
toddlers and children, 189
treatment, 189
youth with, 189
The Anxiety Disorders Interview Schedule for Children (ADIS-C), 6
Anxiety Disorders Interview Schedule for Children and Adolescents (ADIS-C/P), 214
Anxiety Disorders Interview Schedule for DSM-IV, Child and Parent Versions (ADIS-IV), 41
Anxiety Disorders Interview Schedule of DSM-IV – Child version (ADIS-C PTSD) scale, 195, 196, 218
Anxiety Problems DSM-Oriented scale, 193
Anxiety-provoking task, 193
Anxious/Depressed Syndrome scale, 193
Apnoea, 336
Applied behavior analysis (ABA), 152
Apter 4-questions screening, 238, 239
Aspiration, 416
Assessment
    anxiety disorders (*see* Anxiety disorders)
    checklists, 4, 5
    childhood, history, 1
    general psychopathology, 5, 6
    mental health-based, 1
    neuropsychological (*see* Neuropsychological assessment)
    observations, 3, 4
    psychological tests, 1
    specialized mental health scales, 6, 7
    structured interviews, 2, 3
    toilet training (*see* Toilet training)
Assessment methods, communication disorder
    CCC-2, 317
    CDI, Macarthur-Bates, 318, 319
    CELF-5, 316, 317
    DISCO, 320
    dynamic assessment, 324
    LDS, 318
    PLS-5, 323–324
    PPVT-4, 321, 322
    SCDC, 321
    SSI-4, 323
    TOCS, 322, 323
    TOPL-2, 319
Assessment tools, ASD
    adaptive behavior skills, 160, 161
    assessment battery, 157
    cognitive abilities, 159, 160
    communication abilities, 159–161
    comprehensive diagnostic evaluation, 157
    diagnostic interviews, 157, 158
    executive functioning, 161, 162
    issues with eating and drinking, 162
    motor skills, 161
    observation scales, 158, 159
    rating scales, 158, 159
    sleep difficulties, 162
    theory of mind, 162
    updated/modified, 157
Assessment, pediatric acute pain
    fear, 368, 369
    location, pain
        APPT, 368
        the Eland Color Tool, 368
    pain intensity
        faces scales, 366
        FPS-R, 366, 367
        NRS, 367
        numerical rating scales, 367
        Poker Chip Tool, 365, 366
        test-retest reliability, 366
        VAS, 367
        Wong-Baker FACES Pain Scale, 367
Assessment, pediatric chronic pain
    pain quality, intensity, frequency and duration, 369, 370
    physical functioning
        functional disability, 370, 371
        sleep, 371, 372
    psychosocial factors
        anxiety and depression, 372
        fear, pain-related, 372
        optimism, 374
        pain acceptance, 373
        pain catastrophizing, 372
        pain self-efficacy, 373, 374
        parent responses, to child's pain, 373
        valued life goals, 374
    the PROMIS tools, 374
Assessment, pediatric feeding disorders
    baseline evaluation, 426
    caregiver training evaluation, 427
    direct observation
        avoidant/restrictive food intake disorder, 422
        feeding difficulties and mismanagement, 422
        home baseline, 421–422
        intensive day-treatment, 422
        interview, 422

Assessment, pediatric feeding disorders (cont.)
    outpatient services, 422
        SEEDS, 423
        standardized outcome baseline, 422
    functional analysis, 424–425
    goal evaluation, 427–428
    initial admission, 423
    interdisciplinary team
        behavior analysts, 420
        behavior-analytic approach, 419
        doctoral-level behavior analysts and licensed psychologists, 421
        feeding therapists, 420, 421
        licensed psychologists, 420
        physician's, 420
        recommending treatment, 420
        registered dietician, 420–421
        speech-language pathologist, 420
    intervention evaluation, 426–427
    preference assessments, 423–424
    reinforcement assessment, 425–426
    typical vs. atypical feeding, 418–419
Assessment, pica
    behavior plan, 294
    behavioral, 294
    ethical issues, 297
    FBA, 294
    individual's safety, 297
    individuals assessment measures
        ASD-CC, 296
        BPI, 296
        Conners CBRS, 296
        QABF, 295
        STEP, 295
    of severity
        dangerous, 297
        life-threatening, 297
        mild, 297
        moderate, 297
        severe, 297
    screening practices, 298
Assessment, social skills
    diagnostic assessment test, 302
    MTSS model, 303
    role-play, 309
    SDOs and FBAs, 311 (see also Social skills)
Attention assessment
    definition, 115
    orienting, 115
    orthogonal components, 115
    selection, 115
    simple attention tasks, 115–116
    sustained attention, 116–117
    unitary process, 115
    visual attention, 115
Attention-deficit hyperactivity disorder (ADHD), 83, 86, 88, 103, 228, 229, 316, 318, 321, 340
    ASD, 141–143
    assessment
        professional guidelines, 133

vs. screening, 133–134
symptoms, 132, 133
children with ID, 129
comorbid conditions, 128
diagnosis
    brain stem, role, 129
    "catecholamine hypothesis", 130
    CPT-3, 130–131
    DSM-II, 130
    DSM-III, 131
    DSM-5, 20, 131
    EEGs, 130
    "hyperactive child syndrome", 130
    ICD classification systems, 131
    psychological measures, 130
educational assessment, 143
etiology, 129
impairment, 129
medical specialty assessments
    ENT/otolaryngologist, 139, 140
    genetic testing, 139
    neurological, 138
on intellectual function, 128
postnatal lead exposure, 128
prevalence rate, 127
psychological assessment, 140, 141
screening
    ABC, 137
    CBCL, 136
    and common instruments, 136
    computerized/pencil, 135
    CPRS, 137
    CPTs, 137, 138
    CTRS, 136
    educational screening, 134
    medical screening, 135
    NICHQ Vanderbilt Assessment Scales, 137
    paper instruments and checklists, 135
    psychological screening, 135
tobacco use, 128
treatment rates, 128
youth with FASD, 128
youth with ID, 141
Atypical AN, 393
Atypical BED, 393
Atypical BN, 393
Auditory Consonant Trigrams, 119
Auditory/Verbal and one Visual/Nonverbal subtests, 112
Autism
    and ADHD (see Attention deficit hyperactivity disorder (ADHD))
    ASD (see Autism spectrum disorder (ASD))
    disability specific assessments, 141
    DSM-5, 131
Autism screening
    developmental screening tool, 154
    ESAT, 155
    evidence, 154

Index

FYI, 155
M-CHAT, 154, 155
parameters, 152
recommended screening measures, 155
Autism spectrum disorder (ASD)
  assessment
    adaptive behavior, 156
    best practices, 164
    CCC-2, 317
    CDI, 319
    cognitive ability/intelligence, 156
    DISCO, 320
    language, 156
    observational measures, 156
    PPVT-4, 322
    process of, 152
    SCDC, 321
    self-report measures and interviews, 156
    tools (see Assessment tools, ASD)
    TOPL-2, 319
  clinical practice, 151
  diagnosis
    challenges, 164, 165
    comorbidity, 165
    comprehensive diagnostic evaluation, 163
    developmental trajectory, 163
    implications, 166
    multidisciplinary teams, 163, 164
    school/primary care physician, 162
    using multiple sources, 163
  DSM-5, 20, 141
  early diagnosis, 154
  and FASD, 142
  and ID, 142
  motor deficits, childhood disorders, 469
  as neurodevelopmental disorder, 151
  prevalence of, 151
  screening (see Autism screening)
  and SLI, 317
  social impairment, 142
  and SPCD, 314
  symptomology (see Autism symptomology)
  time sampling, 3
  toileting problems, 456
Autism Spectrum Disorder – Comorbid for Children Scale (ASD-CC), 296
Autism Spectrum Disorder – Diagnostic for Children (ASD-DC), 296
Autism symptomology
  adolescence, 153
  adulthood, 153–154
  age and development, 152
  eye contact, 152
  infants and toddlers, 152
  school-age children, 153
Autism-tics, attention-deficit/hyperactivity disorder, and other comorbidities inventory (A-TAC), 237, 238
Avoidant/restrictive food intake disorder (ARFD), 292

B

Baiting, 294
Barret Impulsiveness Scale, 183
BASC-3 Behavioral and Emotional Screening System (BESS), 306, 307
BASC-3-Student Observation System, 253
Battelle Developmental Inventory, Second Edition (BDI-2), 76–77, 459, 460
Bayley Scales of Infant and Toddler Development, Third Edition (Bayley-III), 61, 62, 77–78, 460, 476, 477
BEARS acronym, 443
Beck Depression Inventory, 175
Beery-Buktenica Developmental Test, 121
The Beery-Buktenica Developmental Test of Visual-Motor Integration (Beery VMI), 474
Behavior Assessment System for Children (BASC), 25
Behavior Assessment System for Children – Second Edition (BASC-2), 104
Behavior Problem Inventory (BPI), 461
Behavior Rating Inventory of Executive Functioning (BRIEF), 104
Behavior rating scales
  advantages, 305
  BESS, 306, 307
  broadband, 305
  central tendency effect, 305
  criterion scoring, 305
  description, 304
  halo effects, 305
  informant discrepancies, 305
  leniency/severity, 305
  narrowband, 305
  normative scoring, 305
  SAEBRS, 306
  SEBS, 307
  SIBS, 307
  SSIS-SEL, 305, 306
Behavioral assessment, SIB, 265, 284
Behavioral avoidance task (BAT), 199–201
Behavioral observation, 199
  BAT (see Behavioral avoidance task (BAT))
  parent–youth interaction tasks, 200
  physiological anxious arousal, 200
  self-reported level of distress, 200
  social evaluative tasks, 200
Behaviorism, 294
Behavioural insomnia
  description, 334
  limit-setting type (BIC-LST), 334
  prevalence of, 334
  sleep-onset association (BIC-SOA) type, 334
  types, 334
Bellevue Index of Depression, 175
Bigorexia, 396
Bilingualism, 315
Binet-Simon intelligence test, 60
Binge eating disorder (BED)
  diagnostic features, 399–402
  distress and disgust, 392

Binge eating disorder (BED) (cont.)
  ED-related behaviors, 392
  prevalence, 392
  psychological factors, 396, 397
Bipolar At-Risk Criteria, 183
Bipolar disorder
  adult literature, 180
  anxiety and social dysfunction, 171
  Barret Impulsiveness Scale, 183
  behaviors, 171
  biological factors and environmental events, 170
  Bipolar At-Risk Criteria, 183
  CBCL-MS, 180–181
  CBQ, 181
  CDRS-R, 181
  characteristics, 171, 172
  Child Mania Rating Scale-Parent, 181
  childhood and adolescence, 171
  children and adolescents, 180
  ChIPs, 181
  comorbidity, 171–173
  criteria, 172
  depression symptoms, 171
  development, 170
  diagnosis, 170
  GBI-R, 181
  Kiddie-SADS, 182
  MDQ-A, 182
  measures for children and adolescents, 174, 180
  vs. mood dysregulation disorder, 171
  mood lability issues, 171
  neuroimaging, 182–183
  onset, 173, 174
  pediatric, 169
  and personality disorders, 172
  psychological and physical trauma, 170–171
  symptoms, 169–172
  violence/bizarreness descriptors, 171
  YMRS, 182
Blood pressure, 434
Body mass index (BMI), 434, 441
Borderline personality disorder (BPD), 340
Bottom-up model, 17, 25, 26
Brain tumors, 103
Bronchopulmonary dysplasia, 416
Brown-Peterson Task (BPT), 119
Bruininks-Oseretsky Test of Motor Proficiency, Second Edition (BOT-2), 474, 475
Bulimia nervosa (BN)
  diagnostic features, 399–402
  distress and disgust, 392
  ED-related behaviors, 392
  prevalence, 392
  psychological factors, 396, 397

C

California Verbal Learning Test for Children (CVLT-C), 111–112
Callous-unemotional (CU) traits, 247
Cardiac arrhythmia, 405
Cardiometabolic risk (CMR), 439
Caregiver stress, 417
Cattell-Horn-Carroll (CHC) theory of intelligence, 59, 64, 105
CDC recommends, 442
Center for Epidemiologic Studies Depression Scale, 175
Centers for Disease Control (CDC), 433
Cerebral palsy (CP), 138, 416, 440, 469, 470
Challenging behaviors
  pica, 294–296
  SIB, 264
  toileting problems, assessment, 461
Checklists
  CBCL, 5
  Hopkins Symptom Checklist, 5
Child and Adolescent Memory Profile (ChAMP), 113, 114
Child and Adolescent Psychiatric Assessment (CAPA), 2, 40
Child Anxiety Impact Scale-Parent Version (CAIS-P), 6
Child Anxiety Sensitivity Index (CASI), 198
Child Assessment Schedule (CAS), 2
Child Behavior Checklist (CBCL), 5, 6, 17, 136, 213, 237, 238, 461
Child Behavior Checklist-Mania Scale (CBCL-MS), 180–181
Child Bipolar Questionnaire (CBQ), 181
Child Depression Scale, 176
Child Mania Rating Scale-Parent, 181
Child Posttraumatic Cognitions Inventory, 216
Child PTSD Symptoms Scale (CPSS), 216
Child Tourette's Syndrome Impairment Scale (CTIM), 237
Child Trauma Screening Questionnaire, 216
Child's Reaction to Traumatic Events Scale (CRTES), 215
Child's reading abilities, 107
Childhood
  cancer, 416
  definitions of, 332
  disorders, 104
  infancy and toddlerhood, 332
Childhood PTSD Interview (CPI), 214
Children
  assessment scales, 6
  CAPA, 2
  CBCL, 5
  checklists, 4
  DICA, 2
  differential diagnosis, 8
  DISC, 3
  ISCA, 2
  Kiddie-SADS/K-SADS, 2
  mental health-based assessments, 1
  observations, 4
  psychopathology, 6
  RCADS, 7
  SCARED, 6
Children's Automatic Thoughts Scale (CATS), 198

Index

Children's Color Trails Test (CCTT), 115
Children's Communication Checklist-Second Edition (CCC-2), 317
Children's Depression Inventory (CDI), 7, 175–176
Children's Depression Rating Scale-Revised Version (CDRS-R), 177, 181
Children's Depression Scale (CDS), 177
Children's Depression Screener (ChIlD-S), 176, 177
The Children's Fear Scale (CFS), 368
Children's Interview for Psychiatric Syndromes (ChIPs), 40, 181
Children's Memory Scale (CMS), 112–113
Children's Paced Auditory Serial Addition Task (CHIPASAT), 119
Children's PTSD Inventory (CPTSD-I), 214
Children's Revised Impact of Events Scale (CRIES), 215, 216
The Children's Report of Sleep Patterns (CRSP), 371
The Children's Sleep Habits Questionnaire (CSHQ), 371, 380
Children's Yale-Brown Obsessive Compulsive Scale (CY-BOCS), 198
Chronic pain
 assessment (*see* Assessment, pediatric chronic pain)
 common pediatric pains, 363
 costs, 363
 definition, 363
 prevalence rates, 363
 symptom, 363
 in youth, 363
The Chronic Pain Acceptance Questionnaire-Adolescent version (CPAQ-A), 373
Clinical assessment, 13, 24, 29
Clinical Assessment of Behavior (CAB), 25
Clinical Evaluation of Language Fundamentals, fifth edition (CELF-5), 316, 317
Clinician-Administered PTSD Scale for Children and Adolescents (CAPS-CA), 214, 215
Cognitive tics, 227
Cognitive-behavioral therapy (CBT), 190
Color-Word Interference Test, 118
Committee on Quality Issues (CQI), 403
Communication
 adequacy, 313
 description, 313
 disorders, 314
 factors, 313
 functionality, 313
 SPCD, 314
Communication disorders
 bilingualism, 315
 challenging behavior, 315
 characterization, 313
 comprehensive assessment, 316 (*see also* Assessment methods, communication disorder)
 diagnoses, 314
 difficulties, 314
 SLI, 313
 speech sound disorder, 315
 stuttering, 314–316

Communication skills, 313, 314, 316–318, 321, 324
Communicative Development Inventory, 318, 319
Co-morbid
 ASD, 131
 children with ADHD, 128, 131
 CTRS, 136
 medical and psychological disorders, 135
 sleep disorders, 139
 symptoms, ASD, 142
Comorbid mental disorders, 397
Complex tics, 227
Computer-adaptive tests (CATs), 91
Conduct disorder (CD)
 causes, 246
 conduct problems and aggression, 245
 CU traits, 248, 249
 definition, 245
 for diagnosis, assessment
  behavior rating scales, 250
  behavioral observation, 252, 253
  interviews, 251, 252
  methods, 250
 DSM-5, 246
 etiology, 247
 and ODD, 251
 prevalence, 246
 rebelliousness, levels, 248
 subgroup, children with CD, 247
 symptoms, types, 245
 for treatment planning, assessment
  age of onset, 255
  callous-unemotional traits, 255, 256
Conners Comprehensive Behavior Rating Scales (CBRS), 296
Conners' Continuous Auditory Test of Attention (CATA), 117
Conners' Continuous Performance Test, third edition (CPT-3), 116, 131
The Conners' Parent Rating Scale (CPRS), 137
The Conners' Teachers Rating Scale (CTRS), 136
Contextual Assessment of Social Skills (CASS), 309, 311
Continuous performance tests (CPTs), 137, 138
Contributory factors, 436
Curriculum-based measurement (CBM)
 materials, 92
 mathematics probes, 94
 pre-reading, 92, 93
 procedures, 91, 92
 reading, 93
 writing probes, 94
Cushing syndrome, 435, 437, 444

D

DABS, *see* Diagnostic Adaptive Behavior Scale (DABS)
Danish register study, 392
DDST-II, *see* Denver Developmental Screening Test II (DDST-II)
Declarative memory systems, 111

Deinstitutionalization, 17
Delayed Recognition (DR), 112
Delayed sleep phase syndrome (DSPS)
    criteria, 336
    description, 336
    diagnosis, 337
    potential consequences, 336
    prevalence, 337
Delis-Kaplan Executive Function System (D-KEFS), 118
Delis-Kaplan Executive Function System's Trail Making Test (D-KEFS TMT), 115, 116
Denver Developmental Screening Test II (DDST-II), 79
Depression, 207
Depression Indicator Assessment Battery, 177
Depression Observation Schedule (DOS), 177
Depression Self-Rating Scale for Children (DSRSC), 177, 178
Depression Symptom Checklist, 178
Design Memory subtest, 114
Design Recognition and Picture Recognition subtests, 114
Developmental behavior scales
    ASQ-3, 78–79
    Bayley-III, 77–78
    BDI-2, 76–77
    DDST-II, 79
    MSEL:AGS, 78
Developmental coordination disorder (DCD)
    "clumsy", 471
    description, 471
    individuals with DCD, 471
    skill level, 471
Developmental Coordination Disorder Questionnaire 2007 (DCDQ'07), 479
Developmental disabilities (DD), 65, 66, 127, 375, 416
    ADHD, in children (see Attention deficit hyperactivity disorder (ADHD))
    ASD, 439
    CP, 440
    FASD, 439
    ID, 440 (see also Pain)
    and obesity, 438
    SIB, 276, 282
    toileting problems, assessment (see Toileting problems)
Developmental functioning, motor skills
    aim, 476
    Bayley-III, 476, 477
    BDI-2, 476
    DIAL-4, 477
    ESI-R, 477, 478
    MAP, 478
    motor functioning, 476
    MSEL:AGS, 478
Developmental Indicators for the Assessment of Learning, Fourth Edition (DIAL-4), 477
Diabulimia, 395, 396
Diagnosis
    assessment methods, 8
    CBCL, 6
    checklists, 5
    differential diagnosis, 8
    DSM, 2
    DSM-III, 7
    history, mental health, 7
    identification, mental health, 8
    observations, 3
Diagnosis, pica
    ASD-CC, 296
    behavioral interventions, 290
    DSM-5, 291, 292
    DSM-III, 292
    DSM-IV, 292
    medical records, 294
Diagnostic Adaptive Behavior Scale (DABS), 76
Diagnostic and Statistical Manual of Mental Disorders, Fifth Edition (DSM-5), 228
    academic problems, 85
    ADHD, 86
    educational diagnoses, 85
    environmental factors, 84
    intellectual disability, 85
    neurodevelopmental disorders, 85
    SLD, 86
    social-emotional functioning, 85
    sources, 84
Diagnostic Infant and Preschool Assessment (DIPA), 217
Diagnostic Interview for Children and Adolescents (DICA), 2, 41, 196
Diagnostic Interview for Children and Adolescents-Revised (DICA-R), 214
Diagnostic Interview for Social and Communication Disorders (DISCO), 320
Diagnostic Interview Schedule for Children (DISC), 3, 6, 39
Diagnostic Interview Schedule for Children Version IV (DISC-IV), 196
Diagnostic interview, ASD, 157, 158
Diagnostic Statistical Manual (DSM)
    history, 16
    innovations, third version, 16
    revised version, 16
Diagnostic systems
    biological markers, models
        endophenotypes/genetic "markers", 27
        RDoC, 27–29
    categorical criteria models
        DSM-5, 19, 20
        ICD-10, 21
        ICD-11, 23
    children and adolescents, 14
    classification, 18
    classification model, 14
    deinstitutionalization, 17
    dimensional approach, 16
    dimensional criteria models
        advantages, 24
        ASEBA, 25
        clinical assessment, 24
        dimensional assessment systems, 24
        disadvantages, 24

empirical syndromes, 24
"internalizing" and "externalizing", 24
SDQ, 26
statistical techniques, 24
syndrome, 24
factors, 15
functions, 13
mortality and morbidity, in children, 14, 15
power of diagnosis, 14
psychiatric disorders, historical evolution, 18
psychopathological classifications, 15
validation, 17
Differential ability scales (DAS), 62–63
Digit Span, 105
Direct behavior ratings (DBRs), 308–311
Direct behavioural observation, 345
Direct Observation Form from the Achenbach System, 253
Display oral-motor skill deficits, 417
Disruptive mood dysregulation disorder (DMDD)
DSM-5, 20
Down syndrome (DS), 416, 438, 439
Down Syndrome Growing Up Study (DSGS)
growth, 439
DSM-5 changes, 48
Dynamic assessment, 324
Dynamic risk factor
obesity, 436–437
Dysgraphia, 470
Dyssomnias
insomnia
behavioural, 334
definition, 334
prevalence, in older children and adolescents, 335
psychophysiologic, 334, 335
narcolepsy
age of onset, 335
characterization, 335
DSPS (*see* Delayed sleep phase syndrome (DSPS))
paediatric, 335, 336
SDB (*see* Sleep-disordered breathing (SDB))
sleep-related movement disorders (*see* Restless leg syndrome (RLS))
symptoms, 335
Dysthymic Checklist, 178

E
Early Childhood Traumatic Stress Screen (ECTSS), 218
Early diagnosis, ASD, 152, 154
Early Screening Inventory-Revised (ESI-R), 477, 478
Early Screening of Autistic Traits (ESAT), 155
EAT (Eating Among Teens), 441
Eating Activity in Teens (EAT) study, 399
Eating disorder not otherwise specified (EDNOS), 393
Eating disorders (ED)
AA, 394, 395
ADHD, 392
AN (*see* Anorexia nervosa (AN))

assessment
anorexigenic family, 405
blood tests, 403
cardiac arrhythmia, 405
comorbid medical, 402
EKG, 403
externalizing behaviors, 402
GBD, 402
guidelines, 404, 405
junior MARISPAN, 405
Maudsley approach, 405
neuropsychological impairment, 402
outpatient treatment, 405
primary care provider, 403
professional organizations and practice guidelines, 403
psychological disability, 402
Refeeding syndrome, 405
and recovery process, 405
revisit Katelyn's story, 403
risk of mortality, 402
SCOFF, 403
and screening tools, 403, 404
self-harming behaviors, 405
skilled application, 402
symptoms, 402
treatment plan, 405
BED (*see* Binge eating disorder (BED))
bigorexia, 396
BN (*see* Bulimia nervosa (BN))
Diabulimia, 395, 396
DSM-5, 20
etiology
anorexigenic family, 396
assessment, 396
genetic factors, 398
neurobiological factors, 397–398
psychological factors, 396
sociocultural and environmental factors, 398–399
FAT, 394, 395
features, 391
LOC-ED, 395–396
muscle dysmorphia, 396
ON, 394
OSFED (*see* Other specified feeding and eating disorders (OSFED))
persons with developmental disabilities, 392–393
RED-S, 394, 395
research, 393
reverse anorexia, 396
screening, 391
EDNOS, 402
The Eland Color Tool, 368
Encopresis
diagnostic features, 453
individuals meet criteria, 454
POTI, 456
Endocrine disorders, 437

Enuresis
  diagnostic features, 453
  POTI, 456
Environmental assessment, 444
The Essay Composition, 109
Evidence-based assessments, 191
Evidence-based treatment, 190
Executive functioning (EF)
  development, 117
  functional neuroimaging studies, 117
  higher-order cognitive domains, 117
  inhibition, 117, 118
  protective- and risk-factors, 117
  shifting, 119–120
  updating, 118–119
  working memory, 117
Exogenous obesity, 434, 435
Externalizing behavior problems, 207
Externalizing syndrome, 16

F
Faces Pain Scale-Revised (FPS-R), 366, 367
Faces scales, 366, 376
Family-based behavioral treatment (FBT), 439
The Fear of Pain Questionnaire, Child Report (FOPQ-C), 372
Female athlete triad (FAT), 394, 395
Fetal alcohol spectrum disorder (FASD), 439
Fetal alcohol syndrome disorder (FASD), 128, 142, 143
Fifth edition of the DSM (DSM-5)
  ADHD, 20
  ASD, 20
  autistic spectrum, 19
  child-adolescent population, changes, 19
  criticism, 20
  description, 19
  DMDD, 20
  eating disorders, 20
  neurodevelopment disorders, 19
  psychosocial and environmental factors, 19
Fine motor
  ABAS-II, 477
  and adaptive behaviors, 471
  BOT-2, 474
  CP, 469
  DCD, 471
  dysgraphia, 470
  GDD and ID, 468
  MAP, 478
  motor domain, 477
  Movement ABC-2 Performance Test, 475
  MSEL:AGS, 478
  PDMS-2, 476
  skills, 467
  standardized measures, 472
  tasks, 473
  visual-motor/adaptive scale, 477
First Year Inventory (FYI), 155
Fluid Reasoning Index, 105

Fragile X Clinical and Research Consortium (FXCRC), 439
Fragile X syndrome (FXS), 439
Full-scale intelligence quotient (FSIQ) score, 65, 106
Functional analysis, SIB assessment
  "attention" condition, 275
  automatic reinforcement, 278
  behavioral assessment, 272
  care provider attention, 276
  escape from demands, 276–278
  individuals with SIB, 274
  limitations, 279, 280
  methodology, 275
  outcomes, 276, 277
  potential reinforcing events, 273
  school setting, 279
  social positive reinforcement, 276
  subtype classification, 278, 279
  tangible condition, 276
  test conditions and control condition, 275
  tissue damage/trauma, 275
  type of attention, 276
Functional Assessment Observation (FAO), 269
Functional Assessment Screening Tool (FAST), 268
Functional behavioral assessments (FBAs), 294, 295, 304, 311
The Functional Disability Inventory (FDI), 370
Functional magnetic resonance imaging (fMRI), 182

G
Gastroesophageal reflux, 416
Gate control theory, 362
General Behavior Inventory-Revised (GBI-R), 181
General Conceptual Ability (GCA) score, 62
General Memory Index (GMI), 114
Generalized anxiety disorder, 190, 199
Genetic disorders, 438
Global burden of disease (GBD), 402
Global developmental delay (GDD), 468, 469
Global Tic Rating Scale (GTRS), 234–235
Glucocorticoid or steroid medications, 435
Glucocorticoids, 435
Glucose metabolism, 434
Gross motor
  and adaptive behaviors, 471
  BOT-2, 474
  CP, 469
  GDD, 468
  GMFM, 475
  motor domain, 477
  motor impairments, 469
  Movement ABC-2 Performance Test, 475
  skills, 467
  standardized measures, 472
  tasks, 473
  test-retest reliability, 478
  visual-motor/adaptive scale, 477
Gross Motor Function Classification System (GMFS), 470
Gross Motor Function Measure (GMFM), 475

H

Health Assessment Questionnaire (HAQ), 7
History
    childhood assessment, 1
    mental health assessment, 5
    mental health diagnosis, 7
Hopkins Motor and Vocal Tic Scale (HMVTS, 236
Hopkins Symptom Checklist, 5
HRT Standard Deviation (SD), 116
Hypercortisolism, 435
Hypothalamic pituitary adrenal (HPA) axis activity, 193
Hypothyroidism, 435, 437, 444

I

ICD-11, 23
Individualized Numeric Rating Scale (INRS), 377, 378
Individuals with Disabilities Education Act
    (IDEA), 84, 106
    ADHD, 88
    diagnostic evaluations, 86
    intellectual disability, 87
    SLD, 87, 88
    special education services, 86
Inflammatory markers, 172
Informant-based measures, motor functioning
    DCDQ'07, 479
    Movement ABC-2 Checklist, 479
    Vineland-3, 479, 480
Insomnia
    behavioural, 334
    defined, 334
    prevalence, in older children and adolescents, 335
    psychophysiologic, 334, 335
Intellectual and developmental disabilities (I/DD), 263
Intellectual disability, 105
Intellectual disability (ID), 59, 71, 105, 438, 440, 468
    and ADHD, 129, 141
Intellectual functioning
    neuropsychological assessment
        ADHD, 105
        Cattell-Horn-Carroll theory, 105
        crystallized intelligence, 105
        developmental disorders, 104
        diagnosis and functional outcomes, 104
        Fluid Reasoning Index, 105
        FSIQ, 106
        Picture Span, 105
        Processing Speed Index, 105
        Verbal Comprehension Index, 105
        Visual Puzzles, 106
        Visual-Spatial Index, 105
        Wechsler intelligence batteries ranking, 104
        WISC-V, 104–105
        WJ-IV COG and SB5, 105
        working memory, 105
        Working Memory Index, 105
Intelligence testing
    assessment tools, 60
    Bayley scales of infant and toddler development, 61, 62
    CHC theory, 59
    childhood assessments, 59
    differential ability scales, 62–63
    history
        assessment, 60
        Binet-Simon intelligence tests, 60
        intelligence quotient, 61
        mental age, 60
        Stanford-Binet intelligence scales, 61
        Wechsler-Bellevue intelligence scale, 61
    Kaufman brief intelligence test, 64
    Leiter international performance scale, 63
    Mullen scales of early learning, 64
    neurodevelopmental disability, 59
    Peabody Picture Vocabulary Test, 65
    Stanford-Binet intelligence scales, 65, 66
    Universal nonverbal intelligence test, 66, 67
    Wechsler intelligence scale for children, 67
    Wechsler preschool and primary scale
        of intelligence, 68
    Woodcock-Johnson test of cognitive abilities, 68, 69
Internalizing disorder, 16
International Classification of Diseases (ICD),
    16, 399
    atheoretical and scientific perspective, 16
    history, 15, 16
    ICD-11, 23
    ICD-9, 18
    tenth version of the ICD (*see* ICD-10)
International Olympic Committee (IOC), 395
Interobserver agreement (IOA), 464
Interview
    children with disabilities
        ABAS-3, 45, 46
        adaptive behavior, 44
        modifications of procedures, 44
        report writing, 46, 47
    description, 35
    for children
        adaptive behavior, 44
        DSM-5, 42, 43
        highly structured interviews, 39, 40
        initial interview, 36–38
        psychometrics, structured interviews, 42
        selection, procedures, 43
        semi-structured interviews, 40–42
        structured interviews, 38, 39
        unstructured interviews, 38
    unstructured and structured, 35
Interview Schedule for Children and Adolescents
    (ISCA), 2, 41
Intolerance of Uncertainty Scale for Children
    (IUSC), 199
Inventory of Callous-Unemotional Traits
    (ICU), 256

J

Judgment of Line Orientation (JOL), 121
Junior MARISPAN, 405

K

Kaufman brief intelligence test (KBIT), 64
Kiddie Schedule for Affective Disorder and Schizophrenia (Kiddie-SADS), 179, 182
Kiddie Schedule for Affective Disorders and Schizophrenia for School-Aged Children, 214

L

Language Development Survey (LDS), 318
Learning, 113
Learning and memory assessment
 ChAMP, 113, 114
 clinical assessment, 111
 CMS, 112–113
 CVLT-C, 111–112
 definition, 111
 procedural memory system, 111
 process approach, 111
 quantitative, 111
 recognition trials, 111
 systems approach, 111
 type of information, 111
 unitary construct, 111
 verbal and visual, 111
 verbal and visual information, 111
 WRAML2, 114
Leiter international performance scale, 63
Liebowitz Social Anxiety Scale for Children and Adolescents (LSAS-CA), 199
Loss of control ED (LOC-ED), 395–396

M

Macarthur-Bates Communicative Development Inventory (CDI), 318, 319
Major depression
 Beck Depression Inventory, 175
 Bellevue Index of Depression, 175
 CDI, 175–176
 CDRS-R, 177
 CDS, 177
 Center for Epidemiologic Studies Depression Scale, 175
 Child Depression Scale, 176
 in children and adolescents, 172
 ChlID-S, 176, 177
 comorbidity, 172–173
 Depression Indicator Assessment Battery, 177
 Depression Symptom Checklist, 178
 diagnosis, 170
 differential diagnosis, 172
 DOS, 177
 DSM-III and IV criteria, 180
 DSRSC, 177, 178
 Dysthymic Checklist, 178
 in functional skills, 172
 Kiddie-SADS, 179
 Matching Familiar Figures Test, 180
 measures for children and adolescents, 174
 onset, 173, 174
 PIC, 178
 RCADS, 178–179
 SMFQ, 179–180
 suicidal behavior, 172
 symptoms, 169–171
Major depressive disorder, 103
Matching Familiar Figures Test, 180
Math Problem-Solving, 110
Matrix Reasoning, 105
Maudsley approach, 405
Medical assessment, 445
Medicalization, 13
Memory Validity Profile, 104
Mental health disorders, 437
Mental health symptoms
 and obesity, 440–441
Miller Assessment of Preschoolers (MAP), 478
Mini-International Neuropsychiatric Interview for Children and Adolescents (MINI-KID), 40
Modified Checklist for Autism in Toddlers (M-CHAT), 154, 155
Monogenic obesity, 435, 436
Monogenic syndromes
 Down syndrome, 438
 DS, 438, 439
 fragile X, 438
 FXS, 439
 PWS, 438
 Williams syndrome (WS), 438, 439
Mood Disorder Questionnaire-Adolescent Version (MDQ-A), 182
Mood disorders
 adolescent, 180
 childhood, 171, 173
 differential diagnosis, 182
 MDQ-A, 182
 pediatric, 169
 risk factor, range of anxiety-related conditions, 173
 symptoms, 170, 172, 174
 types, 174
Mood dysregulation disorder *vs.* bipolar disorder, 171
Motivation Analysis Rating Scale (MARS), 267
Motivational Assessment Scale (MAS), 267, 268
Motor Coordination (MC), 121
Motor deficits
 childhood disorders
  ASD, 469
  CP, 469, 470
  dysgraphia, 470
  GDD and ID, 468
  genetic disorders, 470
  language disorders, 469
 fine (*see* Fine motor)
 gross (*see* Gross motor)
Motor functioning, 471, 472, 475
 See also Motor skills
Motor skills
 and adaptive behaviors, 470–471
 assessment, 472, 476, 479
  comprehensive, 471

Index

developmental functioning, measures (see Developmental functioning, motor skills)
developmental screening, 471
informant-based measures (see Informant-based measures, motor functioning)
measures, described, 473
parents/caregivers interview, 472
performance-based measures (see Performance-based assessment, motor skills)
standardized measures, 472
deficits (see Motor deficits)
motor milestones, 467
Motor tic, Obsessions and compulsions, Vocal tic Evaluation Survey (MOVES), 235
Motor tics, 227, 228
Movement Assessment Battery for Children (Movement ABC-2), 475
Movement Assessment Battery for Children Checklist (Movement ABC-2 Checklist), 479
Mullen scales of early learning (MSEL), 64–65
Mullen Scales of Early Learning: American Guidance Service Edition (MSEL:AGS), 78, 478
Multidimensional Anxiety Scale for Children-Second Edition (MASC-2), 197
Multimethod assessment, 193
Multiple sleep latency test (MSLT), 344
Multi-tiered system of supports (MTSS) model, 90, 91, 98, 303, 310
Muscle dysmorphia, 396

N
Narcolepsy
  age of onset, 335
  paediatric, 335, 336
  symptoms, 335
National Child Traumatic Stress Network, 212
National Comorbidity Survey Replication Adolescent Supplement (NCS-A), 397
National Eating Disorders Association, 405
National Health and Nutrition Examination Survey (NHANES), 433, 438
National Health Interview Survey (NHIS), 438, 440
The National Institute of Mental Health (NIMH), 17
National Institutes of Mental Health Research Domain Criteria (RDoC), 399–401
National Survey of Children's Health (NSCH), 438
Neurobiological factors
  ED, 397–398
Neurodevelopmental disability, 59
Neurodevelopmental disorders, 103, 104
Neuropsychological assessment
  academic achievement (see Academic achievement assessments)
  applications, 103
  attention (see Attention assessment)
  brain-behavior relationships, 103
  childhood disorders, 104
  cognitive functions, 103
  EF (see Executive functioning (EF))

intellectual functioning, 104–106
learning and memory (see Learning and memory assessment)
neurodevelopmental disorders, 103, 104
neuroimaging, 103
neuropsychological evaluation, 121–122
noncredible responding, 104
pediatric neuropsychologists, 103
presence and location of brain damage, 103
types of childhood psychopathology, 103
types of memory, 103
VS and VC, 120, 121
Neuropsychological evaluation, 121–122
NICHQ Vanderbilt Assessment Scales, 137
Night Eating Questionnaire (NEQ), 394
Night eating syndrome (NES), 391, 393, 394
Non-communicating Children's Pain Checklist-Postoperative Version (NCCPC-PV), 377
Nonverbal assessment methods, 63
Numerical Operations subtests, 110
Numerical Rating Scale (NRS), 367
Nutritional assessment, 443, 444
NYU Child and Adolescent Stressors Checklist, 216

O
Obesity
  assessment
    accurately diagnose, 442
    medical, 445
    primary exogenous obesity, 443–444
    primary monogenic obesity, 444
    psychological assessment tools, 444, 445
    risk factors, 442
    secondary obesity, 444
  CDC, 433
  comorbid disease conditions, 434
  and DD, 438
  definition, 434
  health consequences and medical expenditures, 433
  and mental health symptoms, 440–441
  monogenic syndromes, 438–439
  preschool- and elementary-aged children, 433
  prevention and intervention strategies, 445
  primary/secondary, 434–436
  risk factors
    and contributory, 436
    antipsychotic medications, 437
    biological, nutritional and environmental, 436
    disorders and cardiometabolic diseases, 437
    dynamic risk factor, 436–437
    endocrine disorders, 437
    mental health disorders, 437
    nutritional counseling, 436
    psychiatric symptoms, 437
    static risk factor, 436, 437
    types of interventions, 436
  screening, 441–442
  severity, 434
  WHO, 433

Observations
    child/adolescent's behavior, 3
    method, usage, 4
    multiple behaviors, 4
    target behaviors, 3
    time-sampling method, 3
Obsessive-compulsive disorder (OCD), 190, 198–199, 228, 229, 397
Obstructive sleep apnoea (OSA), 336, 338, 340
Oppositional defiant disorder (ODD), 397
    children with CD, 247
    conduct problems and aggression, 245
    diagnostic criteria, 245
    prevalence, 246
Optimism, 374
Oral aversions, 417
Orthorexia nervosa (ON), 394
Other specified feeding and eating disorders (OSFED)
    distress/impairment, 393
    DSM-5, 393
    EDNOS, 393
    NES, 393, 394
    PD, 393, 394
    prevalence, 393
    and UFED, 393

P
Pain
    acute (*see* Acute pain)
    biopsychosocial model, 359–362
    children with developmental disabilities, 375
        attitudes, 378–379
        beliefs, 379
        caregivers, 378, 379
        case study, 379, 380
        experienced pain, 375
        expression, pain, 375
        impacting, 375
        observational reports, 376–378
        pain-related education, 379
        prevalence rates, 375
        self-reports, 376
        unmanaged pain, 375
        unrecognized and untreated pain, 375
    chronic (*see* Chronic pain)
    definition, 359
    gate control theory, 362
Pain acceptance, 372, 373
The Pain Catastrophizing Scale for Children (PCS-C), 372
Pain self-efficacy, 372–374
Panic disorder, 190
Parasomnias
    insomnia and nocturnal awakenings, 337
    non-REM (NREM)
        N3 stage, 337
        night terrors, 338
        nocturnal enuresis, 338
        somniloquy, 337

    REM, 338
    sleepiness, 337
Parent Tic Questionnaire (PTQ), 235
The Patient-Reported Outcomes Measurement Information System (PROMIS®), 374, 381
Peabody Developmental Motor Scales, Second Edition (PDMS-2), 475, 476
Peabody Picture Vocabulary Test (PPVT), 65
Peabody Picture Vocabulary Test, Fourth Edition (PPVT-4), 321, 322
Pediatric Anxiety Rating Scale (PARS), 198
Pediatric bipolar disorder, 169, 170, 173, 180–182
    diagnostic practices, 172
    symptoms, 171
Pediatric Emotional Distress Scale (PEDS), 217, 218
Pediatric feeding disorders
    assessment (*see* Assessment, pediatric feeding disorders)
    diagnosis and prevalence
        calories and nutrition, 416
        caregiver stress, 417
        child's growth, 415
        complex and dynamic operant behavior chain, 415
        developmental disabilities, 416
        eating, 415
        financially burdensome to healthcare systems, 417
        food refusal, 415
        genetic disorders, 416
        healthcare providers, 415
        liquid dependency, 416
        liquid dependency and rely exclusively, 415
        macro- and micronutrients, 416
        medical conditions, 416
        physical and emotional health concerns, 417
        strain on caregivers, 416
        tube feedings, 416
        types of feeding difficulties, 416
    etiology, 417–418
Pediatric mood disorders, 169
Pediatric neuropsychologists, 103
Pediatric pain
    assessment
        age and cognitive ability, 364
        behavioral, 364
        biopsychosocial model, 363
        family context, 364
        functions, 363
        measures, 359–361
        outcome domains, 363
        parental influences, 365
        parents of youth, 365
        physiological, 364
        self-reports, 364
        sex and gender differences, 365
    evidence-based, 359
    history, 359
The Pediatric Pain Profile (PPP), 378
The Pediatric Quality of Life Inventory – Generic Core Scales (PedsQL), 370, 371
Peer-preferred social skills, 301, 302

Performance deficits, 302
Performance-based assessment, motor skills
    AIMS, 473, 474
    Beery VMI, 474
    BOT-2, 474, 475
    GMFM, 475
    Movement ABC-2, 475
    PDMS-2, 475, 476
    tasks, 472
Persistent (chronic) motor and vocal tic disorder (PMVTD), 228
    diagnosis, 228
Personality disorders, 172
Personality Inventory for Children (PIC), 178
Pervasive developmental disorder, 103
Phonemic coding, 107
Phonic tics, 227
Pica
    assessment (see also Assessment, pica)
        behavioral, 294
        clinical forms, 290
        concerns, 293
        life-threatening item, 293, 294
        signs and symptoms, 293
    behavioral interventions, 290
    classes, 289
    culturally normative forms, 290–291
    description, 292
    diagnosis, 291, 292
    etymology, 291
    history, 291
    prevalence, 292, 293
    self-injurious behavior, 289
Picture Memory subtests, 114
Picture Span, 105
Poker Chip Tool, 365, 366
Polysomnography (PSG)
    advantages, 344
    features, 343
    "gold standard", sleep assessment, 342
    limitations, 344
    MSLT, 344
    standardised methods, 343
Posttraumatic stress (PTS) symptoms, 207
Posttraumatic stress disorder (PTSD)
    ADIS-C/P, 214
    assessment, 208
    assessment tools
        children and adolescents, 219, 220
        young children, 220
    broadband assessment tools, 213–216
    CAPS-CA, 214–215
    children and adolescents with cognitive delays, 218
    children's responses, 208
    clinical assessment, 212–213
    cognitive developmental level, 207
    CPI, 214
    CPTSD-I, 214
    diagnosis, 208
    diagnostic criteria, 209–210
    DICA-R, 214
    DSM-5 criteria
        adolescents and children over 6 years old, 208, 209
        children 6 years old and younger, 209
        specifiers, 209
    epidemiological studies, 207
    etiology and prognosis
        peritrauma, 211
        posttrauma, 212
        pretrauma, 210, 211
    Kiddie Schedule for Affective Disorders and Schizophrenia for School-Aged Children, 214
    nascent coping skills, 207
    natural/man-made disaster, 208
    negative impact trauma, 207
    psychosocial, biological, behavioral, and cognitive functioning, 207
    PTS symptoms, 208
    rating scales (see Rating scales)
    traumatic events, 207
    in young children
        DIPA, 217
        DSM-5 criteria, 216
        PAPA, 217
        trauma assessment tools, 217–218
Prader-Willi syndrome (PWS), 435, 438
Prader-Willi Syndrome Association website (PWSA), 438
Premonitory Urge for Tics Scale (PUTS), 236–237
Prenatal alcohol exposure (PAE), 143
Preschool Age Psychiatric Assessment (PAPA), 217
Preschool Language Scale, Fifth Edition (PLS-5), 323, 324
Primary exogenous obesity
    biological assessment, 443
    environmental assessment, 444
    nutritional assessment, 443, 444
Primary index scores, 106
Primary monogenic obesity, 444
Primary obesity, 434–436
Procedural memory system, 111
Processing Speed Index, 105
Profile of Toileting Issues (POTI), 456, 457
Progress monitoring
    behavioral and emotional strengths, 306
    broadband measures, 310
    definition, 304
    SDOs, 307
    SSIS-SEL, 306
Prosocial behaviors, 308
Provisional tic disorder, 228
Proxy Report Questionnaire for Parents and Teachers (PRQPT), 238
Psychological assessment
    ADHD symptoms, 135, 140, 141
    children with cerebral palsy (CP), 138
Psychological assessment tools, 444, 445
Psychological factors
    ED, 396

Psychotic symptoms, 438
PTSD Alternative Algorithm (PTSD-AA), 217
Purging disorder (PD), 393, 394

Q
Questions About Behavioral Function (QABF), 295

R
Rapid restraint analysis (RRA)
  SIB, 283, 284
Rating scales
  advantages, 231
  assessment of behavior, 231
  CTIM, 237
  GTRS, 234–235
  HMVTS, 236
  individual engages, 231
  MOVES, 235
  multi-informant approach, 231
  normative data, 231
  PTQ, 235
  PUTS, 236–237
  RVBTRS, 232, 233
  STSS, 232
  TODS, 233–234
  TS-CGI, 233
  TSGS, 234
  TSSL, 236
  YGTSS, 231, 232
Rating scales, PTSD
  checklist, 215
  Child Posttraumatic Cognitions Inventory, 216
  Child Trauma Screening Questionnaire, 216
  CPSS, 216
  CRIES, 215, 216
  CRTES, 215
  NYU Child and Adolescent Stressors Checklist, 216
  STEPP, 215
  TSCC, 216
  UCLA Posttraumatic Stress Disorder-Reaction Index, 215
Reading comprehension, 107
Reading rate/fluency, 107
Refeeding syndrome, 405
Reinforcer Assessment for Individuals with Severe Disabilities (RAISD), 423
Relative energy deficiency in sport (RED-S), 394, 395
Reports
  behavioral observations section, 47
  clinical formulation/conclusions section, 47
  conclusion section, 47
  organization, 46
  procedures section, 46
  recommendations, 47
  referral Information section, 46
  test results and interpretations, 47
  writing, 46

Research Domain Criteria (RDoC)
  aims, 27
  arousal and regulatory systems, 27
  assumptions, 27
  depression analysis, 27
  domains, matrix, 27, 28
  mental disorders, mechanisms of, 27
  negative valence system, 27
  NIMH's, 17
  positive valence systems, 27
  potential biological reductionism, 29
Response to intervention (RtI)
  academic progress, 134
  behavioral needs, 134
  "early intervention and assessment", 134
  special education, 134
  tiers, 134
Restless leg syndrome (RLS)
  diagnosis, 337
  prevalence, 337
  as Willis-Ekbom disease, 337
Reverse anorexia, 396
Revised Child Anxiety and Depression Scale (RCADS), 7, 178–179
Revised Children's Manifest Anxiety Scale-Second Edition (RCMAS-2), 197
Revised Face, Leg, Activity, Cry, and Consolability (r-FLACC) scale, 377
Reynolds Child Depression Scale (RCDS), 176
Rey-Osterrieth Complex Figure Test-Copy (ROCFT-C), 121
Rush Video-Based Tic Rating Scale (RVBTRS), 232, 233

S
Sample developmental history questionnaire, 49–54
Scales of Independent Behavior – Revised (SIB-R), 75
Schedule for Affective Disorders and Schizophrenia for School-Age Children (K-SADS), 40, 196
SCOFF, 403
SCOFF and EDI screening tools, 395
The Screen for Child Anxiety Related Emotional Disorders (SCARED), 6, 197
Screening Tool for Early Predictors of Posttraumatic Stress Disorder (STEPP), 215
Screening Tool of Feeding Problems (STEP), 295
Secondary obesity, 434–436, 444
Seizure disorder, 103
Selected disorder-specific assessments, 198–199
  anxiety disorders
    generalized anxiety disorder, 199
    obsessive-compulsive disorder, 198–199
    social anxiety disorder, 199
Selective mutism, 190
Self-injurious behavior (SIB)
  automatic reinforcement, 264
  behavioral assessment, 265, 284
  descriptive analysis
    A-B-C method, 271, 272
    direct observation, 268–270

Index

scatterplot, 271
settings, 268
functional analysis (*see* Functional analysis, SIB assessment)
indirect assessments
    commonly used methods, 265, 266
    correlation coefficient, 267
    FAST, 268
    informants, 266
    MARS, 267
    MAS, 267
    primary advantage, 265
    primary limitation, 266
    reliability, 267
    secondary limitation, 266
    structured interviews, 268
protective equipment, 283, 284
as reflexive behavior, 263
response products, 281, 282
and self-restraint, 264
severity, 263
social attention, 264
socially mediated negative reinforcement, 264
topographies, 263
Self-Injury Trauma (SIT) scale, 282
Sensory tics, 227
Sentence Writing Fluency subtest, 110
Separation anxiety disorder, 190
Shapiro Tourette Syndrome Severity Scale (STSS), 232
Short Mood and Feelings Questionnaire (SMFQ), 179–180
Short-gut syndrome, 416
Simple attention tasks, 115–116
Single muscle contraction, 227
Sleep
    normative sleep patterns, childhood, 332–333
    role, 331
Sleep assessment
    actigraphy, 345, 346
    direct behavioural observation, 345
    objective tools, 342
    PSG, 342–344
    questionnaires, sleep, 347
    sleep diaries, 346, 347
    smartphone applications, 346
    subjective measures, 342
    videosomnography, 344, 345
Sleep assessment questionnaires, 347
Sleep diaries, 346, 347
Sleep disorders
    physical health risks, 331
    in severity with age, 331
Sleep disruptions, 371
Sleep in children
    with medical disorders, 341
    with psychiatric disorders
        ADHD, 340
        anxiety, 339
        autism, 341
        bipolar disorder, 339
        BPD, 340
        brain development and information processing, 338
        depression, 338, 339
        in mental retardation and neurologic conditions, 341
        psychosis, 340
Sleep problems
    assessment tool, childhood, 342–343 (*see also* Sleep assessment)
    during childhood
        classification, 333
        dyssomnias, 333 (*see also* Dyssomnias)
        factors, 333
        ICSD, 333
        parasomnias, 333 (*see also* Parasomnias)
    in primary care, assessment, 347
Sleep-disordered breathing (SDB)
    complications, 336
    disorders, in childhood, 336
    prevalence, 336
Sleep-related eating disorder (SRED), 394
Smartphone applications, 346
Social (pragmatic) communication disorder (SPCD), 314
Social and Communication Disorders Checklist (SCDC), 321
Social anxiety disorder, 190, 199
Social Phobia and Anxiety Inventory (SPAI), 199
Social skills
    assessments
        diagnostic, 304
        FBA, 304
        function of the behavior, 304
        instruments, 304
        progress monitoring, 304
    behavioral excesses, 302
    context-driven behavior, 310
    description, 301
    diagnostic assessment test, 302
    informed consent, 309
    measures, 304
        behavior rating scales (*see* Behavior rating scales)
        DBRs, 308, 309
        direct, 304
        indirect, 304
        role-play assessments, 309
        SDOs, 307, 308
    monitoring test, 302
    peer-preferred, 301, 302
    screening test, 302
    short term and long term outcomes, 301
    social competence, children's, 301
    social skills deficit, 302
    teacher-preferred, 301, 302
    universal screeners, 302 (*see also* Universal screeners)
Social skills deficit, 302
Social Skills Improvement System-Social Emotional Learning (SSIS-SEL), 305, 306
Social skills performance assessment (SSPA), 309, 311
Social, Academic, and Emotional Behavior Risk Screener (SAEBRS), 306

Sociocultural and environmental factors
    ED, 398–399
Somniloquy, 337
Sorting Test, 118
Special education
    children with ID, 134
    documentation, 135
    "other health impairment", 143
    RtI, 134
Specific language impairment (SLI), 313, 317, 322, 325
Specific learning disability (SLD), 86–88, 106
Specific learning disorder, 104
Standard mortality ratio (SMR), 402
Stanford-Binet Intelligence Scales, 61, 65, 66
Stanford-Binet Intelligence Scales, Fifth Edition (SB5), 105, 156
Starting Early: Eating and Developmental Skills (SEEDS), 423
State-Trait Anxiety Inventory (STAI), 197, 198
Static risk factor
    obesity, 436, 437
Stigmatizing Attitudes and Beliefs About Bulimia Nervosa (SAB-BN), 399
Stomach and bowl symptoms, 172
Story Memory Delayed Recall, 114
Story Memory Delayed Recognition subtests, 114
Strengths and difficulties questionnaire (SDQ), 26
Structured interviews
    CAPA, 2
    CAS, 2
    description, 2
    DICA, 2
    DISC, 3
    ISCA, 2
    Kiddie-SADS/K-SADS, 2
    standardization of questions, 3
Student Externalizing Behavior Screener (SEBS), 307
Student Internalizing Behavior Screener (SIBS), 307
Stuttering Severity Instrument-Fourth Edition (SSI-4), 323
Sustained attention, 116–117
The Swanson, Nolan, and Pelham Rating Scale (SNAP), 6, 138
Sympathetic adrenal medullary (SAM) system, 193
Synaptopathy, 144
Systematic direct observations (SDOs)
    advantages, 308
    dimensions, behavior, 307
    and FBAs, 311
    methods, 307
    momentary time sampling, 308
    partial-interval recording, 308
    social skills, assessment, 304
    whole-interval recording, 307

T

Target behaviors, 3, 4
Teacher Telephone Interview: Selective Mutism and Anxiety (TTI-SM), 193
Teacher-preferred social skills, 301, 302
Tenth version of the ICD (ICD-10)
    axes, 21
    criteria with adults, 21
    description, 21
    disorders, groups of, 21–23
    and DSM-IV, 18
    vs. DSM-IV and DSM-5, 21
    and DSM-5, 18
    emotional disorders, 21
    history, 16
    multiaxial classification, 21
    OCD, 21
Test of Childhood Stuttering (TOCS), 322, 323
Test of Everyday Attention for Children (TEA-Ch), 116, 118, 120
Test of Pragmatic Language, Second Edition (TOPL-2), 319
Tic disorders
    characteristics and difficulties, 229–230
    PMVTD, 228
    prevalence estimates, 228
    provisional, 228
    rating scales (*see* Rating scales)
    Tourette's disorder, 228
    treatment, 230
Tics
    and tic disorders, 227, 228
    Apter 4-q, 238, 239
    A-TAC, 237, 238
    characteristics and difficulties, 229–230
    comorbidities, 228–229
    definition, 227
    difficulties, 229–230
    DSM-5, 228
    motor tic, 228
    PRQPT, 238
    single muscle contraction, 227
    types, 227
Time-sampling method, 3
Toilet training
    ABA-based toileting procedures, 462
    age norms, 454
    Bayley-III, 460
    BDI-2, 459
    behavioral interventions, 461
    caregiver factors, 455
    challenging behaviors, 463
    child's progress and training effectiveness, 455
    domain-level interview, 457
    early assessment and intervention, 455
    IOA procedure, 464
    monitoring, 463
    prerequisite skills, 455, 456
    reinforcement procedures, 462
Toileting problems
    adaptive functioning, 453
    assessment
        adaptive behavior (*see* Adaptive behavior)
        ASQ-3, 460, 461
        baseline data, 455
        Bayley-III, 460
        BDI-2, 459–460

caregiver factors, 455
challenging behaviors, 461
children with intellectual and developmental disabilities, 455
clinical interview, 454
cultural factors, 454
developmental measure, 459
individuals with ASD, 456
medical, 454
POTI, 456, 457
prerequisite skills, 455, 456
behavioral Interventions, 461, 462
monitoring progress
ABA-based toileting procedures, 462
challenging behaviors, 463
IOA procedure, 464
measurement procedures, 463
permanent product recording, 463
procedural integrity, 464
time sampling, 463
treatment progress, 462
Tourette syndrome, 173
Tourette Syndrome Global Scale (TSGS), 234
Tourette Syndrome Severity Scale, 232
Tourette Syndrome Symptom List (TSSL), 236
Tourette Syndrome-Clinical Global Impression (TS-CGI), 233
Tourette's disorder, 228
Tourette's Disorder Scale (TODS), 233–234
Tourette's syndrome (TS)
diagnosis, 228
and PMVTD, 228
STSS, 232
treatment, 230
TSGS, 233, 234
TSSL, 236
Trail Making Test – Part A (TMT-A), 115
Trail Making Test – Part B (TMT-B), 115, 118
Trail Making Test (TMT), 118
Trauma assessment tools
PTSD
ECTSS, 218
PEDS, 217
TESI-PR-R, 217
TSCYC, 218
YCPS, 218
Trauma Symptom Checklist for Children (TSCC), 216
Trauma Symptom Checklist for Young Children (TSCYC), 218
Traumatic brain injury, 103, 105
Traumatic Events Screening Inventory Parent Report Revised (TESI-PR-R), 217
Tube feedings, 416
Typical *vs.* atypical feeding, 418–419

U
UCLA Posttraumatic Stress Disorder-Reaction Index, 215
Universal Nonverbal Intelligence Test (UNIT), 66, 67

Universal screeners
definition, 302
goal, 302
MTSS model, 303
sensitivity, 303
specificity, 303
Unspecified feeding or eating disorder (UFED), 393

V
Verbal Comprehension Index, 105
Verbal Delayed (VD), 112
Verbal Fluency Test (VFT), 118, 119
Verbal Immediate (VI), 112
Verbal Memory, 113
Videosomnography
advantage, 344
description, 344
limitations, 344
validity, 344, 345
video studies, 344
ViM index, 114
Vineland Adaptive Behavior Scales, Third Edition (Vineland-3), 45, 46, 72–73, 457, 458, 479, 480
Visual Analogue scales (VAS), 367, 369
Visual Delayed (ViD), 113
Visual Immediate (ViI), 113
Visual memory, 113, 114
Visual Perception (VP), 121
Visual Puzzles, 106
Visual/Nonverbal domain, 113
Visual-Motor Integration (VMI), 121
Visual-motor processing demands, 115
Visual-Spatial Index, 105
Visuoconstruction (VC) functioning, 120, 121
Visuospatial (VS) functioning, 120, 121
Vocal tics, 227

W
The Wechsler Individual Achievement Test – Third Edition (WIAT-III), 106–111
Wechsler intelligence batteries ranking, 104
Wechsler Intelligence Scale for Children (WISC), 67
Wechsler Intelligence Scale for Children – Fifth Edition (WISC-V), 105, 156
Wechsler Preschool and Primary Scale of Intelligence (WPPSI), 68
Wechsler-Bellevue Intelligence Scale, 61
Wide Range Assessment of Memory and Learning, 2nd Edition (WRAML2), 114
Williams syndrome (WS), 438, 439
Willis-Ekbom disease, 337
Wisconsin Card Sorting Test (WCST), 120
Woodcock-Johnson IV Tests of Cognitive Abilities (WJ-IV COG), 105
Woodcock-Johnson Test of Cognitive Abilities, 68, 69

The Woodcock-Johnson Tests of Achievement – Fourth
    Edition (WJ-IV ACH), 107–111
Working memory, 105, 117
Working Memory Index, 105
World Health Organization (WHO), 433
Wound surface areas (WSA), 282

Y

Yale Global Tic Severity Scale (YGTSS), 231, 232
Young Child PTSD Screen (YCPS), 218
The Youth Life Orientation Test (YLOT), 374
Young Mania Rating Scale (YMRS), 171, 182
Youth Risk Behavior Surveys (YRBS), 441

Printed by Printforce, the Netherlands